Oxygen

Gregory C. Kane • Michael Baram
Urvashi Vaid
Editors

Oxygen

Evidence-Based Strategies for Delivery in Respiratory Failure

Springer

Editors
Gregory C. Kane
The Korman Respiratory Institute
and the Division of Pulmonary, Allergy
and Critical Care
The Department of Medicine at the Sidney
Kimmel Medical College of Thomas
Jefferson University
Philadelphia, PA, USA

Michael Baram
The Korman Respiratory Institute
and the Division of Pulmonary, Allergy
and Critical Care
The Department of Medicine at the Sidney
Kimmel Medical College of Thomas
Jefferson University
Philadelphia, PA, USA

Urvashi Vaid
The Korman Respiratory Institute
and the Division of Pulmonary, Allergy
and Critical Care
The Department of Medicine at the Sidney
Kimmel Medical College of Thomas
Jefferson University
Philadelphia, PA, USA

ISBN 978-3-032-18933-2 ISBN 978-3-032-18934-9 (eBook)
https://doi.org/10.1007/978-3-032-18934-9

This Springer imprint is published by the registered company Springer Nature Switzerland AG
The registered company address is: Gewerbestrasse 11, 6330 Cham, Switzerland

For Jean, thanks for fueling my fire. And for Dylan, Mary Bridget, Brian, and Brogan, who fill my life with meaning.

Gregory C. Kane

This is dedicated to all the mentors who inspired us to push ahead and ask more questions.

Michael Baram

For my husband Ajit and our daughter Aanya: my past, present, and future; thank you for your love and unconditional support.

Urvashi Vaid

Contents

Contributors

Douglas R. Adams Department of Anesthesiology and Perioperative Medicine, Sidney Kimmel Medical College of Thomas Jefferson University, Philadelphia, PA, USA

Michael Baram The Korman Respiratory Institute and the Division of Pulmonary, Allergy and Critical Care, The Department of Medicine at the Sidney Kimmel Medical College of Thomas Jefferson University, Philadelphia, PA, USA

Susanna Betti Internal Medicine, Thomas Jefferson University Hospital, Philadelphia, PA, USA

Padmanabh Bhatt Department of Pulmonary, Allergy and Critical Care Medicine, Philadelphia, PA, USA

The Korman Respiratory Institute and the Division of Pulmonary, Allergy and Critical Care, The Department of Medicine at the Sidney Kimmel Medical College of Thomas Jefferson University, Philadelphia, PA, USA

Christina J. Carrero Thomas Jefferson University Hospital, Philadelphia, PA, USA

Shourjo Chakravorty The Korman Respiratory Institute and the Division of Pulmonary, Allergy and Critical Care, The Department of Medicine at the Sidney Kimmel Medical College of Thomas Jefferson University, Philadelphia, PA, USA

Sohiel Deshpande Division of Hematology, The Department of Medicine at the Sidney Kimmel Medical College of Thomas Jefferson University, Philadelphia, PA, USA

Michael Dong The Korman Respiratory Institute and the Division of Pulmonary, Allergy and Critical Care, The Department of Medicine at the Sidney Kimmel Medical College of Thomas Jefferson University, Philadelphia, PA, USA

Nathaniel R. Evans III Division of Thoracic Surgery, The Department of Surgery at the Sidney Kimmel Medical College of Jefferson University, Philadelphia, PA, USA

Ibukun Fakunle Department of Pulmonary, Critical Care, and Allergy, Thomas Jefferson University Hospital, Philadelphia, PA, USA

Tyler R. Grenda Division of Thoracic Surgery, The Department of Surgery at the Sidney Kimmel Medical College of Jefferson University, Philadelphia, PA, USA

Ritu Grewal The Korman Respiratory Institute and the Division of Pulmonary Allergy and Critical Care, Thomas Jefferson University and the Sidney Kimmel Medical College, Philadelphia, PA, USA

Robert Hilton The Korman Respiratory Institute and the Division of Pulmonary, Allergy and Critical Care, The Department of Medicine at the Sidney Kimmel Medical College of Thomas Jefferson University, Philadelphia, PA, USA

Gregory C. Kane The Korman Respiratory Institute and the Division of Pulmonary, Allergy and Critical Care, The Department of Medicine at the Sidney Kimmel Medical College of Thomas Jefferson University, Philadelphia, PA, USA

Simrin Kooner Penn State Health, Milton S. Hershey Medical Center, Hershey, PA, USA

Daniel Kramer The Korman Respiratory Institute and the Division of Pulmonary, Allergy and Critical Care, The Department of Medicine at the Sidney Kimmel Medical College of Thomas Jefferson University, Philadelphia, PA, USA

Mackenzie Kramer The Korman Respiratory Institute and the Division of Pulmonary, Allergy and Critical Care, The Department of Medicine at the Sidney Kimmel Medical College of Thomas Jefferson University, Philadelphia, PA, USA

Margaret Kreher Department of Family Medicine, Division of Palliative Care, Thomas Jefferson University, Philadelphia, PA, USA

John C. Madara Medical Intensive Care Unit, Hershey Medical Center, Penn State Health, Milton S. Hershey Medical Center, Hershey, PA, USA

Lauren McDonnell The Korman Respiratory Institute and the Division of Pulmonary and Critical Care, Thomas Jefferson University, Philadelphia, PA, USA

Christopher O'Hara Northwestern Medicine Regional Medical Group – McHenry Hospital, McHenry, IL, USA

Olugbenga Okusanya Division of Thoracic Surgery, The Department of Surgery at the Sidney Kimmel Medical College of Thomas Jefferson University, Philadelphia, PA, USA

David Oxman The Korman Respiratory Institute and the Division of Pulmonary, Allergy and Critical Care, The Department of Medicine at the Sidney Kimmel Medical College of Thomas Jefferson University, Philadelphia, PA, USA

Rafael Perez The Korman Respiratory Institute and the Division of Pulmonary, Allergy and Critical Care, The Department of Medicine at the Sidney Kimmel Medical College of Thomas Jefferson University, Philadelphia, PA, USA

Tara Rakiewicz Division of Hematology, The Department of Medicine at the Sidney Kimmel Medical College of Thomas Jefferson University, Philadelphia, PA, USA

Ruben Rhoades Division of Hematology, The Department of Medicine at the Sidney Kimmel Medical College of Thomas Jefferson University, Philadelphia, PA, USA

Sanaa Rizk Division of Hematology, The Department of Medicine at the Sidney Kimmel Medical College of Thomas Jefferson University, Philadelphia, PA, USA

Saikou Saidy The Korman Respiratory Institute and the Division of Pulmonary, Allergy and Critical Care, The Department of Medicine at the Sidney Kimmel Medical College of Thomas Jefferson University, Philadelphia, PA, USA

Louis Samuels Thomas Jefferson University, Jefferson-Einstein Medical Center Philadelphia, Sidney Kimmel School of Medicine, Philadelphia, PA, USA

Neeraj Sinha The Korman Respiratory Institute and the Division of Pulmonary, Allergy and Critical Care, The Department of Medicine at the Sidney Kimmel Medical College of Thomas Jefferson University, Philadelphia, PA, USA

Christine Stead ELSO, Ann Arbor, MI, USA

Katherine Stull The Korman Respiratory Institute and the Division of Pulmonary, Allergy and Critical Care, The Department of Medicine at the Sidney Kimmel Medical College of Thomas Jefferson University, Philadelphia, PA, USA

Urvashi Vaid The Korman Respiratory Institute and the Division of Pulmonary, Allergy and Critical Care, The Department of Medicine at the Sidney Kimmel Medical College of Thomas Jefferson University, Philadelphia, PA, USA

Frances Mae West Department of Pulmonary, Allergy and Critical Care Medicine, Philadelphia, PA, USA

The Korman Respiratory Institute and the Division of Pulmonary, Allergy and Critical Care, The Department of Medicine at the Sidney Kimmel Medical College of Thomas Jefferson University, Philadelphia, PA, USA

Jacob Woodroof Division of Thoracic Surgery, The Department of Surgery at the Sidney Kimmel Medical College of Thomas Jefferson University, Philadelphia, PA, USA

Part I

Origins and Discovery of Oxygen

The Emergence of Oxygen on Earth

1

Gregory C. Kane

> *To be big and multicellular requires huge amounts of energy, and it takes oxygen to generate that sort of power. Every other way of breathing is simply too feeble. We need oxygen because we need its spectacular reactivity. Without it humans could never have existed.*
>
> —Gabrielle Walker, author of An Ocean of Air

We need oxygen (O_2) because, as has been said, we are big and multicellular. In short, we need its remarkable reactivity; we need it for life itself—reactivity that can create energy for life and the cellular activities that lead to new protein formation and organism growth and that enable the complex functions that permit homeostasis of the human organism. Without sufficient oxygen, our planet would have remained energetically impotent and incapable of creating the complex life forms that currently inhabit the Earth, including humans. This chapter will review how oxygen came to be part of our Earth's atmosphere; interestingly, this was not always the case.

Our pale blue dot, our Earth, which was formed approximately 4.6 billion years ago [1], is the only planet we know of with sufficient levels of oxygen to support complex mammalian life. However, the Earth did not have significant levels of oxygen in its atmosphere from the outset. The process of oxygen accumulation in the atmosphere did not begin in earnest until about 2.6 billion years ago [2]. In the relatively short interval afterward, many geologists and geochemists point to the "Great Oxidative Event" as the first substantial increase in the Earth's atmospheric oxygen, perhaps driven by cyanobacteria [4]. This process began with the earliest microbial life on Earth, cyanobacteria, which used photosynthesis to transform carbon dioxide (CO_2) and water (H_2O) into oxygen and carbohydrates (or glucose) [3]. Photosynthesis can be carried out by select bacteria, algae, and plants in the

G. C. Kane (✉)
The Korman Respiratory Institute and the Division of Pulmonary, Allergy and Critical Care, The Department of Medicine at the Sidney Kimmel Medical College of Thomas Jefferson University, Philadelphia, PA, USA
e-mail: gregory.kane@jefferson.edu

G. C. Kane et al. (eds.), *Oxygen*, https://doi.org/10.1007/978-3-032-18934-9_1

presence of sunlight, carbon dioxide, and water. As a result of this process, oxygen was liberated into the atmosphere.

How is it that scientists were able to establish the timing of these events and identify the presence of significant levels of oxygen? The answer lies in red rocks or "red beds." If you have been fortunate enough, you may have seen some of the most magnificent deposits of red rocks or red beds on the surface of the Earth at Red Rocks Amphitheatre in Colorado, Bryce Canyon in Utah, or Sedona in Arizona. These beautiful rock formations, found in the United States but also across the globe, are evidence of oxygen in the atmosphere and the resultant oxidation of iron-rich rock—literally turning the rocks to a beautiful shade of deep red. This process can be analyzed using carbon dating to estimate the historical time of significant increases in oxygen within the Earth's atmosphere.

Using an analysis of red rock identified in the Republic of Gabon, David Canfield and colleagues identified an increase in oxygen levels starting around 2.3 billion years ago that lasted for 200 million years and stimulated a sequence of critical events that further catalyzed the advancement of life forms on this planet [5]. These events were critical in the yet-to-come evolution of life on this planet, but it was not until 700 million years ago that oxygen levels in the atmosphere began to rise to levels approaching the current 21%. Sponges were some of the first multicellular organisms to inhabit the Earth [6], appearing around 700 million years ago and presaging the Cambrian Age of 541 million years ago to 485 million years ago when the Earth's explosion of life occurred, as recorded through fossils that demonstrate animals with mineralized shells and backbones [7]. This would soon be followed by the emergence of complex plant life on land [8]. With a balance of these forces, oxygen could be maintained in the atmosphere for the continued evolution of land-based animals that use oxygen for energy.

Our planet's atmosphere maintains an astonishing balance of oxygen (O_2) and carbon dioxide (CO_2) levels through a natural process involving plants and their energy strategy using photosynthesis, as well as animals and their energy strategy of respiration. Plants utilize the process of photosynthesis in the presence of sunlight, with carbon dioxide (CO_2) and water, to produce glucose for growth and oxygen [9]. This oxygen is then released into the atmosphere, replenishing the oxygen supply essential for most animal life forms. Animals, on balance, utilize oxygen during cellular respiration to generate energy from food, releasing CO_2 back into the atmosphere as a by-product. This CO_2 is then absorbed by plants, completing the cycle. This reciprocation ensures a dynamic equilibrium between atmospheric oxygen and CO_2 levels, sustaining life on Earth. Surprisingly, however, the actual content of oxygen and carbon dioxide in the atmosphere is quite disparate. While oxygen constitutes 21% of atmospheric gas, carbon dioxide represents just 0.04% of the air we breathe. Despite this difference, the two gases maintain a relatively balanced exchange of one for the other.

A quick discussion of how the relatively low concentration of carbon dioxide plays an outsized role as a greenhouse gas would be helpful for the reader. This is generally because CO_2 is an asymmetric molecule, and as such, it vibrates or oscillates in response to ultraviolet energy reflected back from the Earth into the atmosphere, retaining that energy at the Earth's surface and in the atmosphere. Simple nitrogen (N_2) and oxygen (O_2) are not capable of the type of vibration that CO_2 can exhibit (Fig. 1.1). Other gases in the atmosphere can play the same role of reflecting energy back to Earth, such as methane (CH_4), nitrous oxide (N_2O), and even water vapor (Fig. 1.2).

It is also important to acknowledge that human activities such as deforestation and burning fossil fuels can disrupt the reciprocal exchange of oxygen for carbon dioxide by either depleting the capacity for plant life to utilize CO_2 or generating excess CO_2 through fossil fuel consumption that can contribute to the rising concentration of CO_2, which then contributes to global warming. Based on data from the National Oceanic and Atmospheric Administration (NOAA), which has monitored CO_2 levels since 1958, the global average atmospheric CO_2 was **419.3** parts per million in 2023 ("ppm" for short)—a new record high and approximately 33% higher than in 1958. Figure 1.3 displays the rising CO_2 concentration records over the past 65 years (available from the NOAA in September 2024).

One might expect and yet be pleasantly surprised that the National Oceanic and Atmospheric Administration (NOAA) also measures the O_2 content in the atmosphere. This, too, is changing, but the pace of change relative to the total amount of oxygen in the atmosphere is relatively minor. Reports from the NOAA indicate that between the early 1990s and 2005, the O_2 content of the atmosphere dropped by 0.00248% of its initial amount. Thus, the percentage of oxygen in the atmosphere remains approximately 21%. Experts indicate that the change is most likely explained by the global combustion of fossil fuels over this period since combustion of complex hydrocarbons requires oxygen and cannot occur in the absence of oxygen (Fig. 1.4). Oxygen and nitrogen atmospheric data is collected at Mauna Loa, Hawaii. Despite earlier comments in this chapter underscoring the remarkable balance of oxygen and CO_2 in the atmosphere, this data indicates that there is, indeed, a slight imbalance between photosynthesis and respiration/combustion on our planet at the current time [10].

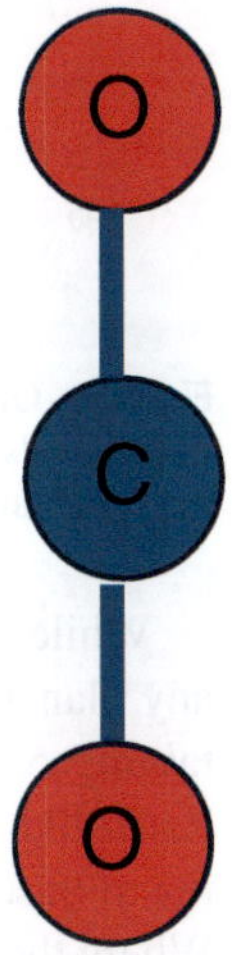

Fig. 1.1 A schematic of CO_2 gas, with carbon in the central position and two oxygens attached via a covalent bond

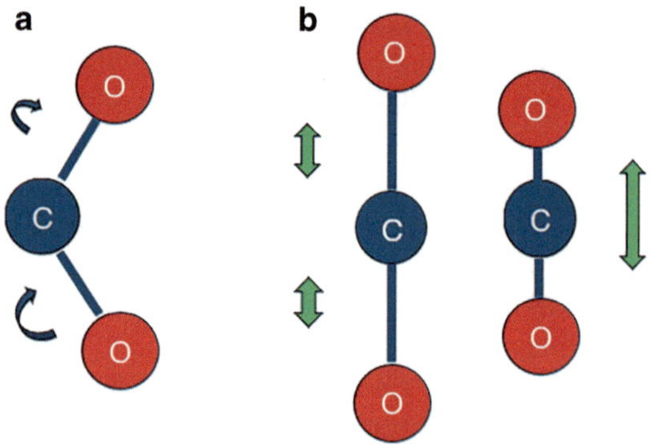

Fig. 1.2 A schematic of the different ways in which CO_2 gas can vibrate when reflected energy from the Earth's surface encounters it in the atmosphere. Panel (**a**) Lateral bending around the carbon atom. Panel (**b**) Symmetric or asymmetric stretching of the linear molecule

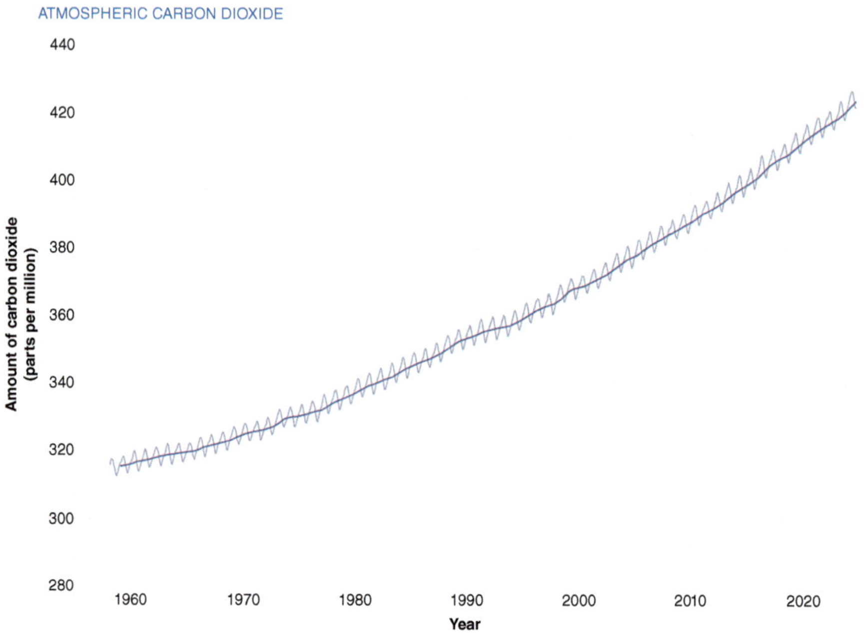

Fig. 1.3 Graphic data from the National Oceanic and Atmospheric Administration showing the rising levels of CO_2 gas in the Earth's atmosphere. (Graphic in the public domain and courtesy of the National Oceanic and Atmospheric Administration, accessed March 15, 2025)

While in reality, the search has really just begun, scientists have not yet identified any planets with an oxygen-rich atmosphere that would permit breathable air containing oxygen. While this represents a major disappointment for those seeking Earth-like planets throughout our universe, there is perhaps some cause for optimism based on the fact that some of these planets at least seem to contain water. Where there is water, there is the possibility of free oxygen if the planet were to be

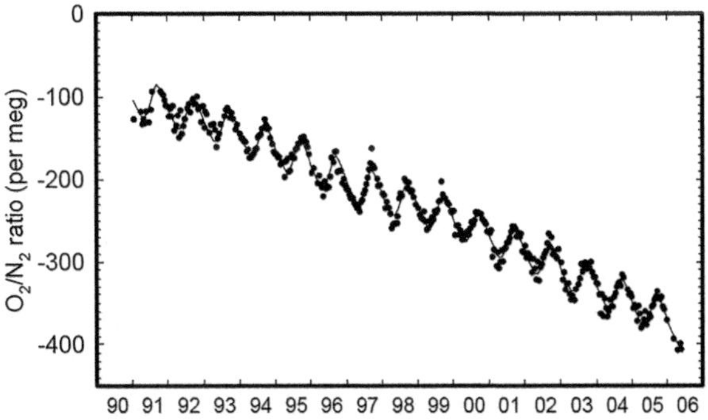

Fig. 1.4 Oxygen and nitrogen atmospheric data

maintained in what has been described as a habitable zone—meaning the right distance from the sun with the right temperatures to support a gaseous atmosphere and the potential for life [11]. While we intensify our quest to find a planet with breathable air containing oxygen as well as a habitable zone to support the possibility of human life, one thing is certain—we had better get working on preserving this planet simultaneously because the possibility of identifying an alternate planet and getting there will likely take some time!

References

1. Age of the Earth. U.S. Geological Survey. 1997. Archived from the original on 23 December 2005. Retrieved 2006-01-10.
2. Rye R, Holland HD. Paleosols and the evolution of atmospheric of oxygen: a critical review. Am J Sci. 1998;298(8):621–72.
3. Bekker A, Holland HD, Wang P, Iii DR, Stein HJ, Hannah JL, Coetzee LL, Beukes NJ. Dating the rise of atmospheric oxygen. Nature. 2004;427:117–20. https://doi.org/10.1038/nature02260.
4. Holland HD. When did the Earth's atmosphere become oxic? A reply. Geochem News. 1999;100:20–2.
5. Canfielda DE, Ngombi-Pembab L, Hammarlunda EU, Bengtsonc S, Chaussidond M, Gauthier-Lafayee F, Meunierb A, Riboulleauf A, Rollion-Bardd C, Rouxelg O, Asaelg D, Pierson-Wickmannh A-C, El Albanib A. Oxygen dynamics in the aftermath of the Great Oxidation of Earth's atmosphere. Proc Natl Acad Sci. 2013;110:16736–41.
6. Hentschel U, Piel J, Degnan SM, Taylor MW. Genomic insights into the marine sponge microbiome. Nat Rev Microbiol. 2012;10:641–54.
7. Briggs DEG. The Cambrian explosion. Curr Biol. 2015;25(19):R864–8. ISSN 0960-9822. https://doi.org/10.1016/j.cub.2015.04.047. (https://www.sciencedirect.com/science/article/pii/S0960982215004984).
8. Puttick MN, Morris JL, Williams TA, Cox CJ, Edwards D, Kenrick P, Pressel S, Wellman CH, Schneider H, Pisani D, Donoghue PCJ. The interrelationships of land plants and the nature of the ancestral embryophyte. Curr Biol. 2018;28(5):733–45.e2. ISSN 0960-9822. https://doi.org/10.1016/j.cub.2018.01.063.
9. https://www.sciencedirect.com/science/article/pii/S0960982218300964. Accessed 1 Dec 2024.
10. https://www.climate.gov/news-features/understanding-climate/climate-change-atmospheric-carbon-dioxide. Accessed 1 Dec 2024.
11. https://science.nasa.gov/universe/exoplanets/discovery-alert-a-super-earth-in-the-habitable-zone/. Accessed 1 Dec 2024.

The Discovery of Oxygen and the Dawn of Respiratory Physiology: The Genius of Joseph Priestley and Antoine Lavoisier

2

Gregory C. Kane

Knowing that oxygen entered the atmosphere 3 billion years ago is a modern construct. Prior to the eighteenth century, humans did not even know that oxygen was a unique gas. It was just as remarkable to establish that this unique gas was present in the atmosphere and was essential for life. Again, investigative science led the way with a number of simple and elegant experiments.

Joseph Priestley was a polymath who began his illustrious career as a religious pastor, but it very soon became apparent that he had a myriad of skills, and he engaged in a variety of important areas of investigation of the physical sciences and the properties that governed the world around him [1]. His worldview was heavily influenced, however, by his religious vocation, perhaps like many in this age of science, where the religious life provided a pathway to education in the sciences. Born three-quarters of a century before Gregor Mendel and initially a pastor, when his flock deserted him, he moved on to education and proved to be quite effective as a teacher. Science, however, continued to pull at his sleeves. In 1772, he published "The History and Present State of Discoveries Relating to Vision, Light, and Colors". That same year, quite remarkably, he published his "Experiments and Observations on Different Kinds of Air", which appeared in *Philosophical Transactions* and received the gold medal from the Royal Society, and he was elected a member of this prestigious organization [1].

While oxygen may have entered the Earth's atmosphere more than 2.6 billion years ago, it was not until the eighteenth century that the Greek concepts of air, earth, fire, and water were investigated further to increase our understanding of the constituents of breathable air [2]. Perhaps as a harbinger of the scientific age that

G. C. Kane (✉)
The Korman Respiratory Institute and the Division of Pulmonary, Allergy and Critical Care, The Department of Medicine at the Sidney Kimmel Medical College of Thomas Jefferson University, Philadelphia, PA, USA
e-mail: gregory.kane@jefferson.edu

G. C. Kane et al. (eds.), *Oxygen*, https://doi.org/10.1007/978-3-032-18934-9_2

would come in the nineteenth and twentieth centuries, several innovative instigators simultaneously explored the existence of a specific component of air that was capable of producing fire, but it was Joseph Priestley who published his findings first and who, therefore, gains the credit for his discovery of oxygen, which Priestley referred to as dephlogisticated air in the annals of science. Phlogiston would loosely translate as *burning up* from the root *phlox*, which means *flame.*

The genius of Joseph Priestley with regard to identifying distinct components of the air that we breathe lies in a trifecta of scientific experiments, which clearly established a unique and specific component of the air that we breathe, as it relates to its ability to promote combustion and extend the life of animals. The first of these three experiments is remarkably elegant in its design and implications. When a candle is placed in a bell jar with an experimental mouse, Priestley observed that the creature's survival is shortened, as if the burning of the candle removed a specific substance that was necessary to the survival of the mouse (see Fig. 2.1). The second is just as elegant but opens the door to another area of scientific inquiry. When a plant is also placed in the bell jar with the flame and the mouse, the survival of the mouse is extended, as if the plant contributes something to the breathable air that is also unique and enables the survival of the mouse. Finally, when sunlight is aimed at mercury oxide, a new and unique component of gas appears to be released into the atmosphere and captured in the bell jar. The substance that is released contributes to extending life and enriching the respiration of Joseph Priestley himself and of the mouse. Taking together, these three experiments would establish a new understanding of a specific component of the air that we breathe, which would ultimately be referred to as oxygen [2].

Figures 2.1, 2.2, and 2.3 show the elegance of the basic experiments by Priestley and Lavoisier, which contributed to understanding that a specific element of air was responsible for sustained respiration.

If there are any weaknesses to Priestley's contribution, it was twofold. First, Priestley, a former pastor, tried to refer to the religious properties of this gas, which perhaps prevented him from describing the significance of his findings in purely scientific terms. He referred to this component as "dephlogisticated air," but it would be left to Antoine Lavoisier, working in mainland Europe, to take these concepts further and describe the process of respiration and the role that oxygen plays in it.

Lavoisier was a French nobleman and chemist who accelerated our entry to the age of the chemical revolution of the 1700s, paving the way for the industrial revolution of the next 200 years [3]. Moreover, it would be Lavoisier who would give that component of air capable of combustion the name *oxygene* in French, or oxygen in English. Working essentially in parallel but independently of Priestley, Lavoisier also established that there was a component of air generated from mercury oxide. What Lavoisier added to the conversation, beyond the name and the recognition that oxygen was a unique component of the air we breathe, was that oxygen could be depleted from the air, leaving an inert component that did not contribute to combustion [4, 5]. Yet one last figure in chemistry of this era was Carl Wilhelm Scheele from Sweden (which then included parts of mainland Europe

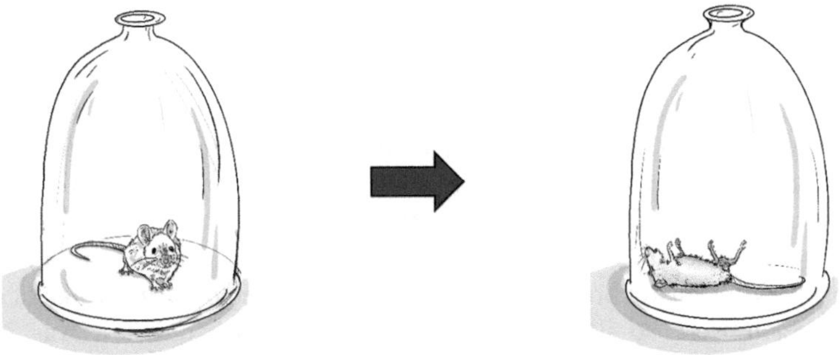

Fig. 2.1 A mouse enclosed in a small bell jar will only survive for about 10 minutes. (Figure Credit: Michael Natter, MD)

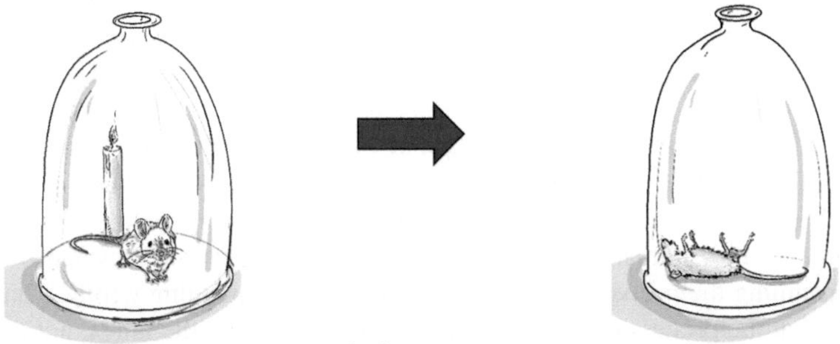

Fig. 2.2 A mouse in a small bell jar with a candle will die more rapidly (even if it has food and water). (Figure Credit: Michael Natter, MD)

Fig. 2.3 A mouse in a small bell jar with a live plant will live (as long as it has food and water, and the plant has water). (Figure Credit: Michael Natter, MD)

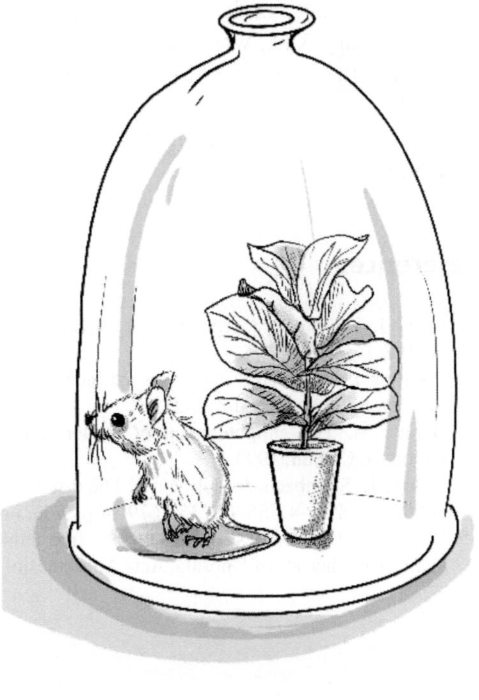

where Scheele resided and performed his work [6]). Scheele received less notoriety for his work, again in parallel with Priestley and Lavoisier, perhaps because he was known not to regularly take laboratory notes—a cautionary tale for all of today's investigators [7]. Lavoisier's wife, it has been reported, is credited with a major role in Lavoisier's discoveries and achievements [7].

In my final analysis, we should cede credit to the discovery of an independent component of the air we breathe to Joseph Priestley based upon his troika of experiments, which were so illuminating when linked together, but it was Antoine Lavoisier who nearly simultaneously made the same discoveries *and* provided a nomenclature for the new gaseous entity, which was a component of air. He also identified and described the three gases involved in respiration (oxygen, nitrogen, and carbon dioxide) and further made the analogy that breathing is much like the combustion of coal [8]. He offered the groundbreaking quote that ushered in the age of respiratory physiology: "*La respiration n'est qu'une combustion lente de carbone et d'hydrogène, qui est semblable en tout à celle qui s'opère dans une lampe ou dans une bougie allumée, et que, sous ce point de vue, les animaux qui respirent sont de véritables corps combustibles qui brûlent et se consument.*" Translated into English, this would read: "Respiration is nothing but a slow combustion of carbon and hydrogen, similar in all respects to that of a lamp or a lighted candle, and from this point of view, animals which breathe are really combustible substances burning and consuming themselves" [8, 9]. Lavoisier only got one thing wrong. That is, he thought that the process of combustion occurred entirely in the lungs, not realizing perhaps that oxygen might be transported from the lungs to trillions of cells through the circulatory system [9]. It would be early in the next century when the cell theory, put forward by Schwann, Schleiden, and Virchow, would add clarity and lead to our current understanding of energy production at the cellular level [10]. Or perhaps, Lavoisier was not familiar with the hypotheses of Galen, a Greek physician of the second century A.D., who is credited with describing that some blood goes to the lungs from the right side of the heart and that air is absorbed into the pulmonary veins [11]. Lavoisier, however, did demonstrate his remarkable genius further by hypothesizing that oxygen might be used therapeutically more than 100 years before John Scott Haldane [12].

References

1. Corry J. The life of Joseph Priestley: LL.D., F.R.S., &c., with critical observations. Wilkes Graft & Co.; 1804.
2. Priestley J. Discoverer of oxygen national historic chemical landmark. American Chemical Society. Retrieved 21 May 2021.
3. Beretta M. The enlightenment of matter. The definition of chemistry from Agricola to Lavoisier. Canton; 1993.
4. George L. Sternbach, Joseph Varon. The discovery and rediscovery of oxygen. J Emerg Med. 2005;28(2):221–4. ISSN 0736-4679. https://doi.org/10.1016/j.jemermed.2004.10.012.
5. Severinghaus JW. Priestley, the furious free thinker of the enlightenment, and Scheele, the taciturn apothecary of Uppsala. Acta Anaesthesiol Scand. 2002;46:2–9.

6. Frost RI. The northern wars. War, state and society in northeastern Europe 1558–1721. Longman; 2000. p. 133–4. ISBN 978-0-582-06429-4.
7. Berger K. Trailblazing pharmacist is remembered for discovering several elements. Pharm Times. 2021;87(12). https://www.pharmacytimes.com/view/trailblazing-pharmacist-is-remembered-for-discovering-several-elements. Accessed 8 Dec 2024.
8. Lavoisier A. Traité Élémentaire de Chimie, présenté dans un ordre nouveau, et d'après des découvertes modernes. 1st ed. Paris: Cuchet, Libraire, retrieved 2012-04-15 via Gallica; 1789.
9. West JB. The collaboration of Antoine and Marie-Anne Lavoisier and the first measurements of human oxygen consumption. Am J Physiol Lung Cell Mol Physiol. 2013;305(11):L775–85. https://doi.org/10.1152/ajplung.00228.2013. Epub 2013 Oct 4. PMID: 24097559.
10. Ribatti D. An historical note on the cell theory. Exp Cell Res. 2018;364(1):1–4.
11. Aird WC. Discovery of the cardiovascular system: from Galen to William Harvey. J Thromb Haemost. 2011;9(Suppl 1):118–29. https://doi.org/10.1111/j.1538-7836.2011.04312.x. PMID: 21781247.
12. Haldane JS. The therapeutic administration of oxygen. Br Med J. 1917;1:181–3.

"We Are All on Fire": Understanding the Biochemistry of Human Metabolism: Including Aerobic and Anaerobic Pathways for Generating Energy

3

Gregory C. Kane and Urvashi Vaid

Introduction

"I'm on fire" is the fourth single on Bruce Springsteen's 1985 album *Born in the USA* and one of ten hits from this iconic album [1]. How fitting that Springsteen's hit song captures the sentiment of Antoine Lavoisier and notable biochemist Nick Lane [2, 3]. We are all indeed "on fire," though the process of cellular respiration produces heat but not light. Perhaps lovers on a Friday night might "glow," but the reality of cellular respiration in the human organism is that heat is generated, but there is no visible flame or spark. Cellular respiration, however, is the essence of what keeps us warm and how we, as warm-blooded, complex mammalian organisms, maintain an ideal temperature for cellular activity and survival and support the cellular activity for growth, locomotion, and thought.

Many readers of this chapter may have a recollection of biochemistry that is cloaked in angst and fear, but at its core, cellular respiration is a process in which food sources such as the six-carbon carbohydrate substrate, glucose, are simply broken down in the presence of oxygen to generate water and carbon dioxide (CO_2). In this process, adenosine triphosphate (ATP), the cellular purveyor of energy, created mainly in the mitochondrial matrix, serves as the "power pack of life" and is formed to be used as the energy source for the essential cellular activities of life. These essential cellular activities include molecule and ion transport across membranes, muscle contraction for locomotion and circulation, nerve impulse propagation and signaling, substrate phosphorylation, chemical synthesis, and assembling of proteins and nucleic acids. The structure of ATP is a nucleoside

G. C. Kane · U. Vaid (✉)
The Korman Respiratory Institute and the Division of Pulmonary, Allergy and Critical Care, The Department of Medicine at the Sidney Kimmel Medical College of Thomas Jefferson University, Philadelphia, PA, USA
e-mail: urvashi.vaid@jefferson.edu

G. C. Kane et al. (eds.), *Oxygen*, https://doi.org/10.1007/978-3-032-18934-9_3

triphosphate, consisting of a nitrogenous base (adenine), a ribose sugar, and three linked phosphate groups. Energy is released from ATP to be used in the essential cellular processes, as each of the linked phosphate groups are detached.

To understand cellular respiration, it is fitting to start with the words and contributions of Antoine Lavoisier. Quite prescient was Lavoisier in stating that the process of respiration is like the combustion of coal [4–6]. Springsteen got it right and so should today's students. As discussed in Chap. 2, Lavoisier was a visionary, but he did not get everything perfectly correct. What he did get right was that the process of energy production in the cell is indeed analogous to the combustion of coal. Coal has been used by humans on this planet for more than 3000 years [7]. The main differences between the burning of coal and the burning of glucose are that for coal, the energy currencies include heat, steam, and, during the past 150 years, electricity. In cellular respiration, the energy currency is ATP. And as food is broken down, heat is generated. There is one additional similarity and one additional difference that the reader may already be contemplating. First, in burning coal and in burning glucose, there is a requirement to add energy at the start to initiate the process. Just as creating a flame often requires a pilot light or an initial spark from striking flint with another hard stone, the first step of breaking down glucose requires two ATP molecules to be *consumed,* producing the first three-carbon substrate in the sequence of cellular energy production or phosphoglyceraldehyde. This reaction is depicted in Fig. 3.1. This is analogous to the use of a match to light a fire, which then triggers the release of energy. How remarkable that both processes, one in the cell and the other in a furnace, require a first spark to ultimately release the energy flame. The additional difference, however, is quite divergent from the combustion of coal. While the combustion of coal absolutely requires the presence of oxygen, the combustion of glucose can occur in an anaerobic pathway without oxygen. This feebler approach to cellular respiration results simply in the generation of fewer ATP molecules, just two in fact, and generates lactic acid, which can build up rapidly. For humans, the rapid buildup of lactic acid will abruptly limit ongoing exercise until the oxygen debt can be "repaid."

While Lavoisier imagined an invisible flame in the lungs, this invisible flame is actually located within each and every cell in a decentralized fashion throughout the body, and this requires that both glucose and oxygen can be delivered to the trillions of cells, where the breakdown of glucose is going to generate water (H_2O) and carbon dioxide (CO_2). To do this, we rely on our circulatory system of arteries, veins,

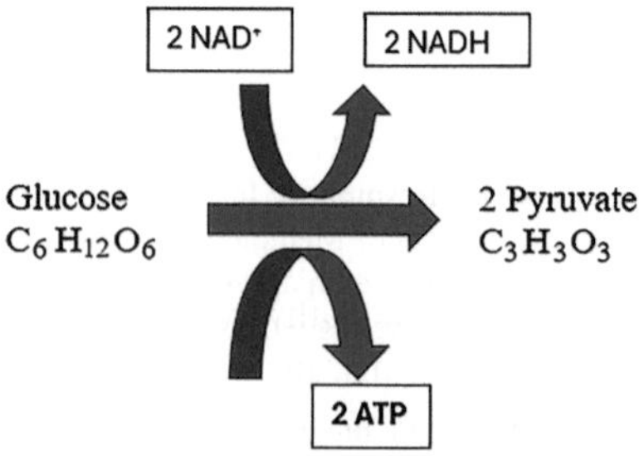

Fig. 3.1 Breakdown of the 6-carbon glucose to form pyruvate, generating a net gain of two ATP molecules in the glycolysis pathway

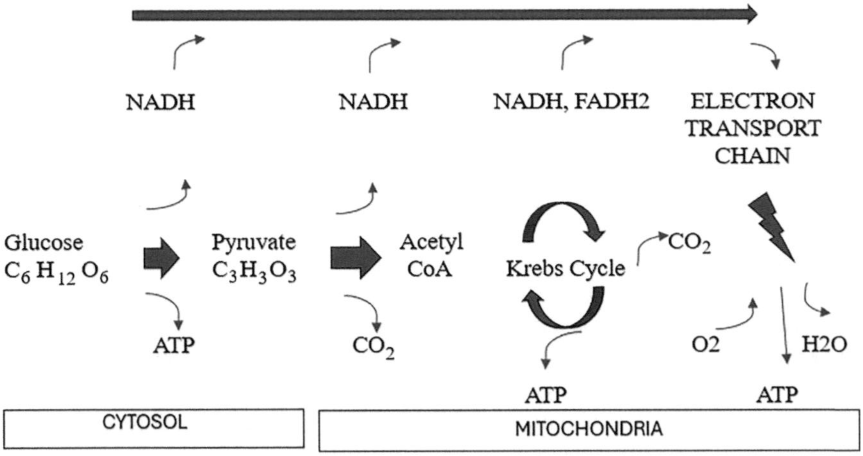

Fig. 3.2 The three stages of cellular metabolism for energy production: glycolysis, the citric acid (TCA or Krebs) cycle, and the electron transport chain

and capillaries as they course to each cell in our bodies. Lavoisier himself described this process as no different than the combustion of coal, and we should think of it this way in a most practicable and straightforward manner.

When cells have adequate access to oxygen, this process is described as aerobic metabolism. In the absence of oxygen, this is referred to as anaerobic metabolism, and there is quite a difference, mainly in the amount of energy derived from the reactions. The presence of oxygen is necessary to provide a robust level of energy for successful homeostasis. Thirty-six ATP (net gain) is usually expected from aerobic metabolism, but the exact amount can vary from 32 to 36 in the presence of oxygen through the steps outlined in Fig. 3.2.

In this book, we will focus on the energy production roles of cellular respiration, but we will defer our discussion of the generation of the building blocks of life for a separate time, as this is beyond the focus of a book dedicated to understanding how and why oxygen is so important to the human organism and how and why delivering oxygen during pathophysiologic disturbances created by diseases needs to be overcome with supplemental oxygen and often supplemental oxygen aided by enhanced pressure to maintain the cellular supply of the very energy source necessary to maintain homeostasis and health.

This process is perhaps quite analogous to the burning of hydrocarbons in power plants to generate electricity to power our homes, cars, and appliances.

Stage I: Glycolysis

This metabolic pathway was the first to be mapped out and is highly conserved in living organisms, including prokaryotes [8]. It is also referred to as the Embden–Meyerhof–Parnas pathway after the scientists who contributed to its discovery.

Meyerhof firmly believed that all living organisms must be governed by the laws of chemistry and physics and devoted his life to understanding "the energetics of cell processes" [9].

Any simple sugar can serve as a substrate for the glycolysis pathway (glucose, galactose, or fructose). The process of cellular respiration begins with glycolysis, in which the six-carbon substrate glucose is broken down into two three-carbon pyruvate molecules, utilizing two ATP molecules for the phosphorylation process but generating four ATP, thus resulting in a net gain of two ATP molecules (see Fig. 3.1). Importantly, this can occur in the presence *or the absence* of oxygen. This pathway occurs in the cytosol of the cell and comprises ten reactions. Pyruvate generated via glycolysis is then either converted to lactic acid or enters the mitochondria to power the Krebs cycle (see below). The process of excess generation of lactic acid in times of low oxygen supply-to-demand ratios, as in vigorous and prolonged exercise, is called fermentation. It is akin to the process used in making beer using yeast.

Glycolysis not only generates our energy currency (ATP) but also glycolytic intermediates that propel other biosynthetic pathways. Its primary function is to feed the next stage of cellular respiration, but in the absence of oxygen, it performs the life-sustaining role of providing ATP for cellular survival. Consider its importance in ATP generation for cells like erythrocytes that lack mitochondria!

It is interesting to note that an autosomal recessive genetic mutation of the enzyme involved in glycolysis (pyruvate kinase) can result in an inability to generate ATP and thus cause cell swelling and damage, leading to hemolytic anemia and splenomegaly. On a more macabre note, arsenic poisoning deters ATP synthesis since arsenic serves in place of phosphate, thus halting cellular respiration [10].

Anaerobic glycolysis is clinically relevant in cancer biology as well. Warburg made the observation in the 1920s that tumor cells consume glucose and generate lactate at much higher rates than normal tissue, even in the presence of oxygen (the Warburg effect). This finding laid the foundation for positron emission tomography (PET) scans that detect highly metabolic tissue by measuring the tissue's consumption of radiolabeled glucose injected into a patient. This increase in glycolysis is thought to help generate metabolic intermediates for anabolic pathways required in rapidly dividing cells.

Stage II: The Krebs Cycle or the TCA or the Citric Acid Cycle

The next step in cellular respiration is the feeding of acetyl-CoA generated by the oxidative metabolism of pyruvate formed after glycolysis, into the Krebs cycle, or the tricarboxylic acid (TCA) or the citric acid cycle. Interestingly, this step of conversion of pyruvate to acetyl-CoA is the only one that directly utilizes oxygen, though the subsequent steps are reliant on the entry of acetyl-CoA to move forward.

Sir Hans Krebs received the Nobel prize for his discovery of the eponymous Krebs cycle, or the citric acid cycle. He was a biochemist and a trained physician—thus a true clinician-scientist [11].

The Krebs cycle comprises a series of eight enzymes and occurs in the nutrient-rich mitochondrial matrix (Fig. 3.3). Each molecule of acetyl-CoA entering this cycle will result in 12 ATP molecules. As we mentioned, this is an oxygen-dependent stage.

The cycle is truly circular in that every molecule of acetyl-CoA entering follows the same path, producing two molecules of carbon dioxide, three molecules of NADH, one molecule of $FADH_2$, and one molecule of ATP or GTP. Since each glucose molecule produces two molecules of acetyl-CoA, this output is doubled. This may not seem very energy-efficient, going by the number of ATP produced, but one must recognize the potential of the electron carriers NADH and $FADH_2$ that enter the next stage and help generate the bulk of ATP through oxidative phosphorylation (the next stage featured later in this chapter).

Clinically, the pyruvate dehydrogenase complex, which is responsible for the conversion of pyruvate to acetyl-CoA, thus feeding the Krebs cycle, can be deficient or encoded aberrantly due to genetic mutations, resulting in neurodegenerative disorders and lactic acidosis. A deficiency of the active form of thiamine can mimic

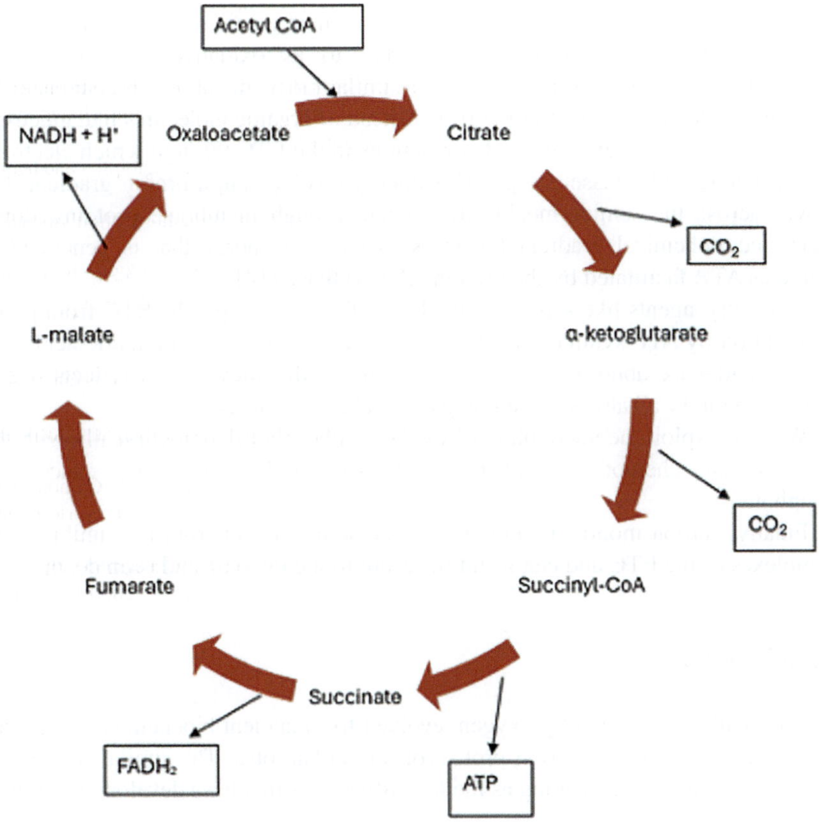

Fig. 3.3 The citric acid cycle simplified

this and manifests as wet beriberi if chronic (high-output heart failure) or dry beriberi if acute (peripheral neuropathy) [12].

Stage III: Oxidative Phosphorylation Comprising the Electron Transport Chain (ETC) and Chemiosmosis

The final stage of cellular respiration is divided into two parts: the ETC and chemiosmosis. An electrochemical gradient created by redox reactions in the electron transport chain located in the inner mitochondrial membrane leads to the creation of ATP and water by a process of oxidative phosphorylation. No wonder the mitochondria is referred to as the "powerhouse" of the cell!

This stage likely evolved from prokaryotic fermentation of highly reduced organic molecules, creating an acidic environment, resulting in the first membrane-associated H+ pumps. These early electron-transport-driven and ATP-derived H+ pumps set the stage for the more complex ETC [13]. The discovery of the ETC is credited to the biochemist Albert Lehninger in 1961.

The ETC comprises a series of four protein complexes and two redox reactions. These are responsible for creating an electrochemical gradient and resulting in ATP formation. This whole process is referred to as oxidative phosphorylation. Interestingly, chloroplasts in plants have a similar biochemical process but use light to generate electrons that enter the ETC instead of organic molecules like glucose.

The protein complexes and redox reactions in the ETC through which electrons flow generate and release energy. This energy results from a proton gradient that moves across the semipermeable membrane through membrane proteins, down their electrochemical gradient (chemiosmosis). The energy that is generated is stored as ATP, facilitated by the protein ATP synthase [14].

Clinically, agents like aspirin (salicylic acid) can uncouple the ETC from phosphorylation by ATP synthase, overheating the cell and generating lactic acid. The classic acid–base abnormality seen in patients with salicylic acid reflects this—acute respiratory alkalosis and anion gap metabolic acidosis.

We also exploit the uncoupling of oxidative phosphorylation clinically with the use of certain chemotherapy agents (such as doxorubicin for breast cancer and lymphoma).

Finally, carbon monoxide and cyanide poisoning result from the inhibition of complexes of the ETC and can result in severe tissue hypoxia and even death.

Conclusions

The fire within us, fueled by oxygen, evolved from ancient biochemical processes that are highly conserved from prokaryotes to eukaryotes. The similarities across living organisms are as striking as the few differences that have developed. Cellular respiration remains the driving force for all our metabolic and anabolic processes, without which we cannot survive. Most importantly, this process relies on oxygen—any other form of respiration and metabolism would be just too ineffectual. From glycolysis to the citric acid cycle to oxidative phosphorylation, the generation of ATP underlies our ability to fuel the complexity of the human body. And the mitochondria live up to their name—powerhouses of the cell!

References

1. Buskin R. Bruce Springsteen 'Born In The USA' – Classic Tracks. Sound on Sound. Retrieved March 4, 2012. Recorded with Max Weinberg and Roy Bittan, this moodily atmospheric, synth-based rockabilly track would be added to the album and released as its fourth single; 2010.
2. Chouchani ET, Kazak L, Spiegelman BM. New advances in adaptive thermogenesis: UCP1 and beyond. Cell Metab. 2019;29(1):27–37.
3. Lane N. Transformer: the deep chemistry of life and death. New York: W. W. Norton & Company; 2022.
4. Beretta M. The enlightenment of matter the definition of chemistry from Agricola to Lavoisier. Canton Mass., SHPUSA; 1994.
5. Sternbach GL, Varon J. The discovery and rediscovery of oxygen. J Emerg Med. 2005;28(2):221–4. ISSN 0736-4679. https://doi.org/10.1016/j.jemermed.2004.10.012.
6. Severinghaus JW. Priestley, the furious free thinker of the enlightenment, and Scheele, the taciturn apothecary of Uppsala. Acta Anaesthesiol Scand. 2002;46:2–9.
7. Qiu M, et al. Earliest systematic coal exploitation for fuel extended to ~3600 B.P. Sci Adv. 2023;9:eadh0549. https://doi.org/10.1126/sciadv.adh0549.
8. Kierans SJ, Taylor CT. Glycolysis: a multifaceted metabolic pathway and signaling hub. J Biol Chem. 2024;300(11):107906. https://doi.org/10.1016/j.jbc.2024.107906. Epub 2024 Oct 22. PMID: 39442619; PMCID: PMC11605472.
9. Chandel NS. Glycolysis. Cold Spring Harb Perspect Biol. 2021;13(5):a040535. https://doi.org/10.1101/cshperspect.a040535. PMID: 33941515; PMCID: PMC8091952.
10. Chaudhry R, Varacallo MA. Biochemistry, Glycolysis [Updated 2023 Aug 8]. In: StatPearls [Internet]. Treasure Island: StatPearls Publishing; 2025. Available from: https://www.ncbi.nlm.nih.gov/books/NBK482303/.
11. Berlin N. Hans Krebs: the formation of a scientific life 1900–1933, vol 1. JAMA. 1992;268(23):3379–80. https://doi.org/10.1001/jama.1992.03490230109044.
12. Alabduladhem TO, Bordoni B. Physiology, Krebs cycle [Updated 2022 Nov 23]. In: StatPearls [Internet]. Treasure Island: StatPearls Publishing; 2025. Available from: https://www.ncbi.nlm.nih.gov/books/NBK556032/.
13. Alberts B, Johnson A, Lewis J, et al. The evolution of electron-transport chains. In: Molecular biology of the cell. 4th ed. New York: Garland Science; 2002. Available from: https://www.ncbi.nlm.nih.gov/books/NBK26849/.
14. Ahmad M, Wolberg A, Kahwaji CI. Biochemistry, electron transport chain. [Updated 2023 Sep 4]. In: StatPearls [Internet]. Treasure Island: StatPearls Publishing; 2025. Available from: https://www.ncbi.nlm.nih.gov/books/NBK526105/.

4 Positron Emission Tomography (PET) Scanning: How Tissue Metabolism With and Without Aerobic Oxygen Metabolism Helps Find Cancerous Tumors

Gregory C. Kane

In the early 1920s, Otto Warburg, a Nobel laureate, made a startling discovery, which was initially thought to provide the potential of a therapeutic role in cancer management but ultimately became a revolutionary approach to identifying whether findings on computerized tomography (CT) scan might be cancerous.

Warburg's studies revealed that cancer cells lack the proper metabolic machinery for generating ATP via oxidative glycolysis due to a lack of appropriately functioning mitochondria. The effect of this evolutionary sleight of hand is that to avoid cell death or necrosis, cancer cells are consigned to utilize the anaerobic pathway for energy production, as outlined in Chap. 3. The practical effect of this defect is that "cell for cell" or "gram for gram," each unit of cancerous tissue must use 16–18 times as much glucose to generate a mole of ATP as would normal tissue of the same size or measure. Warburg hypothesized that this mutated form of cellular respiration was the root cause of carcinogenesis. However, it later became clear that the mutation leading to altered respiration was in parallel with the oncogenes that led to uncontrolled cellular growth [1]. As a result, this effect has not been utilized for successful therapy but leads to marked signal enhancement when radiolabeled glucose (fluorodeoxyglucose (FDG)) is used together with cross-sectional imaging. In the process, cancerous tumors have significant uptake that can be quantitated visually, "lighting up tumors" wherever they might hide, with a few notable exceptions that will be described. Recognizing that respiration is like the combustion of coal, this increased signal detected on FDG positron emission tomography (PET) imaging recognizes the wildfire of malignant tumors in ways that were previously

G. C. Kane (✉)
The Korman Respiratory Institute and the Division of Pulmonary, Allergy and Critical Care, The Department of Medicine at the Sidney Kimmel Medical College of Thomas Jefferson University, Philadelphia, PA, USA
e-mail: gregory.kane@jefferson.edu

G. C. Kane et al. (eds.), *Oxygen*, https://doi.org/10.1007/978-3-032-18934-9_4

undetectable. All of this is due to the differential ability of normal tissue to more successfully use oxygen in metabolism than cancerous tissue or lesions.

The details of PET scanning are relatively commonplace in modern medicine, where a nuclear scan utilizes a radioisotope, which can, in the case of PET scanning, be attached to a glucose molecule and demonstrate a standardized uptake value (SUV), which measures how much radiotracer is taken up by tissues in the body, such as malignant cancers. Fluorodeoxyglucose (FDG) is commonly used as the radiotracer to detect cancer. The FDG PET emits radiation that can be detected by a nuclear medicine camera and can even be quantified (Fig. 4.1) based upon differential tissue uptake of this radiolabeled glucose molecule. The physiology can also be recognized by the concentration of PET-avid radiotracer in the brain since the brain has a high metabolic rate normally (Fig. 4.1) as well as the presence of a concentration of PET-avid signal in the urinary bladder since glucose and radiolabeled glucose are both excreted through the kidneys and then concentrate in the bladder (see Fig. 4.2).

Understanding the important biochemistry of the Krebs cycle or oxidative metabolism has provided one of the most important imaging tools of modern medicine and represents yet another iterative enhancement in imaging, which continues to advance the early diagnosis and management of cancer patients [2]. How interesting that the eponymous "Krebs cycle's" key reactions were described by the

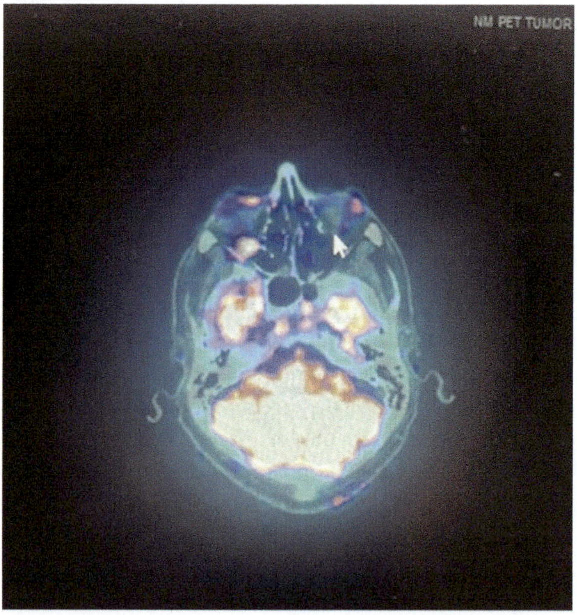

Fig. 4.1 Imaging the base of the brain as a part of a PET scan. This demonstrates the uniform, intense, and elevated SUV throughout the brain, attributable to the natural elevated glucose metabolism of the brain for thought and human functioning. PET scan, therefore, is not considered generally helpful for the diagnosis of brain tumors or metastases. Alternate radiotracers may be used to discern brain function. In this figure, the eyes and sinuses are visualized at the top portion of the figure, and the base of the brain is viewed in the posterior portion of the cross-sectional image

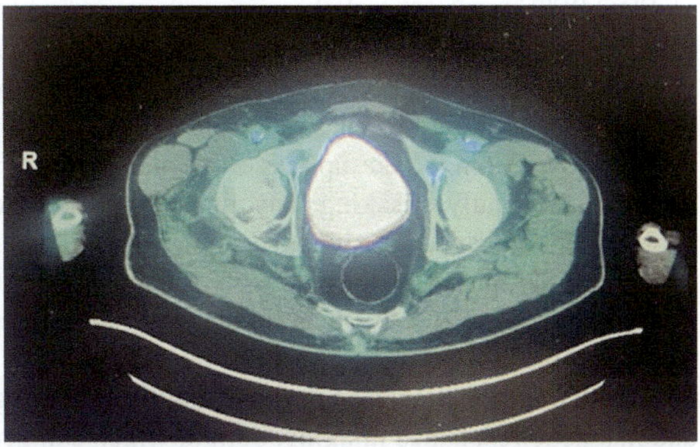

Fig. 4.2 PET scan images of the bladder. Fluorodeoxyglucose (FDG), used as the radiotracer, is excreted through the bladder, limiting the effectiveness of PET scanning for the diagnosis of bladder tumors

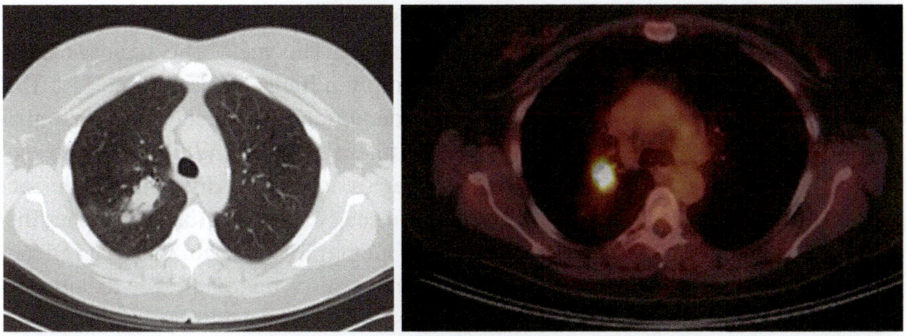

Fig. 4.3 In this figure, a complex right-upper-lobe nodular mass is detected on CT scan (left panel), and the likelihood of cancer is indicated based on the positive PET scan (right panel). The finding of increased FDG PET uptake is not diagnostic of cancer but can be used to guide therapy and the need for biopsy and can also help detect potential metastatic sites that could also serve as an important site for biopsy. The SUV of this lesion was 7.9, strongly suggesting carcinoma. In this case, there were no metastatic sites. This patient, who underwent treatment before the introduction of immunotherapy, has been a long-term survivor with no recurrence at 10 years

British-German physician scientist Sir Hans Krebs, who was a mentee of Otto Warburg in his early years.

FDG PET imaging aids the approach to diagnosing and treating malignancies through the confirmation of increased PET-avid activity within the lesion. Moreover, it can help establish whether the patient is free or not of metastatic foci of disease, as the scanning includes the liver and bones, as well as all tissues from the base of the brain to the mid-thigh, on traditionally created scanning protocols [4]. Figure 4.3 shows a PET-positive right-lung mass. The absence of metastatic disease facilitated prompt referral for resection. The reader can appreciate how the traditional CT image on the left clearly reveals a lobular mass in the left lung. However, the bright yellow PET-avid uptake in the right panel provides not only confirmation of cancer suspicion, but the absence of distant disease revealed by the lack of other foci of abnormal uptake suggests that treatment for early-stage disease through resection can be carried out (see Fig. 4.3 above).

FDG PET imaging may help confirm the presence of a tumor in unusual lesions, lead to the upstaging of suspected cancers and alteration in the treatment program, and predict long-term survival [3]. It can also lead to the differentiation of unusual tumors, such as slow-growing carcinoid tumors [3], which, because they are more slowly growing, may take up less FDG and emit a lower SUV intensity on PET imaging. Generally speaking, any finding of increased PET signal on PET-CT should be confirmed by biopsy, as it will change the therapeutic approach. Figure 4.4 demonstrates the relatively reduced uptake in the lesion located in the left lung that proved to be a carcinoid tumor—a tumor with a lower potential for metastatic disease.

Unlike traditional mechanisms of imaging, including computerized tomography and magnetic resonance imaging, both of which can generate two-dimensional and complex three-dimensional images of the brain, head and neck, chest, thorax, abdomen, and pelvis; PET adds a physiological assessment of tissues based on the degree of uptake of glucose, representing metabolic activity. This metabolic activity can be related to carcinogenesis, inflammation, or simply a high metabolic rate [5]. The areas in which PET scans can be helpful include not only cancer detection but also cancer staging, treatment monitoring, and treatment targeting. While there are pitfalls, when used as part of early detection strategies, it can help differentiate cancerous and noncancerous abnormalities and facilitate early treatment through separating cancerous tumors from noncancerous lesions. One pitfall is recognizing that inflammatory processes at inflammatory lesions may also reveal PET-avid uptake. Figure 4.5a, b shows uptake that suggested possible cancer, but biopsies confirmed sarcoidosis. It is also important to acknowledge that not all cancers display PET avidity on PET scanning. The ground-glass lung cancer noted in Fig. 4.6 showed no

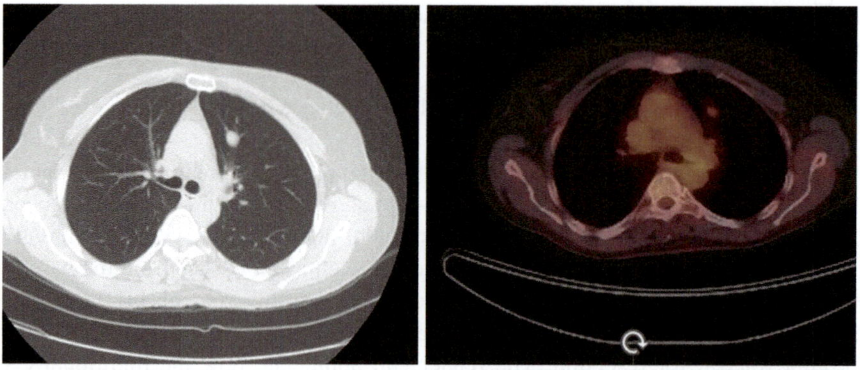

Fig. 4.4 Evaluation of the lung fields demonstrates a hypermetabolic 1.3 × 1.3 round nodule in the left upper lobe, which has an SUV max of 1.40, increasing to 1.69 on the delayed images (an increase of 21%). This increase in metabolic activity over time suggests malignancy, but the overall low SUV offers a clue to the presence of a slow-growing carcinoid tumor, which was diagnosed in this patient at resection. The reader will recognize that the orientation of these scans places the viewer at the feet of the patient, and thus, the left lung lesion is noted on the right side of the panel

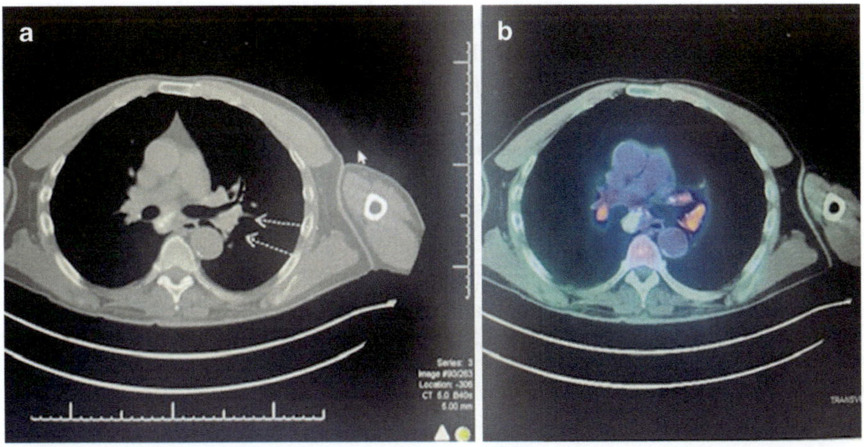

Fig. 4.5 (**a**, **b**) CT images of a patient with mediastinal adenopathy (right) and corresponding PET scan images at the same level showing left hilar PET-avid uptake (left panel), as well as right infra-hilar uptake adenopathy, which was ultimately diagnosed as sarcoidosis, reminding clinicians that positive PET lesions may be attributable to inflammatory or infectious etiologies (not calcified subcarinal mediastinal adenopathy situated between and below the major bronchi, which is not hypermetabolic). The SUV at the right hilum was 4.2, and the SUV at the left hilum was 4.8. Biopsies of multiple corresponding sites confirmed granulomatous inflammation without infection and with no evidence of cancer

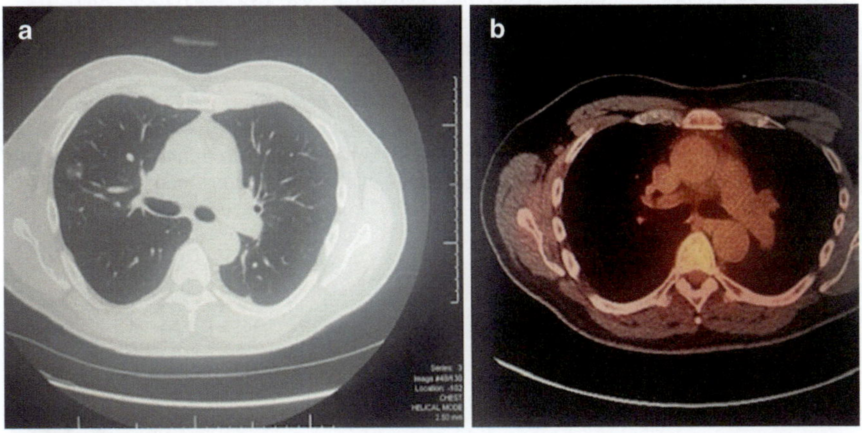

Fig. 4.6 (**a**, **b**) The right lateral ground-glass opacity (see panel **a**) noted in a nonsmoker was slowly growing (there were three solid densities within the lesion that were consistent with blood vessels). The corresponding PET scan of this lesion was negative for PET-avid FDG uptake (see left panel **b**). Based on growth, the lesion was noted to be cancerous at biopsy and was resected

PET uptake. Nonetheless, this lesion proved to have elements of invasive cancer, which were suggested by growth in the overall dimension of the lesion.

The utility of this technology is made possible by the ability of PET scans to exploit alterations in oxygen utilization at the local tissue level in ways that would amaze Otto Warburg were he alive today. Krebs himself would probably not necessarily be amazed, given the remarkable details of his discoveries. The classical iconic status of the Krebs cycle among premedical students in college biochemistry classrooms "has earned little love or real understanding," according to Nick Lane, but its impact has been more substantially extended through its applications in PET scanning [6]. Oncologists, surgeons, and physicians from multiple backgrounds are, indeed, aware of the power of PET scanning for enhanced detection and improved diagnosis of cancer.

References

1. Hsu PP, Sabatini DM. Cancer cell metabolism: Warburg and beyond. Cell. 2008;134(5):703–7. https://doi.org/10.1016/j.cell.2008.08.021. PMID 18775299. S2CID 17778749.
2. Gregory DL, Hicks RJ, Hogg A, Bins DS, Shum PL, Milner A, Link E, Ball DL, MacManus MP. Effect of PET/CT on management of patients with non–small cell lung cancer: results of a prospective study with 5-year survival data. J Nucl Med. 2012;53(7):1007–15. https://doi.org/10.2967/jnumed.111.099713.
3. Russ D, Barta J, Evans N, Kane GC. Anatomic distribution and clinical features of pulmonary carcinoids: a single-institutional study. Ann Thorac Surg Short Rep. 2024;3:299–303.
4. Griffeth LK. Use of PET/CT scanning in cancer patients: technical and practical considerations. Bayl Univ Med Cent Proc. 2005;18(4):321–30. https://doi.org/10.1080/08998280.2005.11928089. PMID: 16252023; PMCID: PMC1255942.
5. Lane N. Transformer: the deep chemistry of life and death. New York: W. W. Norton & Company; 2022.
6. Khurana A. Don't forget the Krebs Cycle. ASCO Daily New published June 24, 2024. https://dailynews.ascopubs.org/do/don-t-forget-krebs-cycle-new-findings-cancer-metabolism. Accessed 29 Dec 2024.

Part II

The Physiology of Respiration

Gas Laws

5

Urvashi Vaid

Introduction

Inhaling a gas that fuels our cellular processes (oxygen (O_2)) and exhaling metabolic waste in the form of a gas (carbon dioxide) is fundamental to life. Therefore, it behooves us to understand the physical principles and laws that govern the behavior of these gases. These gas laws were identified during experiments in the seventeenth, eighteenth, and nineteenth centuries and ideally hold true in a closed system at a standard temperature and pressure. Though these conditions are not replicated in the human body, gas laws play a fundamental role in our understanding of pulmonary physiology and, thus, are worth a deep dive. As Jacques Charles famously said, *"The properties of gases govern not only our environment but our very lives."* In this chapter, we will use gas laws to illustrate key physiological phenomena and outline clinical applications with the focus on oxygen as a gas.

Gas Laws: Definitions and Clinical Applications

1. *Boyle's Law*

Robert Boyle published a seminal book detailing his experiments around reducing the pressure of air with the help of an air pump developed by him and Robert Hooke in 1660, called *New Experiments Physico-Mechanicall, Touching the Spring of the Air, and Its Effects* [1]. This experiment allowed observations of physiology at normal and low barometric pressures and challenged the notion at the time that a

U. Vaid (✉)
The Korman Respiratory Institute and the Division of Pulmonary, Allergy and Critical Care, The Department of Medicine at the Sidney Kimmel Medical College of Thomas Jefferson University, Philadelphia, PA, USA
e-mail: urvashi.vaid@jefferson.edu

G. C. Kane et al. (eds.), *Oxygen*, https://doi.org/10.1007/978-3-032-18934-9_5

vacuum was impossible. It was the second edition of this book, published in 1662, that outlined what became known as Boyle's law, namely, the inverse relationship between the volume of a gas and the pressure it exerts. The seminal experiments were described well by Boyle and included pouring mercury into J-shaped tubes made of sealed glass at the short end and open at the long end. As mercury was poured in, the air trapped in the short end kept getting compressed. The height of the column of mercury was thus an expression of the pressure of the air trapped in the short end of the J-tube (Fig. 5.1) [2].

Boyle's law states that the volume of a gas is inversely proportional to the pressure exerted by it, given a constant temperature.

$$P \alpha 1/V \text{ or } P \cdot V = k$$

(where k is the temperature-dependent constant)

For the same gas, if conditions are changed (either pressure or volume), given a constant temperature, the changes will be predictable and are expressed as:

$$P_1 \cdot V_1 = P_2 \cdot V_2$$

The most significant application of this law, as it pertains to gases, and specifically oxygen, is the effect of altitude on atmospheric pressure. As altitude increases, atmospheric pressure decreases. Based on Boyle's law, the volume of gas would thus increase in a closed system. Many of us have experienced this as we try and open a bag of pretzels in an airplane cabin and note the rush of air from the expanded bag. Consider a patient with a pneumothorax or chronic obstructive pulmonary disease COPD with a noncommunicating bulla ascending in a commercial flight, where cabin pressures are approximately equal to atmospheric pressures at an altitude of

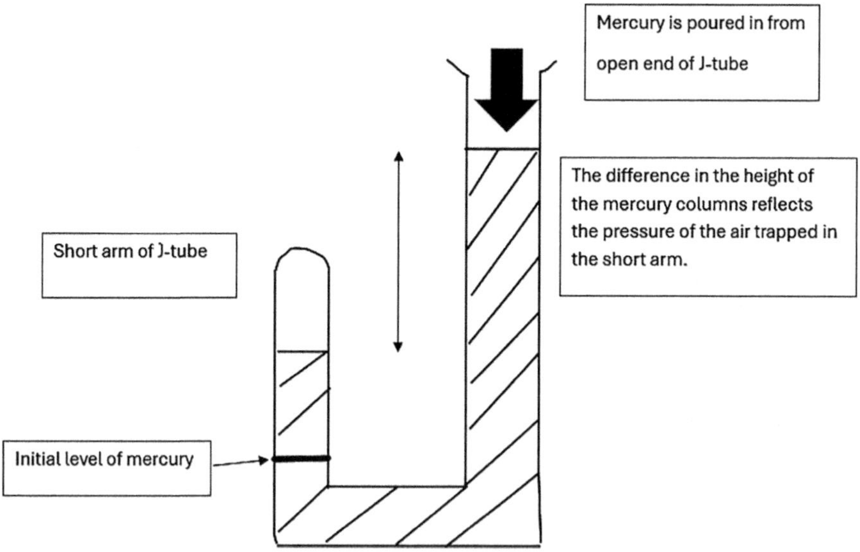

Fig. 5.1 Boyle's original experiment

8000 feet. The volume of that closed extraparenchymal air is expected to increase by up to 30% [3]. This can naturally increase the risk of rupture of the bulla and potentially result in a tension pneumothorax in commercial or medical evacuation flights.

Similarly, consider a scuba diver who descends into the depths of the oceans and inhales compressed air. On the descent, intrathoracic air pressure increases from breathing the compressed air. Upon ascending from such depths, the compressed air re-expands, but if it happens too quickly while the diver holds their breath, it can result in barotrauma, pneumothorax and pneumomediastinum, for example, where air tears into the pleural space, causing hypoxia (due to the loss of surface area for gas exchange due to rapid lung alveolar collapse/atelectasis) and hypotension (due to a rise in intrathoracic pressure, impeding venous return to the heart and thus precipitously dropping cardiac output) [4].

Finally, the principles of Boyle's law allow us to measure intrathoracic lung gas volumes accurately using body plethysmography. This technique measures lung volumes of a patient sitting in an airtight chamber. As the patient breathes, the volume in the patient's thorax and thus the chamber changes, as does the pressure defined by Boyle's law. Since we can measure the change in pressure and know what the starting volume of the chamber is, the total lung capacity, including air trapped in noncommunicating spaces like bullae, can be measured accurately [5].

2. *Charles's Law*

Charles's law, formulated by the French scientist Jacques Charles in 1787 and further elaborated by Joseph Lois Gay-Lussac, states that the volume of a gas is directly proportional to the absolute temperature, given a constant pressure and fixed mass of gas. In his experiments, Jacques Charles filled five balloons with equal volumes of various gases. He then increased the temperature of the balloons and noted that the volume of each balloon increased by the same amount. He thus came upon the relationship we now know of as:

$$V \alpha T \text{ or } V / T = k$$

(where k is the constant)

If temperature is the only condition changed, the corresponding unknown can be calculated using:

$$V_1 / T_1 = V_2 / T_2$$

Fundamentally, as gases warm, they expand. When one takes a deep breath in, that air is warmed and expands in volume.

Conversely, at lower temperatures, volume decreases. This occurs at high altitudes and, with the additional pressure changes, results in the rarefaction of air (lower inhaled partial pressure of O_2) and therefore hypoxia.

The volume/temperature relationship was also found to be very useful when designing thermometers and thermodynamic devices using hydrogen.

Storage of gases at high pressures and lower temperatures enables us to use smaller volumes, thus enabling more efficient storage.

Charles's law is evident in the design of hot air balloons, in the engineering of internal combustion engines, and especially in meteorology, predicting weather patterns and environmental modeling.

The culinary world takes advantage of this relationship as well, using steam and pressure as a cooking technique.

3. *Gay-Lussac's Law or the Third Gas Law*

Joseph Lois Gay-Lussac was a product of the French and Chemical Revolutions. His keen interest in the properties of gases led him to publish what is now known as Charles's law since Jacques Charles had arrived at this law 15 years prior to him. Gay-Lussac went on to experiment further by ascending over 7000 m above sea level in balloons filled with hydrogen in the early 1800s! His keen observations of pressure, temperature, and humidity at those altitudes led to the law as we know it to this day.

Gay-Lussac's law states that given a constant volume, the pressure of a given mass of a gas and the absolute temperature of a gas are directly proportional to each other.

$$P \alpha T \text{ or } P / T = k \text{ where } k \text{ is a constant}$$

With constant volumes, changes in pressure can be calculated for corresponding changes in temperature if the baseline variables are known.

$$P_1 / T_1 = P_2 / T_2$$

This law is applicable to the storage of gases in cylinders and underlies the importance of the pressure relief valve to prevent explosions.

In addition, consider cooking chicken in a pressure cooker. As the liquid becomes water vapor, given the cooker is at a fixed volume, the water vapor pressure keeps increasing as the temperature rises, resulting in a much faster cooking time.

If you have checked your car tire pressure before and after a drive, you might notice that it is higher after the drive—another example of the heat generated by friction from driving raising the pressure in the tire since the volume is fixed.

If we put Boyle's, Charles's, and Gay-Lussac's laws together mathematically, we get an important relationship that can help reliably predict the behavior of gases:

$$P_1 \cdot V_1 / T_1 = P_2 \cdot V_2 / T_2$$

4. *Avogadro's Law*

Amedeo Avogadro discovered his law when contemplating how to reconcile Gay-Lussac's law and Dalton's law (see later). Avogadro's law states that at the same temperature and pressure, equal volumes of gases contain the same number of molecules. It would later be established that 6.023×10^{23} is Avogadro's number.

The space occupied by one mole of an ideal gas is called molar volume. This is 22.4 L, given a standard temperature and pressure.

Consider a balloon filled with 500 mL of helium and another filled with 500 mL of hydrogen. At the same temperature and pressure, these two balloons will contain the same number of molecules of the gas.

This law is combined with the previous three to derive the ideal gas law (see the next section in this chapter).

5. *Ideal Gas Law*

The ideal gas equation was first stated in 1834 by Benoit Paul Emile Clapeyron, a French engineer and one of the founders of thermodynamics. This relationship describes ideal gases and their behavior. A gas consists of several molecules colliding randomly with each other. In order to predict the behavior of a gas, one has to make certain assumptions: First, we must assume that the volume of the gas particles is negligible in comparison to its container; second, that the gas particles are of equal size and are not bound by intermolecular forces with the other gas particles; third, that the gas particles are in constant random motion as per Newton's law of motion; and finally, that all gas particle collisions are perfect and do not result in a loss of energy.

No gas is ideal, but most gases at room temperature approach these assumptions.

The ideal gas law is a combination of four laws (Boyle's, Charles's, Gay-Lussac's, and Avogadro's) and is mathematically depicted as:

$$P \cdot V = n \cdot R \cdot T$$

where P = pressure, V = volume, n = number of moles of the gas, R is the ideal gas constant, and T is the absolute temperature in Kelvin.

An important example of how this law is used in medicine is that it helps determine the amount of oxygen available in a cylinder. Assumptions made are that the temperatures inside and outside the cylinder remain constant. This is useful when we know what the rate of oxygen consumption is for a patient before we transport the patient to allow for sufficient volume in the cylinder during transportation [6].

6. *Dalton's Law*

John Dalton had a deep interest in meteorology. It was his keen observations of the weather, wind velocity, and barometric pressure that led him to his experiments on gases, specifically water vapor. It was he who discovered that air was not a chemical solvent but a mechanical system composed of multiple particles, all exerting pressure independently.

Outlined in 1803 in his publications and lecture "On the Absorption of Gases by Water and Other Liquids," Dalton's law of partial pressures states that at constant temperature and volume, the sum of the partial pressures of each gas in a mixture of non-reacting gases is equal to the total pressure exerted by the mixture of gases [7].

$$P_{\text{total}} = P_1 + P_2 + P_3 \ldots.$$

The change in partial pressure of gases as altitude increases is well explained by Dalton's law. As altitude increases, the partial pressure of oxygen decreases, thus resulting in less oxygen being inhaled with every breath (remember the FiO_2 still remains 21%) and can result in hypoxia and high-altitude pulmonary edema (HAPE) or high-altitude cerebral edema (HACE) [6]. This law is also used in the derivation of the alveolar gas equation, which helps us determine what the alveolar partial pressure of oxygen is expected to be at different altitudes (or depths) based on the barometric pressure.

Finally, this law, along with Henry's law (see below), governs how much anesthetic gas will be delivered to alveoli for patients undergoing general anesthesia. Changing the concentration of the anesthetic gas will influence the depth of anesthesia achieved [8].

7. *Henry's Law*

William Henry was a chemist who experimented with gases and their solubility in water under varying pressure, leading to his law being published in 1803 in *the Philosophical Transactions of the Royal Society of London* [9].

Henry's law states that given a constant temperature, the amount of dissolved gas in a liquid is directly proportional to the partial pressure of the gas in equilibrium with the liquid.

$$P = K \cdot M$$

where P is the partial pressure of the gas, K is Henry's constant of proportionality, and M is the molar concentration of the gas.

What this means is that under higher pressures, a larger quantity of gas can dissolve or be absorbed by the liquid.

Decompression sickness can be explained by Henry's law. As scuba divers move deeper and the barometric pressure rises, the partial pressures of inspired gases like nitrogen increase, and thus, a larger volume is dissolved in blood. If the scuba diver ascends too quickly without making the requisite safety stops, this gas will bubble out of the blood, resulting in decompression sickness or "the bends" [4]. Think of the bubbles that escape from a soda can as you open it—it is the sudden loss of pressure on opening the can that allows the dissolved gas (carbon dioxide) to escape as a gas.

Conclusions

Understanding the application of gas laws to human physiology is fundamental to unraveling the pathophysiology of disorders developing at various barometric pressures and for the therapeutic administration of oxygen and anesthetic gases. Table 5.1 summarizes these laws and their medical significance. The patient and their health care provider can marvel at the discovery of these laws and their everyday application—possibly strengthening their understanding of the "why" behind these phenomena.

Table 5.1 Gas laws and their major medical significance [10]

Gas law	Equation	Fixed variable	Major medical significance
Boyle's law	$P_1V_1 = P_2V_2$	Temperature	Altitude and its effects on the availability of oxygen and resultant hypoxia
Charles's law	$V_1/T_1 = V_2/T_2$	Pressure	Storage of gases in containers
Gay-Lussac's law	$P_1/T_1 = P_2/T_2$	Volume	Storage of gases in containers
Ideal gas law	$PV = nRT$	None	Calculating volume of O_2 and/or anesthetic gases available in a cylinder/closed system
Dalton's law	$P_{total} = P_1 + P_2 + P_3 + \ldots$	Temperature and volume	Diving and decompression sickness

P = pressure
V = volume
T = temperature in Kelvin
n = number of moles of the gas
R = ideal gas constant

References

1. West JB. Robert Boyle's landmark book of 1660 with the first experiments on rarified air. J Appl Physiol. 2005;98:31–9. https://doi.org/10.1152/japplphysiol.00759.2004.
2. Distillations Magazine, courtesy. https://www.sciencehistory.org/stories/magazine/full-boyle/.
3. Hu X, Cowl CT, Baqir M, Ryu JH. Air travel and pneumothorax. Chest. 2014;145(4):688–94. https://doi.org/10.1378/chest.13-2363.
4. Bove AA. Diving medicine. Am J Respir Crit Care Med. 2014;189(12):1479–86. [PubMed].
5. Sharma P, Sankari A. Body plethysmography. [Updated 2025 Jun 2]. In: StatPearls [Internet]. Treasure Island (FL): StatPearls Publishing; 2025. Available from: https://www.ncbi.nlm.nih.gov/books/NBK615301/.
6. Tenny KM, Cooper JS. Ideal gas behavior. [Updated 2024 May 6]. In: StatPearls [Internet]. Treasure Island (FL): StatPearls Publishing; 2025. Available from: https://www.ncbi.nlm.nih.gov/books/NBK441936/.
7. Dalton J. On the absorption of gases by water and other liquids, vol. 6. 2nd ed. Memoirs of the Literary and Philosophical Society of Manchester; 1805. p. 271–87.
8. Savioli G, Ceresa IF, Gori G, Fumoso F, Gri N, Floris V, Varesi A, Martuscelli E, Marchisio S, Longhitano Y, Ricevuti G, Esposito C, Caironi G, Giardini G, Zanza C. Pathophysiology and therapy of high-altitude sickness: practical approach in emergency and critical care. J Clin Med. 2022;11(14):3937. https://doi.org/10.3390/jcm11143937. PMID: 35887706; PMCID: PMC9325098.
9. Rosenberg RM, Peticolas WL. Henry's law: a retrospective. JCE. 2004;81(11). https://doi.org/10.1021/ed081p1647.
10. Chandan G, Cascella M. Gas laws and clinical application. [Updated 2023 Aug 28]. In: StatPearls [Internet]. Treasure Island (FL): StatPearls Publishing; 2025. Available from: https://www.ncbi.nlm.nih.gov/books/NBK546592/.

The First Clinical Uses of Supplemental Oxygen

6

Gregory C. Kane

> *When you really listen to another person from their point of view, and reflect back to them that understanding, it's like giving them emotional oxygen.*
>
> *Stephen Covey*

We closed Chap. 2 with the discovery of oxygen but also looked forward to the work of John Scott Haldane, who first proposed the utilization of oxygen as a therapeutic modality, even if he was not the first one to actually report the therapeutic application. Indeed, this heralded the era of respiratory therapy and the first century of using oxygen as a therapeutic modality in both health and disease [1].

Haldane, the Scottish respiratory physiologist and hero of the Great War, received his medical education in Edinburgh, the great center of European thought and science, which had arisen in the seventeenth and eighteenth centuries but was still very much relevant through the nineteenth century when Haldane pursued his medical education [2]. His contributions included the therapeutic use of oxygen for medical reasons, the development of an early type of gas mask and the oxygen tent [3, 4]. In an ironic twist of fate, Haldane died of pneumonia in 1936, having been treated with his own invention. He died in an oxygen tent. This was quite fitting as Haldane has often been credited with his bravery, having performed numerous experiments on himself over his remarkable career [4]. His experimental work would include traveling into coal mines to understand what was killing coal miners (this turned out to be carbon monoxide), working on submarines to prevent decompression illness, and other investigations. He also passed along his scientific method to his son J.B.S

G. C. Kane (✉)
The Korman Respiratory Institute and the Division of Pulmonary, Allergy and Critical Care, The Department of Medicine at the Sidney Kimmel Medical College of Thomas Jefferson University, Philadelphia, PA, USA
e-mail: gregory.kane@jefferson.edu

G. C. Kane et al. (eds.), *Oxygen*, https://doi.org/10.1007/978-3-032-18934-9_6

Haldane, a polymath in his own right and a gifted scientist, who also contributed to the fields of physiology, genetics, biochemistry, and statistics.

In 1911, while on an expedition to Pike's Peak, Colorado, just 35 years after Colorado had become a state, Haldane investigated cyanosis at extreme elevations, becoming aware of the adverse effects of low levels of ambient oxygen. Noting that humans with pneumonia did not fare well at elevation, he wrote that "alveolar oxygen pressure may be a matter of decisive importance…at Cripple Creek (altitude of about 10,000 feet above sea level) in the Rocky Mountains, I found that this was so well recognized that all cases of pneumonia were put in the train and sent down to the prairie level" [4].

He went further, stating, "It is well known that the administration of oxygen often produces at least temporary benefit in cases of serious interference with the respiratory or circulatory functions." Haldane would go on to promote the use of this therapeutic intervention in the Great War (1914–1917) [2, 4].

While Haldane is often credited with popularizing the use of oxygen as a therapy, the first recorded clinical series was published in 1890 [6]. In this report, Dr. Albert N. Blodgett described a woman of nervous temperament with an unremitting severe cough, fever, and tachycardia, who was the subject of his observations. Consistent with clinical bacterial pneumonia, she had evidence of cyanosis, anorexia, and herpes labialis. Cases such as these were considered universally fatal in the 1800s, and it was in this setting that continuous inhalation of oxygen was provided with a favorable outcome. It is not difficult for a physician from any era of Medicine to find that the application of new lifesaving therapies can be a profoundly moving and emotional experience for the treating physician, especially in critical, life-threatening cases and in early cases of treating previously fatal conditions. This emotional response is connected to the deep sense of responsibility for the patient's survival and the often dramatic nature of the patient's recovery against the expectations of the times. In Blodgett's experience, we are not left to simply use our imaginations when it comes to offering hope where there was once little or none. He states this in his treatise in clinical terms:

> When I directed the continuous administration of the gas [oxygen], I did so under the positive conviction that the patient was irrevocably doomed, and the best result that I looked for, was simply relief to the sensation of suffocation, and not any curative action… At this time, I had only employed the gas in the manner ordinarily directed, that is, two or three gallons at a time, several times daily. I now directed its use without cessation, and to my great surprise, the patient not only obtained the relief desired, but was enabled to carry on the function of respiration. The amount of gas employed was not far from two hundred gallons in twenty-four hours. [5]

If calculations were correct, this would have amounted to only approximately 0.5 L per minute, much lower than the typical flow rates used today, but the effect must have been impressive all the same. Perhaps the benefit was in addressing pulmonary hypertension. Thus, in a little over 100 years since Priestley and Lavoisier completed their groundbreaking studies, oxygen was being employed clinically. By today's standards, this interval between milestones of scientific advancement would have been considered quite substantial, but given the pace of Medicine in the 1800s, the reader might be more understanding of the relatively slow uptake of the use of this important therapeutic modality. Finally, Blodgett's successful application of oxygen at a relatively low flow rate might herald future considerations for administering oxygen at lower levels than may have become standard in the 1980s and 1990s.

Shockingly, in oxygen administration, once noted to be safe in cases of pneumonia, some clinicians went a little too far in using oxygen for a variety of conditions and administered it via a variety of orifices, including the rectum [12].

Beyond the impact of oxygen in terms of relieving the hypoxia in the tissues, it was Haldane who understood and commented on the impact of carbon dioxide (CO_2) clearance and thus may have been among the first physicians to understand this important reciprocal relationship [13]. In particular, it was Dalton's law that established that in a fixed volume, the addition of a third gas, such as carbon dioxide (CO_2), would necessarily require a decrease in the partial pressure of the first gas, such as oxygen [14].

By the early twentieth century, oxygen could be delivered up to a concentration of 40–60% via oxygen tents for cases of pneumonia, as reviewed by Dr. Robert S. Palmer, and nasal cannula oxygen delivery was simply considered too feeble for the complex patients of this era who might have been suffering from bacterial pneumonia in the setting of rheumatic heart disease [10]. Thus, in the early part of the past century, oxygen tents were preferred. All the same, by the midpoint of the past century, supplemental oxygen became the standard adjunctive therapy for acute respiratory failure as well as medical procedures performed in the hospital setting [13].

Today, supplemental oxygen delivered passively can be administered via nasal cannula, a simple face mask, a face tent, or a venturi mask [7]. Table 6.1 outlines the types of passively delivered oxygen defined as delivered without positive pressure such as positive end–expiratory pressure (PEEP). It would not be until the early twenty-first century that a new modality of administering oxygen via cannula would be developed, namely, the high-flow nasal cannula (HFNC), which would be highly popularized in the COVID-19 era in the early 2020s [15].

In parallel with the use of oxygen, physicians understood that respiratory failure could be due to either hypoxemia or hypercapnia. Hypercapnia represented a unique challenge, as it would require the application of some type of support to enhance the

Table 6.1 Devices used in simple supplemental oxygen therapy [8–11]

Modality	Flow rate per minute	Fraction of inspired oxygen (FiO_2) (%)	Indications
Nasal cannula	1–6 L	0.24–0.40	Non-severe respiratory distress, procedures without sedation
Simple face mask	5–10 L	0.35–0.50	When higher FiO_2 is required and in patients who are mouth breathers
Venturi mask	2–15 L	0.24–0.50	In circumstances where a specific FiO_2 is desired (i.e., Chronic Obstructive Pulmonary Disease)
Non-rebreather mask	10–15 L	0.60–0.90	Carbon monoxide poisoning or severe hypoxemia

movement of air into and out of the thorax. While there were rarely used prototypes, such methods were not employed widely until the first successful negative-pressure ventilator, developed by the Boston engineer Philip Drinker, was employed clinically in 1928 [16]. His "iron lung" represented a major advance and was powered by electricity, making prior hand-powered facsimiles, which were used in isolated circumstances, obsolete. Drinker's machine weighed nearly a ton and was soon eclipsed by a lighter and more easily manufactured device developed by J.H. Emerson, also of Massachusetts, just a few years later, in the early 1930s [17, 18]. This modality became the preferred approach to support victims of polio, who suffered from paralyzed respiratory muscles and other chronic respiratory conditions.

Today, the therapeutic use of oxygen includes passive delivery and devices as outlined above, as well as more active methodologies that employ the use of positive pressure, either through high-flow nasal cannula, noninvasive ventilation, or intubation and mechanical ventilation (Table 6.2). Extracorporeal membrane oxygenation (ECMO), first utilized in the early 1970s, involves an alternate methodology altogether, wherein it uses an external pump and a process of membrane oxygenation to achieve oxygen and carbon dioxide exchange [19, 20]. Surprisingly, this sophisticated method still requires simple diffusion of oxygen, even though it is facilitated by bringing oxygen into close contact with the membrane oxygenator [19]. It would be important to state here that the evolution of contemporary ECMO owes its development to the groundbreaking work of John Gibbon, whose heart–lung machine enabled the first open heart surgery, performed at Jefferson Hospital in Philadelphia in 1953 [21]. Figure 6.1 shows Dr. Gibbon pictured with his patient, *Cecelia Bavolek, and his heart–lung machine, which would revolutionize cardiac surgery and serve as a forerunner for ECMO.*

Noting the remarkable advancement that ECMO represents (discussed in a subsequent chapter), it will be exciting to envision new and revolutionary techniques that may be less invasive but more effective in the delivery of oxygen in critical care settings. All of these new developments stand on the shoulders of the greats of the

Table 6.2 Devices used to deliver supplemental oxygen therapy with pressure, such as positive end–expiratory pressure (PEEP) [15, 16]

Modality	Flow rate per minute	FiO_2 (%)	Indications (examples)
High-flow NC	20–80 L	0.21–1.0	Acute hypoxic respiratory failure, procedures without sedation
CPAP[a]	5–10 L	0.35–0.50	Heart failure and sleep apnea
Bi-level with nasal mask	2–15 L	0.24–0.50	In circumstances where a specific FiO_2 is desired (i.e., COPD)
Bi-level with face mask	10–15 L	0.60–0.90	Carbon monoxide poisoning or severe hypoxia
AVAPS[b]	0–15 L	0.24–0.90	COPD and neuromuscular disease

[a]Continuous positive airway pressure delivered via a well-fitting nasal mask or face mask
[b]Average volume–assured pressure support is a technique that is highly valuable in patients with chronic respiratory failure from conditions such as neuromuscular disease

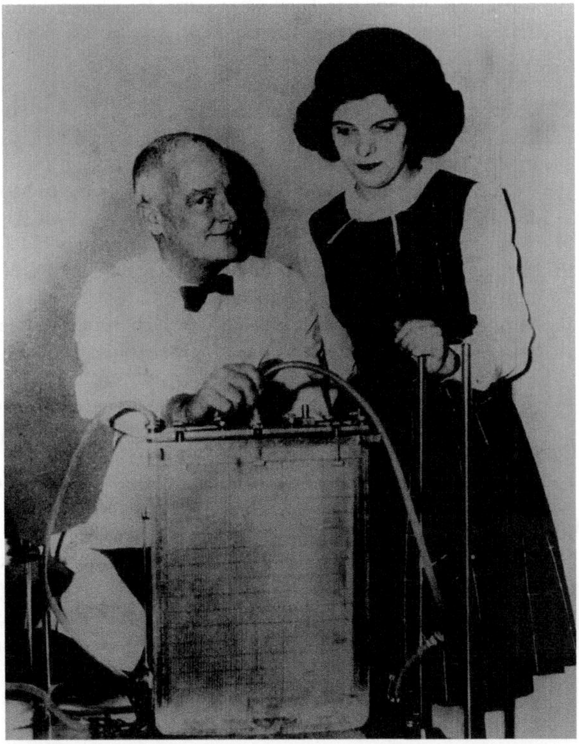

Fig. 6.1 Dr. John H. Gibbon Jr. (left) and Cecelia Bavolek in 1963 with the machine he invented and used to perform a lifesaving surgery in 1953 by correcting an atrial septal defect. (Photo courtesy of the Siegman Archives at Thomas Jefferson University, Philadelphia)

nineteenth and twentieth centuries, who first used oxygen to create new survival opportunities for diseases of that age and of today and imagined ways to bypass the lungs altogether to facilitate medical and surgical treatments.

References

1. Haldane JS. The therapeutic administration of oxygen. Br Med J. 1917;1:181–3.
2. Douglas CG. John Scott Haldane. 1860–1936. Obit Not Fell R Soc. 1936;2(5):114–39. https://doi.org/10.1098/rsbm.1936.0009. JSTOR 769132.
3. Acott C. JS Haldane, JBS Haldane, L Hill, and A Siebe: a brief resume of their lives. South Pac Underwater Med Soc J. 1999;29(3):161–5.
4. Blue plaque tribute to scientific pioneer. Oxford Mail. 4 May 2009. Accessed 11 Dec 2024.
5. Blodgett AN. The continuous inhalation of oxygen in cases of pneumonia otherwise fatal, and in other diseases. Boston Med J. 1890;123:481–5.
6. Palmer RS. Oxygen therapy in the treatment of pneumonia and postoperative pulmonary complications. N Engl J Med. 1929;200(7):330–2. https://doi.org/10.1056/NEJM192902142000705.
7. Rengasamy S, Nassef B, Bilotta F, Pugliese F, Nozari A, Ortega R. Administration of supplemental oxygen. N Engl J Med. 2021;385:17. https://doi.org/10.1056/NEJMc2113496.
8. Hardavella G, Karampinis I, Frille A, Sreter K, Rousalova I. Oxygen devices and delivery systems. Breathe (Sheff). 2019;15(3):e108–16.
9. Gibson RL, Comer PB, Beckham RW, McGraw CP. Actual tracheal oxygen concentrations with commonly used oxygen equipment. Anesthesiology. 1976;44:71–3.

10. Wexler HR, Aberman A, Scott AA, Cooper JD. Measurement of intratracheal oxygen concentrations during face mask administration of oxygen: a modification for improved control. Can Anaesth Soc J. 1975;22:417–31.
11. Speir WA Jr, Kaplan HM, Wier MA, Ellison LT. Oxygen concentration delivered by Venturi masks with in-line humidification. JAMA. 1971;216:879–80.
12. Kellogg JH. Oxygen enemata as a remedy in certain diseases of the liver and intestinal tract. JAMA. 1888;11:258–62. [Google Scholar].
13. Haldane JS. The therapeutic administration of oxygen. Br Med J. 1917;1(2928):181–3. https://doi.org/10.1136/bmj.1.2928.181. PMID: 20768466; PMCID: PMC2348015.
14. Henry WC. Memoirs of the life and scientific researches of John Dalton. London; 1854.
15. Matthay MA. Saving lives with high flow nasal cannula. N Engl J Med. 2015;372:2225–6. https://doi.org/10.1056/NEJMe1504852.
16. Nishimura M. High-flow nasal cannula oxygen therapy devices. Respir Care. 2019;64:735–42.
17. Drinker P, Shaw LA. An apparatus for the prolonged administration of artificial respiration: I. Design for adults and children. J Clin Invest. 1929;7(2):229–47.
18. Hodes HL. Treatment of respiratory difficulty in poliomyelitis. In: Poliomyelitis: papers and discussions presented at the Third International Poliomyelitis Conference. Philadelphia: Lippincott; 1955. p. 91–113.
19. Mehta S, Hill NS. Noninvasive ventilation. Am J Respir Crit Care Med. 2001;163(2):540–77. https://doi.org/10.1164/ajrccm.163.2.9906116. PMID: 11179136.
20. Badulak JH. Veno venous extracorporeal membrane oxygenation. Gas exchange, the membrane lung, and the ventilator. ATS Scholar. 2020. https://doi.org/10.34197/ats-scholar.2020-0077VO.
21. Bartlett R, Arachichilage DJ, Chitlur M, Hui SR, Neunert C, Doyle A, Retter A, Hunt BJ, Lim HS, Saini A, Renné T, Kostousov V, Teruya J. The history of extracorporeal membrane oxygenation and the development of extracorporeal membrane oxygenation anticoagulation. Semin Thromb Hemost. 2024;50(1):81–90. https://doi.org/10.1055/s-0043-1761488. Epub 2023 Feb 7. PMID: 36750217.

7 Do No Harm

Gregory C. Kane

Why then, can one desire too much of a good thing?

Shakespeare, Author of As You Like It, 1623

Too much of anything is bad, too much good whiskey is barely enough.

Mark Twain

Blodgett's description of the first successful use of oxygen in a patient with pneumonia was prescient for several apparent reasons but for one subtle reason as well [1]. His eloquent description of the impact of oxygen therapy is remarkable, especially when one considers the limited flow rate of oxygen he provided, especially by today's standards, and that this flow rate of approximately just half a liter per minute may have only raised the fraction of inspired oxygen (FiO_2) by 1% at most. Blodgett's descriptive report should give the modern physician some pause because it underscores that just a very small amount of oxygen can have clinical benefits. One wonders whether we should have taken heed of Blodgett's hidden message that "too much of a good thing could be bad."

As such, it is not surprising that Julius H. Comroe, MD, described apparent toxicity from the administration of oxygen as early as 1945 [2], publishing his results in the *Journal of the American Medical Association*, and 40 years later, Ron Crystal, MD, and colleagues noted early alveolar changes that account for alterations in pulmonary histopathology, which can occur in human volunteers with as little as 17 hours of exposure to an atmosphere with 95% oxygen [3]. Crystal's work showed

G. C. Kane (✉)
The Korman Respiratory Institute and the Division of Pulmonary, Allergy and Critical Care, The Department of Medicine at the Sidney Kimmel Medical College of Thomas Jefferson University, Philadelphia, PA, USA
e-mail: gregory.kane@jefferson.edu

G. C. Kane et al. (eds.), *Oxygen*, https://doi.org/10.1007/978-3-032-18934-9_7

that while bronchoalveolar lavage–derived inflammatory cells were not elevated, there were abnormalities noted in recovered macrophages that could be associated with increased pulmonary fibrosis over time. These findings included increased levels of fibronectin and increased levels of macrophage-derived growth factor for fibroblasts. This important work, and that of others in the field, set the stage for subsequent clinical trials, which ultimately demonstrated that the treatment of patients with profound lung failure from the acute respiratory distress syndrome (ARDS) would have improved outcomes when fractional inspired levels of oxygen delivery were modulated to 60% or less [4–6].

In clinical care, especially among acutely ill adults, excess oxygen can impact outcomes, including survival. For example, in a meta-analysis of critically ill patients following cardiac arrest, stroke, traumatic brain injury, and even after cardiac surgery, higher arterial oxygen partial pressure (PaO_2) values correlated with higher mortality [7, 8]. The work of Helmerhorst and colleagues provided a further specific definition of the potential harms of excess oxygen, as defined by the arterial oxygen partial pressure, noting that severe hyperoxia (PaO_2 >200 mmHg) in ICU patients led to higher mortality rates and fewer ventilator-free days when compared to mild or normal hyperoxia [8]. In this study, normoxia was defined in a very appropriate way based upon PaO_2 from 60 to 100 mmHg and mild hyperoxia from 101 to 200 mmHg. As a result, the ARDS network, a collaborative of the National Institutes of Health and the National Heart, Lung, and Blood Institute, has issued a protocol outlining the goal for PaO_2 in ARDS as being 55–80 mmHg and acceptable O_2 sats of 88–95%, with a lung protective strategy that limits ventilator-induced injury as well [9].

The discussion thus far has focused on relatively high levels of inspired oxygen, which result in substantial increases in the partial pressure of arterial oxygen, but it is important that we take this discussion further, focusing on the literature from the past decade, which has established that oxygen provided via nasal cannula, even in relatively common conditions, has potential adverse effects in a variety of routine conditions.

In 2015, Stub and colleagues from the Heart and Diabetes Institute in Melbourne, Australia, challenged a long-held approach to treating patients with symptomatic coronary artery disease and myocardial infarction (MI) by comparing the application of oxygen in patients admitted with myocardial infarction who were not hypoxic to the administration of air! The *Annals of Medicine* rarely offer such an elegant and simple study, challenging historical dogma, as oxygen had been provided to patients with angina as early as 1900 and even up to 100% in the middle of the twentieth century [10–12]. In the clinical trial by Stub and his group, 441 patients with confirmed ST-segment elevation MI (STEMI) underwent primary endpoint analysis after randomization to the administration of air or oxygen. The group receiving oxygen had an increased rate of recurrent myocardial infarction, which was surprisingly high at 5.5% compared to that of the group receiving air, which was 0.9% ($P = 0.006$). There was also a substantial increase in the incidence of cardiac arrhythmias (40.4% versus 31.4%; $P = 0.05$). The differences in outcome persisted at 6 months, with the oxygen patients having more substantial MIs as defined by the infarct size on cardiac magnetic resonance imaging (MRI). Only 139 of the subjects had available data for this portion of the analysis. The authors concluded that the administration of oxygen may *increase* early myocardial injury. As a student, I was taught that oxygen was one of the cornerstones of therapy for patients with acute myocardial infarction, applying this therapy with a logical goal of limiting the infarct size and mitigating myocardial injury. How amazing it was to learn, from Stub's straightforward randomized protocol, that this simple and seemingly beneficial therapy of supplemental oxygen could actually be associated with a worse outcome. Perhaps prompted by this publication, Derek Chu and others performed an extensive meta-analysis, published in *The Lancet* in 2018, which called into question the application of oxygen in other relatively straightforward clinical applications. Chu examined the outcomes of more than 16,000 patients across 25 different randomized clinical trials with sepsis, critical illness, stroke, trauma, myocardial infarction, cardiac arrest, and emergency surgery. In those subjects who received oxygen consistent with a conservative administration strategy versus a more liberal administration strategy, hospital mortality was lower at 30 days [13]. Based on this publication, a new standard has been established in general hospital care for limiting the use of oxygen and more closely monitoring O_2 saturations, avoiding hyperoxia in a variety of routine non-respiratory care circumstances. While there certainly may be exceptions, it is clear that the era of routine administration of oxygen for acutely ill adults is in the past. Outcomes are maximized by avoiding oxygen in certain diagnoses where there is no evidence of hypoxemia, limiting oxygen therapy by not initiating its use in patients that have O_2 saturations of 93% or above and stopping oxygen in those patients with saturations of 96% or above. This strategy helps avoid hyperoxia based on peripheral arterial O_2 saturation [14]. See Fig. 7.1

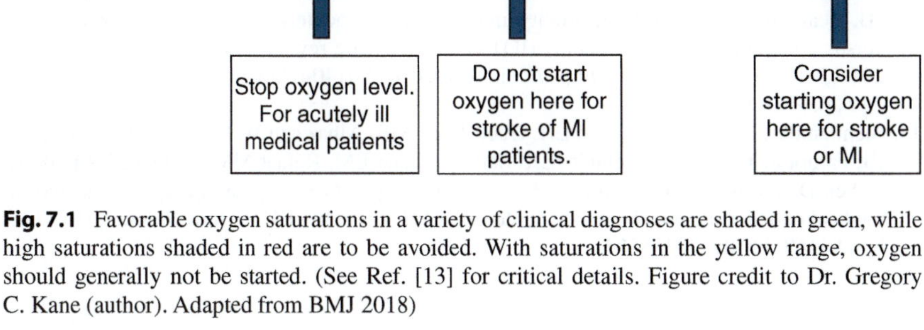

Fig. 7.1 Favorable oxygen saturations in a variety of clinical diagnoses are shaded in green, while high saturations shaded in red are to be avoided. With saturations in the yellow range, oxygen should generally not be started. (See Ref. [13] for critical details. Figure credit to Dr. Gregory C. Kane (author). Adapted from BMJ 2018)

for a graphic display of the current recommendations from the British Medical Society.

In summary, confirming the findings of important physician scientists of the twentieth century, namely, Comroe and Crystal, we have learned through the ARDS network that limiting hyperoxia is associated with improved outcomes in sick ICU patients with respiratory failure. Even the simple application of low-flow oxygen via nasal prongs in many diagnoses appears to have deleterious effects on mortality and should be avoided.

References

1. Blodgett AN. The continuous inhalation of oxygen in cases of pneumonia otherwise fatal, and in other diseases. Boston Med J. 1890;123:481–5.
2. Comroe JH Jr, Dripps RD, Dumke PR, Deming M. Oxygen toxicity: the effect of inhalation of high concentrations of oxygen for twenty-four hours on normal men at sea level and at a simulated altitude of 18,000 feet. JAMA. 1945;128:710–7.
3. Davis WB, Rennard SI, Bitterman PB, Crystal RG. Pulmonary oxygen toxicity- early pulmonary alveolar changes induced by Hyperoxia. N Engl J Med. 1983;309:878–83. https://doi.org/10.1056/NEJM198310133091502.
4. Mustafa MG, Tierney DF. Biochemical and metabolic changes in the lung with oxygen, ozone, and nitrogen dioxide toxicity. Am Rev Respir Dis. 1978;118:1061–85.
5. Sackner MA, Landa J, Hirsch J, Zapata A. Pulmonary effects of oxygen breathing: a 6-hour study in normal men. Ann Intern Med. 1975;82:40–3.
6. Helmerhorst HJ, Roos-Blom MJ, van Westerloo DJ, et al. Association systematic review, meta-analysis, and meta-regression of cohort studies. Crit Care Med. 2015;43:1508–19. https://doi.org/10.1097/CCM.0000000000000998.
7. Kilgannon JH, Jones AE, Shapiro NI, et al. Association between arterial hyperoxia following resuscitation from cardiac arrest and in-hospital mortality. JAMA. 2010;303(21):2165–71. https://doi.org/10.1001/jama.2010.707.
8. Helmerhorst HJ, Arts DL, Schultz MJ, et al. Metrics of arterial hyperoxia and associated outcomes in critical care. Crit Care Med. 2017;45(2):187–95. https://doi.org/10.1097/CCM.0000000000002084.
9. http://www.ardsnet.org/files/ventilator_protocol_2008-07.pdf. Accessed 9 Mar 2025.
10. Steele C. Severe angina pectoris relieved by oxygen inhalations. BMJ. 1900;2:1568.
11. Stub D, Smith K, Bernard S, Nehme Z, AVOID Investigators, et al. Air versus oxygen in ST-segment-elevation myocardial infarction. Circulation. 2015;131(24):2143–50. https://doi.org/10.1161/CirculationAHA.114.014494.
12. Russek HI, Regan FD, Naegele CF. One hundred per cent oxygen in the treatment of acute myocardial infarction and severe angina pectoris. JAMA J Am Med Assoc. 1950;144(5):373–5.
13. Chu DK, Kim LH, Young PJ, Zamiri N, Almenawer SA, Jaeschke R, Szczeklik W, Schünemann HJ, Neary JD, Alhazzani W. Mortality and morbidity in acutely ill adults treated with liberal versus conservative oxygen therapy (IOTA): a systematic review and meta-analysis. Lancet. 2018;391(10131):1693–705. https://doi.org/10.1016/S0140-6736(18)30479-3. Epub 2018 Apr 26. PMID: 29726345.
14. Siemieniuk RAC, Chu DK, Kim LH, Güell-Rous MR, Alhazzani W, Soccal PM, Karanicolas PJ, Farhoumand PD, Siemieniuk JLK, Satia I, Irusen EM, Refaat MM, Mikita JS, Smith M, Cohen DN, Vandvik PO, Agoritsas T, Lytvyn L, Guyatt GH. Oxygen therapy for acutely ill medical patients: a clinical practice guideline. BMJ. 2018;363:k4169. https://doi.org/10.1136/bmj.k4169. PMID: 30355567.

Fundamentals of Using Oxygen via Nasal Cannula in Health and Disease

8

Mackenzie Kramer and Urvashi Vaid

Introduction

The nasal cannula was first introduced by Wilfred Jones as a patient interface for oxygen delivery in the 1940s. Now, more than 1.5 million adults in the United States receive long-term oxygen therapy (LTOT) to improve their quality of life and prolong survival [1]. Identifying which patients receive a mortality benefit remains a balance of evidence-based guidelines and an understanding of pulmonary physiology. This concept will be expanded upon later.

In 1917, Haldane described the therapeutic potential of providing supplemental oxygen and understood that the concentration of oxygen delivered was important [2]. In the 1930s, Alvan Barach suggested using long-term oxygen therapy in the home for chronic pulmonary disease and invented the meter mask, which provided the ability to vary the O_2 concentration; however, the technology was not yet available for mass production. Over subsequent years, the development of oxygen delivery systems in hospitalized settings became widely utilized. In the 1960s, the benefits of using continuous low-flow oxygen continued to expand. In the 1980s, randomized landmark clinical trials in patients with chronic obstructive pulmonary disease (COPD) and severe, chronic hypoxemia were published, which established the foundation to use long-term oxygen therapy (LTOT) in select patient populations. This chapter will outline the indications for and the mechanisms of oxygen delivery via nasal cannula, focusing on physiology. Later chapters will focus on oxygen delivery devices and high-flow oxygen delivery.

M. Kramer · U. Vaid (✉)
The Korman Respiratory Institute and the Division of Pulmonary and Critical Care, The Department of Medicine at the Sidney Kimmel Medical College of Thomas Jefferson University, Philadelphia, PA, USA
e-mail: Mackenzie.Kramer@jefferson.edu; Urvashi.Vaid@jefferson.edu

G. C. Kane et al. (eds.), *Oxygen*, https://doi.org/10.1007/978-3-032-18934-9_8

Indications for Oxygen Therapy

Indications for the Use of Oxygen in Acute Settings

Previous chapters of this book have outlined the discovery of oxygen, its first therapeutic use in modern medicine, and the pitfalls of using supplemental oxygen. Oxygen is used very commonly as an acute therapy when patients complain of shortness of breath and/or have low oxygen saturations, as measured by a pulse oximeter. More than 25% of patients visiting the emergency department receive supplemental oxygen [3]. Many times, the flow of oxygen seems to have a calming effect on the anxious patient. As described in Chap. 12, hypoxemia is an extraordinarily strong stimulus, causing peripheral chemoreceptors to fire impulses that travel centrally to the medullary respiratory centers to increase both alveolar and minute ventilation. This pathway results in patients increasing their respiratory rates and then their tidal volumes in the presence of hypoxemia. The application of supplemental oxygen increases the partial pressure of alveolar oxygen and thus the supply of oxygen to the tissues, thereby reducing hypoxia. The benefit of oxygen is associated with risk. Recent literature shows that mortality is increased when oxygen is provided to hospitalized patients in the absence of hypoxemia [4]. Current recommendations for initiating oxygen therapy acutely vary by the underlying indication, for example, restricting oxygen therapy to target saturations of 88–92% in patients with COPD and hypercapnia (detailed in the Chap. 12). Consensus recommendations now target a goal peripheral capillary oxygen saturation between 92% and 96% to mitigate the effects of profound hypoxia and hyperoxia [5]. Table 8.1 summarizes oxygen therapy targets in acute illnesses.

Indications for the Chronic Use of Oxygen

Over the past five decades, medical societies have developed evidence-based guidelines for the indications and delivery of oxygen as a long-term therapy. Current guidelines state that oxygen therapy is indicated for patients with severe, chronic hypoxemia, which is defined as a partial pressure of arterial oxygen (PaO_2) less than or equal to 55 mmHg or a peripheral capillary oxygen saturation (SpO_2) less than or equal to 88%. Additionally, supplemental oxygen therapy is indicated for patients with a PaO_2 of 56–59 mmHg, with evidence of right-sided heart failure, polycythemia, or cor pulmonale [6].

These specific thresholds to determine oxygen therapy were established from landmark randomized controlled trials, specifically the Nocturnal Oxygen Therapy Trial (NOTT) and the Medical Research Council (MRC) trials, which have shown survival benefits and improvement in quality of life when using long-term oxygen therapy (LTOT) in hypoxemic patients with chronic obstructive pulmonary disease and other hypoxemic chronic lung diseases that met the inclusion criteria [7].

NOTT and MRC trials demonstrated that LTOT for at least 15–18 hours per day improves survival in patients with chronic obstructive pulmonary disease (COPD)

Table 8.1 Oxygen saturation targets for acute medical illnesses [5]

Oxygen saturation target	Disease state	Pathophysiologic rationale
Low (88–92%)	Conditions causing chronic hypercapnia, like COPD, obesity hypoventilation syndrome, obstructive sleep apnea, and neuromuscular diseases	Ameliorating hypoxia abolishes the hypoxic vasoconstrictive response and thus worsens Ventilation-Perfusion (V/Q) matching The Haldane effect off-loads more CO_2 into the blood in the presence of O_2 Centrally, the loss of CO_2 as a driver of respiration may be lost, leaving hypoxia as the main driver Absorption atelectasis from too much oxygen delivered to the alveoli results in loss of surface area for gas exchange
Between high and low (90–96%)	Ischemic strokes: Use O_2 if SpO_2 <96% Myocardial infarctions: Use O_2 if SpO_2 <90% or if dyspneic or in heart failure Other acutely ill patients: provide oxygen if SpO_2 <94%	Trials did not show a reduction in mortality or disability with increasing levels of oxygen in these conditions
High (close to 100%)	Conditions such as cluster headaches, carbon monoxide poisoning, pneumothorax, and sickle cell crises	Here, the delivery of higher partial pressures of oxygen to the alveoli helps resolve the underlying conditions faster

and daytime hypoxemia. These studies also included the correlation between survival and the average daily duration of oxygen use. The Registry-Based Treatment Duration and Mortality in Long-Term Oxygen Therapy (REDOX) trial compared a 24-hour versus 15-hour regimen in patients with severe hypoxemia and found no significant difference in mortality at the one-year follow-up [8]. The REDOX trial patient population included patients with COPD (70%) as well as pulmonary fibrosis (12%) and found no difference in all-cause hospitalization, COPD symptoms, or other adverse events between the groups.

In conclusion, the NOTT and MRC randomized clinical trials demonstrated that long-term oxygen therapy improves survival among patients who have COPD and severe resting hypoxemia. The updated official clinical practice guideline for home oxygen therapy in adults with chronic lung disease was published from a multidisciplinary workshop at the American Thoracic Society (ATS) International Conference in 2017, with the goal to optimize home oxygen therapy for adults, and will be discussed throughout this chapter [9].

Considerations While Using Long-Term Oxygen Therapy

Oxygen therapy is used with the goal of maintaining an SpO_2 above 90–92% but below 96–98% to avoid both hypoxemia and hyperoxia. In addition to the deleterious effects of hyperoxia, as discussed in a previous chapter, patients using long-term oxygen therapy experience significant functional, mechanical, and financial limitations, which negatively affect their quality of life. In addition, patients report a significant lack of education related to their oxygen equipment, as well as a restriction of choices in portable versus stationary oxygen equipment by durable medical equipment companies (DME).

Additionally, smoking near oxygen tanks or flowing sources of oxygen, such as nasal cannulas, poses a significant risk of fire and explosion, which can lead to severe burns, inhalational injury, property damage, and even death. Oxygen itself is not flammable but instead is an oxidizer. As an oxidizer, it greatly accelerates combustion, so a small spark from a lighter can ignite clothing, hair, or the oxygen delivery system itself, resulting in catastrophic injury. During the period of 2017–2021, there were roughly 1041 oxygen-related thermal burns annually, with 228 house fires and nearly 96 deaths a year [10]. The American Thoracic Society recommends that all patients receiving home oxygen be provided with comprehensive education on the dangers of smoking near oxygen, and smoking cessation support should be provided as a standard of care.

Prescribing Oxygen Therapy

When a patient meets the criteria for long-term oxygen therapy, the appropriate fraction of inspired oxygen (FiO_2) to prescribe is determined by titrating oxygen to maintain an SpO_2 ≥90% (or a PaO_2 >60 mmHg) at rest. To determine the actual fraction of inspired oxygen that is delivered to the alveoli, providers must consider the interplay of oxygen flow rate, patient respiratory pattern, mouth position, and airway anatomy, among other factors. Another important consideration is the increasing recognition that patients with darker skin pigmentation may have occult hypoxemia. Occult hypoxemia is defined as an arterial oxygen saturation of <88% despite a pulse oximeter saturation reading of ≥92%. A pulse oximeter is a noninvasive tool to measure the oxygen saturation of blood. These devices use absorption spectrophotometry to measure the absorption of two wavelengths of light across the body. There is a higher risk of mortality associated with occult hypoxemia in ICU and surgical patients, so this is not without clinical consequences [11]. It may also prevent these patients from qualifying for home oxygen therapy despite low true arterial oxygen saturations. Oximeters that are validated across a wide range of skin tones are in development to help mitigate this disparity.

Nasal cannulas deliver a pure source of oxygen through simple nasal prongs at a set flow rate, which ranges from 1 to 6 L/min. Due to tubing resistance and increasingly turbulent airflow, there is a marginal improvement in oxygen delivery beyond 6 L/min. Ideally, the fractional concentration of oxygen in inspired gas delivered increases approximately 3–4% per L/min [12]. Room air has a fraction of inspired oxygen at 21%, so, for example, 4 L/min of oxygen via a nasal cannula would correspond to a fractional concentration of oxygen in inspired gas of approximately 36%.

However, the desired fractional concentration of oxygen in inspired gas is not only dependent upon the set flow rate (1–6 L/min) but, additionally, on the volume of ambient air inhaled during breathing. For example, if a patient was experiencing respiratory distress with an increased respiratory rate and/or tidal volume, the fraction of ambient air also increases, in turn, leading to lower levels of fractional concentration of oxygen in the inspired gas. Consider a child breathing a tidal volume of 150 mL per breath at a rate of 20 breaths/minute. The child's total minute ventilation would be 3 L/min. If the child is placed on oxygen via a nasal cannula at 2 L/min, the room air entrained with every breath will lower the FiO_2 dramatically. And if the child becomes increasingly tachypneic, they are more likely to be exchanging air in the dead space regions of the respiratory system rather than in the alveoli where gas exchange can occur. It is important to note that infants and children have a proportionally greater dead space than adults due to the anatomy of their oropharynx.

Additionally, there are unpredictable fractions of inspired gas with oral versus nasal breathing, with studies showing conflicting results. Nasal patency is another limiting factor, and humidification systems are recommended to prevent drying of the nasal mucosa and nasal mucosal bleeding (epistaxis) from prolonged use.

Oxygen Delivery Devices

Continuous-flow oxygen through a nasal cannula is considered the standard prescription for long-term oxygen delivery in hypoxemic patients. Continuous-flow oxygen is delivered at a constant, preset flow rate throughout the entire respiratory cycle, independent of the patient's inspiratory or expiratory phase. Consider a healthy adult breathing 500 mL of tidal volume per breath at a rate of 15/min. The total minute ventilation for this adult would be calculated at 7.5 L/min (0.5 L × 15 breaths). If they are anxious or exercising or develop an illness that drives up their minute ventilation by increasing either their tidal volume and/or their respiratory rate, they may increase their minute ventilation to much higher levels. Maximum flow rates also increase, the maximum inspiratory flow rate being 25–30 L/min at rest but rising to 40–60 L/min for brief periods when the ventilatory demand increases. Continuous-flow oxygen is the initial preferred method of oxygen delivery because it provides a predictable and consistent oxygen supply and allows for the replacement of air in the oropharynx with oxygen, thus lowering the dead space. However, continuous-flow oxygen is inefficient as only a small amount of oxygen delivered to the nose reaches the alveoli. Thus, despite increasing the FiO_2 of the inhaled air, it is limited in its ability to increase the partial pressure of alveolar oxygen. Additionally, the oxygen supply at home may be limited. Consider a full cylinder of oxygen, 680 L in volume and pressurized to 2000 PSI, from which the patient is receiving oxygen at 2 L/min. This cylinder will last for 4 h and 30 min. The DME companies provide information and safety sheets on individual cylinder sizes and flow rates to all patients.

Alternate delivery systems, such as demand oxygen delivery systems, or pulse dose, provide oxygen only during inspiration and are used primarily to conserve oxygen. The chapters following this one outline these other delivery methods and the issue of transportation and portability in greater detail.

Additional considerations include reservoir cannulas, which function by storing oxygen in a reservoir space during exhalation, making that oxygen available as a bolus upon the onset of the next inhalation [13]. Reservoir cannulas are available in different configurations based on patient preference. An Oxymizer®, a mustache configuration, is located directly beneath the nose and tends to be more comfortable to patients; however, it can be more noticeable on the face and leads to other patients rejecting it. The Oxymizer® Pendant, a pendant configuration, utilizes an in-line plastic reservoir that rests on the anterior chest wall. The fluidic mustache reservoir cannula is designed to operate at higher flow rates, thus serving as a conserving device as well as a high-flow device.

Adjustment to Oxygen Prescription

Adjustment of the initial oxygen prescription may be required for exertion, sleep, travel, and acute exacerbations.

Exercise

It is common for patients with chronic obstructive pulmonary disease who qualify for long-term oxygen therapy to experience hypoxemia at rest and further desaturate during exertion. It is, therefore, imperative to determine the oxygen flow rate necessary during exertion and include this in the oxygen prescription for the patient. Additional considerations may be used other than exertional desaturations, including increasing flow rates for other metrics such as dyspnea and exercise improvement. Additionally, the 2020 ATS guidelines support emerging evidence that ambulatory oxygen may improve health-related quality of life in patients with other pulmonary diseases and must be considered in other patient populations, such as those with interstitial lung disease [9].

Exercise Training

It is widely accepted that exercise training within the context of pulmonary rehabilitation improves outcomes of exercise capacity, dyspnea, and health-related quality of life in patients with COPD. Whether the use of oxygen during exercise training in COPD patients without hypoxia may be of additional benefit continues to be in question. A randomized trial of 29 patients with COPD and hypoxemia reported that supplemental oxygen doubled the effect of endurance training compared to exercising in atmospheric air [14]. Supplemental oxygen during exercise has been shown to reduce ventilatory limitation, improving exercise tolerance, but the effect on long-term outcomes such as strength gain remains in question.

As an aside, pro athletes are commonly observed using supplemental oxygen on the sidelines of sporting events. Supplemental oxygen is theorized to delay fatigue by helping clear lactic acid more efficiently and improve endurance by increasing aerobic capacity. While some studies suggest benefits, the extent to which supplemental oxygen improves performance in healthy athletes is still being studied, and there may be a psychological or placebo effect at play. Additionally, supplemental oxygen during physical activity can lead to risks and side effects and should only be used under medical professionals' guidance.

Nocturnal Desaturations

Among patients prescribed long-term oxygen therapy for daytime hypoxemia, clinicians should determine if higher flow rates are necessary for nocturnal desaturations. In the NOTT, for example, oxygen flow rate was increased by 1 L/min during sleep. Additionally, as many as 30% of patients with COPD who do not have daytime hypoxemia will experience desaturations during sleep [15]. Overnight polysomnography can help clarify if obstructive sleep apnea is playing a role and can provide nocturnal monitoring of hypoxemic events.

Air Travel

During air travel, as altitude increases, ambient air in the cabin decreases, leading to a decrease in the partial pressure of oxygen of inspired air, which can lead to hypoxemia in patients with lung disease [16]. The British Thoracic Society (BTS) recommends that if a patient is already on LTOT at <4 L/min, they should increase oxygen to 2 L/min greater than their prescription while in flight [16]. However, for patients with an oxygen requirement of >4 L/min at rest, it may be difficult to ensure adequate supplemental oxygen in flight, and it is generally recommended to avoid air travel. Various methods have been suggested for patients who need specific testing for in-flight hypoxemia. The BTS guidelines suggest using a combination of resting SpO_2 <95% at sea level and risk factors that would increase the likelihood of in-flight hypoxemia to guide the need for further testing [16]. The 6MWT is recommended to improve sensitivity for patients at risk of hypoxemia and reduce the overall number of patients referred to hypoxia altitude stimulation testing [17]. Hypoxia altitude stimulation testing (HAST) is a procedure where patients are exposed to a low-oxygen gas mixture, like the air pressure in a plane cabin, to further assess oxygen needs in flight. Additionally, other altitudes can also be stimulated if ordered by a health care provider. It is crucial to identify which patients are at risk of in-flight hypoxia, simulate in-flight conditions if necessary, and estimate in-flight requirements. The Federal Aviation Administration (FAA) requires a prescription from the clinician, and prior approval from the airline is needed. This topic is elaborated in greater detail in later chapters.

Reassessment

The discontinuation of oxygen among patients who do not benefit from it is an opportunity to improve the safety and value of health care delivery. The American Board of Internal Medicine and Consumer Reports' "Choosing Wisely" campaign recommended that patients recently discharged on home oxygen after hospitalization have a follow-up prior to renewal of the prescription. In a cohort study, only 43.6% of patients had a complete reassessment of oxygen within 90 days of hospital discharge [18]. Additionally, when a complete reassessment did occur, nearly half of the patients were eligible for discontinuation.

Conclusions

Oxygen therapy has a reasonably strong evidence base for improving functional status, quality of life, and mortality in certain diseases like COPD. It seems common sense to deliver the fuel (oxygen) that our cells and tissues so desperately need to ensure survival and repair. The nasal cannula is a commonly used delivery device, with limitations to the quantity of oxygen delivered and portability. Despite this, it is ubiquitous in acute medical settings as the first delivery device for oxygen and in homes for patients on long-term oxygen.

References

1. Jacobs SS, Lederer DJ, Garvey CM, Hernandez C, Lindell KO, McLaughlin S, et al. Optimizing home oxygen therapy. An Official American Thoracic Society Workshop Report. Ann Am Thorac Soc. 2018;15(12):1369–81.
2. Sekhar K, Rao S. John Scott Haldane: the father of oxygen therapy. Indian J Anaesth. 2014;58(3):350.
3. Hale KE, Gavin C, O'Driscoll BR. Audit of oxygen use in emergency ambulances and in a hospital emergency department. Emerg Med J. 2008;25:773–6. https://doi.org/10.1136/emj.2008.059287. PMID: 18955625.
4. Hu DK, Kim LH, Young PJ, et al. Mortality and morbidity in acutely ill adults treated with liberal versus conservative oxygen therapy (IOTA): a systematic review and meta-analysis. Lancet. 2018;391:1693–705. https://doi.org/10.1016/S0140-6736(18)30479-3. PMID: 29726345.
5. Siemieniuk RAC, et al. Oxygen therapy for acutely ill medical patient: a clinical practice guideline. BMJ. 2018;363:k4169. https://doi.org/10.1136/bmj.k4169.
6. Stoller JK, Panos RJ, Krachman S, Doherty DE, Make B. Oxygen therapy for patients with COPD. Chest [Internet]. 2020;138(1):179–87. Available from: https://www.ncbi.nlm.nih.gov/pmc/articles/PMC2897694/.

7. Yusen RD, Criner GJ, Sternberg AL, Au DH, Fuhlbrigge AL, Albert RK, et al. The long-term oxygen treatment trial for chronic obstructive pulmonary disease: rationale, design, and lessons learned. Ann Am Thorac Soc. 2018;15(1):89–101.
8. Ekström M, Andersson A, Papadopoulos S, Kipper T, Pedersen B, Kricka O, et al. Long-term oxygen therapy for 24 or 15 hours per day in severe hypoxemia. N Engl J Med. 2024;391(11):977–88.
9. Jacobs SS, Krishnan JA, Lederer DJ, Ghazipura M, Hossain T, Tan AYM, et al. Home oxygen therapy for adults with chronic lung disease. An Official American Thoracic Society clinical practice guideline. Am J Respir Crit Care Med. 2020;202(10):e121–41.
10. https://www.nfpa.org/education-and-research/research/nfpa-research/fire-statistical-reports/fires-and-burns-involving-home-medical-oxygen.
11. https://www.jwatch.org/na55581/2022/12/28/pulse-oximetry-less-accurate-patients-with-darker-skin.
12. Fuentes S, Chowdhury YS. Fraction of inspired oxygen (FiO2) [Internet]. PubMed. Treasure Island (FL): StatPearls Publishing; 2022. Available from: https://www.ncbi.nlm.nih.gov/books/NBK560867/.
13. Tiep BL, Burns M, Hererra J. A new pendant oxygen-conserving cannula which allows pursed lips breathing. Chest. 1989;95(4):857–60. https://doi.org/10.1378/chest.95.4.857.
14. Neunhäuserer D, Steidle-Kloc E, Weiss G, Kaiser B, Niederseer D, Hartl S, et al. Supplemental oxygen during high-intensity exercise training in nonhypoxemic chronic obstructive pulmonary disease. Am J Med. 2016;129(11):1185–93.
15. Fletcher EC, Miller J, Divine GW, Fletcher JG, Miller T. Nocturnal oxyhemoglobin desaturation in COPD patients with arterial oxygen tensions above 60 mm Hg. Chest. 1987;92(4):604–8.
16. Coker RK, Armstrong A, Church AC, Holmes S, Naylor J, Pike K, et al. BTS Clinical Statement on air travel for passengers with respiratory disease. Thorax. 2022;77(4):329–50.
17. Edvardsen A, Akerø A, Christensen CC, Ryg M, Skjønsberg OH. Air travel and chronic obstructive pulmonary disease: a new algorithm for pre-flight evaluation. Thorax [Internet]. 2012;67(11):964–9.
18. Spece LJ, Epler EM, Duan K, Donovan LM, Griffith MF, LaBedz S, et al. Reassessment of home oxygen prescription after hospitalization for chronic obstructive pulmonary disease. A potential target for deimplementation. Ann Am Thorac Soc. 2021;18(3):426–32.

Hemoglobin: The Ideal Conveyor of Oxygen

9

Sohiel Deshpande and Ruben Rhoades

Introduction

Hemoglobin (Hb) is vital to the transport of oxygen through the body of an organism. Erythrocytes (red blood cells) are the carriers of hemoglobin in vertebrates. Even though the term "blood" has been in use since the times of Plato and Aristotle around 400 BCE, its individual constituents, including the red blood cell, were not identified until about the seventeenth century [1]. Furthermore, it was not until the nineteenth century that the physical characteristics and structure of hemoglobin were discovered. Laurence Bragg and Max Perutz demonstrated the structure of the crystalline form of horse methyl hemoglobin using X-ray crystallography in 1952. Perutz was later awarded the Nobel Prize in Chemistry, along with John Kendrew, for the discovery of the structure of hemoglobin and myoglobin, respectively [2]. In this chapter, we will describe the structure, function, and dynamic interaction of the hemoglobin molecule with oxygen.

Basic Structure of Hemoglobin

The mammalian hemoglobin (Hb) molecule is made up of two components: the *heme* and *globin* moieties. A typical Hb molecule exists as a quaternary structure composed of four distinct globin subunits (Fig. 9.1). Each subunit comprises a polypeptide chain with a bound heme molecule.

Heme is a protoporphyrin complex with a centrally placed ferrous ion (Fe^{2+}), which can be oxidized to bind to an oxygen molecule. Thus, each subunit of

S. Deshpande · R. Rhoades (✉)
Division of Hematology, The Department of Medicine at the Sidney Kimmel Medical College of Thomas Jefferson University, Philadelphia, PA, USA
e-mail: Ruben.Rhoades@jefferson.edu

G. C. Kane et al. (eds.), *Oxygen*, https://doi.org/10.1007/978-3-032-18934-9_9

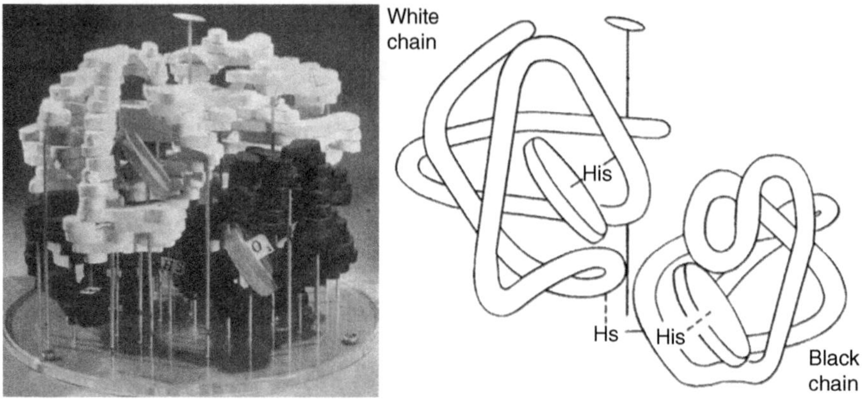

Fig. 9.1 Structure of hemoglobin as described by Perutz and colleagues. (From Perutz et al. [2]. Reproduced with permission from Springer Nature)

hemoglobin is effectively an oxygen-binding site. Heme is synthesized partially in the mitochondria and the cytosol of the erythrocytes and hepatocytes in the human body [3].

The *globin* components are polypeptide chains. Standard convention has historically been to use Greek letters to identify complex protein chains, so each globin chain within the hemoglobin tetramer is indicated by such letters (e.g., α, β, γ, and δ) [4]. The common subunit composition in human Hb comprises two alpha and two beta chains ($\alpha_2\beta_2$), which is termed HbA or normal adult hemoglobin. Two alpha and two gamma chains ($\alpha_2\gamma_2$) give rise to fetal Hb (HbF). To date, more than 200 distinct variants of the Hb molecule have been described. Occasionally, variations in these chains, such as $\alpha_2\beta^S{}_2$ (HbS) in sickle cell disease (SCD), can be a cause of pathology [5]. With this background about the structure in mind, the interactions of Hb with oxygen can be explored in further detail.

Hemoglobin–Oxygen Interaction

Oxygen in mammalian blood exists in two forms: bound to Hb (98%) and dissolved in plasma (2%). Hb is considered to be the most efficient carrier of oxygen in the human body. A Hb tetramer is capable of reversibly binding four molecules of oxygen (one per heme moiety). Through their experiments using magnetism, Linus Pauling and colleagues at the California Institute of Technology were able to draw conclusions about the nature of this interaction. It was known that in the natural unbound state, oxygen has two unpaired electrons, which would contribute to some magnetic effect. However, during their experiments, both oxy- and carboxyhemoglobin (carboxy-Hb) did not demonstrate any magnetism. They thus postulated that gases like oxygen and carbon monoxide (CO) bind to the iron atoms in heme via covalent bonds, in the process, losing their unbound electrons [6].

Fundamental differences in the structure of the hemoglobin molecule were noted on X-ray crystallographic images of the oxy- and deoxy-Hb. It was thus accurately suggested that Hb exists in an equilibrium between two structures: a tense form (T), which has a low affinity to oxygen due to constraints of additional hydrogen bonds and salt bridges, and a relaxed form (R), with an increased affinity to oxygen [7]. Subsequent work has shown that multiple states exist during the T-to-R transition and even possibly beyond ("multi-relaxed states") [8]. Conformational changes that occur within the hemoglobin molecule after the binding of the first oxygen atom allow for better exposure of other binding sites. This progressively increases the affinity of Hb for binding subsequent molecules of oxygen. Conventionally, the oxygen–Hb dissociation curve (Fig. 9.2) has been used to graphically represent the relationship between partial pressure of oxygen (PO_2) and the oxygen saturation (SO_2) [9]. The affinity of oxygen for Hb is often represented by the PO_2 at which Hb is 50% saturated with oxygen (P_{50}).

Allosteric proteins are ligands that, when bound to one site of a protein, influence and affect the binding of other ligands at different sites on the same protein. Thus, the stereochemical changes that occur within the quaternary structure of the Hb molecule when the first oxygen binds to it were described as allosteric effects,

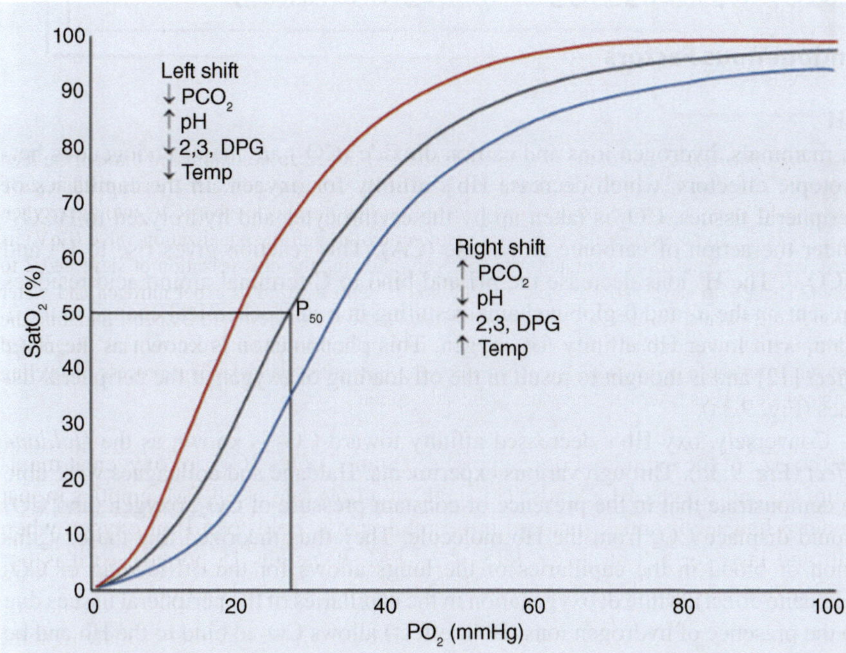

Fig. 9.2 The oxygen–hemoglobin dissociation curve. The center (black) line represents normal conditions. The left-shifted (red) curve represents states of high oxygen affinity for hemoglobin, while the right-shifted (blue) curve represents states of low oxygen affinity for hemoglobin and increased oxygen delivery to tissues. Causes for each type of shift in the dissociation curve are listed. (From Gupta and Somasundaram [9]. Reproduced with permission from Springer Nature)

which allowed oxygen molecules to bind to or dissociate from the Hb molecule efficiently. The phenomenon of "cooperative binding" among the oxygen-binding sites explains the sigmoid shape in the oxygen–Hb dissociation curve, indicating an increased affinity for subsequent oxygen molecules to Hb after the binding of the first oxygen molecule [7, 10, 11] (Fig. 9.2). The Hill coefficient is used as a measure of this cooperativity between ligand binding sites, with values >1 indicating positive cooperativity, as in the case of Hb and oxygen.

Oxygen Delivery to Tissues

Ultimately, oxygenation of tissues is determined by various factors, including the partial pressure of oxygen in arterial blood (PaO_2), saturation of Hb by oxygen (SaO_2), Hb concentration in blood, affinity of oxygen to Hb, and the cardiac output. The loading and off-loading of oxygen from the hemoglobin molecule is a highly dynamic interaction and is influenced by a multitude of factors, both internal and external to the erythrocyte (Fig. 9.2).

Factors Impacting Oxygen–Hemoglobin Affinity

Endogenous Factors

pH

In mammals, hydrogen ions and carbon dioxide (CO_2) are major endogenous heterotopic effectors, which decrease Hb's affinity for oxygen. In the capillaries of peripheral tissues, CO_2 is taken up by the erythrocytes and hydrolyzed to HCO_3^- under the action of carbonic anhydrase (CA). This reaction gives rise to H^+ and HCO_3^-. The H^+ ions decrease the pH and bind to C-terminal amino acid residues present on the α- and β-globin chains, resulting in a stereochemical change to the T state, with lower Hb affinity for oxygen. This phenomenon is known as the *Bohr effect* [12] and is thought to result in the off-loading of oxygen at the peripheral tissues (Fig. 9.3a).

Conversely, oxy-Hb's decreased affinity toward CO_2 is known as the *Haldane effect* (Fig. 9.3b). Through various experiments, Haldane and colleagues were able to demonstrate that in the presence of constant pressure of CO_2, oxygen (and CO) would displace CO_2 from the Hb molecule. They thus theorized that the oxygenation of blood in the capillaries of the lungs allows for the off-loading of CO_2 (Haldane effect), while deoxygenation in the capillaries of the peripheral tissues due to the presence of hydrogen ions (Bohr effect) allows CO_2 to bind to the Hb and be transported back to the lungs. This rapid interplay between the Bohr and the Haldane effects allows for optimal oxygen exchange in the lungs and tissues [13, 14].

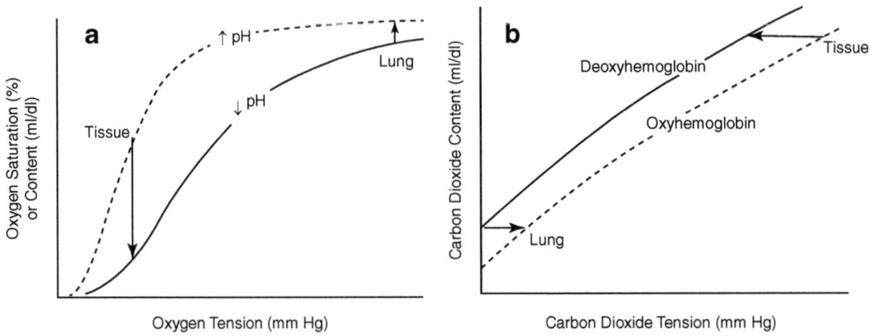

Fig. 9.3 Reciprocal interactions between oxygen (**a**) and carbon dioxide (**b**) binding to hemoglobin—the Bohr effect and the Haldane effect. (From Hsia [14]. Reproduced with permission from the Massachusetts Medical Society)

2,3-Bisphosphoglycerate

Another important endogenous effector is 2,3-bisphosphoglycerate (2,3-BPG or 2,3-DPG) [15]. It is a naturally occurring metabolic by-product of glycolysis, which is the sole method of metabolism in erythrocytes. The negative charges on the surface of 2,3-BPG bind to positively charged amino acids in the β-cleft in deoxy-Hb, which stabilizes it in the T conformation and thus reduces its affinity toward oxygen [8], shifting the oxygen–Hb dissociation curve to the right and increasing P_{50}. Intracellular H^+ ion concentration exhibits an inverse relationship with 2,3-BPG concentrations in erythrocytes, such that a high H^+ ion concentration (low pH) decreases 2,3-BPG [16, 17]. This affords Hb a mechanism for achieving homeostasis in the face of changing intracellular conditions.

Chloride

Chloride (Cl^-) ions play a role in altering the structure and oxygen affinity of Hb. In the T conformation, excess positive charges in the central cavity of Hb repel each other and raise the free energy, leading to increased oxygen affinity [18]. The binding of Cl^- ions to these positive charges, though, lowers the free energy of the T state and, thus, also the oxygen affinity. Therefore, the net effect of Cl^- on Hb is to stabilize the T conformation and shift the oxygen–Hb to the right [18, 19].

Sphingosine-1-Phosphate

Sphingosine-1-phosphate (S1P) is a signaling lipid molecule present in erythrocytes that interacts with various proteins and binds to cell surface receptors [8]. It has been shown to be overexpressed in erythrocytes in SCD [20]. S1P is upregulated in hypoxic conditions and has been shown to induce glycolysis and 2,3-BPG production, thus promoting oxygen release and shifting the oxygen–Hb dissociation curve to the right [21].

Hemoglobin Variants

As discussed earlier, variation in the combinations of globin chains gives rise to variants of Hb. While approximately a thousand Hb variants have been described, a common and naturally occurring variant is *fetal Hb (HbF)*, which comprises two alpha and two gamma chains ($\alpha_2\gamma_2$). Differences in the globin chain structure result in subtle changes in the inter-subunit interfaces of the hemoglobin molecule, leading to variation in its interaction with oxygen. This shifts the oxygen-binding curve to the left (i.e., to a higher oxygen–Hb affinity state). The structure of HbF, which is typically present at the pre-neonatal and early neonatal stages, facilitates maximal binding of oxygen to Hb, especially in situations where its supply is limited. The increased affinity of HbF to oxygen, even at relatively lower partial pressures, allows the transfer of oxygen from the maternal to the fetal Hb via the placenta [22]. The production of HbF declines gradually after birth and is replaced by HbA. However, as discussed below, it has been shown to be beneficial to increase the expression of HbF to compensate for certain hemoglobinopathies such as SCD. The effect of other hemoglobin variants on the oxygen–Hb dissociation curve is shown in Fig. 9.4.

A common pathologic variant of Hb is sickle Hb (*HbS*), which causes SCD. This is a genetic disorder caused by a point mutation (A > T) at codon 6 (rs334) of β-globin [23], leading to a single amino acid substitution (glutamic acid to valine) [24]. This change alters the structure of Hb, such that at low oxygen tension, the erythrocyte polymerizes [25] and forms its characteristic "sickle" form. Polymerized HbS causes microvascular vaso-occlusion and hemolysis and subsequent complications of pain, ischemia, thrombosis, and, ultimately, end-organ damage. It has been shown that HbS polymerizes only in the T conformation [25, 26], leading to attempts to devise therapeutics aimed at shifting the quaternary structure of Hb to the R conformation to prevent polymerization, as described below. HbS erythrocytes have been found to have higher levels of 2,3-BPG and intracellular H^+ [27], which, as

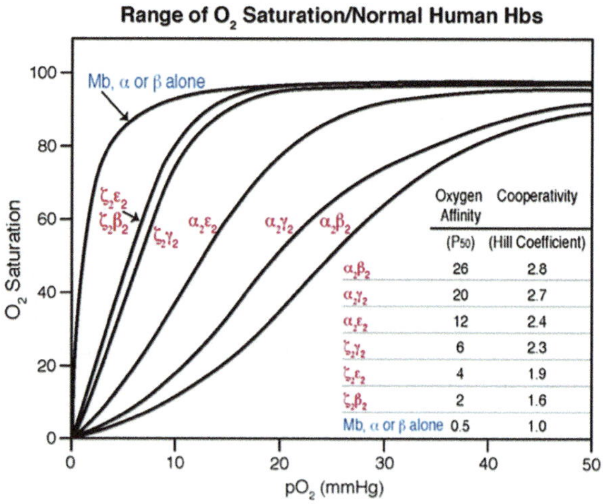

Fig. 9.4 Various hemoglobin variants and the degree of left shift in the oxygen–hemoglobin dissociation curve ($\alpha_2\beta_2$ or HbA is represented by the curve on the right). (From Manning et al. [22])

described above, promote the T conformation of Hb and shift the oxygen–Hb dissociation curve to the right, which, in turn, induces more erythrocyte polymerization and intravascular sickling.

Exogenous Factors

Temperature

Temperature exerts an effect on Hb–oxygen affinity in various ways and is inversely proportional to oxygen affinity for Hb. It directly affects Hb by decreasing oxygen affinity at high temperatures, shifting the oxygen–Hb dissociation curve to the right and increasing the P_{50} [28] (Fig. 9.2). This occurs because the reaction of Hb with oxygen is exothermic [29]—as temperature drops, exothermic conditions are favored to promote equilibrium; thus, oxygen binds more readily to Hb. Conversely, in warm tissues such as muscles in exercise, oxygen is unloaded from Hb to conserve heat [29]. This effect is thought to confer physiological advantages to organisms as Hb is able to effectively release oxygen during times of increased metabolic need, which might occur during fever, exercise, or inflammation. Hypothermia, on the other hand, leads to increased oxygen affinity and difficulty in releasing oxygen to tissues. Changes in temperature also indirectly affect the oxygen binding to Hb. For example, at high temperatures, the CO_2 Bohr effect described above is increased, while the effect of 2,3-BPG is blunted [30].

Altitude

At higher altitudes, decreased atmospheric pressure leads to decreased partial pressure of oxygen in inspired air. Thus, there is impaired loading of oxygen onto the Hb molecule. One adaptive mechanism is the increase of 2,3-BPG in response to hypoxia [31], which thus decreases oxygen affinity for Hb, shifting the oxygen–Hb dissociation curve to the right and raising the P_{50}. The compensatory mechanism for this change is to increase the rate of ventilation, which is not sustainable in situations of extremely high altitudes, and the resultant hyperventilation may lead to respiratory alkalosis. Thus, oxygen supplementation is often required at extremely high altitudes.

Other Allosteric Effectors

Numerous other substances alter the affinity of oxygen for Hb. Among the most potent ones that lower oxygen affinity are inositol hexaphosphate (IHP), propionates, aryloxyalkanoic acids, and nitric oxide (NO) [8]. Similar to 2,3-BPG, IHP is an organic phosphate that binds to the β-cleft in deoxy-Hb and stabilizes it in the T conformation, but it binds with far greater affinity than 2,3-BPG [32]. Propionates such as bezafibrate also stabilize the T state, though via different binding sites compared to 2,3-BPG or IHP [8], and solutions containing both bezafibrate and IHP exert a profound allosteric effect, promoting deoxy-Hb [32]. Aryloxyalkanoic acids, depending on the binding site, can stabilize either the T or R conformation [8].

On the other hand, aromatic aldehydes such as vanillin [33] and furfural [34] increase oxygen affinity for Hb and promote the R conformation. These were thus early targets for drug development to treat SCD [8].

Another molecule that exerts an allosteric effect on Hb is NO. It has a high affinity for Hb, and apart from the usual high-affinity ferrous binding site that Hb uses to scavenge NO from peripheral tissues, there is a secondary binding site on the β-globin chain. NO binds to the cysteine residue Cysβ93—forming S-nitrosothiol (SNO) and S-nitrosohemoglobin [35]. This binding is allosterically regulated. As oxygen binds to Hb, the latter's structure changes from the T to the R conformation, which increases its affinity toward SNO. Conversely, its affinity for SNO is decreased when Hb off-loads the oxygen in the peripheral circulation. In this way, Hb acts as a mode of delivery of NO to the peripheral tissues, which brings about vasodilation and, in turn, increases oxygen supply [36].

Therapeutics

The effectors of oxygen–Hb dissociation, as described above, have been leveraged in the form of therapeutics. The best examples come from SCD, in which deoxy-Hb polymerizes and forms insoluble sickle cells, a state further exacerbated by intracellular factors (elevated 2,3-BPG and H^+) that promote the T conformation of Hb [27]. There is typically a delay time from deoxygenation to polymerization and the appearance of the insoluble fibers of HbS, and delaying the time to polymerization can markedly extend that delay time, allowing HbS erythrocytes to pass through deoxygenated blood without polymerizing [37]. Voxelotor, a small-molecule inhibitor of HbS polymerization, was approved by the FDA in 2019, though it was subsequently taken off the market in 2024 due to safety concerns [38]. It binds to the N-terminus of an α-globin chain and exerts an allosteric effect that promotes the R conformation and shifts the oxygen–Hb dissociation curve to the left [39] (Fig. 9.5). By promoting oxy-Hb, the polymerization of HbS erythrocytes is delayed, leading to less sickling and improvements in hemolysis and anemia [39, 40]. However, the shift in the oxygen–Hb dissociation curve may come at the cost of impaired oxygen

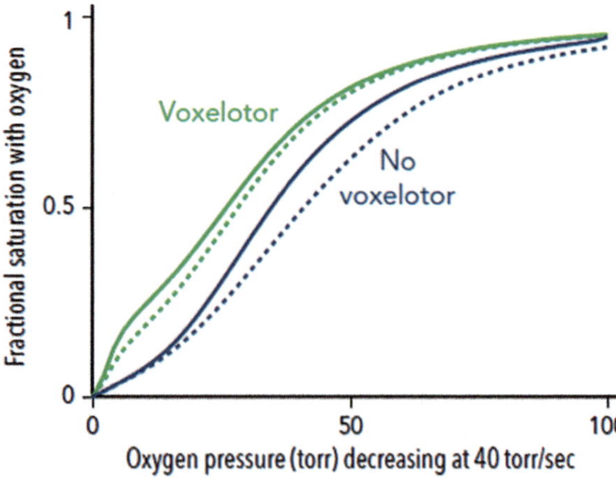

Fig. 9.5 Plot of oxygen saturation vs. dynamic oxygen pressure in sickle hemoglobin (HbS) in the presence or absence of voxelotor, which causes a left shift in the oxygen–hemoglobin dissociation curve by keeping HbS in its oxygenated form and preventing polymerization. (From Henry et al. [41]. Reproduced with permission from The American Society of Hematology)

delivery to tissues, and the net effect of increased oxy-Hb offsets impairment in delivery only at the lowest partial pressures of oxygen [41].

Other means to address polymerization in SCD have included the use of gene therapy to induce Hb variants that do not polymerize as deoxygenated HbS does. An appealing target is HbF induction, which, as described above, has a high affinity for oxygen and a left-shifted dissociation curve. Clinically, high HbF levels lead to fewer sequelae of sickling [42]. Hydroxyurea, an FDA-approved therapy for SCD—and the most widely used therapy for it worldwide—works primarily by suppressing erythropoiesis in the bone marrow and subsequently increasing HbF expression [42]. A newer treatment modality is gene therapy, designed to increase HbF expression. Exagamglogene autotemcel (CASGEVY®) was FDA approved in 2023 for the treatment of severe sickle cell disease. It works via clustered regularly interspaced short palindromic repeats (CRISPR)–Cas9 gene editing of *BCL11A* in patients' hematopoietic stem and progenitor cells (HSPCs) [43]. *BCL11A* is a transcription repressor that downregulates HbF expression [44]. This therapy transduces HSPCs ex vivo, followed by infusion after myeloablative bone marrow conditioning. It has been shown to increase HbF to a mean of >40% and improve anemia and vaso-occlusive episodes [43].

A separate cellular therapy aims at inducing the expression of a novel Hb variant with increased oxygen affinity. Lovotibeglogene autotemcel (LYFGENIA®) was FDA approved in 2023 for severe SCD and works by transducing HSPCs with a lentiviral vector (BB305) encoding a modified β-globin gene, whose product is HbA^{T87Q} [45]. This Hb variant contains a threonine-to-glutamine substitution at position 87 of β-globin within the acceptor hydrophobic pocket and exerts an inhibitory effect on polymerization, thus giving it an oxygen–Hb affinity similar to HbA [46]. After transduction and infusion of the treated HSPCs, HbA^{T87Q} composed approximately 40% of total Hgb, with resultant improvement in anemia and painful vaso-occlusive episodes [45].

Finally, other compounds are being developed that alter oxygen–Hb affinity, including ones that lower 2,3-BPG levels and an aldehyde that binds to α-globin and increases Hb's affinity for oxygen [37].

Acquired Disorders of Hemoglobin–Oxygen Affinity

Carboxyhemoglobin

CO is a by-product of the partial combustion of organic compounds and is toxic to humans due to its competitive inhibition of oxygen. CO binds to Hb with approximately 150–250 times greater affinity than oxygen [47]. Thus, even at very low partial pressures of CO, oxygen binding is impaired due to the high affinity for CO. The effect of a CO molecule binding to Hb also increases the affinity of the remaining oxygen molecules to Hb, shifting the oxygen–Hb dissociation to the left and reducing oxygen delivery to tissues [48, 49], further contributing to the tissue hypoxia that occurs with CO poisoning. Similar to the relationship between oxygen and Hb, the binding of CO induces allosteric effects on Hb, which seem to be pH-dependent. At a pH of 7, three CO molecules are required to fully change Hb to the R form, while at a basic pH of 9, the binding of only one CO molecule can induce a change to the R form [50, 51]. Levels of carboxy-Hb >50% are typically fatal, while levels >20% usually require medical intervention and can rarely be fatal [52]. At high concentrations of carboxy-Hb, symptoms include cardiac abnormalities (arrhythmias, ischemia, and arrest), pulmonary abnormalities (non-cardiogenic pulmonary edema and respiratory arrest), hypotension, seizures, and coma [52].

Methemoglobinemia

Methemoglobin, in which the iron atom in Hb is oxidized from the ferrous (Fe^{2+}) to the ferric (Fe^{3+}) state, is ineffective as an oxygen carrier. Similar to carboxyhemoglobin, methemoglobin shifts the oxygen–Hb dissociation curve leftward, with increased affinity for oxygen and impaired tissue delivery [53]. Transient, low levels of methemoglobin are common, but it can be easily reduced in normal erythrocytes [54] by nicotinamide adenine dinucleotide and hydrogen (NADH) and cytochrome B5 reductase, as well as a nicotinamide adenine dinucleotide phosphate and hydrogen (NADPH)-dependent reductase generated by the hexose monophosphate shunt and aided by methylene blue [54, 55]. It can also be reduced by ascorbic acid [56]. Congenital deficiencies in these enzymes or the glucose-6-phosphate dehydrogenase (G6PD) enzyme can predispose individuals to severe methemoglobinemia and cyanosis. This topic is explored in more detail in Chap. 11.

References

1. Meletis J, Konstantopoulos K. The beliefs, myths, and reality surrounding the word hema (blood) from homer to the present. Anemia. 2010;2010:857657. https://doi.org/10.1155/2010/857657.
2. Perutz MF, Rossmann MG, Cullis AF, Muirhead H, Will G, North AC. Structure of haemoglobin: a three-dimensional Fourier synthesis at 5.5-A. Resolution, obtained by X-ray analysis. Nature. 1960;185(4711):416–22. https://doi.org/10.1038/185416a0.
3. Ponka P, Schulman HM. Regulation of heme biosynthesis: distinct regulatory features in erythroid cells. Stem Cells. 1993;11(Suppl 1):24–35. https://doi.org/10.1002/stem.5530110607.
4. Friedman JM. Structure, dynamics, and reactivity in hemoglobin. Science. 1985;228(4705):1273–80. https://doi.org/10.1126/science.4001941.
5. Marengo-Rowe AJ. Structure-function relations of human hemoglobins. Proc (Bayl Univ Med Cent). 2006;19(3):239–45. https://doi.org/10.1080/08998280.2006.11928171.
6. Pauling L, Coryell CD. The magnetic properties and structure of hemoglobin, oxyhemoglobin and carbonmonoxyhemoglobin. Proc Natl Acad Sci USA. 1936;22(4):210–6. https://doi.org/10.1073/pnas.22.4.210.
7. Monod J, Wyman J, Changeux JP. On the nature of allosteric transitions: a plausible model. J Mol Biol. 1965;12:88–118. https://doi.org/10.1016/s0022-2836(65)80285-6.
8. Ahmed MH, Ghatge MS, Safo MK. Hemoglobin: structure, function and allostery. Subcell Biochem. 2020;94:345–82. https://doi.org/10.1007/978-3-030-41769-7_14.
9. Gupta M, Somasundaram I. Hyperbaric oxygen therapy: principles and applications. 1st ed. Singapore: Springer Nature Singapore; 2023.

10. Perutz MF. Stereochemistry of cooperative effects in haemoglobin. Nature. 1970;228(5273):726–39. https://doi.org/10.1038/228726a0.
11. Perutz MF, Wilkinson AJ, Paoli M, Dodson GG. The stereochemical mechanism of the cooperative effects in hemoglobin revisited. Annu Rev Biophys Biomol Struct. 1998;27:1–34. https://doi.org/10.1146/annurev.biophys.27.1.1.
12. Bohr CH, Hasselbalch K, Krogh A. Ueber einen in biologischer Beziehung wichtigen Einfluss, den die Kohlensäurespannung des Blutes auf dessen Sauerstoffbindung übt. Skandinavisches Archiv Für Physiol. 1904;16(2):402–12.
13. Christiansen J, Douglas CG, Haldane JS. The absorption and dissociation of carbon dioxide by human blood. J Physiol. 1914;48(4):244–71. https://doi.org/10.1113/jphysiol.1914.sp001659.
14. Hsia CC. Respiratory function of hemoglobin. N Engl J Med. 1998;338(4):239–47. https://doi.org/10.1056/NEJM199801223380407.
15. Benesch R, Benesch RE. The effect of organic phosphates from the human erythrocyte on the allosteric properties of hemoglobin. Biochem Biophys Res Commun. 1967;26(2):162–7. https://doi.org/10.1016/0006-291x(67)90228-8.
16. Bellingham AJ, Detter JC, Lenfant C. Regulatory mechanisms of hemoglobin oxygen affinity in acidosis and alkalosis. J Clin Invest. 1971;50(3):700–6. https://doi.org/10.1172/JCI106540.
17. Desforges JF, Slawsky P. Red cell 2,3-diphosphoglycerate and intracellular arterial pH in acidosis and alkalosis. Blood. 1972;40(5):740–6.
18. Perutz MF, Fermi G, Poyart C, Pagnier J, Kister J. A novel allosteric mechanism in haemoglobin. Structure of bovine deoxyhaemoglobin, absence of specific chloride-binding sites and origin of the chloride-linked Bohr effect in bovine and human haemoglobin. J Mol Biol. 1993;233(3):536–45. https://doi.org/10.1006/jmbi.1993.1530.
19. Perutz MF, Shih DT, Williamson D. The chloride effect in human haemoglobin. A new kind of allosteric mechanism. J Mol Biol. 1994;239(4):555–60. https://doi.org/10.1006/jmbi.1994.1394.
20. Sun K, D'Alessandro A, Ahmed MH, Zhang Y, Song A, Ko TP, et al. Structural and functional insight of sphingosine 1-phosphate-mediated pathogenic metabolic reprogramming in sickle cell disease. Sci Rep. 2017;7(1):15281. https://doi.org/10.1038/s41598-017-13667-8.
21. Sun K, Zhang Y, D'Alessandro A, Nemkov T, Song A, Wu H, et al. Sphingosine-1-phosphate promotes erythrocyte glycolysis and oxygen release for adaptation to high-altitude hypoxia. Nat Commun. 2016;7:12086. https://doi.org/10.1038/ncomms12086.
22. Manning JM, Manning LR, Dumoulin A, Padovan JC, Chait B. Embryonic and fetal human hemoglobins: structures, oxygen binding, and physiological roles. In: Hoeger U, Harris J, editors. Vertebrate and invertebrate respiratory proteins, lipoproteins and other body fluid proteins. Subcellular biochemistry, vol. 94. Cham: Springer; 2020. p. 275–96. https://doi.org/10.1007/978-3-030-41769-7_11.
23. Goldstein J, Konigsberg W, Hill RJ. The structure of human hemoglobin. VI. The sequence of amino acids in the tryptic peptides of the beta chain. J Biol Chem. 1963;238:2016–27.
24. Ingram VM. Gene mutations in human haemoglobin: the chemical difference between normal and sickle cell haemoglobin. Nature. 1957;180(4581):326–8. https://doi.org/10.1038/180326a0.
25. Eaton WA, Hofrichter J. Sickle cell hemoglobin polymerization. Adv Protein Chem. 1990;40:63–279. https://doi.org/10.1016/s0065-3233(08)60287-9.
26. Henry ER, Cellmer T, Dunkelberger EB, Metaferia B, Hofrichter J, Li Q, et al. Allosteric control of hemoglobin S fiber formation by oxygen and its relation to the pathophysiology of sickle cell disease. Proc Natl Acad Sci USA. 2020;117(26):15018–27. https://doi.org/10.1073/pnas.1922004117.
27. Poillon WN, Kim BC. 2,3-Diphosphoglycerate and intracellular pH as interdependent determinants of the physiologic solubility of deoxyhemoglobin S. Blood. 1990;76(5):1028–36.
28. Barcroft J, King WO. The effect of temperature on the dissociation curve of blood. J Physiol. 1909;39(5):374–84. https://doi.org/10.1113/jphysiol.1909.sp001345.

29. Weber RE, Campbell KL. Temperature dependence of haemoglobin-oxygen affinity in heterothermic vertebrates: mechanisms and biological significance. Acta Physiol (Oxf). 2011;202(3):549–62. https://doi.org/10.1111/j.1748-1716.2010.02204.x.
30. Hlastala MP, Woodson RD, Wranne B. Influence of temperature on hemoglobin-ligand interaction in whole blood. J Appl Physiol. 1977;43(3):545–50. https://doi.org/10.1152/jappl.1977.43.3.545.
31. Sun K, Liu H, Song A, Manalo JM, D'Alessandro A, Hansen KC, et al. Erythrocyte purinergic signaling components underlie hypoxia adaptation. J Appl Physiol (1985). 2017;123(4):951–6. https://doi.org/10.1152/japplphysiol.00155.2017.
32. Yonetani T, Park SI, Tsuneshige A, Imai K, Kanaori K. Global allostery model of hemoglobin. Modulation of O(2) affinity, cooperativity, and Bohr effect by heterotropic allosteric effectors. J Biol Chem. 2002;277(37):34508–20. https://doi.org/10.1074/jbc.M203135200.
33. Zaugg RH, Walder JA, Klotz IM. Schiff base adducts of hemoglobin. Modifications that inhibit erythrocyte sickling. J Biol Chem. 1977;252(23):8542–8.
34. Xu GG, Pagare PP, Ghatge MS, Safo RP, Gazi A, Chen Q, et al. Design, synthesis, and biological evaluation of ester and ether derivatives of antisickling agent 5-HMF for the treatment of sickle cell disease. Mol Pharm. 2017;14(10):3499–511. https://doi.org/10.1021/acs.molpharmaceut.7b00553.
35. Jia L, Bonaventura C, Bonaventura J, Stamler JS. S-nitrosohaemoglobin: a dynamic activity of blood involved in vascular control. Nature. 1996;380(6571):221–6. https://doi.org/10.1038/380221a0.
36. Stamler JS, Jia L, Eu JP, McMahon TJ, Demchenko IT, Bonaventura J, et al. Blood flow regulation by S-nitrosohemoglobin in the physiological oxygen gradient. Science. 1997;276(5321):2034–7. https://doi.org/10.1126/science.276.5321.2034.
37. Eaton WA, Bunn HF. Treating sickle cell disease by targeting HbS polymerization. Blood. 2017;129(20):2719–26. https://doi.org/10.1182/blood-2017-02-765891.
38. Alkindi S, Al Subhi A, Pathare A. Rapid withdrawal of voxelotor can precipitate sickle cell disease related crisis. Ann Hematol. 2025. https://doi.org/10.1007/s00277-025-06503-x.
39. Oksenberg D, Dufu K, Patel MP, Chuang C, Li Z, Xu Q, et al. GBT440 increases haemoglobin oxygen affinity, reduces sickling and prolongs RBC half-life in a murine model of sickle cell disease. Br J Haematol. 2016;175(1):141–53. https://doi.org/10.1111/bjh.14214.
40. Vichinsky E, Hoppe CC, Ataga KI, Ware RE, Nduba V, El-Beshlawy A, et al. A phase 3 randomized trial of voxelotor in sickle cell disease. N Engl J Med. 2019;381(6):509–19. https://doi.org/10.1056/NEJMoa1903212.
41. Henry ER, Metaferia B, Li Q, Harper J, Best RB, Glass KE, et al. Treatment of sickle cell disease by increasing oxygen affinity of hemoglobin. Blood. 2021;138(13):1172–81. https://doi.org/10.1182/blood.2021012070.
42. Steinberg MH. Fetal hemoglobin in sickle cell anemia. Blood. 2020;136(21):2392–400. https://doi.org/10.1182/blood.2020007645.
43. Frangoul H, Locatelli F, Sharma A, Bhatia M, Mapara M, Molinari L, et al. Exagamglogene autotemcel for severe sickle cell disease. N Engl J Med. 2024;390(18):1649–62. https://doi.org/10.1056/NEJMoa2309676.
44. Bauer DE, Orkin SH. Hemoglobin switching's surprise: the versatile transcription factor BCL11A is a master repressor of fetal hemoglobin. Curr Opin Genet Dev. 2015;33:62–70. https://doi.org/10.1016/j.gde.2015.08.001.
45. Kanter J, Walters MC, Krishnamurti L, Mapara MY, Kwiatkowski JL, Rifkin-Zenenberg S, et al. Biologic and clinical efficacy of LentiGlobin for sickle cell disease. N Engl J Med. 2022;386(7):617–28. https://doi.org/10.1056/NEJMoa2117175.
46. Negre O, Eggimann AV, Beuzard Y, Ribeil JA, Bourget P, Borwornpinyo S, et al. Gene therapy of the beta-hemoglobinopathies by lentiviral transfer of the beta(A(T87Q))-globin gene. Hum Gene Ther. 2016;27(2):148–65. https://doi.org/10.1089/hum.2016.007.
47. Caughey WS. Carbon monoxide bonding in hemeproteins. Ann N Y Acad Sci. 1970;174(1):148–53. https://doi.org/10.1111/j.1749-6632.1970.tb49781.x.

48. Douglas CG, Haldane JS, Haldane JB. The laws of combination of haemoglobin with carbon monoxide and oxygen. J Physiol. 1912;44(4):275–304. https://doi.org/10.1113/jphysiol.1912.sp001517.
49. Collier CR. Oxygen affinity of human blood in presence of carbon monoxide. J Appl Physiol. 1976;40(3):487–90. https://doi.org/10.1152/jappl.1976.40.3.487.
50. Sawicki CA, Gibson QH. Quaternary conformational changes in human hemoglobin studied by laser photolysis of carboxyhemoglobin. J Biol Chem. 1976;251(6):1533–42.
51. Sawicki CA, Gibson QH. The relation between carbon monoxide binding and the conformational change of hemoglobin. Biophys J. 1978;24(1):21–33. https://doi.org/10.1016/S0006-3495(78)85328-4.
52. Wilbur SWM, Williams R, et al. Toxicological profile for carbon monoxide. Atlanta: Agency for Toxic Substances and Disease Registry (US); 2012.
53. Darling RC, Roughton FJW. The effect of methemoglobin on the equilibrium between oxygen and hemoglobin. Am J Physiol-Legacy Content. 1942;137(1):56–68. https://doi.org/10.1152/ajplegacy.1942.137.1.56.
54. Gibson QH. The reduction of methaemoglobin in red blood cells and studies on the cause of idiopathic methaemoglobinaemia. Biochem J. 1948;42(1):13–23. https://doi.org/10.1042/bj0420013.
55. Jaffe ER. The reduction of methemoglobin in erythrocytes of a patient with congenital methemoglobinemia, subjects with erythrocyte glucose-6-phosphate dehydrogenase deficiency, and normal individuals. Blood. 1963;21:561–72.
56. Gibson QH. The reduction of methaemoglobin by ascorbic acid. Biochem J. 1943;37(5):615–8. https://doi.org/10.1042/bj0370615.

A Deadly Snowfall in the City: Carbon Monoxide Poisoning Is a Real Threat to Oxygen Delivery

10

Gregory C. Kane

Clinical Vignette

A 12-year-old boy was transported to a local emergency room (ER) in Philadelphia during the Blizzard of 1996. His mother called 911 after he developed a headache, nausea, and shortness of breath while in the back seat of a running automobile. He had been assisting his father in digging the car out from the recent snowstorm and was placed in the back seat with the car running and the heat on because of the cold. The rear portion of the automobile remained covered in snow at the time of the emergency. His parents were legal immigrants, but English was not their first language.

On arrival in the emergency room, the vital signs on triage showed that his heart rate was 138 per minute, blood pressure was 130/84 mmHg, respiratory rate was 30 per minute, and pulse ox was 96%. The boy was placed on face mask oxygen because of breathlessness and tachycardia. On physical examination, the lungs were clear, cardiac tones were regular without appreciable murmur, and the abdomen was soft. The child was somnolent but arousable and appeared confused. An alert member of the health care team obtained an arterial sample for blood gas measurement, which revealed a pH of 7.29, PCO_2 of 30 mmHg, and PO_2 of 366 mmHg. The carboxy hemoglobin level was 26%, and the measured oxyhemoglobin level was 72%. A diagnosis of carbon monoxide (CO) poisoning was established. Fluids were administered, and the applied face mask oxygen was increased to 100%. The decision was made to manage this patient in the emergency room setting with serial measures of carboxyhemoglobin and close monitoring. There was no evidence of seizures, and the child was monitored closely. Additional laboratory studies at

G. C. Kane (✉)
The Korman Respiratory Institute and the Division of Pulmonary, Allergy and Critical Care, The Department of Medicine at the Sidney Kimmel Medical College of Thomas Jefferson University, Philadelphia, PA, USA
e-mail: gregory.kane@jefferson.edu

G. C. Kane et al. (eds.), *Oxygen*, https://doi.org/10.1007/978-3-032-18934-9_10

admission confirmed a lactate of 3.9 mmol/L and an anion gap of 16. Other routine laboratories were unremarkable, including complete blood count and serum chemistries.

Six hours after presentation and being placed on supplemental oxygen, which was rapidly up-titrated to 100% via a non-rebreather mask, the child's carboxyhemoglobin level had decreased to 4.3%. The child was observed for another 6 h, at which time repeat carboxyhemoglobin was under 1%, and the child was discharged home. There was no further neuropsychiatric testing or sequelae described.

Readers' Note

Between January 6 and January 8, 1996, a large portion of the northeastern United States was blanketed by up to three feet of snow. According to the national weather service, this was one of the greatest snowfalls of the twentieth century (Fig. 10.1).

In the wake of increased cases of carbon monoxide poisoning associated with the Blizzard of 1996, an increase in media campaigns to warn the public has been noted. Experts have highlighted that members of minority groups and non-English speakers are at particular risk, in part because of the language barrier and in part because of their socioeconomic status, which might expose them to faulty heating systems [1]. Public health strategies to address these people are certainly warranted. In the

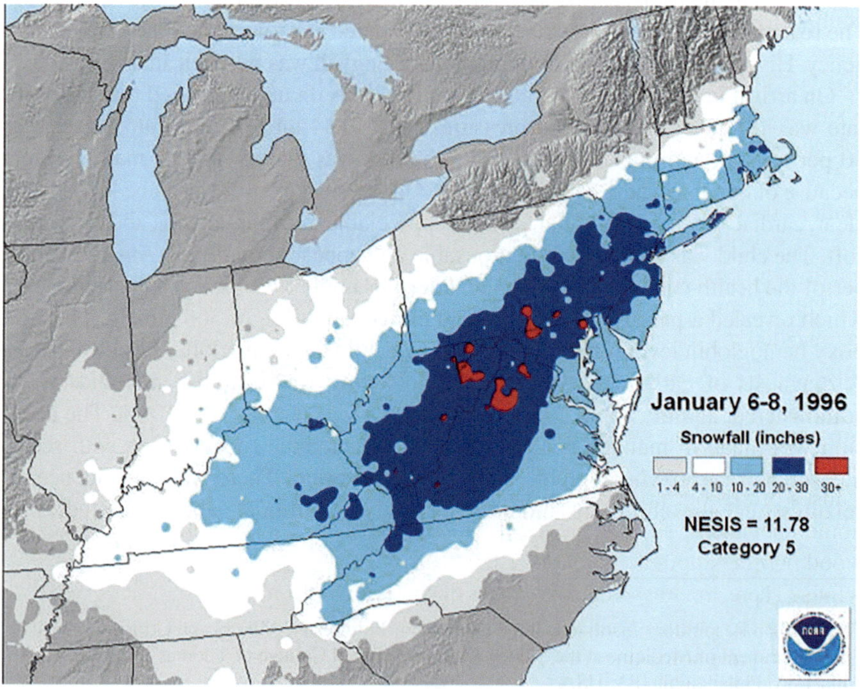

Fig. 10.1 This figure from the National Oceanic and Atmospheric Administration shows the relative snowfall during the Blizzard of 1996. People living in the blue, dark blue, or red zone may have had their cars covered in snow, including covering the tailpipe/exhaust systems. (Accessed February 2, 2025)

case presented, the family did not understand the risk associated with a running vehicle with a tailpipe covered by high drifting snow and carbon monoxide accumulation.

Carbon Monoxide Poisoning

Carbon monoxide (CO) gas poisoning has an impact on the body since CO displaces oxygen from binding sites on the hemoglobin, preventing oxygen from being carried to the peripheral tissues. This impact is further magnified by alterations in the oxyhemoglobin dissociation curve, which limit the release of the reduced amount of oxygen that is still pumped out into the arterial circulation. Carbon monoxide (CO) is undetectable to the human senses; it is tasteless, colorless, and odorless [1]. Unlike a gas leak, which can be detected because of an odorant called mercaptan, which is injected into the natural gas system and has a highly distinctive smell like rotten eggs, carbon monoxide avoids detection unless the environment is outfitted with CO monitors. The two most important ways to avoid or detect carbon monoxide exposure include utilizing a carbon monoxide detector in your home or apartment and understanding that carbon monoxide is a by-product of combustion. It is released into the atmosphere as a result of the incomplete combustion of hydrocarbon fuels such as gasoline, wood, or natural gas. The risk is generally related to combustion that occurs in enclosed spaces without appropriate venting. Standard home heating systems that are in good working order have a lower risk as long as they are properly maintained. Therefore, it is essential to keep the fireplace flue open, avoid the use of non-approved home heating devices and the home gas stove for generating heat, and be mindful that carbon monoxide can accumulate when gas-powered automobiles are running in enclosed spaces (including when they are blanketed in snow) [2]. Homeowners should never move gas grills into the living space for cooking purposes. Electric vehicles do not have any risk of CO generation, but as of this writing, they make up a small fraction of the automobiles in use within the United States. Federal regulations require that carbon monoxide (CO) detectors be installed in every home with a fuel-burning appliance and be located outside each separate sleeping area [3]. Most states have additional regulations as well.

Most cases of carbon monoxide poisoning in the United States are not related to fire exposures. And while the majority have been unintentional, carbon monoxide poisoning continues to be an important cause of suicide in the United States [4]. Causes of carbon monoxide exposure are typically related to incorrectly installed home appliances, such as stoves or hot water heaters, or poorly ventilated gas or wood burning appliances. Cases rise in the northern parts of the United States each winter. There are, however, rare causes of CO poisoning that can be quite surprising, including the circumstances surrounding the case presented in the opening of this chapter [3] and some unexpected scenarios that include swimming under a pontoon boat while the motor is idling, sitting in the cheap seats for a Monster Truck Show, or grilling on a gas grill operated within a small tent enclosure in the winter (when the enclosure may be tightly sealed and poorly ventilated).

The problem with significant exposures to carbon monoxide gas is that carbon monoxide directly competes with oxygen for binding to hemoglobin. Significant exposures occur because of the high volume of CO generation and a small space that is enclosed and/or poorly ventilated. Carbon monoxide has a high affinity to the same ferrous heme–containing proteins that are normally available for oxygen. Importantly, the affinity of hemoglobin for carbon monoxide is more than 200 times as strong as the affinity of hemoglobin for oxygen [5]. Beyond the affinity of hemoglobin for carbon monoxide, there is an additional factor that further inhibits the distribution of oxygen to the peripheral tissues in persons poisoned by carbon monoxide. This shift to the "left" of the oxyhemoglobin dissociation curve leads to a lower availability of oxygen at any specific partial pressure of oxygen in the local tissues. The lower availability created by reduced unloading of the already limited amount of oxygen bound to hemoglobin further exacerbates tissue hypoxia beyond what would be created by the simple presence of carboxyhemoglobin [5]. This is important and is worth emphasizing by thinking about an important example from another chapter. This author experienced severe hypoxia at an altitude of nearly 19,000 feet while climbing Mount Kilimanjaro in 2012. Measured O_2 sats on final approach to the summit were just 66%. This is lower than the oxyhemoglobin level in the presented case of carbon monoxide poisoning. The major difference here is that mountain climbers have a "shift to the right" of their oxyhemoglobin dissociation curves, while for some even more sinister but unclear reason, CO poisoning pushes the curve to the left. It is this process of shifting the curve to the left that further thwarts the delivery of oxygen to the tissues. On the other hand, the limited supply of hemoglobin in climbers is offloaded more effectively to the brain, critical organs, and muscle tissue because of the shift to the right. To use an analogy, it would be like delivering a limited supply of oxygen to patients who are short of breath in bottles that cannot be opened (a shift to the left as seen in CO poisoning) versus delivering that same limited supply but in bottles that are open and ready for consumption (shift to the right as seen in climbers with time to acclimatize).

It remains to be seen whether the reestablishment of oxygen in the deprived brain cells of carbon monoxide poisoning survivors' cells may somehow worsen the injury.

Cases of carbon monoxide poisoning have been documented for over 200 years, including by Napoleon's surgeon in the early 1800s, making this condition a quirk of evolutionary history that has not yet led to biological adaptation. This is likely due to the random and relatively rare nature of its occurrence. Therefore, it may only be recognized and avoided by creating increased awareness in our communities [6]. Table 10.1, adapted from the Federal Emergency Management Agency, outlines commonsense strategies to avoid carbon monoxide poisoning.

Carbon monoxide is known as the "invisible killer" because it is colorless, odorless, and undetectable to the human senses. Breathing in large amounts of carbon monoxide prevents oxygen from reaching your body's tissues, creating symptoms and a risk of death. Table 10.2 displays preventive strategies to avoid CO poisoning [7].

Table 10.1 Steps that can ensure safe use of portable home electricity generators

Advice	Rationale
Use generators outside and away from doors and windows.	If used inside or near entrances, carbon monoxide can accumulate inside the home.
Do not use generators in wet areas.	This can lead to electrocution or electric shock.
Always use appropriate electric cords for connecting to the generator.	Cords other than heavy-duty cords can lead to an electric fire.
Do not refuel the generator while it is running.	Spilling fuel or gasoline on a hot generator can lead to fire.
Make sure your home is outfitted with carbon monoxide detectors.	This will alert residents to potentially harmful levels of carbon monoxide.

A generator is a popular piece of equipment used to generate electricity during power outages and can be deadly when used inside a home. Material is adapted from the Federal Emergency Management Agency [8]

Table 10.2 CO safety measures adapted from the Federal Emergency Management Agency of the US government

Carbon monoxide safety measures
1. Install and maintain CO alarms inside your home to provide early warning of CO.
2. Assure that CO alarms are in a central location, outside each sleeping area, and on every level.
3. Use portable generators outdoors and in well-ventilated areas that are away from all doors, windows, and vents of the home.
4. Make sure that vents from household dryers, furnaces, fireplaces, and stoves are clear of snow and debris.

For more information, access www.usfa.fema.gov

The clinical characteristics of carbon monoxide poisoning are manifest principally by tissue hypoxia and the difficulty of recognizing the presentation without appropriate historical clues. Quite commonly, the clinical signs and symptoms may appear like those of influenza or other nonspecific viral illnesses. Headache and nausea are common to both illnesses early in their course. Furthermore, it does not help that both of these conditions peak in the winter months, making the clinical diagnosis even more difficult [8, 9]. Table 10.3 outlines the possible presenting symptoms for persons affected by carbon monoxide. It is important to recognize that symptoms may vary from minor to profound, depending on the degree and duration of exposure [1, 9, 10]. It is of interest that up to 13% of persons in a major carbon monoxide exposure event in a public high school reported in the literature had no symptoms at the time of evaluation despite real exposure [11]. This could be related to the intensity of the exposure and whether it was sustained or intermittent (such as from walking in and out of a room that was the main source). People with levels of 30% or greater are likely to experience a coma, and levels approaching 40–50% carry a high mortality rate [12].

Table 10.3 Symptoms reported by patients presenting with carbon monoxide poisoning

Symptom	Reported frequency
Headache	>90%
Dizziness	>75%
Weakness	>50%
Nausea	40–50%
Changes in mentation, such as confusion	>40%
Dyspnea	>40%
Changes in vision	>25%
Chest pain	Up to 10%, depending on the age
Coma	6%
Abdominal pain	5%
Muscle cramping	5%

Treatment of Carbon Monoxide Poisoning

The principles of treatment for CO poisoning are supportive, plus utilizing supplemental oxygen to speed the clearance and exhalation of carbon monoxide. In severe cases, hyperbaric oxygen (HBO) delivery can be used to speed up the clearance of CO by increasing the gradient for excretion. The first step after recognition is removal from the cause of CO exposure. In most ER environments, this has already been accomplished. The next key step is administering oxygen in increased concentrations or amounts. This helps in two ways. First, increased delivered oxygen will increase the amount of oxygen delivered via the serum. This impact will be small as the added benefit when the hemoglobin's ability to carry oxygen is limited is marginal and may be only another 10–15%. Second, and most importantly, higher concentrations of dissolved oxygen create a diffusion gradient that enhances the process of offloading CO despite the greater affinity of hemoglobin for CO over oxygen. The higher concentration of oxygen delivered by masks in the ER changes the dynamic and helps speed up the clearance of CO by a factor of five- to sixfold, speeding up recovery. Studies have, however, shown less reliable kinetics in clinical practice [11].

For severe cases, there is a therapy that can be employed, called hyperbaric oxygen (HBO) therapy. Placing the affected patient in a hyperbaric chamber with 2 ATM of pressure can increase the partial pressure of oxygen in the bloodstream from 663 mmHg to more than 1200 mmHg. The increased pressure of oxygen forces CO off the hemoglobin more readily than normobaric oxygen (NBO), allowing the patient to exhale CO even more quickly, restoring the blood oxyhemoglobin more rapidly. Based on published data, this approach using hyperbaric therapy is reserved for high levels of CO poisoning or patients with advanced complications, such as seizures.

Figure 10.2 may help the reader visualize the benefit of hyperbaric oxygen treatment, which multiplies the amount of oxygen molecules in the serum by up to ten times. Surprisingly, the neurological benefit of routine normobaric administration

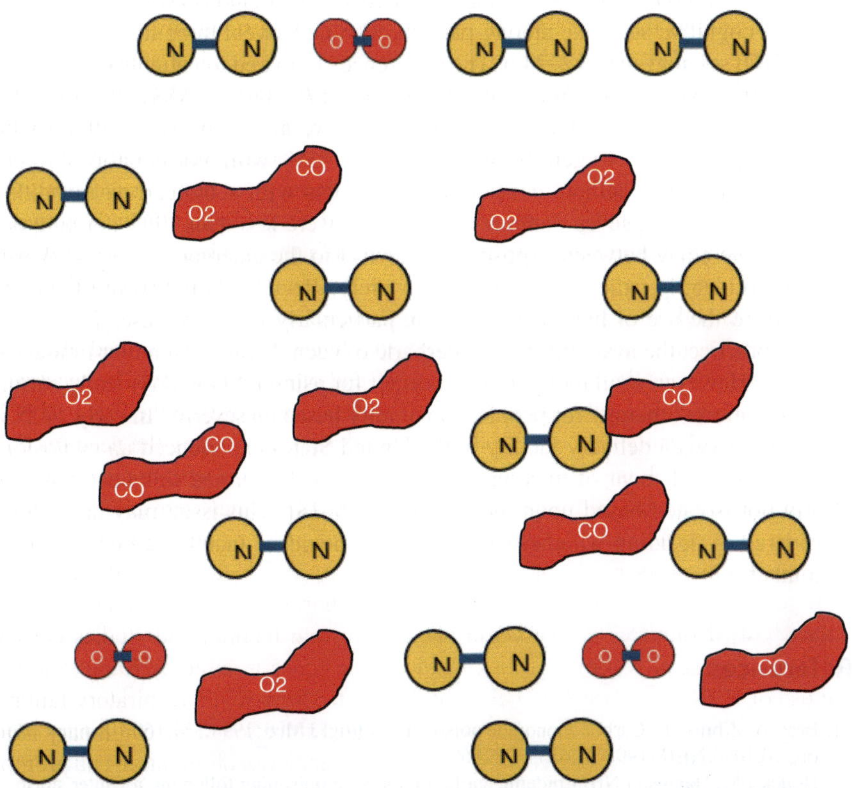

Fig. 10.2 A schematic of oxygen and nitrogen dissolved in serum among various red blood cells (shown as biconcave discs). In this schematic, one can imagine the improvement in CO excretion kinetics, which would come from increasing the number of oxygen molecules in the serum (shown as O_2 in the serum) through the use of a hyperbaric oxygen chamber. N = nitrogen, O = oxygen, and the biconcave discs are red blood cells with about 55% of binding sites bound to CO

of oxygen has not been shown consistently to create a neuropsychiatric benefit [13], perhaps because trials have investigated patients with varying severity of disease and manifestations. A relatively recent systematic review examined findings from six randomized clinical trials (RCTs) reported between 1989 and 2010. This meta-analysis indicated that compared with patients treated with normobaric oxygen (NBO), the use of hyperbaric oxygen (HBO) resulted in a lower incidence of neuropsychological sequelae, including headache, memory deficits, measures of concentration, sleep disturbance, and other delayed neurological sequelae. An important cautionary note is required here because the results did not reach statistical significance as the reported confidence intervals overlapped with 1.0 [14]. Unfortunately, there has been only one high-quality randomized and blinded clinical trial examining hyperbaric oxygen therapy. This prospective trial, published more than two decades ago at a single center, was carried out by experienced clinician scientists in the field of carbon monoxide poisoning. Their results demonstrated a lower incidence of cognitive sequelae among patients who underwent three hyperbaric oxygen (HBO) sessions over 12–24 h. The difference compared to patients treated with normobaric oxygen was impressive (25% vs. 46%; $P = 0.007$). Moreover, the rates of persistent cognitive sequelae at 12 months were also improved in those who received hyperbaric oxygen (HBO) (18% vs. 33% with normobaric oxygen; $P = 0.04$) [13]. The authors considered all patients with acute carbon monoxide poisoning, including seven patients whose levels were less than 10%, pointing out that the time delay between exposure and arrival to the emergency room makes it difficult to identify patients who may be severely affected. Currently, most experts recommend the use of hyperbaric oxygen, particularly in severe cases [1, 15]. In clinical practice, the availability of hyperbaric oxygen therapy is a major limitation to its use. However, availability within a center for using HBO will typically permit rapid initiation of therapy for people who qualify based on severity. In early 2025, a hyperbaric oxygen delivery facility in the United States experienced an explosion, which adds an element of uncertainty to the use of HBO, and this occurrence is clearly not isolated based upon the literature [16–18]. This issue may have to be considered in deciding whether such facilities should be maintained or increased in number.

References

1. Ernst A, Zibrak JD. Carbon monoxide poisoning. N Engl J Med. 1998;339:1603–8. https://doi.org/10.1056/NEJM199811263392206.
2. Houck PM, Hampson NB. Epidemic carbon monoxide poisoning following a winter storm. J Emerg Med. 1997;15:469–73.
3. https://www.law.cornell.edu/cfr/text/24/3280.211. Accessed 2 Feb 2025.
4. Shin M, Bronstein AC, Glidden E, Malone M, Chang A, Law R, Boehmer TK, Strosnider H, Yip FSO. Morbidity and mortality of unintentional carbon monoxide poisoning: United States 2005 to 2018. Ann Emerg Med. 2023;81(3):309. Epub 2022 Dec 28.
5. Rodkey FL, O'Neal JD, Collison HA, Uddin DE. Relative affinity of hemoglobin S and hemoglobin a for-carbon monoxide and oxygen. Clin Chem. 1974;20:83–4.
6. Roughton FJW, Darling RC. The effect of carbon monoxide on oxyhemoglobin dissociation curve. Am J Phys. 1944;141:17–31.
7. Walker E, Hay A. Carbon monoxide poisoning. BMJ. 1999;319(7217):1082–3. https://doi.org/10.1136/bmj.319.7217.1082. PMID: 10531079; PMCID: PMC1116882.
8. www.usfa.fema.gov. Accessed 2 Feb 2025.
9. Kales SN. Carbon monoxide intoxication. Am Fam Physician. 1993;48:1100–4.
10. Myers RAM, Snyder SK, Emhoff TA. Subacute sequelae of carbon monoxide poisoning. Ann Emerg Med. 1985;14:1163–7.
11. Burney RE, Wu SC, Nemiroff MJ. Mass carbon monoxide poisoning: clinical effects and results of treatment in 184 victims. Ann Emerg Med. 1982;11:394–9.
12. Penney D, Benignus V, Kephalopoulos S, Kotzias D, Kleinman M, Verrier A. Carbon monoxide. In: WHO guidelines for indoor air quality: selected pollutants. Geneva: World Health Organization; 2010.
13. Weaver LK, Howe S, Hopkins R, Chan KJ. Carboxyhemoglobin half-life in carbon monoxide-poisoned patients treated with 100% oxygen at atmospheric pressure. Chest. 2000;117:801–8.

14. Weaver LK, Valentine KJ, Hopkins RO. Carbon monoxide poisoning: risk factors for cognitive sequelae and the role of hyperbaric oxygen. Am J Respir Crit Care Med. 2007;176:491–7.
15. Lin CH, Su WH, Chen YC, Feng PH, Shen WC, Ong JR, Wu MY, Wong CS. Treatment with normobaric or hyperbaric oxygen and its effect on neuropsychometric dysfunction after carbon monoxide poisoning: a systematic review and meta-analysis of randomized controlled trials. Medicine (Baltimore). 2018;97(39):e12456. https://doi.org/10.1097/MD.0000000000012456. PMID: 30278526; PMCID: PMC6181555.
16. https://www.kbtx.com/video/2025/03/12/arrests-made-after-5-year-old-boys-death-hyperbaric-chamber-explosion/. Accessed 14 Mar 2025.
17. Sheffield PJ, Sheffield RB, Sheffield JC. Review of recent clinical hyperbaric chamber fires (1992-2011) UHMS: ASM (abstract E86). UHM; 2012. p. 1014–5.
18. Jain KK. Hyperbaric chambers: equipment, technique, and safety. In: Textbook of hyperbaric medicine. Cham: Springer; 2017. https://doi.org/10.1007/978-3-319-47140-2_7.

Methemoglobinemia

11

Tara Rakiewicz and Sanaa Rizk

Introduction

We have described hemoglobin (Hgb) as the ideal conveyor of oxygen as the ferrous irons in their natural state constitute four binding sites, each capable of binding to an oxygen molecule, forming a "tetramer" resembling a drone with four carrying sites, each holding an oxygen molecule. While this elegant process appears to work in a ubiquitous fashion across all humans and many animal species, there is the possibility that, at times, hemoglobin simply cannot bind to oxygen. This can occur when the hemoglobin is already bound to carbon monoxide (see Chap. 10) or in the setting of methemoglobin (MHb), which has an alternate structure, leaving it incapable of binding to oxygen. In its normal state, blood is constituted by 1% of methemoglobin, which is auto-reduced to its appropriate hemoglobin state. This precarious balance can be altered by genetic conditions or certain drugs, resulting in a much larger proportion of methemoglobin, which markedly diminishes the oxygen-carrying capacity of human blood [1].

Consider the following case report by Kane and Lunenfeld [1]. A middle-aged man was admitted to the hospital with head and neck cancer, a history of alcohol abuse, and vomiting blood. The gentleman was initially stable hemodynamically, with a heart rate of 70 beats per minute and a stable blood pressure. An initial physical examination was unremarkable, and laboratories confirmed mild anemia with a hemoglobin of 9.3 g/dl, adequate platelets, and normal renal function. An endoscopy was performed and involved the use of topical cetacaine spray, one of the many medications that can trigger an unexpected imbalance in the ratio of methemoglobin and hemoglobin. Indeed, during the endoscopy, the patient developed

T. Rakiewicz · S. Rizk (✉)
Division of Hematology, The Department of Medicine at the Sidney Kimmel Medical College of Thomas Jefferson University, Philadelphia, PA, USA
e-mail: Tara.rakiewicz@jefferson.edu; Sanaa.rizk@jefferson.edu

G. C. Kane et al. (eds.), *Oxygen*, https://doi.org/10.1007/978-3-032-18934-9_11

Table 11.1 Factors suggesting methemoglobinemia in a patient

A "saturation gap," which means that the PO_2 is high relative to the pulse oximetry reading or calculated O_2 saturation
Chocolate brown color arterial blood drawn for blood gas measurement
Use of a drug that may promote methemoglobinemia: see Table 11.2
Normal cardiopulmonary exam in a patient with respiratory distress
Normal FAST exam in a patient with respiratory distress

hypoxemia, as revealed by pulse oximetry monitoring, and subsequent respiratory distress; there were no obvious pulmonary or cardiac abnormalities detected.

Blood gas was obtained, and staff noted its "chocolate" brown color. Perhaps most importantly, the measured blood gas using co-oximetry showed a PO_2 of 117 mmHg despite a measured O_2 saturation of less than 25%. This paradoxical finding, which cannot be easily explained by the traditional oxyhemoglobin dissociation curve, points to a mismatch between PO_2 and calculated SaO_2 being preserved while pulse oximetry is reduced, which has been dubbed the "oxygen saturation gap." It suggests that hemoglobin may be abnormal due to carbon monoxide poisoning, methemoglobinemia, or sulf-hemoglobinemia [2]. Indeed, the diagnosis of methemoglobinemia, well-established on blood gas measured with co-oximetry, may be missed on a blood gas that calculates the oxyhemoglobin saturation based solely on the PaO_2 unless one recognizes that the pulse oximetry reading typically between 80 and 90% suggests an alternate problem. Table 11.1 outlines the clinical findings that may suggest a diagnosis of methemoglobinemia.

The Structure of Hemoglobin and Changes with Methemoglobinemia

Hemoglobin (Hgb) is made of four individual polypeptides with dedicated heme groups, making two alpha and two beta subunits. There is a component of a ferrous iron atom of each heme group that oxygen is able to reversibly bind to. However, oxygen is only able to bind reversibly because iron is in its ferrous (Fe^{2+}) state. This allows for appropriate oxygen binding in the lungs and subsequent dissociation and delivery throughout the body's tissues, as referenced with the dissociation curve. Oxygen can bind to ferrous iron reversibly, given the structure of Hgb's heme group, complete with a distal and proximal histidine; the ferrous iron is attached to the proximal histidine [3].

Methemoglobin (MHb) is a variation of the classic hemoglobin molecule. Instead of the reduced, ferrous (Fe^{2+}) state, the iron atom of a subunit's heme group is fixed in the ferric (Fe^{3+}), oxidized state. Ferric (Fe^{3+}) iron is not able to bind with oxygen, and this change in structure for the globin molecule has dramatic consequences. The oxygen dissociation curve of hemoglobin is shifted to the left, increasing the affinity of MHb for oxygen. This becomes problematic as the increased affinity leads to a lack of oxygen delivery to vital tissues, resulting in a functionally hypoxic state. Essentially, MHb carries less oxygen and binds more tightly to the limited oxygen, prohibiting appropriate oxygen delivery and inducing a state of "functional

Table 11.2 Drugs that have been linked to methemoglobinemia [14]

Acetanilid	Dinitrophenol	Paraquat
Alloxan	Exhaust fumes (combustion)	Phenacetin
Aniline	Ferricyanide	Phenazopyridine
Arsine	Flutamide	Phenol
Benzene drugs	Hydroxylamine	Phenytoin
Benzocaine, lidocaine, prilocaine, and bupivacaine	Metoclopramide hydrochloride	Primaquine phosphate
Chlorates	Methylene blue	Rifampin
Chloroquine	Naphthalene	Silver nitrate
Chlorates	Nitrates	Sodium valproate
Chromates	Nitric oxide	Smoke inhalation
Clofazimine	Nitrofurantoin	Sulfasalazine
Dapsone	Nitroglycerine	Sulfonamides
Dimethyl sulfoxide	Sodium nitroprusside	Trinitrotoluene

anemia," with a "dual deficiency" of reduced oxygen-carrying capacity and reduced release of that oxygen to the tissues [4].

The reduction–oxygenation process of iron continuously occurs in normal red blood cells' metabolism. While this process does happen naturally in the normal, healthy population, it occurs at a rate less than 1% [4]. This can occur for a variety of reasons, including auto-oxidation after oxygen delivery, reactions with various free radicals that exist in the blood, or potential interaction with exogenous chemicals. While these oxidation reactions continuously occur, the red blood cell enzyme cytochrome b5 reductase (Cyb5R) carries out a reduction–oxygenation reaction with methemoglobinemia. It functions to oxidize Nicotinamide adenine dinucleotide hydrogen (NADH) to Nicotinamide adenine dinucleotide (NAD) and reduces the ferric iron, converting it back to ferrous iron [5]. In fact, this enzyme was previously named methemoglobin reductase; it accounts for 99% of the daily MHb reduction. Other pathways have also been shown to be involved in the reduction of methemoglobin, including a non-physiologically active Nicotinamide adenine dinucleotide phosphate (NADPH) methemoglobin reductase that relies on G6PD generation of NADPH, glutathione, and ascorbic acid.

Etiology of Methemoglobinemia

MHb can be caused by a variety of reasons; however, they can broadly be categorized into either congenital or acquired.

Congenital

Cytochrome b5 reductase deficiency is inherited in an autosomal recessive manner, either homozygous or a compound heterozygote for a pathologic variant. This deficiency is ultimately caused by mutations in the CYB5R3 gene, located on chromosome 22q 13-qter, which codes for the cytochrome b5 reductase enzyme; to date, over 78 different mutations have been found to cause cytochrome b5 reductase deficiency [6, 7]. There are two different isoforms of Cyb5r, and as mutations can occur in either, this results in two different disease types:

Type 1 disease results from mutations in the erythrocyte-specific isoform, which functions normally to reduce methemoglobin back to a functional hemoglobin. Missense variants are the most common mutation and lead to an unstable enzyme solely in the erythrocytes. Type 1 disease is the most common and causes methemoglobinemia alone; it accounts for about 90% of Cyb5r3 variants. Clinical presentations include cyanosis, dyspnea, headaches, or fatigue. Generally, those affected by type 1 disease have MHb concentrations that range from 10% to 35%, and most are asymptomatic, even at these levels.

Type 2 disease is a result of mutations in the more generalized isoform of Cyb5r, which is embedded in the endoplasmic reticulum and functions in a variety of metabolic reactions in other tissues, outside of erythrocytes. Type 2 disease has more far-reaching consequences, given the isoform's systemic processes, thought to be potentially involved in the myelination metabolism of the nervous system. Not only does it result in methemoglobinemia, but it is also accompanied by developmental delay or intellectual disability, with other neurologic manifestations that ultimately lead to a failure to thrive. This accounts for about 10% of Cyb5r3 disease variants.

Another cause of congenital methemoglobinemia is hemoglobin M disease. This is inherited in an autosomal dominant pattern, and instead of a mutation in the enzyme that reduces methemoglobin, these mutations occur in the globin portion of the structure. There have been at least 13 different Hgb M variants described; variants can be secondary to changes in either alpha, beta, or gamma globin genes. The resulting changes in the amino acid sequence often force a substitution of either the proximal or distal histidine in the heme pocket, often for a tyrosine. This is a significant change, as the tyrosine can form a complex with iron and phenolate that resists reduction from the ferric (Fe3+) back to the ferrous (2+) state, ultimately preventing the reduction of MHb [8]. The multiple globin variants present with different phenotypes and can all lead to cyanosis in affected individuals. Generally, the alpha globin variants will present with cyanosis at birth, while the beta globin variants will become evident later in the first year of life. Hemolytic anemia can also be present in some subset of variants.

Deficiency in cytochrome b5 is one of the rarest forms of hereditary methemoglobinemia. Cytochrome b5 acts as the substrate for the Cyb5r3 enzyme to appropriately reduce MHb back to Hgb; when present, it acts as the electron donor to MHb in the reduction–oxidation reaction. There are few documented reports of these patients, and the diagnosis can be challenging to confirm. Cases that do confirm this genetic loss of functional protein are often associated with cyanosis and ambiguous genitalia due to a homozygous variant in the CYB5A gene [8, 9].

Acquired

There are many possible etiologies for acquired MHb, mostly attributed to medication use or toxic ingestion. These drugs or exposures subsequently cause either a direct oxidation or an indirect oxidation of hemoglobin via metabolites to the ferric state (3+). Additionally, several recreational drugs have been implicated in acquired MHb, including amyl nitrite (poppers) or nitrous oxide (laughing gas). Among the notorious classes of drugs that can cause MHb are topical anesthetics like lidocaine; hard drugs like cocaine, heroin, and fentanyl are often "cut" or diluted with these agents and can lead to very high levels of MHb. Aside from topical anesthetics, some other prominent drugs that have been implicated include dapsone, rasburicase, nitrofurantoin, phenytoin, rifampin, sulfasalazine, and metoclopramide. For a full list of casual agents, please refer to Table 11.2.

Those who are most at risk for acquired MHb are individuals with a heterozygous variant of CYB5R3, as they are more susceptible to drug-induced insults. Additionally, newborns and infants are an at-risk population, given the reduced baseline activity of the Cyb5r3 enzyme.

Clinical Presentations

Methemoglobinemia should be a consideration on the differential diagnosis for patients who are presenting with cyanosis or hypoxia measured on a pulse oximeter that is not responsive to supplemental oxygen treatment. While it can happen in any age group, special consideration should be made for infants or adults. Often, patients will also present with chocolate-colored blood. A patient's presentation varies on the severity of MHb present in the blood; please see Table 11.3 for approximate MHb% and general symptoms. It is important to note that the severity of symptoms and degree of MHb can vary depending on a multitude of different factors, including the drug or toxic exposure amount and rate, as well as the patient's underlying comorbidities and whether they carry a variant of Cyb5r3.

Pulse oximetry is the standard approach for the measurement of oxygen levels in a patient, used either intermittently or continuously. This device measures oxygen

Table 11.3 Symptoms at MHb percentage [4]

MHb (%)	Symptoms
<15	Asymptomatic
15–30	Cyanosis, anxiety, lightheadedness, fatigue, headache
30–50	Tachypnea, confusion, syncope
50–70	Seizures, arrhythmias, metabolic acidosis, coma
>70	Death

concentration by passing two waves of light, red and near-infrared, through a part of the patient's body to a photodetector. Oxygenated hemoglobin and deoxygenated hemoglobin absorb red and infrared light differently, which allows for distinction between the two. The pulse oximeter measures the absorption of light in arterial blood over the course of a cardiac cycle and calculates the ratio between oxygenated and unoxygenated blood; this is used to report a percentage of bound hemoglobin. An oxygenation level that is clinically accepted as normal is 94% peripheral oxygen saturation (SpO_2) or greater. At times, this may be lower (>88%) depending on the patient and other medical comorbidities, i.e., chronic obstructive pulmonary disease. It is important to understand the mechanism of peripheral oxygen saturation measurements using a pulse oximeter when considering methemoglobinemia. MHb absorbs both red and near-infrared light at a similar degree, leading to inaccuracies in the ability to calculate an appropriate ratio. In fact, as MHb's absorption of red light is similar to deoxygenated blood, once the levels of MHb are high enough, the patient's SpO_2 will trend toward 85% [10]. This is because the ratio of absorption of red and near-infrared light approaches 1.

Another way to measure blood oxygen concentration is from a sample of arterial blood with a blood gas, measuring the partial pressure of oxygen in the blood (SaO_2). While the SpO_2 is falsely low and unresponsive to supplemental oxygen, the SaO_2 measurement has an inverse issue. An arterial blood gas (ABG) is a calculation based on the serum pressure of oxygen, and the test assumes that all hemoglobin is normal—either oxygenated or deoxygenated. The gap between a patient's decreased SpO_2 and falsely normal SaO_2 is known as the "saturation gap" and can be a clue into MHb or other hemoglobinopathies as the etiology. When suspecting methemoglobinemia, a co-oximetry, which is an actual measurement of each type of hemoglobin, should be obtained. Instead of using two waves of light to pass through blood and give a percentage of oxygen, a co-oximetry passes blood through multiple different wavelengths and allows for the distinction between various types of hemoglobin, including MHb and carboxyhemoglobin, which is necessary for a diagnosis.

When considering the diagnosis of congenital methemoglobinemia or attempting to differentiate congenital methemoglobinemia from acquired, there is additional testing after confirmation of the increased MHb levels. The gold standard to differentiating these two is the cytochrome b5 reductase enzyme activity measurement. After identifying decreased Cyb5r3 activity, confirmation of congenital MHb is recommended with next-generation sequencing (NGS). Sending for NGS will also identify variants of the CYB5R3 gene, either labeled as pathogenic, likely pathogenic, or of undetermined significance.

Treatment

Just as the degree of symptoms of MHb can vary, so can treatment. Some patients may improve with simply the removal of the offending agent and supportive care; at other times, patients may require treatment with antidotal agents and high amounts of supplemental oxygen. Oftentimes, treatment depends on the patient's age, severity of symptoms, etiology of MHb, and associated comorbidities.

After diagnosis of acquired methemoglobinemia and the removal of the offending agent, supportive care can be started with intravenous hydration as well as high amounts of supplemental oxygen [4]. The additional oxygen helps deliver oxygen to tissues, as well as improves the metabolism of MHb. Further treatment considerations are offered generally in patients who have 20% MHb and are symptomatic, with the threshold increased to 30% MHb in those who are asymptomatic. Special consideration should be made on an individualized basis for patients who are asymptomatic but have increased risk factors for impaired oxygenation at baseline, including heart and lung disease, or baseline anemia.

The most used treatment of significant, acute methemoglobinemia is methylene blue (MB), an agent that is also used in ifosfamide-induced encephalopathy, as well as other types of shock. In the setting of MHb, MB acts as an antidotal agent at a different pathway from Cyb5r3, instead acting on the normally non-physiologically active NADPH methemoglobin reductase. MB accepts an electron from NADPH, which then reduces ferric iron (3+) back to its ferrous (2+) state [11]. The preferred dose to use is 1–2 mg/kg (of actual body weight) infused over 5–30 minutes [12]; clinicians can repeat the dose 1 h later if MHb remains >30% or if the patient has persistent symptoms. Should more than two doses be required, it is recommended that consultation be made with a toxicologist or the poison control center be contacted for further recommendations. For patients who have ingested long-acting culprit toxins/agents, i.e., dapsone, repeated doses may be required. There are significant possible side effects to be aware of when using this medication, of which a prominent one is the discoloration of bodily fluids after administration; patients will often have blue coloration of the skin or blue/green urine. While this is benign and will improve after metabolism, further side effects include hypersensitivity reactions, possible central nervous system depression, and serotonin syndrome, and, should it extravasate from an IV, MB is a known vesicant. Additionally, at high doses or in patients with G6PD deficiency and infants, MB may cause a paradoxical MHb and hemolysis. Careful consideration should be made prior to the use of MB to ensure that it is appropriate for the clinical scenario. For severe cases of MHb that are refractory to MB, there have been published case reports of positive treatment with the use of exchange therapy or the use of hyperbaric oxygen [8]. Blood transfusions can be considered in those patients who also have anemia.

Another accepted treatment of MHb includes ascorbic acid, or vitamin C, which acts by reducing excess oxidative stress. It is given via infusion at 1–10 g every 6 h until MHb levels normalize 13. While ascorbic acid and MB have not been compared head-to-head in clinical trials, MB is generally preferred in the setting of acute, severe symptomatic MHb, given its fast onset and dramatic improvements with a few doses. Ascorbic acid takes a longer time to be effective, generally >24 h, but does not have the significant side effects seen with MB. Ascorbic acid is usually indicated first in patients with a known G6PD deficiency or who are at a high risk of serotonin syndrome.

In the management of patients with a congenital form of methemoglobinemia, oftentimes, they do not require treatment. These patients will generally be diagnosed in infancy or childhood and have circulating MHb levels of about 10–30%, often asymptomatic even at rates of MHb nearing 40%. Treatment is usually pursued solely for cosmetic reasons, secondary to cyanosis. Options for treatment include methylene blue, either with or without ascorbic acid; ascorbic acid only; or, potentially, riboflavin (B2). However, it is important to note that these treatments are not always effective and can be problematic with a potential for the development of nephrolithiasis (chronic ascorbic acid use) or hemolysis (methylene blue in G6PD deficiency).

Conclusions

Methemoglobinemia can be challenging to identify but simple in terms of diagnostic and treatment algorithms. Understanding the pathophysiology behind the disease and the abnormalities seen on initial blood work, including a blood gas and vital sign examination, can be a critical clue to the diagnosis of MHb. Definitive diagnosis includes a blood gas with co-oximetry for detecting specific types of altered hemoglobin. Treatment varies depending on the patient's symptoms, ranging from observation to intervention with medications, such as methylene blue (MB) or ascorbic acid (Vit C). Detailed medication history, in addition to recreational drug history, is warranted in all patients for whom MHb is on the differential. Special consideration is made for infants or children presenting with cyanosis, as they can have congenital MHb.

References

1. Lunenfeld E, Kane GC. Methemoglobinemia: sudden dyspnea and oxyhemoglobin desaturation after esophagoduodenoscopy. Respir Care. 2004;49(8):940–2. PMID: 15271232.
2. Akhtar J, Johnston BD, Krenzelok EP. Mind the gap. J Emerg Med. 2007;33(2):131–2. https://doi.org/10.1016/j.jemermed.2006.11.016. Epub 2007 Jun 5. PMID: 17692762.
3. Marengo-Rowe AJ. Structure-function relations of human hemoglobins. Proc (Bayl Univ Med Cent). 2006;19(3):239–45. https://doi.org/10.1080/08998280.2006.11928171. PMID: 17252042; PMCID: PMC1484532.
4. Ludlow JT, Wilkerson RG, Nappe TM. Methemoglobinemia. 2023 Aug 28. In: StatPearls [Internet]. Treasure Island: StatPearls Publishing; 2025. PMID: 30726002.
5. Wright RO, Lewander WJ, Woolf AD. Methemoglobinemia: etiology, pharmacology, and clinical management. Ann Emerg Med. 1999;34(5):646–56. https://doi.org/10.1016/s0196-0644(99)70167-8. PMID: 10533013.
6. Online Mendelian Inheritance in Man, OMIM®. MIM Number: 250800: Entry – #250800 – Methemoglobinemia due to deficiency of methemoglobin reductase – OMIM. Baltimore: Johns Hopkins University; 20 Jan 2010.
7. Gupta V, Kulkarni A, Warang P, Devendra R, Chiddarwar A, Kedar P. Mutation update: variants of the CYB5R3 gene in recessive congenital methemoglobinemia. Hum Mutat. 2020;41(4):737–48. https://doi.org/10.1002/humu.23973.

8. Iolascon A, Bianchi P, Andolfo I, Russo R, Barcellini W, Fermo E, Toldi G, Ghirardello S, Rees D, Van Wijk R, Kattamis A, Gallagher PG, Roy N, Taher A, Mohty R, Kulozik A, De Franceschi L, Gambale A, De Montalembert M, Forni GL, Harteveld CL, Prchal J, SWG of red cell and iron of EHA and EuroBloodNet. Recommendations for diagnosis and treatment of methemoglobinemia. Am J Hematol. 2021;96(12):1666–78. https://doi.org/10.1002/ajh.26340. Epub 2021 Sep 23. PMID: 34467556; PMCID: PMC9291883.
9. Hegesh E, Hegesh J, Kaftory A. Congenital methemoglobinemia with a deficiency of cytochrome B5. N Engl J Med. 1986;314(12):757–61. https://doi.org/10.1056/NEJM198603203141206.
10. Chan ED, Chan MM, Chan MM. Pulse oximetry: understanding its basic principles facilitates appreciation of its limitations. Respir Med. 2013;107(6):789–99. https://doi.org/10.1016/j.rmed.2013.02.004. Epub 2013 Mar 13. PMID: 23490227.
11. Nappe TM, Pacelli AM, Katz K. An atypical case of methemoglobinemia due to self-administered benzocaine. Case Rep Emerg Med. 2015;2015:670979. https://doi.org/10.1155/2015/670979. Epub 2015 Mar 19. PMID: 25874137; PMCID: PMC4383305.
12. Methylene Blue. Lexi-Drugs. UpToDate Lexidrug. UpToDate Inc. https://online.lexi.com. Accessed 28 Feb 2024.
13. Ascorbic Acid. Lexi-Drugs. UpToDate Lexidrug. UpToDate Inc. https://online.lexi.com. Accessed 28 Feb 2024.
14. Rehman HU. Methemoglobinemia. West J Med. 2001;175(3):193–6. https://doi.org/10.1136/ewjm.175.3.193. PMID: 11527852; PMCID: PMC1071541.

The Control of Breathing

12

Ibukun Fakunle and Urvashi Vaid

Introduction

An interest in how one breathes and the fundamental need to breathe to stay alive dates back many millennia, but the scientific work that elucidated the mechanisms of breathing and its control is very recent, dating back 80–85 years. An initial interest in breathing was pioneered by the Chinese and Hindu civilizations, who took a deep dive into the way we breathe and described long, deep breaths emanating from the abdomen. This has evolved into what we know today as meditation, which has scientifically proven benefits. Later, the Greeks linked the heart, the lungs, and the skin by postulating that the heat generated by the heart had to be cooled by the air we breathe. It was only in the eighteenth century that respiratory physiology advanced with the advent of a deeper understanding of chemistry, Joseph Priestley's discovery of oxygen, Lavoisier's understanding of the difference between combustion and respiration, and the discovery of the anatomy of the circulatory system and its receptors. Finally, further experiments on animals and humans localized the medulla as the key area controlling respiration and recognized the importance of higher inhaled CO_2 concentrations resulting in an increase in total ventilation [1]. In this chapter, we focus on the fine-tuned negative feedback loops that unconsciously and continually modulate respiration to maintain normal pH, provide life-sustaining oxygen to tissues, and remove excess acid, thus maintaining homeostasis at all times.

I. Fakunle
Department of Pulmonary, Critical Care, and Allergy, Thomas Jefferson University Hospital, Philadelphia, PA, USA
e-mail: Ibukun.Fakunle@jefferson.edu

U. Vaid (✉)
The Korman Respiratory Institute and the Division of Pulmonary, Allergy and Critical Care, The Department of Medicine at the Sidney Kimmel Medical College of Thomas Jefferson University, Philadelphia, PA, USA
e-mail: Urvashi.Vaid@jefferson.edu

G. C. Kane et al. (eds.), *Oxygen*, https://doi.org/10.1007/978-3-032-18934-9_12

Hox genes play a critical role in the determinism of ensuring that humans have lungs and where we have them [2]. Hox genes encode transcription factors that dictate what and where specific structures develop in the body. For example, a Hox gene mutation causes the *Drosophila melanogaster* (fruit fly) to develop legs on its head in place of antennae. Just as humans are predetermined to have lungs to breathe and live, lung function is subject to control, at least in part, by the very gases that it exchanges. Let us follow the path a fetus takes from gestation to birth.

A fetus receives oxygen and nutrient-rich blood from its mother through the umbilical vein [3]. So it was thought that fetuses did not need to breathe in the traditional sense. We now understand, however, that fetuses do breathe. In the third trimester, for about 30% of the time, mammalian fetuses make intermittent episodic breathing movements because of diaphragmatic activity. These movements make repetitive changes to intrathoracic pressure similar to postnatal life. And these movements by exerting mechanical forces on the lungs are crucial to the growth of the lungs [4].

Mass effects on the intrathoracic space, such as diaphragmatic hernia and pleural effusion, can restrict lung growth by causing structural obstruction and impairing normal fetal breathing movements. Similarly, lesions that paralyze the diaphragm can do the same. In animal models, sectioning the phrenic nerve nullified fetal breathing movements and inhibited lung growth [4].

Prior to the advent of surfactant replacement therapy and advancements in assisted ventilation, respiratory distress syndrome was a leading cause of neonatal morbidity and mortality. Nowadays, with more equipped neonatal intensive care units and improved survival of extremely preterm neonates, we encounter disordered lung growth, or bronchopulmonary dysplasia [4].

It follows that since episodic fetal breathing is necessary for lung growth and this activity becomes more pronounced in the third trimester, babies born prematurely would not have gained the optimal benefit of this "breathing practice" prior to delivery and thus develop bronchopulmonary dysplasia.

Upon delivery and exposure to the elements, the baby must breathe air to supply oxygen to its tissues. The mechanical and sensory stress of delivery is thought to trigger the first breath, and as CO_2 levels build in the blood, they stimulate central chemoreceptors to increase ventilation. Interestingly, the tidal volume remains roughly 6 ml/kg from birth to maturity, but a newborn has a much higher respiratory rate [5].

It is now thought that a neural network called the central pattern generator exists within the ventral brain stem and generates the respiratory rhythm. This generator generates rhythmic output in the absence of rhythmic input and so also dictates our rhythmic motions of walking, talking, and chewing. Two coupled anatomically distinct rhythm generators, the pre-Bötzinger complex and the retrotrapezoid nucleus/respiratory group, are responsible for driving inspiration and expiration, respectively (the pacemakers of respiration!). And one of the two dominates by producing a faster rhythm [6, 7].

Respiratory Centers

The respiratory centers comprise three areas in the brain: the dorsal respiratory group of neurons in the nucleus of the tractus solitarius, the ventral group of neurons in the medulla, and the pontine group of neurons in the pons.

The dorsal neuronal group's role is predominantly inspiratory, and the ventral medullary neurons are predominantly expiratory. The pre-Bötzinger complex mentioned earlier resides in the rostral half of the ventral medulla. The pontine neurons regulate the output from the medulla and are divided into the pneumotaxic center (inhibiting respiration) and the apneustic center (prolonging inhalation).

The Role of Oxygen in Controlling Breaths

The lungs and chest wall exist in a dynamic pressure–volume relationship with the atmosphere. Under normal circumstances, the pressure in the pleural space is always negative relative to the pressure in the alveoli. This is to maintain a slightly positive transpulmonary pressure, which maintains alveolar distension, preventing the lungs from recoiling or deflating.

At the end of expiration, the pressure within the alveoli is near zero. That is, it is nearly equal to the atmospheric pressure. At the start of inspiration, upon receiving a signal from the pre-Bötzinger complex, the diaphragm and external intercostal muscles contract to expand and lift the rib cage. The pressure within the alveoli becomes negative relative to the atmosphere to draw air in. That is, normal breathing is a negative-pressure ventilation system. And the pressure in the pleural space becomes even more negative to allow the lungs to expand.

As earlier described, the rhythm of breathing is dictated by the central pattern generator in the ventral brain stem, which can produce rhythmic output without rhythmic input. That said, there are modulating factors involved in the breathing process. This is particularly salient because of the cellular metabolic activity and the drive to maintain homeostasis.

Much has been described about the effect of carbon dioxide on the brain stem. In a bid to maintain homeostasis, whenever there is an increase in the blood content of carbon dioxide (and thus a lowering of the pH, or "respiratory acidosis"), there is a resultant increase in the rate and volume of breathing. This raises the question: Are there other gaseous elements that may affect the rate and volume of breathing, particularly when the blood content of carbon dioxide is normal?

Indeed. Oxygen also regulates breathing. This effect is particularly notable when the blood content of carbon dioxide is increased and the blood content of oxygen is low.

As a refresher, oxygen delivery to any tissue depends on the engine of the body, which is the heart; its output (heart rate × stroke volume); and the amount or content of oxygen in the blood. The content of oxygen in the blood itself is made up of the majority bound to hemoglobin (Hb) and the minority that is free oxygen dissolved in blood.

There are peripheral chemoreceptors called carotid and aortic bodies, which reside in the bifurcation of the carotid arteries bilaterally and the aortic arch, respectively. These bodies, the carotid more so than aortic, sense oxygen content and oxygen tension as arterial blood flows by the chemoreceptors. In response, the bodies increase their firing rate, via the glossopharyngeal nerve in the case of carotid bodies and the vagus nerve in the case of aortic bodies, to trigger the reticular formation in the medulla and thus increase minute ventilation (respiratory rate × tidal volume) [8].

Note that since oxygen delivery dictates oxygen tension, both anemia and a fall in cardiac output can induce an increase in the firing rate in the aortic and carotid bodies to ultimately result in increased minute ventilation.

Interestingly, in animal studies, when the carotid and aortic bodies have been removed or denervated, hypoxia directly depresses the central respiratory center [9].

Reflex Mechanisms of Respiratory Control

Accompanying the peripheral chemoreceptors are receptors present around and within the substance of the lung. These include mechanoreceptors and juxtacapillary receptors, among others. They are not directly responsive to changes in oxygen tension but respond instead to stretch, pulmonary venous congestion, lung injury, and other insults. Slow-adapting stretch spindles respond to changes in lung volume, whereas fast-adapting irritant receptors respond to chemical triggers and foreign bodies. Ultimately, they also contribute to breath control, and we will detail a few important examples.

The Hering–Breuer reflexes, also called the pulmonary stretch reflexes, arise from the stimulation of mechanoreceptors. In the Hering–Breuer inflation reflex, sustained inflation of the lung decreases the frequency of respiration, i.e., taking a slow deep breath in reduces your respiratory rate. The stretch receptors in the airway smooth muscle sense the deep breath and transmit impulses via the vagus to the inspiratory off switch in the brain stem respiratory center, which then decreases the rate of respiration. These receptors are slow-adapting. In conscious adults, large tidal volumes (800–1500 ml) are required to elicit this reflex. In infants, this reflex is more important, as it is activated within their normal tidal volume ranges. It helps prevent large tidal volumes and alveolar overdistension. In the Hering–Breuer deflation reflex, abrupt deflation increases the respiratory rate. This may be a result of decreased stretch receptor activity. Thus, an abrupt deflation in the lung from the pneumothorax, for example, will result in hyperpnea. Also, this reflex is responsible for periodic sighs that prevent atelectasis (alveolar collapse).

Another important example of how stretch reflexes play a role in the control of breathing is demonstrated by the pharyngeal dilator reflex. In this reflex, negative pressure in the upper airway causes contraction of the pharyngeal dilator muscles. Impulses are transmitted from the nose, mouth, and the upper airways via the trigeminal, laryngeal (branch of the vagus), and glossopharyngeal nerves. This is a very important reflex, especially during sleep, as it prevents the upper airway from collapsing and causing obstructive sleep apnea.

Irritant receptors in the respiratory system play a role in protecting the lung parenchyma. Chemical or mechanical irritation of the airways can result in sneezing, coughing, and/or hyperpnea and elevated blood pressure. The impulses are transmitted via the vagus nerves from the airways and the trigeminal and olfactory nerves from the nasal mucosa.

Reflexes arising from the pulmonary vascular receptors (J receptors) also play a protective role. Receptors in the pulmonary circulation are called J receptors or juxta-pulmonary–capillary receptors. These unmyelinated nerve fibers are stimulated by lung injury, large inflation, acute pulmonary vascular congestion, and pulmonary embolism among others. Increased stimulation of these receptors by pulmonary vascular congestion results in tachypnea and may contribute to the feeling of dyspnea or shortness of breath. Decreased stimulation of these receptors as in pulmonary embolism leads to decreased ventilation locally in the area affected by the embolus

Finally, reflexes arising from muscles and tendons and from pain can control breathing. Ventilation can be increased by the stimulation of receptors in the muscle, tendons, and joints, especially during exercise and when the respiratory workload is excessive. Somatic pain causes hyperpnea (deep and high RR), whereas visceral pain causes apnea or decreased ventilation [10, 11]. Figure 12.1

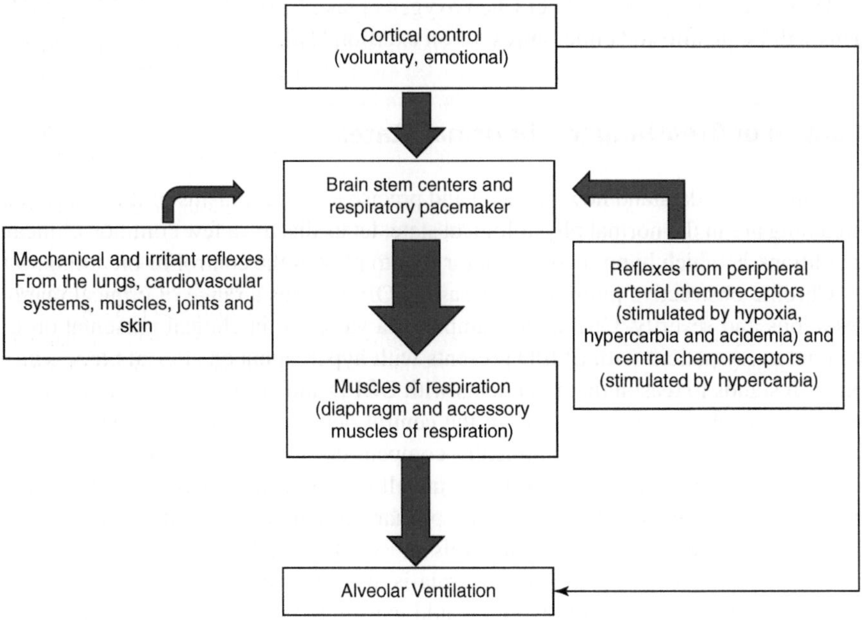

Fig. 12.1 The organization and reflex control of breathing

summarizes the organization of the respiratory control system and the various components and feedback loops that control breathing.

Oxygen Uptake Across Alveoli

To take effect on receptors, the nervous system, and ventilation, oxygen must first enter the blood.

Under normal conditions at rest, as blood flows through the pulmonary capillaries, oxygen is taken up by the red blood cells in the vessels interfacing with the alveoli. This process occurs within one-third of the time it takes blood to get from the start of the capillary to the end of the capillary. So the uptake of oxygen is very effective. The partial pressure of oxygen (PaO_2) in the blood rises rapidly to approximately that of the alveolar oxygen, as oxygen is taken up from the alveoli, binding to hemoglobin and, more importantly, dissolving in the blood to generate a "back pressure" in the plasma. This explains how oxygen is a perfusion-limited gas because its movement from the alveoli to the blood is limited by the pressure generated by itself in the blood.

Oxygen can also become diffusion-limited in situations where the diffusion properties of the lungs are impaired—such as in interstitial lung disease, in which the interstitium is thickened; pulmonary capillary thickening; and emphysema. In these situations, the partial pressure of oxygen in the blood does not reach that of the alveoli by the end of the capillary, and so it is limited by the diffusion properties of the lungs.

Hypoxia is the resultant effect when oxygen uptake across the alveoli is impaired. This will be manifested either at rest or on exertion [12].

Control of Breathing in Abnormal States

Now that we understand how nuanced and precise the mechanisms of the control of breathing are in the normal physiological state, let us discuss a few common clinical conditions in which hypoxia has a major role to play in the control of breathing.

Chronic obstructive pulmonary disease (COPD) spans a range of clinical manifestations and severity. One such example of a variation in clinical presentation is that not every patient with COPD presents with hypercapnia on arterial blood sampling. It stands to reason that in patients with COPD and chronic hypercapnia, there is a new threshold for ventilation in the central nervous system. This occurs provided renal function can metabolically compensate to bring the pH closer to the normal range and that the pH of the extracellular fluid in their brain is also near normal. Thus, hypoxemia becomes the primary modulator of ventilation. This is why it is recommended that high levels of supplemental oxygen be avoided in chronic hypercarbia because if hypoxemia is abolished in these patients, a fall in minute ventilation may result, which would worsen hypercapnia. Interestingly, this theory has since been downplayed. Targeting higher levels of oxygenation in patients with COPD and hypercarbia is now known to eliminate the pulmonary vasculature's hypoxic vasoconstrictive response. This can worsen the V/Q mismatch by preventing the redirection of blood from poorly ventilated alveoli to well-ventilated alveoli. Additionally, the Hb–CO_2 dissociation curve is postulated to shift to the right in the presence of O_2, thus off-loading CO_2 into the blood, increasing its levels (the Haldane effect). Finally, excess oxygenation can result in absorptive atelectasis, thus decreasing the alveolar surface area for gas exchange. As a result, consensus recommendations for hypercapnic patients with COPD target an O_2 saturation of 88–92% [13].

In the event of obstruction of pulmonary blood flow by a blood clot (acute pulmonary embolism), ventilation–perfusion mismatch is the mechanism by which hypoxia occurs. In cases of massive or high-risk pulmonary embolism causing right ventricle failure, an ineffective right ventricle unable to pump blood forward through the main pulmonary artery into the lungs for gas exchange will result in hypoxia by restricting pulmonary vascular perfusion to ventilated areas (dead space) and increasing perfusion out of proportion to ventilation in the ventilated areas ($Q \ggg V$, which is shunt physiology), hence a severe ventilation–perfusion mismatch.

In addition, right ventricle failure in high-risk pulmonary embolism is characterized by a dilated chamber with acutely elevated pressures, which result in flattening of the interventricular septum and impairment of the structure and function of the left ventricle. The left ventricle relies on the right ventricle to provide blood, which, after oxygenation in the lungs, will be pumped through systemic circulation; a failed right ventricle will impair systemic circulation. If the degree of blood flow in the setting of massive pulmonary embolism is substantial, PEA can result because of the failed filling of the left ventricle, leading to cardiac arrest and death if not rapidly reversed.

As discussed earlier, hypoxia sensed by the peripheral chemoreceptors will signal to the central medullary respiratory centers to increase ventilation.

Atmospheric pressure has an inverse relationship with altitude. Therefore, at higher altitudes, even though the fraction of oxygen in the atmosphere (FiO_2) remains 21%, there is a reduction in the partial pressure of oxygen relative to sea level. This is known to us by our understanding of the alveolar gas equation [$PAO_2 = FiO_2 \times (P_{atm} - P_{H2O}) \times PaCO_2/0.8$] (see Chap. 39).

If a bare-faced human (one not using supplemental oxygen) journeys up a mountain such as Kilimanjaro, which boasts an elevation of 19,342 feet above sea level, they will experience a reduction in the partial pressure of oxygen in inspired air and, subsequently, alveolar air. This, in addition to other effects of high altitude, such as a rightward shift of the oxygen dissociation curve, facilitates off-loading of oxygen from the hemoglobin to the tissues. Enhanced off-loading can help make up for the lower venous oxygen content at least in part.

The carotid and aortic bodies sense this reduction in oxygen content created by alveolar hypoxia and increase their action potential to the glossopharyngeal and vagus nerves, respectively, to trigger the respiratory centers in the brain stem to increase ventilation. Thus, hypoxia causes respiratory alkalosis at high altitudes.

And finally, a rare genetic disease is caused by a mutation that results in insensitivity centrally to changes in PCO_2. This disease is known as Ondine's curse, or congenital central hypoventilation syndrome, and causes the person to be dependent on conscious breathing controlled by the cerebral cortex. Thus, when asleep, the affected person tends to slow down or stop breathing [13].

Conclusion

Triggered by a tireless central respiratory pacemaker, our breathing is under the control of an intricate set of feedback loops, working to maintain oxygenation and acid–base homeostasis. If hypoxia, hypercarbia, or acidemia develops, the peripheral chemoreceptors sense this and send signals via the ninth and tenth cranial nerves to the central chemoreceptors to modulate the output to the muscles of respiration, thus increasing minute ventilation. Centrally, chemoreceptors can respond directly to acidemia by way of a high partial pressure of CO_2 ($PaCO_2$) in arterial blood with a similar result. All this reverses in the conditions of alkalemia. Without this level of precision, our cells and tissues would not be provided with the requisite levels of oxygen nor would they be able to perform their metabolic roles in an efficient and productive manner.

References

1. Fitzgerald RS, Cherniack NS. Historical perspectives on the control of breathing. Compr Physiol. 2012;2(2):915–32. https://doi.org/10.1002/cphy.c100007. PMID: 23798292.
2. Kappen C. Hox genes in the lung. Am J Respir Cell Mol Biol. 1996;15(2):156–62. https://doi.org/10.1165/ajrcmb.15.2.8703471.
3. Harriet Lane Service (Johns Hopkins Hospital), Anderson CC, Kapoor S, Mark TE. The Harriet Lane handbook: a manual for pediatric house officers. 23rd ed. Philadelphia: Elsevier; 2024.
4. Kitterman JA. The effects of mechanical forces on fetal lung growth. Clin Perinatol. 1996;23(4):727–40. PMID: 8982567.
5. Adamson SL. Regulation of breathing at birth. J Dev Physiol. 1991;15(1):45–52. PMID: 1908494.
6. Hooper SL. Central pattern generators. In: Encyclopedia of life sciences. Wiley; 1999–2010. https://doi.org/10.1038/npg.els.0000032. ISBN 978-0-470-01590-2.
7. Smith JC, Ellenberger HH, Ballanyi K, Richter DW, Feldman JL. Pre-Bötzinger complex: a brainstem region that may generate respiratory rhythm in mammals. Science. 1991;254(5032):726–9. https://doi.org/10.1126/science.1683005. PMC 3209964. PMID 1683005.
8. Lahiri S, Nishino T, Mokashi A, Mulligan E. Relative responses of aortic body and carotid body chemoreceptors to hypotension. J Appl Physiol Respir Environ Exerc Physiol. 1980;48(5):781–8. https://doi.org/10.1152/jappl.1980.48.5.781.
9. Gourine AV, Funk GD. On the existence of a central respiratory oxygen sensor. J Appl Physiol (1985). 2017;123(5):1344–9. https://doi.org/10.1152/japplphysiol.00194.2017.
10. Ganong WF, Barrett KE. Ganong's review of medical physiology. 26th ed. New York: McGraw-Hill Education; 2019.
11. Hall JE, Hall ME. Guyton and Hall textbook of medical physiology. 14th ed. Philadelphia: Elsevier; 2021.

12. West JB, Luks AM. West's respiratory physiology: the essentials. 11th ed. Philadelphia: Wolters Kluwer; 2021.
13. Brinkman JE, Toro F, Sharma S. Physiology, respiratory drive. [Updated 2023 Jun 5]. In: StatPearls [Internet]. Treasure Island: StatPearls Publishing; 2025. Available from: https://www.ncbi.nlm.nih.gov/books/NBK482414/.

Part III

Chronic Respiratory Failure

Principles of Outpatient Use for Patients with Chronic Lung Diseases, Including COPD and Pulmonary Fibrosis

13

Rafael Perez

Introduction

Long-term oxygen therapy (LTOT), also called home oxygen therapy, originated around the middle of the twentieth century [1]. Dr. Alvan Barach, known in the United States for promoting oxygen therapy in the hospital setting during the 1920s, pioneered supplemental oxygen in the ambulatory setting in patients with stable chronic hypoxemia. He and others studied lung gas exchange during the Second World War, driven by the need to develop the technology for continuous oxygen delivery at high altitudes. Scientists learned much about the predominance of ventilation-to-perfusion abnormalities in human disease, most notably in chronic obstructive disease (COPD). Small clinical studies followed in the United States and Europe to investigate the potential benefits of supplemental oxygen in individuals with COPD and hypoxemia.

Pioneering Studies that Established the Benefits and Standards of Supplemental Oxygen

In 1965, Dr. Thomas Petty was allowed to "try out" a new trans-filling liquid oxygen delivery system from the space age. He and colleagues carried out a trial to assess the benefits of supplemental O_2 in subjects with severe COPD, who had evidence of cor pulmonale and polycythemia [2]. Six subjects were stabilized for 1 month in a clinical research unit, where they were provided with nutrition,

R. Perez (✉)
The Korman Respiratory Institute and the Division of Pulmonary, Allergy and Critical Care, The Department of Medicine at the Sidney Kimmel Medical College of Thomas Jefferson University, Philadelphia, PA, USA
e-mail: rafael.perez@jefferson.edu

G. C. Kane et al. (eds.), *Oxygen*, https://doi.org/10.1007/978-3-032-18934-9_13

exercise, bronchodilator therapy, and management of comorbidities, especially congestive heart failure. They underwent right-heart catheterization after the month of optimal COPD management. All had elevated mean pulmonary arterial pressures. Chromium-51-tagged studies showed expanded red cell mass. The subjects were then placed on oxygen by nasal cannula for 1 month, maintaining oxygen saturations above 90%. Repeat right-heart catheterization on room air showed decreased mean pulmonary arterial pressures in four of the six subjects, and chromium-51-tagged studies showed a decline in red cell mass. Another similarly designed study by Abraham in the United Kingdom found that supplemental oxygen decreased pulmonary hypertension in individuals with advanced chronic bronchitis [3].

The studies by Petty, Abraham, and others showed that supplemental oxygen in individuals with COPD ameliorated the pathophysiology of chronic hypoxemia and improved exercise ability and quality of life. Other studies during the 1970s focused on the effects of oxygen supplementation in alleviating pulmonary hypertension and improving exercise tolerance in COPD, which established the parameters of the levels and duration of oxygen therapy [1]. In short, these studies showed that oxygen supplementation to maintain a blood oxygen tension of more than 55 mmHg for an optimal duration of 15–18 h/day decreased pulmonary hypertension and improved exercise tolerance in individuals with COPD. However, more rigorous longitudinal studies were needed to better understand the long-term outcomes of using LTOT, especially the effects on mortality.

Two seminal trials in the 1970s form the basis for prescribing LTOT today. The British Medical Research Council (BMRC) performed the "Long-term domiciliary oxygen therapy in chronic hypoxic cor pulmonale complicating chronic bronchitis and emphysema" study at three treatment centers in the United Kingdom [4]. Sixty-six men and 21 women were prospectively assigned in a 1:1 fashion to 15 h of supplemental oxygen to keep blood oxygen tension higher than 60 mmHg or to no oxygen therapy. The subjects had advanced airflow limitation, with a low forced expiratory volume in one second (FEV1), less than 1.2 L/s, and a resting PaO_2 between 40 and 60 mmHg on room air. They were followed up for 5 years with baseline and yearly measures of pulmonary pressures by right-heart catheterization and changes in red cell mass by the tagged chromium-51 technique. There were no differences in the mean pulmonary artery pressure between the oxygen-treated and control subjects, but pulmonary vascular resistance increased "much more" in the control group. Red cell mass decreased in the oxygen treatment group and increased slightly in the control group. Most notably, supplemental oxygen, mostly around 2 L/min by nasal cannula for at least 15 h a day, decreased the mortality rate immediately in the women subjects. However, men did not see a decreased mortality until 500 days into the trial. Secondary outcomes like exercise tolerance or hospitalizations were not different between those on supplemental oxygen and those on no oxygen therapy.

The "Continuous or nocturnal therapy in hypoxemic chronic obstructive pulmonary disease" trial, referred to as the nocturnal oxygen therapy trial (NOTT), was a 3-year study performed in North America around the same time as the study in the

United Kingdom [5]. Six treatment centers in the United States and Canada enrolled 203 individuals with COPD, with an average FEV1 of 30% predicted and hypoxemia defined as a blood oxygen tension of less than 60 mmHg on room air. The subjects were randomized prospectively to receive continuous oxygen therapy (COT) or nocturnal oxygen therapy (NOT). The goal was to maintain a blood oxygen tension between 60 and 80 mmHg while on oxygen. Laboratory and quality-of-life measures were performed throughout the study, but right-heart catheterization was done only at baseline and 6 months. On average, individuals in the COT group used oxygen for 17.7 h, with over one-half using oxygen for 19 h. Subjects in the NOT group used supplemental oxygen for an average of 12 h. Like the study in the United Kingdom, there was no significant change in the mean arterial pressure. Still, pulmonary vascular resistance and hematocrit decreased in the COT group compared to the NOT cohort. Importantly, mortality was twice as high in the NOT group starting at 12 months into the trial.

Supplemental Oxygen and "Moderate Oxygen Desaturation" in COPD

The BMRC trial and NOTT established the standards for oxygen prescription today. The standards and how to prescribe home oxygen therapy are detailed in Chap. 14. It is notable, though, that these trials showing a benefit on mortality were performed in subjects with severe COPD. Whether oxygen supplementation in individuals with less severe COPD and moderate oxygen desaturation at rest or with exertion showed similar results was unknown. A study called "A Randomized Trial of Long-Term Oxygen for COPD with Moderate Desaturation," referred to as the long-term oxygen therapy (LTOTT) trial, addressed this question [6]. It was a randomized, unmasked, parallel trial that recruited 738 subjects with stable COPD from 42 centers in the United States. They had moderate oxygen desaturation between 89% and 93% by pulse oximetry on room air at rest or exertional oxygen desaturation between 80% and 90%. The subjects were randomized 1:1 to receive oxygen therapy or no oxygen therapy. Participants in the oxygen treatment group used oxygen continuously at 2 L/min if they had moderate oxygen desaturation at rest. Those with only exertional oxygen desaturation had supplemental oxygen titrated to maintain an SpO_2% of 90 or greater and used oxygen only with exertion and sleep during the trial. The primary outcome was to determine if treatment with supplemental oxygen in individuals with COPD and moderate oxygen desaturation resulted in a longer time to death or first hospitalization. There was no difference in the primary outcome between the groups throughout 1–6 years. Also, there were no differences in secondary outcomes, including quality-of-life measures, lung function, or exercise by the 6-min walk test.

The LTOTT trial and four other studies comprising 1002 subjects contributed to a systematic review and meta-analysis focused on the mortality benefit in people with COPD and moderate oxygen desaturation [7]. All of the trials analyzed were randomized, controlled, and parallel-group. The definition of moderate oxygen desaturation varied among the studies, so the review's authors defined moderate desaturation as a resting PaO_2 on room air above 55 mmHg, the threshold of hypoxemia up to which supplemental oxygen has a mortality benefit. The primary outcome measure was the overall mortality at 3 years. The analysis was of high quality and low bias. It was able to leverage data from the combined 1002 participants to demonstrate that continuous or nocturnal oxygen therapy had no benefit on mortality or secondary measures such as COPD exacerbations, hospitalizations, or quality-of-life measures.

The implications of distinguishing between "severe" and "moderate" oxygen desaturation in COPD are profound. Stable individuals with COPD and moderate oxygen desaturation may avoid the cost and inconvenience of wearing supplemental oxygen, even when oxygen saturations decrease transiently into the severe range. The official 2020 American Thoracic Society "clinical practice guideline on home oxygen therapy for adults with chronic lung disease" suggests not prescribing supplemental oxygen for stable individuals with COPD and moderate resting oxygen desaturation [8]. Notably, the guideline does not prohibit or discourage prescribing supplemental oxygen for those who cross the severe hypoxemia threshold with exertion or sleep. The prescription of supplemental oxygen in the face of only moderate oxygen desaturation in stable COPD is discussed in Chap. 14.

Tobacco Smoking During the Use of Supplemental Oxygen

Chronic obstructive pulmonary disease along the chronic bronchitis–emphysema spectrum is mostly the result of tobacco smoking, and ongoing smokers seeking assessment for supplemental oxygen is common. Up to 30% of individuals with COPD who qualify for supplemental oxygen continue to smoke [9]. The issues around smoking while using supplemental oxygen primarily revolve around safety and prevention of burn injuries. Some providers and practices will not prescribe supplemental oxygen to ongoing smokers for safety reasons. How and if supplemental oxygen is prescribed for smokers is detailed in Chap. 14. Ultimately, the question is whether or not supplemental oxygen benefits smokers who qualify for long-term oxygen therapy.

There has not been, nor will there ever be, a randomized clinical trial on the effectiveness of oxygen therapy in smokers who qualify for supplemental oxygen. Such a study would breach the three ethical principles of "respect for persons," "beneficence," and "justice," as outlined in the 1979 Belmont Report on the moral principles and guidelines on the protection of human subjects participating in research [10]. Notably, the original BMRC trial and NOTT did not address the impact of smoking on mortality or other factors that influenced the outcomes, but a later inquiry found that 43% of the subjects in the BMRC trial and 38% in the NOTT were smokers during the studies [11].

Smoking changes the lung structure and function in such ways that one can reasonably assume that the benefits of supplemental oxygen are decreased in smokers. Studies in the mid-twentieth century explored the deleterious effects of tobacco smoking on overall health in general and lung disease in particular. These studies formed the basis for the 1964 Surgeon General's report on smoking and health [12]. One study by Motley and Kuzman in 1958 enrolled 141 current smokers (11% women) with either no obvious lung impairments or varying severity of emphysema or pulmonary fibrosis [13]. They abstained from smoking for 4–6 h before pulmonary lung function or arterial blood gas testing. The study subjects underwent repeated testing after smoking two cigarettes. Only individuals with "very severe" emphysema demonstrated decreased arterial oxygen tension and saturation at rest after smoking, but all groups demonstrated decreased oxygen uptake on treadmill exercise. The investigators found that acute smoking decreased lung compliance and increased the elastic work of breathing in all groups, including those with normal lung function. The take-home point is that each smoking session creates susceptibility to lung injury that harms lung mechanics as well as gas exchange. Ironically, supplemental oxygen, as typically prescribed, may augment the deleterious effects of smoking through added oxidative stress and inflammation. Carpagnano and colleagues demonstrated that even low-dose supplemental oxygen at 28% FiO_2 increased the exhaled breath levels of 8-isoprostane and interleukin-6, as measures of oxidative stress and inflammation, respectively, in healthy nonsmokers and, to a greater degree, in ex-smokers with COPD [14]. One might theorize that the combination of active smoking and oxygen use is more deleterious to lung function than smoking alone.

Electronic Cigarette Use While on Supplemental Oxygen

The proliferation of electronic (e-) cigarettes in recent years as an alternative to smoking or as an aid to quitting smoking presumes that there is a significant harm reduction compared to tobacco smoking. E-cigarettes avoid the generation of carboxyhemoglobin generated by tobacco smoking but cause acute oxidative stress, inflammation, and increased small airway resistance similar to cigarettes [15–17]. Studies on the long-term effects of e-cigarette use on lung function are small and vary greatly in design [16, 18]. Standard lung function testing does not reveal abnormalities, but more detailed lung function measures suggest a persistent increase in airway resistance. Accordingly, it is not known if e-cigarette smoking alone injures the lungs to a degree requiring supplemental oxygen.

Electronic cigarettes vaporize a solution of propylene glycol using a heating element that reaches temperatures of up to 350 °C and can ignite volatile material with oxygen as an accelerant [19]. Burn injuries from e-cigarettes during supplemental oxygen use are few and primarily reported in the lay media but are nonetheless as serious as burn injuries from cigarettes [11, 19]. Using e-cigarettes while on oxygen should be discouraged as strongly as with cigarettes.

Interstitial Lung Disease and Supplemental Oxygen

Individuals with COPD were the subjects used in the clinical trials that established the standards for prescribing supplemental oxygen. These standards apply to all other conditions causing hypoxemia, especially interstitial lung diseases (ILDs). Interstitial lung diseases include idiopathic pulmonary fibrosis, autoimmune-related ILD, chronic hypersensitivity pneumonitis, and other less common diffuse lung diseases that are progressive in many cases to the point that supplemental oxygen becomes part of the management regimen. Up to 40% of individuals with ILD will eventually require supplemental oxygen [20]. Oxygen therapy in ILD is especially challenging because the lung injury provoked by complex inflammatory mechanisms and interstitial remodeling, leading to pulmonary fibrosis, impairs gas exchange to a greater degree than in COPD. The main driver of hypoxemia in both COPD and ILD is damage to alveolar–capillary units, leading to ventilation–perfusion inequalities. Yet an additional diffusion limitation in ILD "blocks" the transfer of oxygen [21]. Higher levels of supplemental oxygen are often needed in advanced ILD compared to COPD, and hypoxemia can be quite profound, especially on exertion. Additionally, many cases of ILD progress despite treatment attempts, and changes in supplemental oxygen levels and oxygen delivery systems are more common than in COPD.

The American Thoracic Society clinical practice guidelines for home oxygen therapy strongly recommend providing oxygen at least 15 h a day for persons with ILD and resting hypoxemia and suggest prescribing oxygen to those with only exertional hypoxemia [22]. The evidence for these recommendations is of low quality, given the lack of randomized clinical trials demonstrating the benefit of supplemental oxygen for significant outcomes such as overall survival, improvement in functional status, and quality of life. A systematic review of retrospective non-randomized studies of persons with mild-to-severe ILD suggested that supplemental oxygen may improve exercise capacity [23]. The review found no improvement in dyspnea, quality of life, or survival domains. An open-label, prospective, randomized crossover trial of supplemental oxygen, focused on health-related quality of life, demonstrated significant improvement in breathlessness and activity levels when the subjects used supplemental oxygen [24]. Two-thirds of the study volunteers favored continuing supplemental oxygen at trial termination, while one-third found carrying and maintaining the oxygen equipment too difficult. A study on physicians' perspectives on prescribing supplemental oxygen in ILD demonstrated a lower threshold for prescribing oxygen than for other chronic lung conditions [25].

Air Travel and Supplemental Oxygen

The partial inspired pressure of oxygen (PiO_2) decreases as the altitude from sea level increases due to the dropping barometric pressure. Cabin pressure in commercial airlines at a cruising altitude of 30,000–40,000 feet simulates an altitude of no more than 8000 feet (2438 m), yielding a barometric pressure of 565 mmHg and a

PiO_2 of 108 mmHg [26]. Individuals with healthy lungs tolerate cabin altitude and pressure quite well at rest, with minimal changes in ventilation and pulmonary vascular blood distribution, and maintain blood oxygen tensions between 55 and 85 mmHg and a blood oxygen saturation >90% [27]. It is not until an altitude of 3000 m is breached that acute changes to hypoxemia induce compensatory hyperventilation and optimal pulmonary vascular changes to transport oxygen across the gas exchange surfaces of the lungs [28]. Persons with significant airway or interstitial abnormalities and impaired gas exchange at low altitudes may not be able to compensate for the hypoxemia, even at airliner cabin pressures. The inability to compensate is undoubtedly true for individuals requiring supplemental oxygen at low altitudes, but it also applies to those with less severe pulmonary disease, who develop significant hypoxemia only during flight. Pulmonary vascular and cardiac comorbidities amplify the deleterious effects of hypoxemia.

The hypoxic challenge test (HCT) is the gold standard for determining which individuals with lung disease qualify for supplemental oxygen during air travel [29]. Also known as the high-altitude simulation test (HAST) [30] or hypoxia inhalation test (HIT) [26], in this procedure patients breathe an oxygen/nitrogen mixture at 15.1% oxygen or sit in a hypobaric chamber at a pressure of 565 mmHg. These challenges take 15–20 min but may last longer if incremental oxygen titration is required to achieve a PaO_2 of ≥55 mmHg or an oxygen saturation >90%. The oxygen desaturation profiles found on hypoxic challenge correlate well with in-flight desaturations at cruising altitudes [26]. Nevertheless, most clinical pulmonary function laboratories do not perform HCT for logistical and cost reasons. Attempts using standard lung function tests to predict significant oxygen desaturation are not very accurate. Bradi and colleagues performed HCT in 24 individuals with COPD and three with cystic fibrosis and compared the results with several published predictive equations, which included ground-level PaO_2 and FEV1 measures [30]. The predictive equations had a poor agreement with HCT. Comparison of HCT with oxygen desaturation profiles on the 6-min walk testing also did not correlate well. Finally, some subjects who did not meet the guidelines for in-flight oxygen had significant oxygen desaturation on HCT. The specific guidelines and caveats for prescribing supplemental oxygen during air travel are discussed in Chap. 14.

Nocturnal Oxygen Therapy

Individuals considered for LTOT are typically tested for supplemental oxygen need while awake in a resting state and during exertion. Test results in the awake state do not predict hypoxemia that may occur with sleep. This is because ventilatory drive decreases, especially during rapid eye movement sleep [31]. Breathing becomes shallower and more rapid with around a 15% decrease in minute ventilation. While this change is well tolerated by healthy individuals, persons with chronic lung diseases may develop significant nocturnal oxygen desaturation. For example, around 40% of people with COPD who qualify for daytime oxygen will also have nocturnal hypoxemia, and notably, a similar proportion without daytime hypoxemia will experience nocturnal oxygen desaturations [32]. Nocturnal hypoxemia is associated with increased COPD exacerbations, development of pulmonary hypertension, and increased mortality [33].

A systematic review of studies exploring nocturnal hypoxemia in ILD reported that most showed an association of nocturnal hypoxemia with decreased survival [34]. A low diffusion capacity and pulmonary hypertension by echocardiography were also associated with nocturnal hypoxemia. It is unknown if ambulatory oxygen desaturation testing predicts nocturnal hypoxemia in ILD. Given the greater severity of hypoxemia in individuals with ILD compared to COPD, it is likely that hypoxemia with sleep is quite common in this group. Assessment and parameters for prescribing nocturnal oxygen are described in Chap. 14.

Summary

The benefits of LTOT, though established mainly in subjects with COPD, apply to all chronic lung conditions that cause pathological hypoxemia of varying severity. This chapter reviews the history and rationale for the parameters by which we regard the benefits of prescribing LTOT. Chapter 14 discusses how oxygen is prescribed and modified for secondary effects such as pulmonary hypertension and polycythemia.

References

1. Petty TL. Historical perspective on long-term oxygen therapy. In: O'Donohue Jr WJ, editor. Long-term oxygen therapy scientific basis and clinical application. New York: Marcel Dekker, Inc.; 1995. p. 1–23.
2. Levine BE, Bigelow DB, Hamstra RD, Beckwitt HJ, Mitchell RS, Nett LM, et al. The role of long-term continuous oxygen administration in patients with chronic airway obstruction with hypoxemia. Ann Intern Med. 1967;66(4):639–50.
3. Abraham AS, Cole RB, Bishop JM. Reversal of pulmonary hypertension by prolonged oxygen administration to patients with chronic bronchitis. Circ Res. 1968;23(1):147–57.
4. Report of the Medical Research Council Working Party. Long term domiciliary oxygen therapy in chronic hypoxic cor pulmonale complicating chronic bronchitis and emphysema. Lancet. 1981;1:681–5.
5. Nocturnal Oxygen Therapy Trial. Continuous or nocturnal oxygen therapy in hypoxemic chronic obstructive lung disease. Ann Intern Med. 1980;93:391–8.
6. Long-Term Oxygen Treatment Trial Research Group, Albert RK, Au DH, Blackford AL, Casaburi R, Cooper JA, et al. A randomized trial of long-term oxygen for COPD with moderate desaturation. N Engl J Med. 2016;375(17):1617–27.
7. Lacasse Y, Casaburi R, Sliwinski P, Chaouat A, Fletcher E, Haidl P, et al. Home oxygen for moderate hypoxaemia in chronic obstructive pulmonary disease: a systematic review and meta-analysis. Lancet Respir Med. 2022;10(11):1029–37.
8. Jacobs SS, Krishnan JA, Lederer DJ, Ghazipura M, Hossain T, Tan A-YM, et al. Home oxygen therapy for adults with chronic lung disease. An official American Thoracic Society clinical practice guideline. Am J Respir Crit Care Med. 2020;202(10):e121–41.
9. Edelman DA, Maleyko-Jacobs S, White MT, Lucas CE, Ledgerwood AM. Smoking and home oxygen therapy—a preventable public health hazard. J Burn Care Res. 2008;29(1):119–22.

10. Nagai H, Nakazawa E, Akabayashi A. The creation of the Belmont report and its effect on ethical principles: a historical study. Monash Bioeth Rev. 2022;40(2):157–70.
11. Lacasse Y, Légaré M, Maltais F. E-cigarette use in patients receiving home oxygen therapy. Can Respir J. 2015;22(2):83–5.
12. Hall W. The 1964 US surgeon general's report on smoking and health. Addiction. 2022;117(12):3170–5.
13. Motley HL, Kuzman WJ, Cigarette smoke. Its effect on pulmonary function measurements. Calif Med. 1958;88(3):211–20.
14. Carpagnano GE, Kharitonov SA, Foschino-Barbaro MP, Resta O, Gramiccioni E, Barnes PJ. Supplementary oxygen in healthy subjects and those with COPD increases oxidative stress and airway inflammation. Thorax. 2004;59(12):1016–9.
15. Vardavas CI, Anagnostopoulos N, Kougias M, Evangelopoulou V, Connolly GN, Behrakis PK. Short-term pulmonary effects of using an electronic cigarette. Impact on respiratory flow resistance, impedance, and exhaled nitric oxide. Chest. 2012;141(6):1400–6.
16. Honeycutt L, Huerne K, Miller A, Wennberg E, Filion KB, Grad R, et al. A systematic review of the effects of e-cigarette use on lung function. NPJ Prim Care Respir Med. 2022;32(1):45.
17. Song Y, Li X, Li C, Xu S, Liu Y, Wu X. What are the effects of electronic cigarettes on lung function compared to non-electronic cigarettes? A systematic analysis. Int J Public Health. 2022;67:1604989.
18. Joshi D, Duong M, Kirkland S, Raina P. Impact of electronic cigarette ever use on lung function in adults aged 45–85: a cross-sectional analysis from the Canadian longitudinal study on aging. BMJ Open. 2021;11(10):e051519.
19. Montoya A, Ozhathil D, Hollowed K, Kahn SA. Burn injury from smoking electronic cigarettes while on supplemental oxygen. J Burn Care Res. 2023;44(2):249–53.
20. Clark KP, Degenholtz HB, Lindell KO, Kass DJ. Supplemental oxygen therapy in interstitial lung disease: a narrative review. Ann Am Thorac Soc. 2023;20(11):1541–9.
21. Yamaguchi K, Mori M, Kawai A, Takasugi T, Oyamada Y, Koda E. Inhomogeneities of ventilation and the diffusing capacity to perfusion in various chronic lung diseases. Am J Respir Crit Care Med. 1997;156(1):86–93.
22. Khor YH, Dudley KA, Herman D, Jacobs SS, Lederer DJ, Krishnan JA, et al. Summary for clinicians: clinical practice guideline on home oxygen therapy for adults with chronic lung disease. Ann Am Thorac Soc. 2021;18(9):1444–9.
23. Bell EC, Cox NS, Goh N, Glaspole I, Westall GP, Watson A, et al. Oxygen therapy for interstitial lung disease: a systematic review. Eur Respir Rev. 2017;26(143):160080. https://doi.org/10.1183/16000617.0080-2016.
24. Visca D, Mori L, Tsipouri V, Fleming S, Firouzi A, Bonini M, et al. Effect of ambulatory oxygen on quality of life for patients with fibrotic lung disease (AmbOx): a prospective, open-label, mixed-method, crossover randomised controlled trial. Lancet Respir Med. 2018;6(10):759–70.
25. Khor YH, Goh NSL, McDonald CF, Holland AE. Oxygen therapy for interstitial lung disease: physicians' perceptions and experiences. Ann Am Thorac Soc. 2017;14(12):1772–8.
26. Kelly PT, Swanney MP, Seccombe LM, Frampton C, Peters MJ, Beckert L. Air travel hypoxemia vs. the hypoxia inhalation test in passengers with COPD. Chest. 2008;133(4):920–6.
27. Lyznicki JM, Williams MA, Deitchman SD, Howe JP, Council on Scientific Affairs, American Medical Association. Medical oxygen and air travel. Aviat Space Environ Med. 2000;71(8):827–31.
28. Mason NP. The physiology of high altitude: an introduction to the cardio-respiratory changes occurring on ascent to altitude. Curr Anaesth Crit Care. 2000;11(1):34–41.
29. Coker RK, Armstrong A, Church AC, Holmes S, Naylor J, Pike K, et al. BTS clinical statement on air travel for passengers with respiratory disease. Thorax. 2022;77(4):329–50.
30. Bradi AC, Faughnan ME, Stanbrook MB, Deschenes-Leek E, Chapman KR. Predicting the need for supplemental oxygen during airline flight in patients with chronic pulmonary disease: a comparison of predictive equations and altitude simulation. Can Respir J. 2009;16(4):119–24.
31. Douglas NJ, White DP, Pickett CK, Weil JV, Zwillich CW. Respiration during sleep in normal man. Thorax. 1982;37(11):840–4.

32. Yoshizaki A, Nagano T, Izumi S, Funada Y, Nakata K, Nishiuma T, et al. Prospective study of nocturnal desaturation in patients receiving home oxygen therapy. Intern Med. 2021;60(19):3071–9.
33. Agusti A, Hedner J, Marin JM, Barbé F, Cazzola M, Rennard S. Night-time symptoms: a forgotten dimension of COPD. Eur Respir Rev. 2011;20(121):183–94.
34. Khor YH, Ng Y, Sweeney D, Ryerson CJ. Nocturnal hypoxaemia in interstitial lung disease: a systematic review. Thorax. 2021;76(12):1200–8.

How to Prescribe Long-Term Oxygen Therapy

14

Katherine Stull and Rafael Perez

Introduction

Long-term oxygen therapy (LTOT) is used for a variety of chronic conditions in which hypoxia contributes to morbidity and mortality. It is prescribed to approximately 1.5 million people in the United States at an annual cost of about 4 billion dollars [1]. The term "LTOT" is often interchanged with "home oxygen therapy," a more general term that includes oxygen use for acute conditions, palliation, or other reasons outside the healthcare setting that are not long-standing. The studies described in Chap. 13 demonstrated the benefits of LTOT and established guidelines for prescribing LTOT in appropriately selected individuals. The guidelines rely heavily on initial studies conducted in subjects with chronic obstructive pulmonary disease (COPD) and later in subjects with interstitial lung disease (ILD) [2].

Nevertheless, the guidelines also apply to individuals with other conditions, accompanied by hypoxia to the level and duration that impedes daily function and decreases survival. These additional conditions include cor pulmonale, heart failure, obesity hypoventilation syndrome, and bronchiectasis. Supplemental oxygen improves blood oxygenation, with anticipated physiological benefits. However, there is a cost associated with obtaining, using, and maintaining oxygen delivery systems in the outpatient setting, typically inside the home and during ambulation outside the home. Both the provider and patient must understand the complexities around the prescription and use of LTOT.

This chapter details how the initial assessment for LTOT is performed and how changes in oxygen needs over time are reassessed. The selection of an appropriate

K. Stull · R. Perez (✉)
The Korman Respiratory Institute and the Division of Pulmonary, Allergy and Critical Care, The Department of Medicine at the Sidney Kimmel Medical College of Thomas Jefferson University, Philadelphia, PA, USA
e-mail: rafael.perez@jefferson.edu

G. C. Kane et al. (eds.), *Oxygen*, https://doi.org/10.1007/978-3-032-18934-9_14

oxygen delivery system based on oxygen requirements, disease severity, and functional status is discussed. The "setup" and delivery of stationary and ambulatory oxygen are reviewed. There are logistical and safety issues to consider when using oxygen inside and outside the home. Specific insurance coverage requirements that the prescribing provider must follow to receive reimbursement are addressed.

Assessment for LTOT

It is essential to note from the outset that the prescription of supplemental oxygen constitutes a significant lifestyle change for the individual who qualifies "by the numbers." An in-depth discussion between the clinician and patient about the pros and cons of using LTOT is a must. Optimal medical treatment of the underlying condition causing hypoxemia should be achieved and maintained. The individual's respiratory environment plays a crucial role in mitigating or eliminating airborne pollutants, particularly tobacco smoke. People respond to a given level of hypoxemia differently and may or may not have accompanying comorbidities, such as heart failure, chronic renal disease, or cognitive impairments. Effects of hypoxemia, such as pulmonary hypertension and polycythemia, may or may not be present. Assessment for qualification for LTOT thus proceeds after thorough history taking, physical examination, and studies that explore the effects of hypoxemia. The provider and informed patient can then use shared decision-making to determine whether supplemental oxygen is appropriate for the individual's quality of life and lifestyle.

The evaluation for LTOT centers on measuring blood oxygen status at rest and during ambulation on a flat indoor surface. Oxygen status is typically measured as percent saturation via pulse oximetry ($SpO_2\%$), which is more practical and comfortable than obtaining serial arterial blood gas (ABG). An $SpO_2\%$ of 88 corresponds to an ABG of 55 mm/Hg, the threshold below which persistent hypoxemia causes bodily harm, as discussed in Chap. 13. The evaluation for LTOT begins with oximetry performed at rest. The individual is placed on continuous supplemental oxygen delivered from a portable oxygen cylinder if the $SpO_2\%$ is ≤ 88. We prefer to adjust the oxygen flow to achieve a saturation of at least 92% because the accuracy of clinical pulse oximeters is within ±2%. Additionally, skin color, poor circulation, and nail polish can also affect pulse oximeter readings [3, 4]. The patient then undergoes ambulation with continuous pulse oximetry. Supplemental oxygen is added or increased if the oxygen saturation drops to 88 or less. There are no time or distance constraints on performing "ambulatory oximetry," but ambulation for 5–6 min is typical. The evaluation is thus dependent on the subjects' mobility and the severity of hypoxemia.

The standard LTOT evaluation involves the patient walking on a flat, uncarpeted surface in an indoor, climate-controlled clinical environment that differs from their home conditions. Fussell and colleagues compared the standard LTOT evaluation with continuous home oximetry in 20 subjects with stable COPD [5]. They found a low correlation between resting and exercise oximetry in the clinic and mean ambulatory SpO_2% under living conditions. There was no correlation between resting and exercise oximetry and time spent with an SpO_2% of ≤88. Other groups have also noted a discordance between the LTOT evaluation in the clinic and continuous oximetry monitoring under real-life conditions, notably uncovering patients who have a negative LTOT evaluation but experience significant oxygen desaturation during certain daily activities and sleep [6, 7]. The studies employ a mix of observational, retrospective, and prospective approaches, demonstrating that oxygen saturations are maintained within the normal range, accompanied by lower average oxygen flows, when evaluated using continuous oxygen monitoring. However, despite the discrepancies in oximetry measures between the standard LTOT evaluation and continuous ambulatory oximetry, there appears to be no difference in health outcomes, such as survival.

The LTOT evaluation does not account for oxygen desaturation during sleep. Lacasse and colleagues studied 128 individuals with COPD who had mild-to-moderate daytime hypoxemia and were not on supplemental oxygen [8]. Thirty-eight percent of the subjects, including 16% who also had sleep apnea, had significant nocturnal oxygen desaturation. Their group later led the double-blind, randomized, placebo-controlled international nocturnal oxygen (INOX) trial in 243 subjects with COPD and nocturnal oxygen desaturation [9]. Recruitment issues left the study underpowered; however, no differences in mortality or need for supplemental oxygen over 3 years were noted between those who received oxygen during sleep and those who received placebo air. Whether oxygen therapy is beneficial for individuals with significant nocturnal oxygen desaturation remains unresolved. Again, it is notable that studies on nocturnal hypoxemia were predominantly performed in individuals with COPD. There is one systematic review that suggests a survival benefit in patients with ILD and nocturnal oxygen desaturation [10].

The oxygen prescription for individuals who have qualifying oxygen desaturation at rest or with exertion may include a recommended oxygen flow rate to use during sleep. However, for patients with advanced lung diseases, like COPD with carbon dioxide (CO_2) retention or ILD with profound hypoxemia, a nocturnal oximetry study helps select the appropriate oxygen flow during sleep.

Oxygen Prescription

The Centers for Medicare & Medicaid Services (CMS) have specific criteria for the evaluation and prescription of supplemental oxygen [11, 12]. The oxygen evaluation for a hospitalized patient must be done within 48 h of discharge to home or a lower level of care. The CMS requirement for outpatients is that the underlying illness causing hypoxemia is treated optimally and is stable. There must be evidence of a face-to-face visit with the prescribing provider within 30 days of the initial oxygen prescription, which documents the following: the primary or secondary qualifying conditions, the alternative treatments that have been tried to improve oxygenation, the results of an arterial blood gas (ABG) or oximetry, whether the patient is mobile in the home environment. The qualifying conditions are noted on the Oxygen Authorization Request Form, CMS-484 (Fig. 14.1), which must accompany every oxygen prescription. This form, along with the face-to-face documentation affirming optimal treatment and patient stability, is submitted to the oxygen vendor (otherwise known as a durable medical equipment (DME) company) for

CMS-484— OXYGEN

SECTION A: Certification Type/Date: INITIAL ___/___/___ REVISED ___/___/___ RECERTIFICATION___/___/___

PATIENT NAME, ADDRESS, TELEPHONE and MEDICARE ID (___) ___-____ Medicare ID	SUPPLIER NAME, ADDRESS, TELEPHONE and NSC or NPI # (___) ___-____ NSC or NPI #______
PLACE OF SERVICE ______ | Supply Item/Service Procedure Code(s):	PT DOB ___/___/___ Sex ___ (M/F) Ht. ___(in) Wt ___
NAME and ADDRESS of FACILITY if applicable (see reverse)	PHYSICIAN NAME, ADDRESS, TELEPHONE and UPIN or NIP # (___) ___-____ UPIN or NPI #______

SECTION B: Information in this Section May Not Be Completed by the Supplier of the Item Supplies.

EST. LENGTH OF NEED (# OF MONTHS): ______ 1-99 (99=LIFETIME) | DIAGNOSIS CODES: ______

ANSWERS	ANSWER QUESTIONS 1-9. (Check Y for Yes, N for No, or D for Does Not Apply, unless otherwise noted.)
a)______mm Hg b)______% c)___/___/___	1. Enter the result of recent test taken on or before the certification date listed in Section A. Enter (a) arterial blood gas PO2 and/or (b) oxygen saturation test; (c) date of test.
❑1 ❑2 ❑3	2. Was the test in Question 1 performed (1) with the patient in a chronic stable state as an outpatient, (2) within two days prior to discharge from an inpatient facility to home, or (3) under other circumstances?
❑1 ❑2 ❑3	3. Check the one number for the condition of the test in Question 1: (1) At Rest; (2) During Exercise; (3) During Sleep
❑Y ❑N ❑D	4. If you are ordering portable oxygen, is the patient mobile within the home? If you are not ordering portable oxygen, check D.
______LPM	5. Enter the highest oxygen flow rate ordered for this patient in liters per minute. If less than 1 LPM, enter an "X".
a)______mm Hg b)______% c)___/___/___	6. If greater than 4 LPM is prescribed, enter results of recent test taken on 4 LPM. This may be an (a) arterial blood gas PO2 and/or (b) oxygen saturation test with patient in a chronic stable state. Enter date of test (c).
	ANSWER QUESTIONS 7-9 ONLY IF PO2 = 56-59 OR OXYGEN SATURATION = 89 IN QUESTION 1
❑Y ❑N	7. Does the patient have dependent edema due to congestive heart failure?
❑Y ❑N	8. Does the patient have cor pulmonale or pulmonary hypertension documented by P pulmonale on an EKG or by an echocardiogram, gated blood pool scan or direct pulmonary artery pressure measurement.
❑Y ❑N	9. Does the patient have a hematocrit greater than 56%?

NAME OF PERSON ANSWERING SECTION B QUESTIONS, IF OTHER THAN PHYSICIAN (Please Print):
NAME______ TITLE______ EMPLOYER______

SECTION C: Narrative Description of Equipment and Cost

(1) Narrative description of all items, accessories and option ordered; (2) Suppliers charge; and (3) Medicare Fee Schedule Allowance for each item, accessory, and option (see instructions on back)

SECTION D: PHYSICIAN Attestation and Signature/Date

I certify that I am the treating physician identified in Section A of this form. I have received Sections A, B and C of the Certificate of Medical Necessity (including charges for items ordered). Any statement on my letterhead attached hereto, has been reviewed and signed by me. I certify that the medical necessity information in Section B is true, accurate and complete, to the best of my knowledge, and I understand that any falsification, omission, or concealment of material fact in that section may subject me to civil or criminal liability.

PHYSICIAN'S SIGNATURE______ DATE ___/___/___
Signature and Date Stamps Are Not Acceptable.
Form CMS-484 (12/18)

Fig. 14.1 The CMS 484 form. This form is available in the public domain. It is required in order for DME companies to supply home oxygen

delivery and setup of LTOT. Notably, patients who received LTOT while hospitalized should be reassessed for continued LTOT within 3 months of discharge.

Individuals evaluated for supplemental oxygen are categorized into one of three CMS coverage groups (Table 14.1). Group I consists of individuals who are prescribed supplemental oxygen based on qualifying arterial blood gas (ABG) or oximetry results. An example is a person with stable COPD or ILD who is functional outside the home setting. Those in the group I category must have a reassessment for continued coverage of supplemental oxygen at 12 months. Group II comprises individuals who do not meet the ABG or $SpO_2\%$ criteria for group I but have a secondary qualifying diagnosis and marginal oxygenation, as outlined in the table. A person with heart failure and a room air $SpO_2\%$ of 89 who is predisposed to dependent edema is an example of this group. Individuals in group II must be reassessed at 3 months following the initial oxygen evaluation to determine if supplemental oxygen is still necessary. Group III describes individuals who do not meet the qualification criteria of the previous groups and is primarily reserved for coverage analysis in clinical trials that include supplemental oxygen in the protocol. It also applies to individuals with cluster headaches, for which intermittent high-flow oxygen has been shown to mitigate the intensity of headache episodes [13].

People who do not qualify for supplemental oxygen at rest or during exertion in the awake state may have qualifying oxygen desaturations during sleep. An individual with a resting $SpO_2\%$ of 89 and a secondary qualifying diagnosis or one who experiences 5 min of oxygen desaturation to ≤88% for a total of 5 cumulative minutes during a minimum of 2 h of recording qualifies for oxygen therapy during sleep by the CMS criteria [12]. This setup only includes a stationary concentrator, not a portable oxygen tank or concentrator. Oxygen may be necessary for patients with sleep apnea, even after successful treatment with a positive airway pressure (PAP) device. Supplemental oxygen is prescribed if qualifying desaturations are noted

Table 14.1 CMS coverage groups for prescribing home oxygen

Group I
$PaO_2 \leq 55$ mmHg or $SpO_2\% \leq 88$ on RA
Reassess at 12 months
Group II
PaO_2 56–59 mmHg or $SpO_2\%$ 89%, with any of the following:
Clinical evidence of cor pulmonale
Electrocardiogram (ECG) evidence of cor pulmonale with P wave >3 mm in lead II, III, or AVF
Dependent edema = CHF
Erythrocythemia with hematocrit >56%
Reassess at 3 months
Group III (N/A):
$PaO_2 \geq 60$ mmHg or $SpO_2\% \geq 90$, with:
Clinical trials using supplemental oxygen
Cluster headaches (must have 5 HA, 15–180 min long)

when there are ten or fewer apneas on treatment. Importantly, oxygen and oxygen equipment used in conjunction with PAP are reimbursed only if the patient qualifies for oxygen through an LTOT evaluation. This setup requires an adapter to allow the oxygen to flow through the constant positive airway pressure (CPAP) mask.

Setting Up Oxygen at Home

Durable medical equipment companies and their subcontractors must meet the CMS accreditation requirements to provide and bill for home oxygen services [14]. Home oxygen is delivered as soon as possible, within 24 h, by a trained technician or respiratory therapist. The equipment setup is done with a focus on education and safety. A typical setup consists of a stationary device, most often an oxygen concentrator. There is also portable equipment, typically small oxygen cylinders or a portable oxygen concentrator (POC). There is a stationary concentrator called a home fill system that allows patients to refill portable tanks rather than depending on delivery. Oxygen concentrators are electrically powered, so larger oxygen cylinders are provided as a backup in case of a power outage. Oxygen from the stationary source is typically delivered through a nasal cannula no longer than 47 feet, limited by the operational capabilities of the standard oxygen concentrator. Resistance to gas flow increases directly with the length of the tube; therefore, patients should be discouraged from connecting extra tubing, which would result in lower oxygen flows than prescribed. The nasal cannula for portable use is limited to 7 feet in length to reduce tripping hazards. Safety centers on the appropriate placement and management of the equipment. People who use oxygen equipment must identify and avoid fire hazards. Oxygen tanks should be secured in the upright position and away from foot traffic. The home should be equipped with functional smoke alarms and fire extinguishers. Signs may be placed on outer doors and windows advising that supplemental oxygen is in use inside the home.

The oxygen vendor typically leaves the patient with information on the use of the equipment and safety precautions. Special attention is paid to smoking inside the home by the patient or others. The burns resulting from smoking while using oxygen are severe and may be deadly [15]. Smokers who use oxygen are warned not to smoke while using supplemental oxygen. Added safety for the person using oxygen may be obtained by connecting a firebreak device in the cannula tube just before it divides into the nasal prongs and another device near the oxygen source [16]. The firebreak device is a thermal fuse that immediately stops oxygen flow through the cannula when combustion is detected. The individual performing the home oxygen setup documents the details of the visit and obtains the patient's signature, attesting to their understanding of using oxygen at home.

Maintenance and performance checks on the oxygen equipment are done by the vendor at intervals recommended by the equipment manufacturer. Home visits for this purpose are conducted every 6–12 months. The vendor should provide a phone number to address any technical problems with the oxygen equipment. Vendor communication with the prescribing provider is crucial if the visiting therapist notes any changes in the client's condition that may necessitate adjustments to the oxygen flow or equipment.

Air Travel with Supplemental Oxygen

The physiology and assessment for using oxygen at airliner cabin altitudes were discussed in Chap. 13. Policies and procedures for delivering oxygen during flight are a collaborative effort between the Federal Aviation Administration (FAA) and the airline industry [17]. Each airline has specific policies to accommodate individuals who require oxygen during their trip. Travelers must provide the airline with advanced notification, preferably several days in advance of travel. Some airlines require medical certification that attests to the need for oxygen and confirms the user's fitness to fly.

Portable oxygen concentrators approved by the FAA are the preferred devices for providing supplemental oxygen during flight and for use after debarkation. Like other durable medical equipment, POCs do not count against carry-on limits. Battery power should be available to last at least one and a half times the flight duration.

Home Oxygen Equipment

The most common home oxygen setup centers on the stationary oxygen concentrator. Oxygen concentrators separate oxygen from the air through a molecular sieve bed using a process called "pressure swing adsorption" [18]. Ambient air is filtered and sieved through a bed of crystalline mineral composed of aluminum silicate, also known as zeolite. The air is forced through the zeolite under pressure via a feed valve (FV), a condition necessary to adsorb nitrogen and water vapor while allowing oxygen to pass through (Fig. 14.2). Pressure is removed when the zeolite bed is fully saturated with nitrogen and water. The release of pressure and a small amount of oxygen diverted back through the sieve expels the nitrogen and some of the water through an exhaust valve (EV). Meanwhile, the system "swings" over to a fresh zeolite bed to continue the air separation process. The system alternates between zeolite beds to continuously generate oxygen and flush out nitrogen.

Oxygen concentrators produce oxygen of around 93% purity because of thermodynamic limitations and the presence of other gases in the air, including noble gases, mainly argon and carbon dioxide, that pass through the zeolite bed. The standard stationary concentrator produces continuous oxygen flow rates up to 5 liters per minute (LPM). Home concentrators with larger molecular sieve beds can generate flows up to 10 LPM.

The stationary concentrator is complemented by portable oxygen, which is most often provided by small gas cylinders carried over the shoulder. The lightest cylinders are made of aluminum and are filled with oxygen to a maximum pressure of 2300 pounds per square inch (psi). The amount of oxygen at this pressure depends

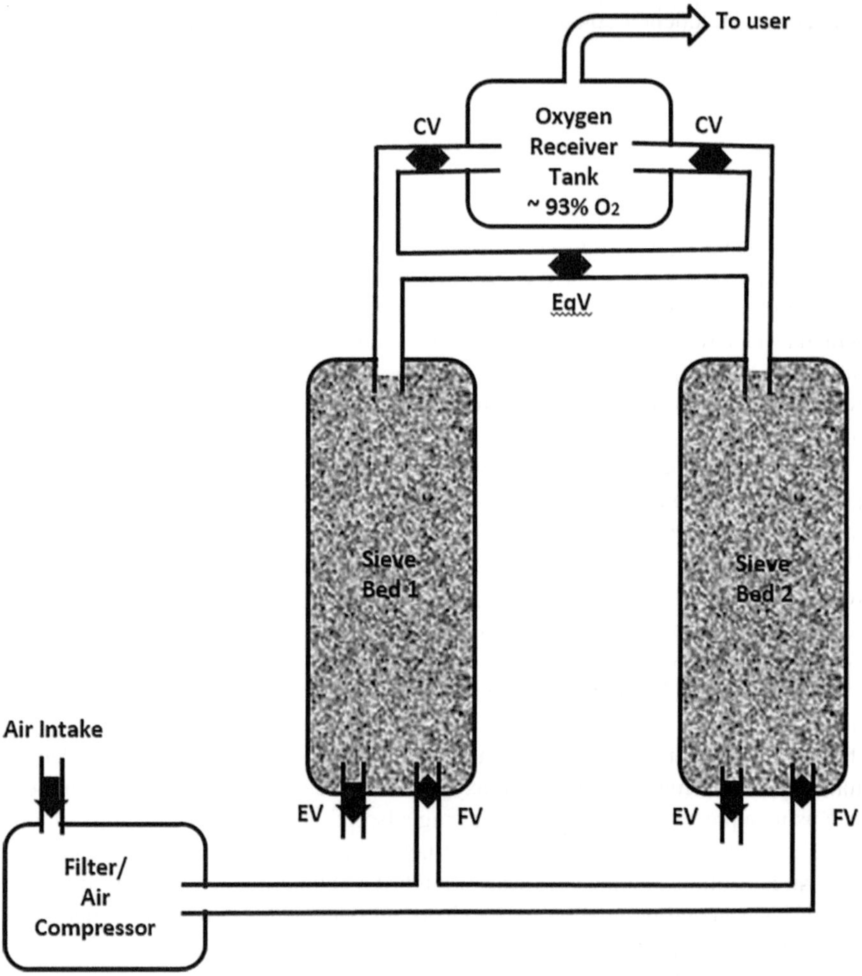

Fig. 14.2 Schematic view of the oxygen concentrator. Filtered air is compressed through the feed valve (FV) into sieve bed 1 (FV to sieve bed 2 is closed). Nitrogen and water are adsorbed in sieve bed 1 under pressure, while oxygen freely passes through the check valve (CV) into the oxygen receiver tank. Some oxygen under pressure is diverted through the equalization valve (EqV) as sieve bed 1 becomes fully saturated with nitrogen, allowing the pressurization of sieve bed 2 to begin. The FV to sieve bed 1 closes, and the bed is depressurized to expel nitrogen and water through the exhaust valve (EV). Almost immediately, the FV to sieve bed 2 opens, initiating the adsorption of nitrogen and water while allowing oxygen to pass into the receiver tank. Regulated oxygen from the receiver tank is connected to the user via a cannula. The process of cycling between sieve beds is termed "pressure swing adsorption"

on the size of the cylinder. For example, a "D tank" holds 360 L of oxygen at maximum psi and weighs 10 pounds. This tank, at a flow rate of 2 LPM, empties in just under 3 h. The "E tank," standard in hospital wards, holds 625 L of oxygen when full and lasts for 5 h at a flow rate of 2 LPM. It weighs 15 pounds, so it is not designed to be carried but may be pulled along on a wheeled carrier.

Portable oxygen cylinders are often too heavy to carry, especially for the most severely debilitated individuals. Smaller tanks may be used to decrease weight, but they empty sooner. This situation means that time and distance away from home are compromised, especially if the person is on continuous-flow oxygen therapy. They are inconvenienced by the need for more tanks between vendor visits and having to take extra tanks with them on longer trips. Oxygen from portable tanks is typically delivered using a continuous-flow regulator. The duration of oxygen delivery is extended by using a regulator that provides a "pulse" of oxygen only with inhalation. The pulse-dose regulator thus extends tank life severalfold depending on the user's activity level and respiratory rate. Pulse-dose regulators are made by various manufacturers, each with its own operating characteristics [19]. Settings on the regulators indicate the amount and flow pattern of oxygen delivered. It is essential to note that the numerical settings on pulse regulators do not directly correspond to the continuous oxygen flow delivered. Continuous oxygen flow partly washes out the anatomical dead space around end-expiration, making more oxygen available with the next inspiration. Pulsed oxygen delivery does not have this effect and may not be an adequate treatment for hypoxemia. Patients considered for pulsed oxygen delivery should undergo ambulatory oximetry using their specific pulsed device to determine if pulse oxygen delivery is appropriate and establish the optimal settings for use at rest and during ambulation.

Another approach to increasing the convenience of oxygen tank portability is the HomeFill system [18]. This system incorporates a compressor and connection for filling portable tanks directly from a stationary oxygen concentrator. The concentrator may be used while the portable oxygen tank is being filled. The HomeFill system accommodates users' levels of activity and reduces the number of tanks kept at home.

Portable oxygen concentrators are smaller versions of the stationary concentrators [18]. The zeolite beds in POCs are smaller, so concentrators that are light enough to carry do not deliver a continuous oxygen flow. Oxygen is instead delivered in a pulse-dose manner. Like pulse-dose regulators, the volume and pattern of each oxygen pulse delivered are controlled by the settings designed by the POC manufacturer. The POC operates on rechargeable batteries and can be directly connected to a standard electrical outlet. There are larger versions of POCs that can deliver continuous oxygen flow, but they are too heavy to carry and are designed to be pulled along by the user. These larger POCs provide continuous oxygen flows up to 3 LPM.

Individuals who require four or more liters per minute (LPM) to maintain acceptable oxygen levels may be set up with a liquid oxygen system [20]. One liter of liquid oxygen contains the equivalent of 860 L of oxygen at atmospheric temperature and pressure, so it lasts longer than compressed oxygen gas cylinders. Liquid oxygen is 100% pure, in contrast to oxygen generated by concentrators. Liquid oxygen at −183 °C is delivered in insulated reservoirs. The oxygen evaporates through a vaporizer coil located outside the reservoir's insulated interior and then travels to the cannula and ultimately to the user, eliminating the need for electricity to operate. The reservoir also has a connection for portable liquid oxygen containers. Like stationary reservoirs, portable liquid oxygen devices do not require electricity to function and are thus spared the added weight of batteries.

Delivery of liquid oxygen is contracted by durable medical equipment vendors, which provide the equipment and expertise to set up home oxygen systems, working with companies that mass-produce liquid oxygen. The transport, setup, and maintenance of liquid oxygen at home are more involved than with a concentrator-based setup. Liquid oxygen evaporates even when not in use and needs to be replenished frequently. The logistics of providing liquid oxygen are costly. As of this writing, the structure of the competitive bidding process mandated by CMS for providing LTOT, combined with thin profit margins, makes it challenging to supply liquid oxygen, and fewer vendors can offer it. It is not currently available to any of the patients within our health system, for example. Improved access to supplemental oxygen, which may facilitate the acquisition of liquid oxygen, is anticipated through the Supplemental Oxygen Access Reform (SOAR) Act, currently under review by Congress [21].

Cannula Designs for Oxygen Delivery to the Airways

The most common approach to administering oxygen in the home setting is via the ubiquitous nasal cannula [22]. The distal end of the standard nasal cannula forms a loop that starts in front of the neck, is taken behind the ears, and ends with soft, flat, curved, or flared nasal prongs inserted into the nares. Oral access is unimpeded, allowing the cannula to be worn continuously. Oxygen cannulas are crush- and kink-resistant, as well as durable. A standard nasal cannula delivers at most 6 L of oxygen per minute. Of note, oxygen delivered by concentrators or liquid systems is completely dry. Dry oxygen is not a problem at flow rates of around 2 LPM since the ambient air humidity usually provides sufficient moisture. Nasal irritation and bleeding may be observed at flow rates of around 4 L/min or more. This problem is mitigated by conducting the oxygen through a water-containing bottle attached to the oxygen source, colloquially referred to as humidification.

Some persons with advanced lung disease require oxygen of 5 LPM or more, exceeding the capabilities of the standard nasal cannula. Higher oxygen flows can be achieved by using cannulas with larger inner diameters, which decrease tube resistance and allow for flow rates of up to 15 LPM. Long-term use of oxygen at a flow rate of 4 L/min or more can be irritating to the nares and upper airways; therefore, these larger-diameter cannulas are more often used in the acute care setting with ample humidification.

Another option for individuals requiring higher oxygen flows is to use cannulas fitted with a reservoir that fills with oxygen during exhalation [19]. The user is then able to entrain oxygen from the reservoir, in addition to receiving the set flow from the nasal prongs. The reservoir may be a round "pendant" located on the cannula just as it begins the loop that terminates at the nares. The reservoir may be shaped as a cylindrical "mustache" located directly under the nose. The reservoirs fill with up to 30 mL of oxygen between inhalations. This approach increases the effectiveness of oxygen delivery by 1.5- to 4-fold, depending on the prescribed flow rate and patient activity. Reservoir cannulas cannot be used with a pulsed regulator, as there is no oxygen flow during exhalation to fill the reservoir. Additionally, these cannulas cannot be used with added humidity, as water would "rain out" in the reservoir, reducing its effectiveness.

A more complex cannula connection to the airways is via the transtracheal catheter (TTC) [19]. The TTC is considered for individuals who require continuous and rapid oxygen flows and experience oxygen desaturation upon movement. Our typical candidate is one with advanced diffuse interstitial lung disease, with a significant component of pulmonary fibrosis. An invasive procedure is needed to place and maintain a TTC, so informed decision-making with the patient is paramount. Placement in the office setting involves endoscopic-guided insertion under local and topical anesthesia, with a week of healing before the patient can use the TTC and several weeks for the catheter tract to mature. The catheter can also be introduced surgically, allowing for immediate use and faster tract maturation. In both techniques, the TTC is placed through the second and third tracheal rings below the cricoid cartilage, with the tip residing in the trachea just above the carina. Here, anatomical dead space is bypassed, and an entrainment effect occurs as oxygen collects in the trachea near the end of expiration. Oxygen flows via the TTC may be decreased by 50% or more compared to nasal delivery.

There are several pros and cons to using a TTC. On the positive side, the duration of the oxygen source is increased. Nasal or skin irritation of the face or ears is avoided. The TTC may be hidden under clothing, enhancing a person's image. Importantly, the procedure is reversible if one cannot tolerate the TTC, and it does not change consideration for lung transplantation. On the negative side, the TTC procedure is costly, and there are infrequent but potential surgical risks, like infection and bleeding. The TTC builds up mucus that requires the user to remove it to clear the channel once or twice a day. The TTC may be dislodged by coughing, requiring removal and replacement.

Advanced Home Oxygen Technologies

High-flow nasal cannula (HFNC) oxygen therapy delivers a blend of oxygen and air with heat and humidity at flow rates of up to 60 L/min [23]. The high flows wash out anatomical dead space and generate a small amount of positive airway pressure that lowers the work of breathing. The heated humidity improves mucociliary function and mucus clearance. Initially designed for use in hospital care for patients with acute respiratory distress, HFNC technology is being investigated for outpatient applications. A crossover study of 30 men with COPD already on LTOT at 2–4 L/min found improvements in respiratory physiology after being placed on HFNC [24]. Application of HFNC for 20 min significantly decreased the respiratory rate, increased tidal volume and end-expiratory lung volume, and accordingly reduced transcutaneous CO_2 levels. A 90-day study of HFNC use in 28 individuals with advanced COPD showed no difference in dyspnea or other upper airway symptoms between standard LTOT and HFNC, used on average for around 7 h daily [25]. However, there was less coughing and wheezing when using HFNC. Sputum became less viscous and eventually decreased in volume. A 12-week crossover study in 29 individuals with hypercapnic COPD compared LTOT alone to LTOT accompanied by nocturnal HFNC, demonstrating significant improvements in symptoms, activity, and quality of life [26].

The long-term benefits of HFNC therapy were explored in a 12-month trial in subjects with COPD and chronic respiratory failure, with several acute exacerbations per year [27]. Subjects were randomized into 100 controls using LTOT alone and 100 test subjects who used HFNC for 6–7 h a day, along with LTOT. Individuals using HFNC experienced less dyspnea, which was significantly better than that of controls, as early as 1 month into the trial. The quality of life remained stable in the test subjects but deteriorated considerably in the controls. Arterial CO_2 tension decreased over the trial period using HFNC, whereas it increased in patients using LTOT alone. There were no significant differences in lung function tests, but the 6-minute walk test improved in those assigned to HFNC and deteriorated in the control subjects. There were no differences in all-cause mortality. Notably, there was a significant reduction in acute exacerbations of COPD (AECOPD) in the HFNC group. The investigators later performed a cost analysis that included the costs of using HFNC at home, as well as information on hospital admission frequency and duration [28]. Their findings indicated cost savings in using HFNC therapy in individuals with COPD and chronic respiratory failure, who have frequent AECOPD.

The use of HFNC oxygen therapy in the home setting has been studied almost exclusively in people with advanced COPD who are already on LTOT. This therapy is well-suited for patients with airway and gas exchange abnormalities, who benefit from improved airway clearance, enhanced ventilation, and reduced work of breathing. As of this writing, there are no specific recommendations or guidelines for the use of high-flow oxygen therapy in the outpatient setting. Further studies on this promising modality, applied to appropriately selected individuals with chronic respiratory failure in COPD and beyond, are needed before its routine implementation can be considered.

Adaptive Oxygen Delivery

Supplemental oxygen assessment and prescription based on the short in-office ambulatory oximetry test do not account for intervals where too much or not enough oxygen is provided to the user. Technologies to monitor and titrate oxygen delivery flows are being developed, with a focus still predominantly on the inpatient setting. One study investigated the efficiency of an automated oxygen delivery device, the $FreeO_2$™ (Oxynov, Quebec, Canada), which monitored and adjusted oxygen flow to achieve targeted oxygen saturation levels in subjects with COPD [29]. The investigators found six- to 35-fold oxygen savings depending on the oxygen saturation target. Another approach used the entrainment of oxygen from an oxygen reservoir device, the OXFO system (OXFO Corporation, Boston, MA, United States), connected to an oxygen cylinder [30]. The system takes oxygen from a pressurized cylinder at a rate sufficient to maintain a reservoir filled with adequate oxygen at ambient pressure, thereby meeting the oxygen requirements for adequate oxygen saturation. Stable hospitalized patients needing supplemental oxygen at two or more LPM by nasal cannula were tested in a crossover fashion using the OXFO system. Oxygen saturations in the system were the same as those of standard oxygen delivery but demonstrated oxygen volume savings of 13-fold, up to 6 LPM.

Adaptive oxygen delivery technologies enable oxygen therapy to be administered more efficiently than standard continuous oxygen flow systems. They do not appear to be inferior to standard oxygen therapy, as they provide appropriate oxygen saturation levels. Further study is needed to refine adaptive oxygen delivery systems for the ambulatory setting, conduct cost-effectiveness analyses, and assess health outcomes that are at least comparable to those of current therapies.

Closing Thoughts

Long-term oxygen therapy, when first prescribed, is an abrupt and profound change in lifestyle for individuals with chronic lung diseases and potentially harmful hypoxemia. However, the physiological benefits of oxygen therapy may be counterbalanced by the user being "tied down" to oxygen delivery equipment and cannulas, leading to noncompliance that negates the benefits of oxygen therapy. Shared decision-making between the prescribing provider and a well-informed patient is critical. Continued monitoring for worsening hypoxemia and its deleterious effects must be recognized with the anticipation that LTOT may change with aging and disease progression.

References

1. Khor YH, Dudley KA, Herman D, Jacobs SS, Lederer DJ, Krishnan JA, et al. Summary for clinicians: clinical practice guideline on home oxygen therapy for adults with chronic lung disease. Ann Am Thorac Soc. 2021;18(9):1444–9.
2. Jacobs SS, Krishnan JA, Lederer DJ, Ghazipura M, Hossain T, Tan A-YM, et al. Home oxygen therapy for adults with chronic lung disease. An official American Thoracic Society clinical practice guideline. Am J Respir Crit Care Med. 2020;202(10):e121–41.
3. McMorrowa R, Mythenb MG. Pulse oximetry. Curr Opin Crit Care. 2006;12:269–71.
4. Cabanas AM, Fuentes-Guajardo M, Latorre K, León D, Martín-Escudero P. Skin pigmentation influence on pulse oximetry accuracy: a systematic review and bibliometric analysis. Sensors (Basel). 2022;22:3402. https://doi.org/10.3390/s22093402.
5. Fussell KM, Ayo DS, Branca P, Rogers JT, Rodriguez M, Light RW. Assessing need for long-term oxygen therapy: a comparison of conventional evaluation and measures of ambulatory oximetry monitoring. Respir Care. 2003;48(2):115–9.
6. Casanova C, Hernandez C, Sanchez A, Garcıa-Talavera I, de Torres JP, Abreu J, Valencia JM, Aguirre-Jaime A, Celli BR. Twenty-four-hour ambulatory oximetry monitoring in COPD patients with moderate hypoxemia. Respir Care. 2006;51(12):1416–23.

7. Zhu Z, Barnette RK, Fussell KM, Michael Rodriguez R, Canonico A, Light RW. Continuous oxygen monitoring—a better way to prescribe long-term oxygen therapy. Respir Med. 2005;99(11):1386–92.
8. Lacasse Y, Sériès F, Vujovic-Zotovic N, Goldstein R, Bourbeau J, Lecours R, et al. Evaluating nocturnal oxygen desaturation in COPD-revised. Respir Med. 2011;105(9):1331–7.
9. Lacasse Y, Sériès F, Corbeil F, Baltzan M, Paradis B, Simão P, et al. Randomized trial of nocturnal oxygen in chronic obstructive pulmonary disease. N Engl J Med. 2020;383:1129–38.
10. Khor YH, Ng Y, Sweeney D, Ryerson CJ. Nocturnal hypoxaemia in interstitial lung disease: a systematic review. Thorax. 2021;76(12):1200–8.
11. Home Oxygen National Determination [Internet]. National Coverage Determination (NCD) Home Use of Oxygen. https://www.cms.gov/medicare-coverage-database/view/ncd.aspx?NCDId=169. Accessed 10 June 2025.
12. Local Coverage Determination [Internet]. https://www.cms.gov/medicare-coverage-database/view/lcd.aspx?lcdid=33797. Accessed 10 June 2025.
13. Robbins MS, Starling AJ, Pringsheim TM, Becker WJ, Schwedt TJ. Treatment of cluster headache: the American headache society evidence-based guidelines. Headache. 2016;56(7):1093–106.
14. DMEPOS scope and conditions [Internet]. https://www.ecfr.gov/current/title-42/chapter-IV/subchapter-B/part-410/subpart-B/section-410.38. Accessed 10 June 2025.
15. Edelman DA, Maleyko-Jacobs S, White MT, Lucas CE, Ledgerwood AM. Smoking and home oxygen therapy – a preventable public health hazard. J Burn Care Res. 2008;29(1):119–22.
16. Mastropieri CJ, Leonard G, Holmes JH. Stop the burn: a smoking and home oxygen safety initiative with use of firebreaks. J Burn Care Res. 2020;41(1):S15.
17. Oxygen and portable oxygen concentrators for medical use by passengers [Internet]. https://www.ecfr.gov/current/title-14/chapter-I/subchapter-G/part-125/subpart-F/section-125.219. Accessed 10 June 2025.
18. Hardavella G, Karampinis I, Frille A, Sreter K, Rousalova I. Oxygen devices and delivery systems. Breathe (Sheff). 2019;15(3):e108–16.
19. Tiep B, Carter R. Oxygen conserving devices and methodologies. Chron Respir Dis. 2008;5(2):109–14.
20. Ramage CM, Kee SS, Bristow A. A new portable oxygen system using liquid oxygen. Anaesthesia. 1991;46(5):395–7.
21. Supplemental Oxygen Access Reform Act (S.3821/H.R. 7928) [Internet]. https://www.congress.gov/bill/118th-congress/senate-bill/3821. Accessed 10 June 2025.
22. Nasal oxygen cannula: a vital tool in oxygen therapy [Internet]. https://newtransmedical.com/article-detail/bydomEGW. Accessed 10 June 2025.
23. Nishimura M. High-flow nasal cannula oxygen therapy in adults: physiological benefits, indication, clinical benefits, and adverse effects. Respir Care. 2016;61(4):529–41.
24. Fraser JF, Spooner AJ, Dunster KR, Anstey CM, Corley A. Nasal high flow oxygen therapy in patients with COPD reduces respiratory rate and tissue carbon dioxide while increasing tidal and end-expiratory lung volumes: a randomised crossover trial. Thorax. 2016;71(8):759–61.
25. Criner GJ, Criner L-YH, George SA, Thomas JK, Jacobs MR. Feasibility of using daily home high-flow nasal therapy in COPD patients following a recent COPD hospitalization. Chronic Obstr Pulm Dis (Miami). 2022;9(1):4–14.
26. Nagata K, Kikuchi T, Horie T, Shiraki A, Kitajima T, Kadowaki T, et al. Domiciliary high-flow nasal cannula oxygen therapy for patients with stable hypercapnic chronic obstructive pulmonary disease. A multicenter randomized crossover trial. Ann Am Thorac Soc. 2018;15(4):432–9.
27. Storgaard LH, Hockey H-U, Laursen BS, Weinreich UM. Long-term effects of oxygen-enriched high-flow nasal cannula treatment in COPD patients with chronic hypoxemic respiratory failure. Int J Chron Obstruct Pulmon Dis. 2018;13:1195–205.
28. Milne RJ, Hockey H-U, Garrett J. Hospital cost savings for sequential COPD patients receiving domiciliary nasal high flow therapy. Int J Chron Obstruct Pulmon Dis. 2022;17:1311–22.

29. Bourassa S, Bouchard P-A, Dauphin M, Lellouche F. Oxygen conservation methods with automated titration. Respir Care. 2020;65(10):1433–42.
30. Wawrzyniak KM, Hooker G, Osorno Upegui SC, Ortega Martínez RA, Bazoberry A, DiBenedetto DJ, et al. A novel device for conservation of supplemental oxygen: a randomized, crossover study of the efficiency and non-inferiority of the OXFO system. J Glob Health Rep. 2024;8:e2024028. https://doi.org/10.29392/001c.124467.

Use of Oxygen After Lung Surgery

15

Tyler R. Grenda and Nathaniel R. Evans III

Introduction

Supplemental oxygen in the perioperative period, commonly delivered via a nasal cannula or a face mask, is relatively routine for the hospitalization period after lung resection. Typically, supplemental oxygen is utilized with a goal of avoiding hypoxemia following lung resection, particularly in the inpatient hospital phase immediately following lung resection. Ideally, patients are discharged without supplemental oxygen. Oxygen needs that persist following discharge is a source of significant patient concern related to lung surgery. In most investigations, authors have focused on lung cancer resection. Published studies have examined the longer-term need for oxygen following lung surgery, demonstrating a range of 3%–15% of patients who may require discharge to home with supplemental oxygen following primary lung cancer resection [1–4]. The concern for this requirement and the impact on quality-of-life measures have motivated some investigators to explore a greater understanding of the need for supplemental oxygen after lung resection [5]. Unfortunately, previous studies that have evaluated the impact of pulmonary function have not yielded a comprehensive picture. The data surrounding the need for supplemental oxygen following lung resection is somewhat limited [6].

Exploring the Evidence

While data regarding the need for postoperative oxygen requirement may be limited, there are extensive guidelines for the expected morbidity and mortality of lung resection in the setting of lung cancer [7]. These guidelines often rely on

T. R. Grenda (✉) · N. R. Evans III
Division of Thoracic Surgery, The Department of Surgery at the Sidney Kimmel Medical College of Thomas Jefferson University, Philadelphia, PA, USA
e-mail: tyler.grenda@jefferson.edu

G. C. Kane et al. (eds.), *Oxygen*, https://doi.org/10.1007/978-3-032-18934-9_15

preoperative physiological performance to identify patients at the greatest risk of undergoing surgical treatment for lung cancer, particularly with regard to the risk of experiencing morbidity and mortality. For example, when the FEV_1 or the DLCO is less than 40% of the predicted normal, there is an increased risk of perioperative mortality [7, 8]. Cardiopulmonary exercise testing may be utilized in specific clinical scenarios to better differentiate candidacy for lung resection [9]. Ventilation–perfusion lung scans (VQ scans) may be utilized in other specific clinical settings to evaluate for postoperative predicted pulmonary function [10]. Unfortunately, these studies do not provide specific data about predicting oxygen usage after treatment.

With the limited data, it is important to consider the patient population when examining the literature on this topic. A majority of data has focused on patients undergoing lung cancer resection and not a broader population of "lung surgery" procedures. As a result, the literature does not generally extend broadly to all lung surgery procedures and may not be reflective of patients with underlying lung disease undergoing pulmonary surgical procedures for benign diagnoses [7].

When considering the use of oxygen following surgery, this includes several phases of care. The postoperative period following surgery for removal of a portion of the lung includes the inpatient hospitalization phase and the subsequent outpatient setting following discharge. The need for supplemental oxygen immediately following lung resection can be secondary to several etiologies such as pain, poor pulmonary toilet, or atelectasis and may be addressed with incentive spirometry and ambulation. A subset of patients may require continued supplemental oxygen beyond the perioperative period, which may be due to the severity of underlying lung disease, exacerbated by the loss of functional lung tissue.

One factor that may contribute to the risk of postoperative hypoxia is the coexistence of lung cancer with underlying lung disease, such as emphysema [11]. Another factor could relate to the intensity of pulmonary toilet with standard post-op measures such as the iCOUGH protocol [12]. When considering supplemental oxygen needs following surgery, it is important to consider the duration of oxygen use following the index procedure. While approximately 15% of patients may require home oxygen use initially following discharge from the index pulmonary surgical procedure, many patients will be liberated from oxygen use within 1 month following discharge [1]. As such, fewer patients have longer-term needs for lifelong use of oxygen following lung resection [13].

With respect to the inpatient setting immediately following lung resection, there is limited data evaluating the utilization and predictors of oxygen requirement following lung resection. There are several perioperative factors related to the immediate inpatient postoperative period that can contribute to post-resection hypoxia, including ventilation–perfusion mismatch, which may influence the immediate need for additional oxygen, which subsequently resolves in the days following surgery [14]. As a result, only a portion of patients requiring delivery of supplemental oxygen following surgery require a longer duration of oxygen therapy as they transition to home or the post-acute care setting following lung resection. It is important to note that some controversy exists regarding routine oxygen therapy following surgery, as hyperoxia may have some negative physiological effects that may need to be considered [14]. At this time, there is no specific standard approach to the use of oxygen in the hospital immediately following lung resection [15, 16].

Most data surrounding oxygen use following surgery has focused on the home or post-acute care setting. While previous reports have noted that up to 15% of patients may require discharge with supplemental oxygen, more contemporary reports across a patient population undergoing lobectomy for lung cancer in a large population using The Society of Thoracic Surgeons General Thoracic Surgery Database reflect that approximately 8.4% of patients will require discharge with supplemental oxygen [1, 2, 16]. In addition, the literature evaluating domiciliary oxygen use following lung cancer surgery has demonstrated that there may potentially be some association with survival [1].

There may be a significant influence on the quality of life in patients requiring home oxygen [17]. Some efforts have evaluated respiratory function following lung cancer surgery, specifically exercise-induced hypoxia [18, 19]. However, current lung surgery risk models do not specifically focus on the prediction of home oxygen use following surgery.

Given that home oxygen utilization may influence the quality of life following surgery, identifying risk factors for requiring home oxygen is needed in order to stratify patients most at-risk for sustained supplemental oxygen needs. Identifying patients most at-risk for home oxygen use, particularly those most likely to require supplemental oxygen for prolonged or indefinite periods of time following discharge from the hospital, is imperative to addressing quality-of-life concerns related to lung surgery. Previous literature has demonstrated several risk factors for oxygen use at home following lung resection, including obesity and pulmonary function test parameters [2]. In addition, smoking status has been associated with supplemental oxygen requirements at the time of discharge [15, 16]. More efforts will be needed to create risk models to guide the discussion regarding the need for supplemental oxygen and how this may influence the quality of life following elective lung surgery [20]. These efforts should also explore whether upper lobe cancer resection in patients with emphysema might actually have improvement due to a lung-reduction effect [21].

Conclusion

In summary, previous literature has identified up to 15% of patients requiring supplemental oxygen following lung surgery, with more modest estimates in more contemporary reports. Given the impact of this requirement on patients' quality of life and the potential impact on survival, additional studies are needed to understand which patients are most likely to require long-term oxygen use and its impact on patient perceptions of their quality of life [22].

While oxygen use may not be specifically addressed, published literature suggests that outcomes after thoracic surgery for lung cancer improved for patients who quit smoking and used incentive spirometry effectively [12, 13, 15].

Careful discussion about the expected outcomes regarding pulmonary function and the possibility for supplemental oxygen needs for extended periods of time following surgery is quite important when considering treatment options for elective lung surgery, particularly for early-stage lung cancer in patients with established emphysema. These efforts will be imperative to ensure that quality of life is included as a part of the discussion regarding treatment for early-stage lung cancer. As continued efforts toward establishing quality-of-life metrics for lung cancer care are implemented, further evaluation of postoperative respiratory function and requirements for supplemental oxygen are needed. [20].

References

1. Nicastri DG, Alpert N, Liu B, et al. Oxygen use after lung cancer surgery. Ann Thorac Surg. 2018;106(5):1548–55.
2. Nicastri DG, Chan H, You N, et al. Effects of smoking, obesity, and pulmonary function on home oxygen use after curative lung cancer surgery. Ann Am Thorac Soc. 2022;19(3):442–50.
3. Yepes-Temiño MJ, Monedero P, Pérez-Valdivieso JR. Risk prediction model for respiratory complications after lung resection: an observational multicentre study. Eur J Anaesthesiol. 2016;33(5):326–33.
4. Amar D, Munoz D, Shi W, Zhang H, Thaler HT. A clinical prediction rule for pulmonary complications after thoracic surgery for primary lung cancer. Anesth Analg. 2010;110(5):1343–8.
5. Yano T, Shoji F, Koga T. Is oxygen supplementation needed after standard pulmonary resection for primary lung cancer? Ann Thorac Cardiovasc Surg. 2006;12(6):393–6.
6. Brocki BC, Westerdahl E, Langer D, Souza DSR, Andreasen JJ. Decrease in pulmonary function and oxygenation after lung resection. ERJ Open Res. 2018;4(1):00055-2017.
7. Colice GL, Shafa S, Griffin JP, Keenan R, Bolliger CT. Physiologic evaluation of the patient with lung cancer being considered for resectional surgery: ACCP evidenced-based clinical practice guidelines (2nd edition). Chest. 2007;132(3 Suppl):161S–77S. https://doi.org/10.1378/chest.07-1359.
8. British Thoracic Society, Society of Cardiothoracic Surgeons of Great Britain and Ireland Working Party. Guidelines on the selection of patients with lung cancer for surgery. Thorax. 2001;56:89–108.
9. Kallianos A, Rapti A, Tsimpoukis S, Charpidou A, Dannos I, Kainis E, Syrigos K. Cardiopulmonary exercise testing (CPET) as preoperative test before lung resection. In Vivo. 2014;28(6):1013–20.
10. Subramanyam P, Sundaram PS. Which is better-a standalone ventilation or perfusion scan or combined imaging to predict postoperative FEV1 in one seconds in patients posted for lung surgeries with borderline pulmonary reserve. Indian J Nucl Med. 2018;33(2):105–11.
11. Licker MJ, Widikker I, Robert J, Frey JG, Spiliopoulos A, Ellenberger C, et al. Operative mortality and respiratory complications after lung resection for cancer: impact of chronic obstructive pulmonary disease and time trends. Ann Thorac Surg. 2006;81(5):1830–7.
12. Cassidy MR, Rosenkranz P, McCabe K, Rosen JE, McAneny D. I COUGH: reducing postoperative pulmonary complications with a multidisciplinary patient care program. JAMA Surg. 2013;148(8):740–5. https://doi.org/10.1001/jamasurg.2013.358.
13. Sullivan KA, Churchill IF, Hylton DA, Hanna WC. Use of incentive spirometry in adults following cardiac, thoracic, and upper abdominal surgery to prevent post-operative pulmonary complications: a systematic review and meta-analysis. Respiration. 2021;100(11):1114–27.
14. Suzuki S. Oxygen administration for postoperative surgical patients: a narrative review. J Intensive Care. 2020;8:79.
15. Mason DP, et al. Impact of smoking cessation before resection of lung cancer: a society of thoracic surgeons general thoracic surgery database study. Ann Thorac Surg. 2009;88(2):362–71.
16. Bilyy A, El-Nakhal T, Kadlec J, Bartosik W, Tornout FV, Kouritas V. Preoperative training education with incentive spirometry may reduce postoperative pulmonary complications. Asian Cardiovasc Thorac Ann. 2020;28(9):592–7. https://doi.org/10.1177/0218492320957158. Epub 2020 Sep 11. PMID: 32915659.

17. Brown LM, Bonnell L, Parsons N, et al. Predictors of discharge with supplemental oxygen after lobectomy for lung cancer. Ann Thorac Surg. 2025;119(1):180–9.
18. Demmy TL, Plante AJ, Nwogu CE, Takita H, Anderson TM. Discharge independence with minimally invasive lobectomy. Am J Surg. 2004;188(6):698–702.
19. Asaji N, Nakagama T, Uehara H. Preoperative Predictors of Exercise-Induced Hypoxemia Following Lung Cancer Surgery. Cureus. 2025;17(6):e86813.
20. Kneuertz PJ, D'Souza DM, Moffatt-Bruce SD, et al. Robotic lobectomy has the greatest benefit in patients with marginal pulmonary function. J Cardiothorac Surg. 2018;13:56. https://doi.org/10.1186/s13019-018-0748-z.
21. Kushibe K. Assessment of pulmonary function after lobectomy for lung cancer—upper lobectomy might have the same effect as lung volume reduction surgery. Eur J Cardiothorac Surg. 2006;29(6):886–90. https://doi.org/10.1016/j.ejcts.2006.02.047.
22. Takemoto S, Shibamoto Y, Hashizume C, Miyakawa A, Murai T, Yanagi T, Sugie C, Nagai A. Changes in pulmonary function and their correlation with dose–volume parameters in patients undergoing stereotactic body radiotherapy for lung cancer. J Radiat Res. 2021;62(2):338–45. https://doi.org/10.1093/jrr/rraa131.

High-Flow Nasal Cannula

16

Gregory C. Kane

High-flow oxygen therapy through a nasal cannula should be considered to be an effective and safe therapy for the treatment of spontaneously breathing patients with acute hypoxemic respiratory failure.

—Michael A. Mathay, MD, Physician and Investigator

Introduction

Early in this century, a new modality emerged for acute hypoxemic respiratory failure (but not cases accompanied by hypercapnia) that would rival noninvasive ventilation (NIV) for the treatment of severe hypoxemic respiratory failure, representing the first major improvement in the use of a simple nasal cannula in more than 100 years [1–3]. This new technique has been referred to as high-flow nasal cannula (HFNC).

One reason for the century-long delay of this innovation may have been related to an inadequate appreciation of how essential proper humidification is when delivering oxygen at unusually high flows that far exceeded any flow rate used successfully with a simple nasal cannula. Rather than delivering 1–10 liters per minute (LPM) of oxygen, this chapter focuses on oxygen delivery at rates of 10–60 LPM. The sinus cavities serve to warm and humidify air as we breathe, among other benefits, and contribute to enhanced mucociliary function [4, 5]. Inadequately humidified air can lead to airway desiccation, or excessive drying of the airway, which negatively impacts the mucociliary blanket and may make expectoration

G. C. Kane (✉)
The Korman Respiratory Institute and the Division of Pulmonary, Allergy and Critical Care, The Department of Medicine at the Sidney Kimmel Medical College of Thomas Jefferson University, Philadelphia, PA, USA
e-mail: gregory.kane@jefferson.edu

G. C. Kane et al. (eds.), *Oxygen*, https://doi.org/10.1007/978-3-032-18934-9_16

more difficult. In this way, just increasing the flow through a simple nasal cannula could have negative effects. Another reason for the delayed development was the failure to imagine that a high-flow device (with proper humidification) could also deliver positive end-expiratory pressure (PEEP), which had previously been the domain of mechanical ventilation through an endotracheal tube (ETT) or via noninvasive ventilation using a full-face mask [6]. PEEP itself was first discovered and described in the early era of intubation and mechanical ventilation for respiratory failure, including for acute respiratory distress syndrome (ARDS) [7, 8]. The idea of providing a high flow and PEEP may not equal the innovation of the first application of PEEP in the 1960s [8], but it still deserves accolades for adding a new, unique, and remarkable tool for clinicians treating hypoxemic respiratory failure for viral and bacterial pneumonia, mixed heart failure and pneumonia, and other causes of hypoxemic respiratory failure. It is not only effective but also enhances patient comfort over conventional oxygen therapy (COT).

Physiological Benefits and Mechanism of Delivery of HFNC

The magic of high-flow nasal cannula (HFNC) therapy lies in its basic physiological advantages. These include the application of PEEP, which contributes to an increased end-expiratory volume, thus improving V/Q matching and reducing shunt, which can then help reduce the respiratory rate and provide the host with added time to heal before respiratory muscle fatigue can occur [9, 10]. Since HFNC does not provide external work (e.g., there is no pressure differential in inspiration or expiration), it would not be expected to be beneficial in hypercapnic respiratory failure or in cases where the work of breathing is excessive. However, relative to simply increasing the flow through a simple nasal cannula, as would be the result of using COT, HFNC enhances mucociliary clearance through an improved humidification system and can wash out dead space, thereby reducing wasted ventilation and improving pH [9, 11]. The benefits of this strategy and HFNC are highlighted in Table 16.1.

The system utilized for HFNC is complicated but is composed of simple components that, when combined, result in high flows of oxygenated and humidified air. Figure 16.1 is a schematic that identifies each of the essential components. Table 16.2 describes the role of each of these components. When the system is working satisfactorily, the result is the delivery of a high fraction (as high as 100%) of fully humidified oxygen to the lungs, with added PEEP, which may be enhanced while

Table 16.1 Physiological benefits of high-flow nasal cannula

Results in the application of PEEP
Enhances mucociliary clearance
Increases end-expiratory volume
Decreases the respiratory rate
Washes out dead space (including CO_2)

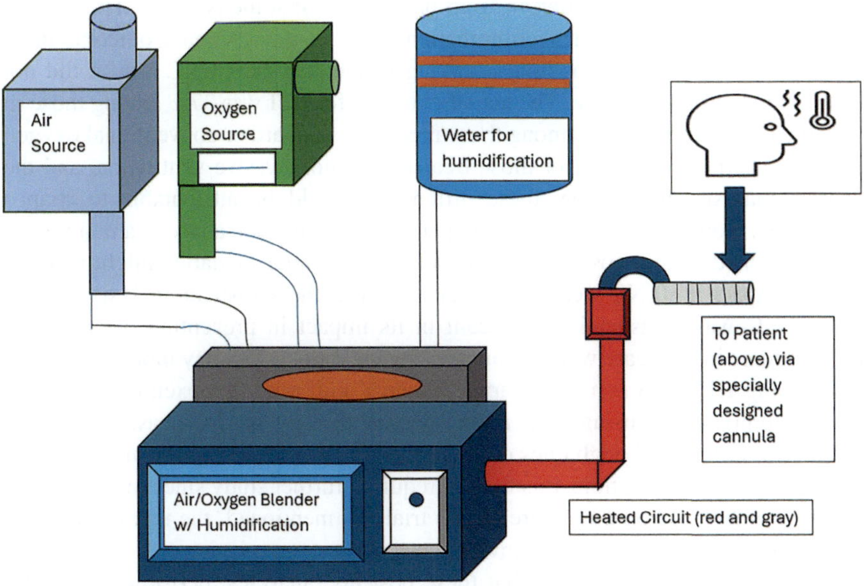

Fig. 16.1 This schematic outlines the components of a high-flow nasal oxygen system, including the oxygen source; a pressurized air source; the water source for humidification; the blender that combines air, oxygen, and humidification; and the heated tubing, ultimately attached to a nasal cannula device (not shown). (This schematic was created by the author)

Table 16.2 An explanation of the components of the high-flow nasal cannula system

Component	Rationale
Oxygen source	Required to generate a high rate of O_2
Water source	Required to allow humidification
Air oxygen blender	Combines humidity and oxygen and is capable of matching O_2 delivery with humidification
Heated circuit	Maintains humidity at body temperature
Novel nasal interface	Can facilitate PEEP, especially when the mouth is closed

the mouth is closed. Such systems can be created with individual components or from a number of commercial vendors. Recognizing the potential for perceived conflict of interest, this author will refrain from describing the commercial options or listing vendors. The provided figure is a simple, generic, non-branded schematic.

Evidence Behind the Use of HFNC

An early and important trial in the use of HFNC was authored by Jean-Pierre Frat and colleagues and featured a comparison of HFNC with COT and noninvasive ventilation in 310 patients who presented with hypoxemic respiratory failure. In this trial, most subjects were suffering from pneumonia of some type [1]. The authors selected the rate of endotracheal intubation (ETI) as their primary outcome measure, and while the rate was lowest among patients in the HFNC arm, it did not reach statistical significance. The actual outcome for ETI was 37% among those in the HFNC arm versus 50% among those receiving standard or conventional oxygen therapy. The rate was 47% for those treated with noninvasive ventilation, and the overall analysis showed that these differences could be attributable to chance ($P = 0.18$). However, when the authors performed a post hoc analysis among those who presented as the most hypoxic subset, which, understandably, might reveal a greater impact if HFNC were a beneficial therapy, the statistical analysis showed that HFNC was statistically significant in its impact in preventing the need for ETI. Leaders in ICU care were encouraged by the reported 90-day mortality benefit when using HFNC in non-hypercapnic patients with acute hypoxemic respiratory failure compared to using face mask oxygen therapy or noninvasive positive-pressure ventilation, though rates on intubation did not differ significantly between the three groups. At the time, this finding required further study since mortality was not the primary outcome measure in this trial. As mentioned, the risk of delaying intubation is real when using noninvasive techniques.

The reader must understand that these post hoc analyses, performed after the fact, did not provide definitive proof of benefit, and further trials would be necessary to make such a claim. Subsequent meta-analyses performed since the Frat trial [12, 13] have shown that HFNC is effective but principally in reducing the need for ETI compared to COT. It is important to note that in several of the systematic reviews, a clear improvement in survival was lacking; however, outcomes were at least as good on high-flow nasal cannula, and patients reported greater comfort and tolerance [12]. A systematic review of patients provided with HFNC after planned extubation showed a lower rate of reintubation, but again, mortality benefit was not demonstrated [14]. Noninvasive ventilation has also proven helpful, and studies clearly delineating a use preference are lacking [15]. One concern raised by Kang et al. for the use of HFNC is that it may delay intubation for hypoxemic respiratory failure, placing patients at risk of mortality related to late intubation. This cautionary note reminds the reader that patients on HFNC require very close observation and prompt intubation once a decision to transition to traditional ventilation via placement of an endotracheal tube has been made [16].

In the era of COVID-19, early studies also showed the benefit of HFNC in reducing the need for airway intubation and mechanical ventilation (34% in the HFNC group versus 51% in the conventional oxygen group) [17]. The authors were careful to examine overall mortality, which was similar between groups [17]. One specific concern in using HFNC, already referenced in general, is relevant for discussion. Some authors have questioned whether the use of high-flow nasal cannula can inappropriately delay the need for mechanical ventilation with intubation [16]. This is of particular importance in COVID-19, where progression from early hypoxic respiratory failure to the need for intubation has been noted to be more rapid than in other types of pneumonia. This phenomenon was addressed by Hernandez-Romieu et al. in a paper published in *Critical Care Medicine* [18]. Their findings did not identify a mortality concern among subjects who were intubated later in their hospital stay. In addition, two retrospective trials have supported the use of HFNC in COVID-19 [19, 20]. Importantly, since pneumonia is a common disease process that can lead to hypoxic respiratory failure, the meta-analysis by Arruda established that HFNC deserves a place in the approach to respiratory failure in COVID-19 [21]. As the literature has evolved around our understanding of the impact of HFNC, we acknowledge that it has the potential to decrease the need to support patients with intubation and mechanical ventilation as they recover from viral or bacterial pneumonias. However, HFNC is just one tool to support patients through such illnesses. Whether we should describe HFNC as "saving lives" may depend on specific diagnoses and time to recovery [3]. Nonetheless, it has become a recognized approach to supporting patients with hypoxemic respiratory failure due to pneumonia.

In order to quantify the risk of delayed intubation and create a score to guide consideration for intubation, researchers have proposed what is known as the ROX index. This index was validated in patients with pneumonia and acute hypoxemic respiratory failure on HFNC and is defined as the ratio of pulse oximetry/fraction of inspired oxygen to respiratory rate. A higher score (>4.88) implied that the need for intubation would be low (that is, the patients were at a low risk of HFNC failure) [22]. A lower score suggested close follow-up, with reassessment in approximately 2 h. This has since been validated in several more studies.

The impact of using HFNC in patients with acute cardiogenic pulmonary edema has been studied less than in other diagnoses, such as pneumonia, but theoretically stands as a feasible approach. The physiological impact of providing PEEP, reducing shunt, and washing out dead space should also be a benefit in cardiogenic pulmonary edema, while treating physicians address the underlying cardiac dysfunction to restore homeostasis [23]. The benefit in acute cardiogenic pulmonary edema would necessarily need to be early in presentation, and so it would be important to conduct trials that focus on a population in the emergency room (ER) [23, 24]. An early trial from Thailand showed no benefit in this population [24]. A follow-up trial, from Ko and colleagues, did show improvement in physiological parameters, such as lactate levels, respiratory rate at 30 min, and blood gas data at 60 min [25]. However, the authors did not note any important differences in rates of intubation, ICU utilization, or mortality benefit. At this time, further investigation is needed before HFNC can be recommended as an important adjunct to early care for patients with acute cardiogenic pulmonary edema. In these cases, CPAP and BiPAP can play a role, and they will be addressed in Chap. 14.

Finally, HFNC has been examined in circumstances of acute exacerbations of COPD. Peng-Lei and colleagues provided a meta-analysis showing no evidence of improved outcomes in terms of endotracheal tube intubation for mechanical ventilation. While they did not report any adverse outcomes, the failure to identify any benefits makes HFNC a poor option for patients with COPD. The authors reported no improvement in rates of intubation (95% confidence interval (CI): 0.49–1.78, $p = 0.84$, overlapping 1.0) and mortality risk (RR 0.91, 95% CI: 0.46–1.79, $p = 0.77$, overlapping 1.0). This study did not report a comparison to COT. This finding actually makes physiological sense, as NIV can provide external work to improve gas exchange and lower elevated levels of P_aCO_2, whereas HFNC does not provide external work as support for breathing [26, 27].

It is important to emphasize that the literature on noninvasive ventilation as compared to intubation with mechanical ventilation for patients with exacerbation of COPD has clearly shown a reduction in the risk of nosocomial infections and even improved outcomes [28, 29]. As such, one could point out by extension that the use of high-flow nasal cannula when reducing the risk for airway intubation and mechanical ventilation may also bring the benefit of reducing nosocomial infections.

Based on the reported data, an approach to treating severe hypoxemic respiratory failure in persons without hypercapnia should begin with the use of a high-flow nasal cannula. Its use can ideally be implemented in the ER, in the hospital wards, or in the ICU, and it holds several unique advantages. Chief among these advantages is the potential to avoid intubating the trachea for mechanical ventilation through placement of an endotracheal tube, together with the attendant benefits created by this strategy, with a reduced risk of nosocomial pneumonia and the avoidance of the need for sedation, which are necessarily part of a more invasive approach. It has been shown to be safe and effective and may lead to reduced need for intubation and mechanical ventilation in selected populations. It has also been shown to have a favorable safety profile while still preserving the opportunity to use mechanical ventilation via an ETT if this becomes necessary. HFNC delivers its benefit not only through greater flows but through the generation of PEEP and washing out dead space, which are unique advantages of this modality compared to conventional oxygen therapy. It is remarkable that a therapy not invented for more than a century after Blodget and others first used nasal cannula–supplied oxygen for pneumonia would be shown to improve upon outcomes so significantly over the traditional delivery of oxygen via nasal prongs [30].

Conclusions and Expert Guidelines

The European Respiratory Society formed a panel of expert clinicians to provide clinical recommendations for the use of HFNC, alongside conventional oxygen therapy (COT) and noninvasive ventilation (NIV). The outcome of convening this panel was eight final recommendations suggesting the use of HFNC [31]:

1. HFNC is preferred over COT in hypoxemic acute respiratory failure (ARF).
2. HFNC is preferred over NIV in hypoxemic ARF.
3. HFNC is preferred over COT during breaks from NIV.
4. Use either HFNC or COT in postoperative patients at a low risk of pulmonary complications.
5. Use either HFNC or NIV in postoperative patients at a high risk of pulmonary complications.
6. Use HFNC over COT in nonsurgical patients at a low risk of extubation failure.

7. Use NIV over HFNC for patients at a high risk of extubation failure unless there are relative or absolute contraindications to NIV.
8. A trial of NIV is required prior to the use of HFNC in patients with COPD and hypercapnic ARF.

In summary, HFNC is an excellent tool for addressing severe hypoxemic respiratory failure due to pneumonia or other causes but not for COPD. HFNC not only provides increased FiO_2 and patient comfort through greater flows and humification but also generates PEEP and washes out dead space, minimizing shunt and reducing the respiratory rate via a comfort-enhancing interface. NIV is still preferred in exacerbations of COPD with elevation of P_aCO_2 because NIV provides external work plus PEEP [29]. All the same, as Dr. Michael Mathay pointed out more than a decade ago, "high-flow oxygen therapy through a nasal cannula should be considered to be an effective and safe therapy for the treatment of spontaneously breathing patients with acute hypoxemic respiratory failure" [3].

References

1. Frat JP, Thille AW, Mercat A, Girault C, Ragot S, Perbet S, et al. High-flow oxygen through nasal cannula in acute hypoxemic respiratory failure. N Engl J Med. 2015;372(23):2185–96.
2. Frat JP, Brugiere B, Ragot S, Chatellier D, Veinstein A, Goudet V, et al. Sequential application of oxygen therapy via high-flow nasal cannula and noninvasive ventilation in acute respiratory failure: an observational pilot study. Respir Care. 2015;60(2):170–8.
3. Matthay MA. Saving lives with high-flow nasal oxygen. N Engl J Med. 2015;372(23):2225–6.
4. Mygind N, Dahl R. Anatomy, physiology and function of the nasal cavities in health and disease. Adv Drug Deliv Rev. 1998;29(1–2):3–12.
5. Williams R, Rankin N, Smith T, Galler D, Seakins P. Relationship between the humidity and temperature of inspired gas and the function of the airway mucosa. Crit Care Med. 1996;24(11):1920–9.
6. Ejiofor BD, Carroll RW, Bortcosh W, Kacmarek RM. PEEP generated by high-flow nasal cannula in a pediatric model. Respir Care. 2019;64(10):1240–9.
7. Pierson DJ, Thomas L. Petty's lessons for the respiratory care clinician of today. Respir Care. 2014;59(8):1287–301.
8. Ashbaugh DG, Bigelow DB, Petty TL, Levine BE. Acute respiratory distress in adults. Lancet. 1967;290(7511):319–23.
9. Helviz Y, Einav S. A systematic review of the high-flow nasal cannula for adult patients. Crit Care. 2018;22:71. https://doi.org/10.1186/s13054-018-1990-4.
10. Groves N, Tobin A. High flow nasal oxygen generates positive airway pressure in adult volunteers. Aust Crit Care. 2007;20:126–31.
11. Hasani A, Chapman T, McCool D, et al. Domiciliary humidification improves lung mucociliary clearance in patients with bronchiectasis. Chron Respir Dis. 2008;5:81–6.
12. Lee CC, Mankodi D, Shaharyar S, Ravindranathan S, Danckers M, Herscovici P, Moor M, Ferrer G. High flow nasal cannula versus conventional oxygen therapy and non-invasive ventilation in adults with acute hypoxemic respiratory failure: a systematic review. Respir Med. 2016;121:100–8.
13. Zhu Y, Yin H, Zhang R, Wei J. High-flow nasal cannula oxygen therapy versus conventional oxygen therapy in patients with acute respiratory failure: a systematic review and meta-analysis of randomized controlled trials. BMC Pulm Med. 2017;17(1):201.

14. Zhu Y, Yin H, Zhang R, Ye X, Wei J. High-flow nasal cannula oxygen therapy versus conventional oxygen therapy in patients after planned extubation: a systematic review and meta-analysis. Crit Care. 2019;23(1):180.
15. Zhao H, Wang H, Sun F, Lyu S, An Y. High-flow nasal cannula oxygen therapy is superior to conventional oxygen therapy but not to noninvasive mechanical ventilation on intubation rate: a systematic review and meta-analysis. Crit Care. 2017;21(1):184.
16. Kang BJ, Koh Y, Lim CM, Huh JW, Baek S, Han M, et al. Failure of high-flow nasal cannula therapy may delay intubation and increase mortality. Intensive Care Med. 2015;41(4):623–32. https://doi.org/10.1007/s00134-015-3693-5.
17. Ospina-Tascón GA, Calderón-Tapia LE, García AF, Zarama V, Gómez-Álvarez F, Álvarez-Saa T, et al. Effect of high-flow oxygen therapy *vs* conventional oxygen therapy on invasive mechanical ventilation and clinical recovery in patients with severe COVID-19: a randomized clinical trial. JAMA. 2021;326(21):2161–71.
18. Hernandez-Romieu AC, Adelman MW, Hockstein MA, Robichaux CJ, Edwards JA, Fazio JC, et al. Timing of intubation and mortality among critically ill coronavirus disease 2019 patients: a single-center cohort study. Crit Care Med. 2020;48(11):e1045. https://doi.org/10.1097/CCM.0000000000004600.
19. Demoule A, Vieillard Baron A, Darmon M, Beurton A, Géri G, Voiriot G, et al. High-flow nasal cannula in critically ill patients with severe COVID-19. Am J Respir Crit Care Med. 2020;202(7):1039–42.
20. Bonnet N, Martin O, Boubaya M, Levy V, Ebstein N, Karoubi P, et al. High flow nasal oxygen therapy to avoid invasive mechanical ventilation in SARS-CoV-2 pneumonia: a retrospective study. Ann Intensive Care. 2021;11(1):37. https://doi.org/10.1186/s13613-021-00825-5.
21. Arruda DG, Kieling GA, Melo-Diaz LL. Effectiveness of high-flow nasal cannula therapy on clinical outcomes in adults with COVID-19: a systematic review. Can J Respir Ther. 2023;59:52–65. https://doi.org/10.29390/cjrt-2022-005. PMID: 36741308; PMCID: PMC9854387.
22. Roca O, Messika J, Caralt B, García-de-Acilu M, Sztrymf B, Ricard JD, Masclans JR. Predicting success of high-flow nasal cannula in pneumonia patients with hypoxemic respiratory failure: the utility of the ROX index. J Crit Care. 2016;35:200–5. https://doi.org/10.1016/j.jcrc.2016.05.022. Epub 2016 May 31. PMID: 27481760.
23. Adhikari P, Bhattarai S, Gupta A, Ali E, Ali M, Riad M, et al. Physiological effects of high-flow nasal cannula therapy and its use in acute cardiogenic pulmonary edema. Cureus. 2021;13(2):e13372.
24. Makdee O, Monsomboon A, Surabenjawong U, Praphruetkit N, Chaisirin W, Chakorn T, Permpikul C, Thiravit P, Nakornchai T. High-flow nasal cannula versus conventional oxygen therapy in emergency department patients with cardiogenic pulmonary edema: a randomized controlled trial. Ann Emerg Med. 2017;70(4):465–472.e2, ISSN 0196-0644. https://doi.org/10.1016/j.annemergmed.2017.03.028.
25. Ko DR, Beom J, Lee HS, You JS, Chung HS, Chung SP. Benefits of high-flow nasal cannula therapy for acute pulmonary Edema in patients with heart failure in the emergency department: a prospective multi-center randomized controlled trial. J Clin Med. 1937;2020:9. https://doi.org/10.3390/jcm9061937.
26. Yang P-L, Yu J-Q, Chen H-B. High-flow nasal cannula for acute exacerbation of chronic obstructive pulmonary disease: a systematic review and meta-analysis. Heart Lung. 2021;50(2):252–61, ISSN 0147-9563. https://doi.org/10.1016/j.hrtlng.2020.12.010.
27. Huan Y, Huang D, Luo J, Liang J. The use of high-flow nasal cannula in patients with chronic obstructive pulmonary disease under exacerbation and stable phases: a systematic review and meta-analysis. Heart Lung. 2023;60:116–26. https://doi.org/10.1016/j.hrtlng.2023.02.016.

28. Guerin C, et al. Face mask NIV reduced nosocomial pneumonia; a prospective epidemiological survey from a single ICU. Intensive Care Med. 1999;23:1024–9.
29. Brochard L, Mancebo J, Wysocki M, et al. Noninvasive ventilation for acute exacerbations of chronic obstructive pulmonary disease. N Engl J Med. 1995;333:817–22.
30. Blodgett AN. The continuous inhalation of oxygen in cases of pneumonia otherwise fatal, and in other diseases. Boston Med J. 1890;123:481–5.
31. Oczkowski S, Ergan B, Bos L, Chatwin M, Ferrer M, Gregoretti C, Heunks L, et al. ERS clinical practice guidelines: high-flow nasal cannula in acute respiratory failure. Eur Respir J. 2022;59(4):2101574.

Noninvasive Ventilation

17

Daniel Kramer

Introduction

Noninvasive ventilation (NIV) was first developed and utilized in the treatment of patients with acute respiratory failure in the 1940s [1]. Since that time, the field has accrued a host of studies demonstrating benefit in select acute etiologies of respiratory failure, particularly acute hypercapnic exacerbations of chronic obstructive pulmonary disease (COPD) and some cases of acute cardiogenic pulmonary edema from congestive heart failure (CHF). There have also been demonstrable benefits from NIV in other select causes of acute hypoxemic and hypercapnic respiratory failure. A more recent development in the world of noninvasive ventilation is the advent of outpatient bi-level and home mechanical ventilation devices and technologies that have allowed for respiratory support for patients with different causes of chronic respiratory failure. Etiologies of outpatient respiratory impairment with potential benefits from outpatient NIV include the following: neuromuscular disease, hypoventilation syndromes, restrictive thoracic disorders, and chronic hypercapnic COPD. This development has spurred the creation of a subspecialty within the fields of pulmonary and sleep medicine, with still a large unmet need for expertise and experience to help manage this unique population of patients. While a variety of devices meet the definition of noninvasive ventilation, this chapter will focus on positive-pressure ventilation.

D. Kramer (✉)
The Korman Respiratory Institute and the Division of Pulmonary, Allergy and Critical Care, The Department of Medicine at the Sidney Kimmel Medical College of Thomas Jefferson University, Philadelphia, PA, USA
e-mail: Daniel.Kramer@jefferson.edu

G. C. Kane et al. (eds.), *Oxygen*, https://doi.org/10.1007/978-3-032-18934-9_17

History of Noninvasive Ventilation

While few hospitals had access to supplemental oxygen in the 1920s to support patients with acute respiratory failure, it was in the late 1920s that the first technology was developed to support patients who needed more respiratory support than supplemental oxygen alone could provide. It was recognized that acute respiratory failure is frequently more complex than mere alveolar gas exchange failure. In severe instances, a critical factor is the mechanical failure of the respiratory pump, which struggles to meet the heightened respiratory demands and essential minute ventilation required to sustain life. The first attempt at addressing this was via the first tank ventilator, otherwise known as the iron lung. The iron lung was first developed in 1927, with its first patient application occurring in 1928. Used initially for patients with polio-induced respiratory muscle failure as well as patients with coal gas poisoning, this technology utilized negative-pressure ventilation to support patients otherwise too weak to breathe spontaneously. While it was a marvel for its time, it was large and cumbersome.

Intermittent positive-pressure ventilation via an anesthesia mask interface in the treatment of acute respiratory failure for conditions such as pneumonia, pulmonary edema, near drowning, and asthma exacerbations was studied by Motley and colleagues at Bellevue Hospital in 1940 [2]. In the 1950s, however, the polio epidemic led to the beginnings of invasive mechanical ventilatory (IMV) support in the form of positive-pressure ventilation, thus overshadowing the study and development of noninvasive techniques. Initially, mechanical ventilation was largely dependent on a tracheostomy interface, with endotracheal tubes becoming more widely available in the 1960s [1]. Throughout the 1950s–1970s, mechanical ventilation became more widespread with further innovation in ventilatory devices and modes. However, as IMV became more universal, there was increasing recognition and understanding of potential complications stemming from endotracheal tubes and tracheostomy devices. Ultimately, this led to a renewed interest in noninvasive ventilation.

Although first tried as early as the 1950s with subsequent use in a few specialized centers, NIV did not become widely available until the 1980s [1]. Continuous positive airway pressure (CPAP) via a nasal mask interface was first introduced in 1981, demonstrating complete resolution of upper airway collapse in patients with obstructive sleep apnea (OSA) [3]. The same group that made this discovery demonstrated the benefits of long-term NIV in a small group of patients with post-infectious muscular weakness and muscular dystrophy [4]. This was followed in the late 1980s with multiple studies showing the potential benefit of NIV in disorders mostly involving neuromuscular weakness and restrictive thoracic disorders [1]. With an influx of studies demonstrating the benefits of long-term NIV and the combined patient and clinician interest in avoiding potential complications of IMV, interest in NIV in managing acute respiratory failure resurfaced. From 1989 to the early 1990s, there were several studies that demonstrated the efficacy of NIV in avoiding IMV in patients with COPD exacerbations, congestive heart failure, and pneumonia [5–10].

With convincing data of efficacy for NIV for certain forms of acute respiratory failure, a rising interest in outpatient NIV developed along with innovation in outpatient NIV technologies. Data has accumulated suggesting significant survival benefit in neuromuscular diseases, Duchenne muscular dystrophy, and amyotrophic lateral sclerosis (ALS) [11, 12]. In addition, a few randomized controlled trials have demonstrated potential benefits in quality of life, hospital readmissions, and mortality in patients with chronic hypercapnia due to severe COPD [13]. These developments have led to the emergence of a subspecialty within pulmonary and sleep medicine for managing patients with chronic respiratory failure with home ventilation.

Physiologic Effects of Noninvasive Ventilation

Noninvasive ventilation (NIV) is a critical therapeutic modality in the management of various respiratory conditions, offering significant physiologic benefits without the need for invasive airways. The benefits of NIV in addressing respiratory derangements derive from similar physiologic effects on the respiratory system seen with invasive ventilation while simultaneously avoiding some of the deleterious effects of an invasive airway. Artificial translaryngeal airways can be uncomfortable and often require sedation for better patient tolerance. Sedation can prolong time on IMV, which can potentially lead to a host of downstream deleterious effects, worsening morbidity and mortality. Importantly, NIV likely reduces the risk of nosocomial infections compared to IMV [14]. In addition, NIV allows for intermittent breaks, which facilitate speaking and swallowing.

One major physiologic benefit of positive-pressure ventilation is the increase in functional residual capacity (FRC). FRC is defined as the volume of air remaining in the lungs after passive exhalation. The FRC behaves as an oxygen reservoir and, when optimized, can aid in alveolar recruitment. This becomes even more important in the setting of respiratory system derangements in acute and chronic lung conditions, as well as in chronic restrictive thoracic disorders. In these conditions, the closing capacity, the lung volume at which small airways collapse, can be increased, requiring a higher FRC to maintain alveolar recruitment [15]. In addition, improving FRC and alveolar recruitment with positive end-expiratory pressure (PEEP) has been demonstrated to improve lung compliance [16]. Maintaining patent small airways and alveolar units while simultaneously improving lung compliance should ultimately improve oxygenation and ventilation and reduce the work of breathing. It has been shown in patients newly intubated on IMV with zero PEEP that FRC drops significantly compared to spontaneous breathing. In this study, FRC was restored with a PEEP of 7.5 cm H_2O and was increased further with a PEEP of 10 cm H_2O, with a 1000 cc increase in FRC at this PEEP level compared to FRC at 0 PEEP [17]. While the study was performed on patients receiving IMV, this effect likely can be extrapolated to NIV. Just as importantly, improved alveolar recruitment and reduced derecruitment will optimize ventilation–perfusion (V/Q) matching, further improving oxygenation and ventilation [18].

Another potential benefit of NIV is the unloading of respiratory muscles, particularly in the setting of increased ventilatory demands and/or increased resistive or elastic forces in the lungs. NIV can unload the respiratory muscles in two ways. First, in patients passively receiving machine-controlled breaths, NIV can reduce the required patient efforts. Second, when a patient is assisted by a ventilator-delivered breath, NIV reduces the muscle load required for a particular tidal volume. In addition, by improving oxygenation and reducing respiratory acidosis and mechanical load, the intensity of output from the Ventilatory Control Center located in the brain stem can be reduced [19]. The combination of these effects can reduce muscle fatigue and offset the protective neural drive to reduce fatigue that can contribute to hypoventilation [20]. However, it is important to note that inappropriate NIV settings can impose increased ventilatory muscle load [21]. This can occur in the setting of ineffective triggering or with cycle asynchronies when the neural and machine-set inspiratory times are disparate.

Positive-pressure ventilation is also employed in managing upper airway collapse in patients with obstructive sleep apnea. Positive pressure, in the form of either PEEP or CPAP alone, can splint open upper airway structures to prevent collapse that would lead to obstructive events [22]. In patients receiving bi-level NIV at night, it is important that the PEEP is set at sufficient pressure to overcome upper airway collapse.

One potential deleterious physiologic effect of NIV occurs in relation to dead space. Contrary to IMV, which reduces anatomic dead space, NIV actually increases dead space. Anatomic dead space constitutes the tubular volume of the airway that does not participate in gas exchange. This starts at the mouth and nostrils and ends distally at the end of the terminal bronchioles before the respiratory bronchioles appear. Because an endotracheal tube bypasses much of the upper airway, dead space is effectively reduced. However, with a noninvasive interface, this dead space will only be increased and depend on the size of the face mask. Kain et al. demonstrated in 1969 that when compared with breathing through a face mask, IMV via an endotracheal tube reduced dead space by about 82 cc's on average [23]. Saatci et al. demonstrated that with a typical full-face mask, anatomical dead space increased from 32% to 42% of the tidal volume [24]. Despite an increase in dead-space ventilation from a facemask interface with NIV, the effective tidal-volume augmentation achieved can often offset this effect and ultimately improve alveolar ventilation.

Use of Noninvasive Ventilation in an Inpatient Setting

While NIV is not appropriate for all patients with acute respiratory failure, its utilization in suitable patients can ultimately ward off the need for IMV and improve outcomes. Relative contraindications are important to take into consideration when deciding whether a patient is a good candidate for NIV. The absolute and relative contraindications are outlined in Fig. 17.1.

Contraindications for Non-Invasive Ventilation

Absolute	Relative
Respiratory arrest	Agitation and/or altered mental status
Cardiac arrest	Inability to protect airway
Uncontrolled vomiting	Excessive secretions
Complete upper airway obstruction	Multi-organ failure
Coma	Shock
	Severe upper GI bleeding
	Facial trauma
	Certain facial deformities
	Severe hemoptysis
	Progressive respiratory failure

Fig. 17.1 Relative and absolute contraindications to noninvasive ventilation

In the following section, we will explore the utility of NIV in specific acute respiratory conditions.

Acute Exacerbations of COPD

In the early 1990s, a landmark randomized controlled trial (RCT) showed that early NIV in patients with acute exacerbations of COPD (AE-COPD) with hypercapnia had a robust effect on preventing invasive mechanical ventilation when compared to those who received usual care without NIV [25]. Subsequent RCTs and meta-analyses further confirmed that NIV in AE-COPD reduces intubation rates, mortality, and hospital length of stay [26–28]. This data ultimately led to clinical practice guidelines recommending the utilization of NIV in patients with AE-COPD with acute or acute-on-chronic respiratory acidosis (pH $\leq$ 7.35) unless the patient is immediately deteriorating (strong recommendation, high certainty of evidence) [29]. NIV can provide significant benefit to these patients by improving alveolar ventilation via augmentation of tidal volumes, reduction in respiratory rates, and subsequent reduction in dynamic hyperinflation. There is also a potential benefit of applied PEEP counterbalancing auto-PEEP, which, if not addressed, can lead to increased respiratory muscle load, ineffective triggering, and worsening dead-space ventilation [30]. These effects ultimately reduce the work of breathing and improve oxygenation and hypercapnia [30, 31].

Acute Cardiogenic Pulmonary Edema

Patients with acute cardiogenic pulmonary edema due to congestive heart failure (CHF) may also benefit from the use of NIV. The pathophysiology of respiratory failure during cardiogenic pulmonary edema includes decreased respiratory system compliance and alveolar flooding due to high capillary hydrostatic pressure from elevated left-sided cardiac filling pressures. Positive-pressure ventilation will help the physiological disturbances of respiratory distress and failure, as described above, but can also have potential beneficial effects on the failing left ventricle. By increasing intrathoracic pressures and reducing the gradient for venous return to the right atrium, positive pressure can reduce preload to both the right and left ventricles [32]. In addition, it can also reduce left ventricular afterload by lowering transmural pressure across the myocardium [30]. It should be noted that increased intrathoracic pressures will elevate right ventricular afterload, and, therefore, positive-pressure ventilation should be used with caution in patients with an acutely failing right ventricle. While RCTs have shown conflicting results, systematic reviews and meta-analyses have consistently demonstrated a reduction in intubations and mortality with the application of CPAP or NIV in this patient population [33]. With the evidence that exists, clinical practice guidelines recommend the use of bi-level NIV or CPAP for patients with acute respiratory failure due to cardiogenic pulmonary edema (strong recommendation, moderate certainty of evidence) [29]. Practically speaking, NIV is most likely to provide benefit in acute heart failure when a patient has increased work of breathing, accessory muscle use, and/or CO_2 retention.

Acute Exacerbations of Asthma

Because of the lack of clear evidence demonstrating benefit for NIV in acute asthma exacerbations, the ATS/ERS 2017 clinical practice guideline did not make a recommendation for or against NIV use in this setting [29]. This may be due to the challenges faced in developing high-quality RCTs in this patient population. However, a 2024 systematic review of eight RCTs and five observational studies found that NIV was associated with reduced intubation rates and time to improvement in accessory muscle use [34]. There were too few deaths to assess for mortality benefit. However, given the potential difficulties in ventilating patients with acute exacerbations of asthma as well as the complications that can be seen with IMV, a trial of NIV is a reasonable approach but must be used with caution on a case-by-case basis.

De Novo Acute Hypoxemic Respiratory Failure

Patients with respiratory distress and/or significant gas exchange issues related to de novo respiratory failure from a variety of diagnoses, such as infectious and noninfectious pneumonia and acute respiratory distress syndrome (ARDS), may be placed on NIV with the hope of warding off the need for IMV. While a large number of clinical trials have been performed assessing outcomes of NIV in this patient population with mixed results, meta-analyses have shown that the risk of intubation and mortality is lower in patients who receive NIV than those treated with conventional oxygen therapy alone [35]. There exists evidence for concern of prolonged periods of vigorous patient respiratory efforts causing self-inflicted lung injury due to large swings in transpulmonary pressures while on NIV [36]. While this phenomenon can be seen with IMV, the presence of an invasive airway allows for the utilization of sedation and paralytics to try to minimize such harm. Additionally, patients with high respiratory drive on NIV can pull larger tidal volumes than would typically be targeted with IMV, where this variable can be more tightly controlled [37]. This further raises concern for the potential for volutrauma with NIV in this patient population. Given that lung-protective ventilation cannot be reliably achieved with NIV, it is likely best reserved for patients with milder respiratory failure combined with a lower respiratory drive [38]. This strategy is supported by an observational study showing that NIV failure was higher in patients with more severe ARDS and higher tidal volumes while on NIV [39]. Given the uncertainty of evidence, clinical practice guidelines from 2017 were unable to offer a recommendation for the use of NIV in de novo acute respiratory failure [29]. In addition, the presence of non-pulmonary organ dysfunction should be factored into decision-making when considering a trial of NIV. If there is significant neurologic or hemodynamic compromise, NIV is likely to fail [38].

A particular patient population with de novo hypoxemic respiratory failure that may benefit from NIV includes patients who are immunosuppressed. Acute respiratory failure in patients who are immunocompromised can have particularly high mortality rates, especially if needing IMV. Studies suggest that early use of NIV in this population could provide a meaningful benefit in outcomes. It was demonstrated in an RCT that the utilization of NIV in patients with a solid organ transplant suffering from acute hypoxemic respiratory failure led to a reduction in intubation rates, complications, ICU length of stay, and mortality compared with the standard of care [40]. Another study demonstrated a mortality benefit with NIV use in patients with bilateral pulmonary infiltrates in a setting of an immunosuppressed state secondary to hematological malignancies, transplantation, or HIV infection [41]. Based on this data, guidelines recommend early NIV for immunocompromised patients with acute respiratory failure (Conditional recommendation, moderate certainty of evidence) [29].

Post-Extubation

Re-intubation after a trial of extubation in the setting of respiratory failure is associated with increased morbidity and mortality [42]. NIV has been studied as a potential bridge to more successful extubation rates in patient populations at elevated risk for re-intubation. It can be used preemptively to prevent the onset of post-extubation respiratory failure or reactively when patients develop this condition. Studies have demonstrated reduced re-intubation rates, post-extubation respiratory failure, and ICU mortality in patients with increased age (>65 years), hypercapnia, congestive heart failure, as well as obesity [43–46]. However, it should be noted that when nonselectively applied preventively or to patients with post-extubation respiratory failure, NIV does not seem to improve re-intubation rates or mortality [47–49]. Based on available data, clinical practice guidelines suggest that NIV be used to prevent post-extubation respiratory failure in high-risk patients (conditional recommendation and low certainty of evidence), while recommending against its use in non-high-risk patients [29].

Use of Noninvasive Ventilation for Chronic Respiratory Failure in the Ambulatory Setting

While the fundamental physiologic principles underlying the use of NIV in acute respiratory failure discussed above remain applicable, its implementation in chronic respiratory failure confers potentially distinct benefits when administered in the outpatient setting. In the outpatient management of chronic respiratory failure, NIV is primarily utilized during sleep, although patients with progressive neuromuscular disorders—such as amyotrophic lateral sclerosis (ALS) or Duchenne muscular dystrophy—may ultimately require diurnal support as their disease advances.

While logistically easier to implement during sleep, the rationale for nocturnal NIV use is also grounded in the characteristic alterations in respiratory physiology that occur during sleep. In particular, rapid eye movement (REM) sleep is associated with marked reductions in skeletal muscle tone, including the intercostal and accessory respiratory muscles, while diaphragmatic function is variably preserved [50]. In patients with underlying diaphragmatic weakness or paralysis, this reduction in compensatory muscle activity can lead to significant hypoventilation. These individuals become especially vulnerable to alveolar hypoventilation, hypercapnia, and subsequent nocturnal hypoxemia.

Moreover, the supine position exacerbates these derangements by increasing upper airway collapsibility due to gravitational influences on the pharyngeal soft tissues [51]. In addition, the supine position can increase diaphragmatic load through cephalad displacement of abdominal contents, especially in obese patients [52]. This effect is most prominent on the dorsocaudal aspect of the diaphragm, compromising its excursion. This can lead to atelectasis and impaired alveolar ventilation in the crucial dorsocaudal regions of the lung that receive a large portion of the blood flow distribution in this position. FRC has also been demonstrated to be reduced during sleep, further placing patients at risk for atelectasis [53]. By resting the respiratory muscles overnight, reducing atelectasis via lung recruitment, and improving or normalizing CO_2 levels in the blood, adequate nighttime NIV may improve daytime gas exchange and symptoms in patients with chronic respiratory failure.

In the following section, conditions associated with chronic respiratory failure with potential benefit from domiciliary NIV will be discussed. While patients with OSA, particularly more severe cases, clearly derive benefit from continuous positive airway pressure (CPAP), this condition will not be explicitly discussed, as this chapter focuses more on bi-level positive-pressure delivery in the setting of acute and chronic respiratory failure. Notably, patients with obesity hypoventilation syndrome (OHS) benefit from bi-level NIV if they fail to improve with CPAP alone [52].

COPD with Chronic Hypercapnia

Acute exacerbations of COPD (AE-COPD) are associated with significant morbidity and mortality and are a leading cause of hospital admissions and the third most common cause of hospital readmissions among Medicare beneficiaries [13, 54]. Particularly, patients with chronic hypercapnic COPD are at higher risk of hospital readmission and death [55]. With clear benefit demonstrated for NIV in patients with AE-COPD with acute hypercapnia, there was emerging interest in studying the potential benefit in severe COPD patients with a history of acute or chronic hypercapnia. Early studies demonstrated mixed results, with most studies showing no benefit of NIV versus usual care [56–58]. However, there was concern that the results were impacted by patient selection and NIV settings that were not intensive enough [13]. Studies were, therefore, performed utilizing the strategy of high-intensity NIV (HI-NIV) in which inspiratory pressures were set on bi-level devices with inspiratory pressures often above 20 cm H_2O. It was felt that HI-NIV was needed to best offset the derangements in respiratory mechanics and gas exchange in this patient population. The HOT-HMV UK trial demonstrated an increased time to readmission or death, mostly driven by a difference in hospital readmissions [59]. Khonlein et al. demonstrated a significant mortality benefit (12% in the HI-NIV group versus 33% in the control group) in stable GOLD 4 COPD patients with chronic hypercapnia [60]. Notably, this trial was unique in that it targeted a reduction in $PaCO_2$. Interestingly, this study demonstrated no difference in exacerbations.

Both the ATS and ERS guidelines recommend domiciliary NIV for severe COPD. However, one notable difference is in guidance regarding whether chronic stable hypercapnia is required. The ERS recommends consideration of NIV if in hospital with acute hypercapnia in the setting of COPD. However, the ATS recommends waiting at least 2 weeks after a hospitalization for AE-COPD to see if the patient has chronic hypercapnia in a fully recovered, stable state [61, 62].

In June 2025, the Centers for Medicare & Medicaid Services (CMS) revised their national coverage determination for the prescription of ambulatory NIV in patients with severe hypercapnic COPD. This update, informed by expert consensus, was prompted by concerns that previous guidelines were overly restrictive and lacked a strong physiologic rationale, thereby limiting access to potentially beneficial therapy [63]. The revised policy is expected to facilitate the prescription of bi-level positive airway pressure (BPAP) devices with backup rates for appropriate patients while curbing the overuse of costly and often unnecessary home mechanical ventilators. This change aims to expand patient access to effective treatment, reduce healthcare expenditures, and potentially lower hospital readmission rates [64, 65].

Neuromuscular Disease and Restrictive Thoracic Disorders

Home noninvasive ventilation (NIV) has shown substantial benefit in patients with neuromuscular diseases (NMD) and restrictive thoracic disorders. Although both groups typically present with reduced vital capacity, the underlying pathophysiology differs significantly. In neuromuscular disorders, respiratory muscle weakness impairs the generation of adequate tidal volumes, even in the presence of a normally compliant respiratory system. In contrast, restrictive thoracic disorders are characterized by reduced respiratory system compliance, which increases the inspiratory load and places excessive demand on otherwise functional respiratory muscles. Both conditions are particularly susceptible to hypoventilation during supine sleep due to the combined effects of altered mechanics and reduced ventilatory drive. Whether the primary issue is insufficient muscular force to meet ventilatory demand or increased load due to a stiff thoracic cage, NIV provides crucial support by unloading the respiratory muscles, enhancing ventilation, and improving gas exchange.

In patients with NMD, NIV can provide symptomatic relief of dyspnea, improve sleep quality, and potentially improve survival [66]. Data have accumulated in more recent years suggesting significant survival benefit in neuromuscular diseases, Duchenne muscular dystrophy, and amyotrophic lateral sclerosis (ALS) [11, 12]. In the United States, NIV is recommended when the forced vital capacity (FVC) is less than 50% of predicted, maximal inspiratory pressure (MIP) or negative inspiratory force (NIF) is less negative than −60 cm H_2O, or when there is evidence of chronic hypercapnia with a $PaCO_2$ of 45 mmHg or higher on arterial blood gas (ABG). However, experts in the field feel these criteria are too strict and lead to late initiation of NIV in patients who would otherwise benefit from earlier initiation [67].

While there are no randomized controlled trials proving the benefit of NIV in restrictive thoracic disorders, the benefit of NIV in NMDs may be able to be extrapolated to this patient population. In addition, there is accumulating data that chronic hypercapnia may have deleterious health effects and that improving, or ideally normalizing, CO_2 levels may improve patient outcomes [68]. The criteria for NIV prescription in restrictive thoracic disorders are the same as for NMD's; however, thoracic disorders must meet two of the above criteria, while NMDs only need to meet one criterion.

Conclusion

In summary, NIV represents a remarkable advance over invasive mechanical ventilation in well-selected patients. Utilized in such circumstances and especially for patients with exacerbations of COPD, heart failure with pulmonary edema, select cases of acute hypoxemic respiratory failure, and post-extubation in high-risk patients. With good implementation in a well-suited patient, they may avoid the need for endotracheal intubation and the complications that stem from an invasive airway. In addition, NIV shows considerable promise in the ambulatory settings for patients with sleep-disordered breathing and chronic respiratory failure related to severe COPD, NMDs, and restrictive thoracic disorders. As technologies for treating and monitoring this high-risk patient population continue to evolve, there will be an ongoing need for practitioners with particular expertise to help achieve the best possible outcomes for these patients.

References

1. Pierson DJ. History and epidemiology of noninvasive ventilation in the acute-care setting. Respir Care. 2009;54(1):40–52.
2. Motley HL, Werko L. Observations on the clinical use of intermittent positive pressure. J Aviat Med. 1947;18(5):417–35.
3. Sullivan CE, Issa FG, Berthon-Jones M, Eves L. Reversal of obstructive sleep apnoea by continuous positive airway pressure applied through the nares. Lancet. 1981;1(8225):862–5.
4. Ellis ER, Bye PT, Bruderer JW, Sullivan CE. Treatment of respiratory failure during sleep in patients with neuromuscular disease. Positive-pressure ventilation through a nose mask. Am Rev Respir Dis. 1987;135(1):148–52.
5. Meduri GU, Conoscenti CC, Menashe P, Nair S. Noninvasive face mask ventilation in patients with acute respiratory failure. Chest. 1989;95(4):865–70.
6. Foglio C, Vitacca M, Quadri A, Scalvini S, Marangoni S, Ambrosino N. Acute exacerbations in severe COLD patients. Treatment using positive pressure ventilation by nasal mask. Chest. 1992;101(6):1533–8.
7. Bott J, Carroll MP, Conway JH, Keilty SE, Ward EM, Brown AM, et al. Randomised controlled trial of nasal ventilation in acute ventilatory failure due to chronic obstructive airways disease. Lancet. 1993;341(8860):1555–7.
8. Meecham Jones DJ, Paul EA, Grahame-Clarke C, Wedzicha JA. Nasal ventilation in acute exacerbations of chronic obstructive pulmonary disease: effect of ventilator mode on arterial blood gas tensions. Thorax. 1994;49(12):1222–4.
9. Brochard L, Isabey D, Piquet J, Amaro P, Mancebo J, Messadi AA, et al. Reversal of acute exacerbations of chronic obstructive lung disease by inspiratory assistance with a face mask. N Engl J Med. 1990;323(22):1523–30.
10. Meduri GU, Abou-Shala N, Fox RC, Jones CB, Leeper KV, Wunderink RG. Noninvasive face mask mechanical ventilation in patients with acute hypercapnic respiratory failure. Chest. 1991;100(2):445–54.
11. Eagle M, Baudouin SV, Chandler C, Giddings DR, Bullock R, Bushby K. Survival in Duchenne muscular dystrophy: improvements in life expectancy since 1967 and the impact of home nocturnal ventilation. Neuromuscul Disord. 2002;12(10):926–9.
12. Ackrivo J, Hsu JY, Hansen-Flaschen J, Elman L, Kawut SM. Noninvasive ventilation use is associated with better survival in amyotrophic lateral sclerosis. Ann Am Thorac Soc. 2021;18(3):486–94.
13. Coleman JM, Wolfe LF, Kalhan R. Noninvasive ventilation in chronic obstructive pulmonary disease. Ann Am Thorac Soc. 2019;16(9):1091–8.
14. Girou E, Schortgen F, Delclaux C, Brun-Buisson C, Blot F, Lefort Y, et al. Association of noninvasive ventilation with nosocomial infections and survival in critically ill patients. JAMA. 2000;284(18):2361–7.
15. Garland A, Hopton P. Airway closure in anaesthesia and intensive care. BJA Educ. 2022;22(4):126–30.
16. Suter PM, Fairley HB, Isenberg MD. Effect of tidal volume and positive end-expiratory pressure on compliance during mechanical ventilation. Chest. 1978;73(2):158–62.

17. Satoh D, Kurosawa S, Kirino W, Wagatsuma T, Ejima Y, Yoshida A, et al. Impact of changes of positive end-expiratory pressure on functional residual capacity at low tidal volume ventilation during general anesthesia. J Anesth. 2012;26(5):664–9.
18. Gattinoni L, Pelosi P, Crotti S, Valenza F. Effects of positive end-expiratory pressure on regional distribution of tidal volume and recruitment in adult respiratory distress syndrome. Am J Respir Crit Care Med. 1995;151(6):1807–14.
19. Mitrouska J, Xirouchaki N, Patakas D, Siafakas N, Georgopoulos D. Effects of chemical feedback on respiratory motor and ventilatory output during different modes of assisted mechanical ventilation. Eur Respir J. 1999;13(4):873–82.
20. MacIntyre NR. Physiologic effects of noninvasive ventilation. Respir Care. 2019;64(6):617–28.
21. Williams K, Hinojosa-Kurtzberg M, Parthasarathy S. Control of breathing during mechanical ventilation: who is the boss? Respir Care. 2011;56(2):127–36; discussion 136.
22. Nicolini A, Banfi P, Grecchi B, Lax A, Walterspacher S, Barlascini C, et al. Non-invasive ventilation in the treatment of sleep-related breathing disorders: a review and update. Rev Port Pneumol. 2014;20(6):324–35.
23. Kain ML, Panday J, Nunn JF. The effect of intubation on the deadspace during halothane anaesthesia. Br J Anaesth. 1969;41(2):94–103.
24. Saatci E, Miller DM, Stell IM, Lee KC, Moxham J. Dynamic dead space in face masks used with noninvasive ventilators: a lung model study. Eur Respir J. 2004;23(1):129–35.
25. Brochard L, Mancebo J, Wysocki M, Lofaso F, Conti G, Rauss A, et al. Noninvasive ventilation for acute exacerbations of chronic obstructive pulmonary disease. N Engl J Med. 1995;333(13):817–22.
26. Plant PK, Owen JL, Elliott MW. Early use of non-invasive ventilation for acute exacerbations of chronic obstructive pulmonary disease on general respiratory wards: a multicentre randomised controlled trial. Lancet. 2000;355(9219):1931–5.
27. Plant PK, Owen JL, Elliott MW. Non-invasive ventilation in acute exacerbations of chronic obstructive pulmonary disease: long term survival and predictors of in-hospital outcome. Thorax. 2001;56(9):708–12.
28. Osadnik CR, Tee VS, Carson-Chahhoud KV, Picot J, Wedzicha JA, Smith BJ. Non-invasive ventilation for the management of acute hypercapnic respiratory failure due to exacerbation of chronic obstructive pulmonary disease. Cochrane Database Syst Rev. 2017;7(7):CD004104.
29. Rochwerg B, Brochard L, Elliott MW, Hess D, Hill NS, Nava S, et al. Official ERS/ATS clinical practice guidelines: noninvasive ventilation for acute respiratory failure. Eur Respir J. 2017;50(2):1602426.
30. Appendini L, Patessio A, Zanaboni S, Carone M, Gukov B, Donner CF, et al. Physiologic effects of positive end-expiratory pressure and mask pressure support during exacerbations of chronic obstructive pulmonary disease. Am J Respir Crit Care Med. 1994;149(5):1069–76.
31. Diaz O, Iglesia R, Ferrer M, Zavala E, Santos C, Wagner PD, et al. Effects of noninvasive ventilation on pulmonary gas exchange and hemodynamics during acute hypercapnic exacerbations of chronic obstructive pulmonary disease. Am J Respir Crit Care Med. 1997;156(6):1840–5.
32. Alviar CL, Miller PE, McAreavey D, Katz JN, Lee B, Moriyama B, et al. Positive pressure ventilation in the cardiac intensive care unit. J Am Coll Cardiol. 2018;72(13):1532–53.
33. Cabrini L, Landoni G, Oriani A, Plumari VP, Nobile L, Greco M, et al. Noninvasive ventilation and survival in acute care settings: a comprehensive systematic review and metaanalysis of randomized controlled trials. Crit Care Med. 2015;43(4):880–8.
34. Homer-Bouthiette C, Wilson KC. Non-invasive ventilation in acute asthma exacerbations: a systematic review. Ann Am Thorac Soc. 2025;22(5):776–84.
35. Ferreyro BL, Angriman F, Munshi L, Del Sorbo L, Ferguson ND, Rochwerg B, et al. Association of noninvasive oxygenation strategies with all-cause mortality in adults with acute hypoxemic respiratory failure: a systematic review and meta-analysis. JAMA. 2020;324(1):57–67.
36. Yoshida T, Fujino Y, Amato MBP, Kavanagh BP. Fifty years of research in ARDS. Spontaneous breathing during mechanical ventilation. Risks, mechanisms, and management. Am J Respir Crit Care Med. 2017;195(8):985–92.

37. Carteaux G, Millán-Guilarte T, De Prost N, Razazi K, Abid S, Thille AW, et al. Failure of noninvasive ventilation for de novo acute hypoxemic respiratory failure: role of tidal volume. Crit Care Med. 2016;44(2):282–90.
38. Munshi L, Mancebo J, Brochard LJ. Noninvasive respiratory support for adults with acute respiratory failure. N Engl J Med. 2022;387(18):1688–98.
39. Bellani G, Laffey JG, Pham T, Madotto F, Fan E, Brochard L, et al. Noninvasive ventilation of patients with acute respiratory distress syndrome. Insights from the LUNG SAFE study. Am J Respir Crit Care Med. 2017;195(1):67–77.
40. Antonelli M, Conti G, Bufi M, Costa MG, Lappa A, Rocco M, et al. Noninvasive ventilation for treatment of acute respiratory failure in patients undergoing solid organ transplantation: a randomized trial. JAMA. 2000;283(2):235–41.
41. Hilbert G, Gruson D, Vargas F, Valentino R, Gbikpi-Benissan G, Dupon M, et al. Noninvasive ventilation in immunosuppressed patients with pulmonary infiltrates, fever, and acute respiratory failure. N Engl J Med. 2001;344(7):481–7.
42. Dadam MM, Pereira AB, Cardoso MR, Carnin TC, Westphal GA. Effect of reintubation within 48 hours on mortality in critically ill patients after planned extubation. Respir Care. 2024;69(7):829–38.
43. Thille AW, Le Pape S. Prophylactic noninvasive ventilation after extubation of obese patients. Am J Respir Crit Care Med. 2025;211(2):146–8.
44. Ferrer M, Sellarés J, Valencia M, Carrillo A, Gonzalez G, Badia JR, et al. Non-invasive ventilation after extubation in hypercapnic patients with chronic respiratory disorders: randomised controlled trial. Lancet. 2009;374(9695):1082–8.
45. Ferrer M, Valencia M, Nicolas JM, Bernadich O, Badia JR, Torres A. Early noninvasive ventilation averts extubation failure in patients at risk: a randomized trial. Am J Respir Crit Care Med. 2006;173(2):164–70.
46. Nava S, Gregoretti C, Fanfulla F, Squadrone E, Grassi M, Carlucci A, et al. Noninvasive ventilation to prevent respiratory failure after extubation in high-risk patients. Crit Care Med. 2005;33(11):2465–70.
47. Esteban A, Frutos-Vivar F, Ferguson ND, Arabi Y, Apezteguía C, González M, et al. Noninvasive positive-pressure ventilation for respiratory failure after extubation. N Engl J Med. 2004;350(24):2452–60.
48. Keenan SP, Powers C, McCormack DG, Block G. Noninvasive positive-pressure ventilation for postextubation respiratory distress: a randomized controlled trial. JAMA. 2002;287(24):3238–44.
49. Su C-L, Chiang L-L, Yang S-H, Lin H-I, Cheng K-C, Huang Y-CT, et al. Preventive use of noninvasive ventilation after extubation: a prospective, multicenter randomized controlled trial. Respir Care. 2012;57(2):204–10.
50. Tabachnik E, Muller NL, Bryan AC, Levison H. Changes in ventilation and chest wall mechanics during sleep in normal adolescents. J Appl Physiol. 1981;51(3):557–64.
51. Dempsey JA, Veasey SC, Morgan BJ, O'Donnell CP. Pathophysiology of sleep apnea. Physiol Rev. 2010;90(1):47–112.
52. Masa JF, Pépin J-L, Borel J-C, Mokhlesi B, Murphy PB, Sánchez-Quiroga MÁ. Obesity hypoventilation syndrome. Eur Respir Rev. 2019;28(151):180097.
53. Hudgel DW, Devadatta P. Decrease in functional residual capacity during sleep in normal humans. J Appl Physiol. 1984;57(5):1319–22.
54. Jencks SF, Williams MV, Coleman EA. Rehospitalizations among patients in the Medicare fee-for-service program. N Engl J Med. 2009;360(14):1418–28.
55. Csoma B, Vulpi MR, Dragonieri S, Bentley A, Felton T, Lázár Z, et al. Hypercapnia in COPD: causes, consequences, and therapy. J Clin Med. 2022;11(11):3180.
56. Casanova C, Celli BR, Tost L, Soriano E, Abreu J, Velasco V, et al. Long-term controlled trial of nocturnal nasal positive pressure ventilation in patients with severe COPD. Chest. 2000;118(6):1582–90.

57. Clini E, Sturani C, Rossi A, Viaggi S, Corrado A, Donner CF, et al. The Italian multicentre study on noninvasive ventilation in chronic obstructive pulmonary disease patients. Eur Respir J. 2002;20(3):529–38.
58. McEvoy RD, Pierce RJ, Hillman D, Esterman A, Ellis EE, Catcheside PG, et al. Nocturnal non-invasive nasal ventilation in stable hypercapnic COPD: a randomised controlled trial. Thorax. 2009;64(7):561–6.
59. Murphy PB, Rehal S, Arbane G, Bourke S, Calverley PMA, Crook AM, et al. Effect of home noninvasive ventilation with oxygen therapy vs oxygen therapy alone on hospital readmission or death after an acute COPD exacerbation: a randomized clinical trial. JAMA. 2017;317(21):2177–86.
60. Köhnlein T, Windisch W, Köhler D, Drabik A, Geiseler J, Hartl S, et al. Non-invasive positive pressure ventilation for the treatment of severe stable chronic obstructive pulmonary disease: a prospective, multicentre, randomised, controlled clinical trial. Lancet Respir Med. 2014;2(9):698–705.
61. Macrea M, Oczkowski S, Rochwerg B, Branson RD, Celli B, Coleman JM, et al. Long-term noninvasive ventilation in chronic stable hypercapnic chronic obstructive pulmonary disease. An official American Thoracic Society clinical practice guideline. Am J Respir Crit Care Med. 2020;202(4):e74–87.
62. Ergan B, Oczkowski S, Rochwerg B, Carlucci A, Chatwin M, Clini E, et al. European Respiratory Society guidelines on long-term home non-invasive ventilation for management of COPD. Eur Respir J. 2019;54(3):1901003.
63. Mokhlesi B, Won CH, Make BJ, Selim BJ, Sunwoo BY, ONMAP Technical Expert Panel. Optimal NIV Medicare access promotion: patients with hypoventilation syndromes: a technical expert panel report from the American college of chest physicians, the American association for respiratory care, the American academy of sleep medicine, and the American thoracic society. Chest. 2021;160(5):e377–87.
64. NCA – Noninvasive Positive Pressure Ventilation (NIPPV) in the home for the treatment of chronic respiratory failure consequent to COPD (CAG-00465N) – decision memo [Internet]. [cited 2025 Jun 24]. Available from: https://www.cms.gov/medicare-coverage-database/view/ncacal-decision-memo.aspx?proposed=N&ncaid=315.
65. Escalating Medicare Billing for Ventilators Raises Concerns | Office of Inspector General | Government Oversight | U.S. Department of Health and Human Services [Internet]. [cited 2025 Feb 13]. Available from: https://oig.hhs.gov/reports/all/2016/escalating-medicare-billing-for-ventilators-raises-concerns/.
66. Shneerson JM, Simonds AK. Noninvasive ventilation for chest wall and neuromuscular disorders. Eur Respir J. 2002;20(2):480–7.
67. Hill NS, Criner GJ, Branson RD, Celli BR, MacIntyre NR, Sergew A, et al. Optimal NIV medicare access promotion: patients with COPD: a technical expert panel report from the American College of Chest Physicians, the American Association for Respiratory Care, the American Academy of Sleep Medicine, and the American Thoracic Society. Chest. 2021;160(5):e389–97.
68. Wilson MW, Labaki WW, Choi PJ. Mortality and healthcare use of patients with compensated hypercapnia. Ann Am Thorac Soc. 2021;18(12):2027–32.

18 Medical Oxygen Production and Supply

Rafael Perez

Introduction

Purified oxygen is produced for industrial, chemical, and medical purposes. Many industries rely on the oxidant and catalytic properties of oxygen in their manufacturing [1]. The steel industry consumes the most commercial oxygen at 65%. Other industries, such as chemical manufacturing and fabrication of ceramics, glass, and metals, use around 24%. Water and wastewater treatment account for 5% of the commercial oxygen produced. Oxygen for medical use makes up 6% of commercial production. A notable difference for medical-grade oxygen is that it has strict regulatory requirements around purity, contaminants, containment specifications, and labeling [2]. The Food and Drug Administration treats medical oxygen as a prescription drug, like all medical gases [3].

Medical oxygen is produced by either cryogenic air separation (CAS) or pressure swing adsorption (PSA). The production method used depends on demand, available energy supply, ease of transportation, and cost. This chapter describes the methods for making medical-grade oxygen by CAS and PSA. The rationale for selecting each method is addressed. Regulatory issues around production, delivery, and consumption are discussed.

R. Perez (✉)
The Korman Respiratory Institute and the Division of Pulmonary, Allergy and Critical Care, The Department of Medicine at the Sidney Kimmel Medical College of Thomas Jefferson University, Philadelphia, PA, USA
e-mail: rafael.perez@jefferson.edu

G. C. Kane et al. (eds.), *Oxygen*, https://doi.org/10.1007/978-3-032-18934-9_18

Cryogenic Air Separation Plants and Oxygen Production and Delivery

Cryogenic air separation plants produce high-purity liquid oxygen, ≥99.5%, at a large scale (Fig. 18.1) [4–6]. The air separation procedure begins with the filtration of dust and other particulates from environmental air. The air is then compressed and undergoes cycles of heating and cooling by molecular sieving through zeolite and activated alumina beds in a process called temperature swing adsorption. This process retains and then expels carbon dioxide, water, hydrocarbons, and other contaminants. The air now contains oxygen, nitrogen, and argon with low levels of contaminants. The cleaned air then undergoes a pre-cooling phase by heat exchange using some of the already made cryogenic gas. The air is then liquefied in large distillation chambers by the Joule–Thomson effect [7], wherein the air is pressurized and rapidly expanded, cooling it to a liquid product. Oxygen, nitrogen, and argon are separated based on their different boiling points. A further post-separation molecular sieving may be applied to remove any remaining contaminants.

Medical-grade liquid oxygen produced by CAS is delivered to the end user in a liquid or gaseous form directly from the primary plant or taken to a storage facility for later distribution [5]. Liquid medical oxygen is delivered to hospitals in tanker trucks designed and certified to transport hazardous gases [8]. The liquid oxygen is pumped into large pressure-regulated storage tanks called vacuum-insulated evaporators located on or near the hospital grounds (Fig. 18.2). The liquid oxygen is

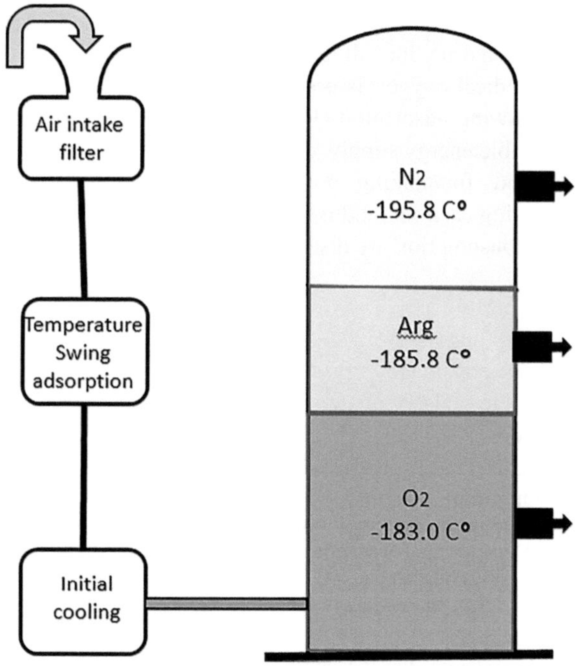

Fig. 18.1 Schematic of the CAS process for the production of liquid oxygen. The initial filtration, adsorption, and cooling stages prepare the now dry and essentially contamination-free air for cryogenic distillation. A series of distillation steps separates oxygen, nitrogen, and argon based on their different boiling points

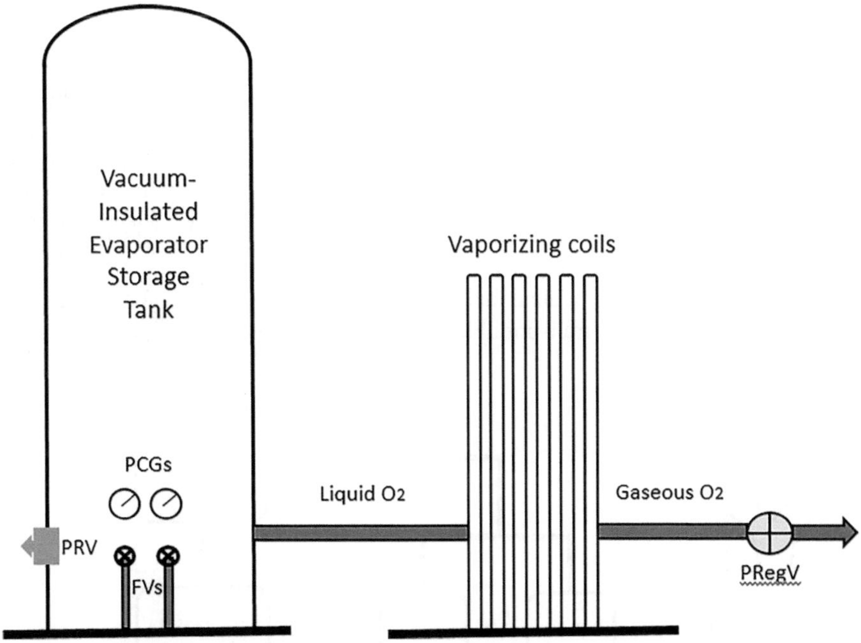

Fig. 18.2 Liquid oxygen delivered to the medical facility is loaded into the storage tank through fill valves (FVs). Oxygen content and pressure are continuously monitored by pressure control gages (PCGs). A pressure relief valve (PRV) dissipates critical increases in pressure as some of the liquid oxygen expands into gas. Liquid oxygen is pumped through vaporizer coils, where it warms and is converted to gaseous oxygen. The oxygen passes into the facility through pressure-regulated valves (PRegV)

channeled through a unit of vaporizing coils and converted to gaseous form. It is then piped into the hospital through pressure-regulated valves.

Some of the liquid oxygen is converted to gaseous oxygen and dispensed in pressurized and appropriately labeled cylinders, clear of contaminants. Compressed gaseous oxygen is used extensively for ambulatory and backup purposes in the home oxygen space. Portable oxygen cylinders in the hospital setting are used for transporting patients within the facility, and large stationary cylinders are stored for backup purposes.

The advantage of producing medical-grade oxygen by CAS is that it can be produced in scalable quantities to meet regional demands and with a purity of ≥99.5%. Moreover, the nitrogen and argon purified by cryogenic distillation are marketed for industrial use. The limitations of a CAS plant are that it requires a high initial investment and a reliable, substantial energy supply. The plant and storage facilities must be built on geologically stable land with a large footprint. Finally, a transportation system to safely deliver oxygen to the end user must be in place.

Pressure Swing Adsorption Plants and Oxygen Production

Pressure swing adsorption plants produce gaseous oxygen at 90–95% purity through molecular sieving, as described in a previous chapter [9, 10]. A PSA plant is essentially a scaled-up version of a home oxygen concentrator. However, there are additional filtration and air-drying steps done to prepare the air for adsorption (Fig. 18.3). The oxygen produced is collected, filtered, and piped directly into a facility's oxygen network. Some of the oxygen may be saved in compressed cylinders as a backup for power outages.

PSA plants are built at medical facilities that require medical oxygen service and do not have access to transportable liquid oxygen because of economic or

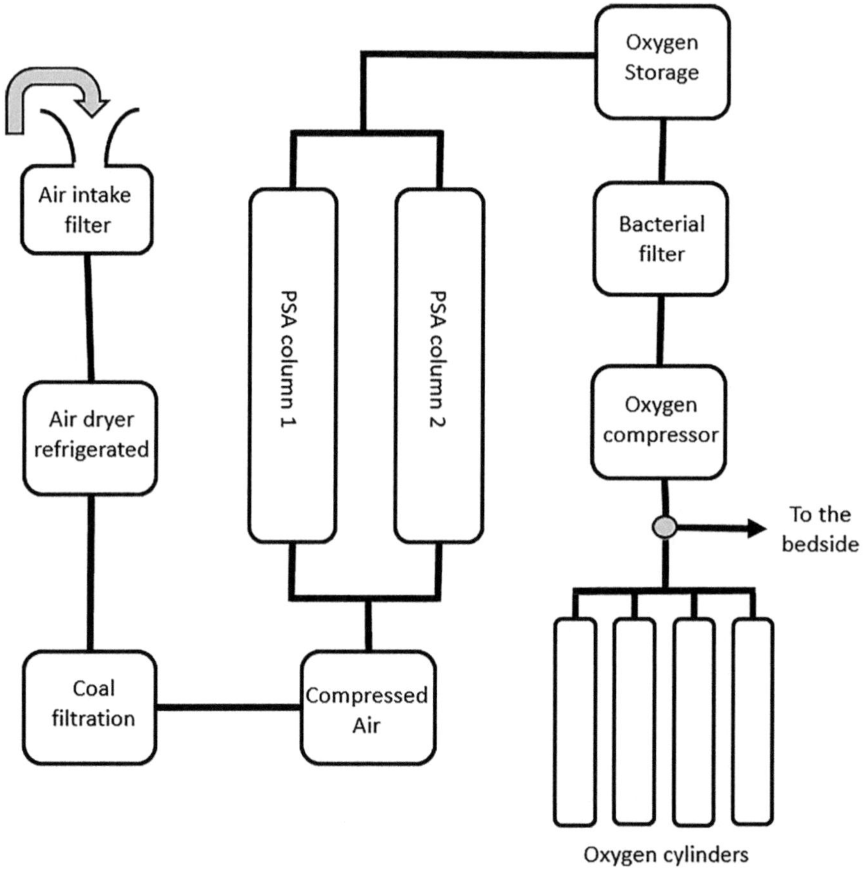

Fig. 18.3 Schematic of the PSA process for producing medical oxygen on-site. Feed air is drawn into the air intake and filtered for particulates. Moisture is removed from the air dryer. Coal filtration removes contaminating hydrocarbons. The air is then compressed and processed by PSA. The purified air is stored and then pulled through a bacterial filter on its way to the bedside or collected in cylinders

transportation barriers. PSA plants are scalable to produce the needed amounts of oxygen and adjustable to a facility's size and the configuration of the space that houses the plant. Their modular design means that they are more easily expanded or relocated.

Regulatory Requirements for Medical Oxygen Production and Delivery

The standards for the safety and efficacy of oxygen and other medical gases are set by the United States Pharmacopeia (USP) [2]. Pharmaceutical-grade medical oxygen must have a purity of 99.5%, which is achieved by CAS but not by PSA. Oxygen produced by PSA must have a purity of 93% +/− 3%. Contaminants must not exceed the following, in parts per million (ppm): carbon dioxide, 300 ppm; carbon monoxide, 5–10 ppm; hydrocarbons, 5 ppm [11]. Quality control is maintained by adhering to Current Good Manufacturing Practices (CGPMs). Batch testing with certificates of analysis is a requirement unique to medical oxygen.

The Food and Drug Administration issues and enforces rules that govern CMPGs, labeling, certification, and safety reporting for oxygen and other medical gases [3]. The Department of Transportation enforces the rules for the transportation of medical oxygen [12]. Medical oxygen is considered a hazardous material during transportation, so personnel responsible for its transport must have hazmat training, and drivers need specialized certification. Transport vehicles and tanker equipment must meet specifications to safely contain and carry liquid oxygen to the point of service. Placards and signage are required on all sides of the tankers warning that hazardous liquid is on board. A shipping manifest displaying the amount of product and demonstrating the chain of custody to the end user is required.

Medical Oxygen Distribution and Availability

Approximately 1.5 million people in the United States use supplemental oxygen at an annual cost of about 2.8 billion dollars [13]. Around 374 million individuals globally need oxygen annually for acute care or long-term therapy [14]. Notably, 82% of these individuals live in low- to middle-income countries (LMICs) lacking the financial and infrastructure resources to produce and supply medical oxygen. Overall, 60% of the world's population does not have ready access to medical oxygen. The 3.5-year COVID-19 pandemic glaringly demonstrated the inequity of medical oxygen, critical for treating the pulmonary complications of severe COVID-19. While high-income countries were able to adjust to the demand for medical oxygen during the pandemic [15], many patients living in LIMICs did not have access to desperately needed medical oxygen [14]. The World Health Organization, through its Access to Oxygen Initiative, is addressing the problem of improving the production of available and sustainable medical oxygen across the world [16].

References

1. EPA. Oxygen supply chain – EPA executive summary [Internet]. [cited 2025 July 30]. Available from: https://www.epa.gov/system/files/documents/2023-03/Oxygen%20Supply%20Chain%20Profile.pdf.
2. FasterCapital. Medical oxygen supply: navigating regulatory challenges in the medical oxygen supply business [Internet]. [cited 2025 July 30]. Available from: https://fastercapital.com/content/Medical-oxygen-supply%2D%2DNavigating-Regulatory-Challenges-in-the-Medical-Oxygen-Supply-Business.html.
3. U.S. Food & Drug. Current good manufacturing practice, certification, postmarketing safety reporting, and labeling requirements for certain medical gases. Fed Regist. 2024;89(118):51738–83.
4. Vinson DR. Air separation control technology. Comput Chem Eng. 2006;30:1436–46.
5. Jha M, Gaur N. Life cycle of medical oxygen from production to consumption. J Family Med Prim Care. 2022;11(4):1231–6.
6. Rao P, Muller M. Industrial oxygen: its generation and use. Center for Advanced Energy Systems, Rutgers, the State University of New Jersey. American Council for an Energy-Efficient Economy; 2007. p. 124–35.
7. Examples.com. Joule-Thomson effect—examples, definition, formula, uses, FAQ's [Internet]. [cited 2025 July 30]. Available from: https://www.examples.com/physics/joule-thomson-effect.html.
8. Jain R, Sharma C. Oxygen supply in hospitals: requisites in the current pandemic. Anesth Essays Res. 2021;15(3):253–6.
9. Jain V, Bhatia V. Out of breath in pandemic – is pressure swing adsorption (PSA) technology a solution for saving lives? J Family Med Prim Care. 2023;12(3):426–9.
10. Carty ML, Bilodeau S. Benchmarking thermodynamic models for optimization of PSA oxygen generators. Multidiscipl Sci J. 2023;6(2):318–41.
11. PHARMACISTPK. Pharmaceutical-grade oxygen (O_2): specifications, testing, and procedures [Internet]. [cited 2025 July 30]. Available from: https://pharmacistpk.com/pharmaceutical-grade-oxygen-o%e2%82%82-specifications-testing-and-procedures/.
12. Code of Federal Regulations. Part 172—Hazardous materials table, special provisions, hazardous materials communications, emergency response information, training requirements, and security plans [Internet]. [cited 2025 July 30]. Available from: https://www.ecfr.gov/current/title-49/subtitle-B/chapter-I/subchapter-C/part-172.
13. Jacobs SS, Lederer DJ, Garvey CM, Hernandez C, Lindell KO, McLaughlin S, et al. Optimizing home oxygen therapy. An official American Thoracic Society workshop report. Ann Am Thorac Soc. 2018;15(12):1369–81.
14. Graham HR, King C, Rahman AE, Kitutu FE, Greenslade L, Aqeel M, et al. Reducing global inequities in medical oxygen access: the Lancet Global Health Commission on medical oxygen security. Lancet Glob Health. 2025;13(3):e528–84.
15. Smith L, Baker T, Demombynes G, Yada P. COVID-19 and oxygen: selecting supply options in LMICs that balance immediate needs with long-term cost-effectiveness. Center for Global Development; 2020. p. 1–7.
16. World Health Organization. Access to oxygen initiative [Internet]. [cited 2025 July 30]. Available from: https://www.who.int/initiatives/oxygen-access-scale-up.

A Deadly Sleep: Obstructive Sleep Apnea and Hypoxemia

19

Michael Dong and Ritu Grewal

Learning Objectives

1. Explain the traditional metrics used to define and quantify obstructive sleep apnea (OSA), including AHI, ODI, and T90.
2. Define hypoxic burden in obstructive sleep apnea and the mechanisms of sympathetic activation that cause multiorgan comorbidity in OSA.
3. Recognize the pathophysiology underlying hypoxic burden and pulmonary disease.
4. Describe the impact of hypoxic burden on pulmonary hypertension, chronic obstructive pulmonary disease, and obesity hypoventilation syndrome.
5. Describe the diagnostic approaches for OSA, including the role of polysomnography, portable sleep monitors, and clinical screening tools.
6. Compare management strategies for OSA, including PAP therapy, behavioral, pharmacologic, dental, and surgical options.

Introduction

Obstructive sleep apnea (OSA) is a prevalent condition characterized by repeated episodes of partial or complete upper airway obstruction during sleep, leading to disrupted sleep and intermittent hypoxia. Obstructive sleep apnea affects an estimated one billion individuals globally, with nearly half exhibiting moderate to severe disease [1]. Clinical heterogeneity is a hallmark, influenced by factors such

M. Dong · R. Grewal (✉)
The Korman Respiratory Institute and the Division of Pulmonary Allergy and Critical Care, Thomas Jefferson University and the Sidney Kimmel Medical College, Philadelphia, PA, USA
e-mail: Ritu.Grewal@jefferson.edu

G. C. Kane et al. (eds.), *Oxygen*, https://doi.org/10.1007/978-3-032-18934-9_19

as advancing age, increased body mass index, sex, race, and the varied conditions that predispose to OSA [2].

Importantly, variability in how OSA is defined and measured plays a major role in this heterogeneity. Standard definitions may fail to fully capture the clinical and pathophysiological spectrum of the disorder. OSA is characterized by recurrent episodes of upper airway obstruction during sleep, either partial (hypopnea) associated with 3% or 4% oxygen desaturation or arousal or complete (apnea), which disrupt normal ventilation and contribute to a range of adverse systemic effects. Episodes of upper airway obstruction during sleep are often accompanied by more profound hypoxemia, with desaturation to 80% or less.

The risk factors and conditions that predispose a patient to OSA share a common mechanism of increasing the collapsibility of the airway and or reducing the resting size during sleep. Obesity is the most significant and prevalent modifiable risk factor. Adipose tissue in the pharynx and tongue narrows the upper airway and predisposes it to dynamic collapse during the respiratory cycle. OSA affects over 40% of individuals with a BMI greater than 30% and up to 60% of those with metabolic syndrome [3]. Male sex is another well-established risk factor, although the underlying biological mechanisms of sex differences are not completely understood. Hormonal influences play a role; for example, progesterone appears to enhance upper airway muscle tone and ventilatory drive, potentially offering premenopausal women some protection, and conversely also increasing the risk of OSA in postmenopausal women [4, 5]. Higher androgen levels, whether endogenous or due to supplementation, may worsen OSA by promoting soft tissue hypertrophy, particularly in the tongue [6]. Additional conditions, such as hypothyroidism, acromegaly, congenital structural abnormalities such as enlarged tonsils, midface hypoplasia, and Down syndrome, to name a few, are associated with a higher prevalence of OSA, likely due to tissue overgrowth and myopathy [7–10].

For clinicians, this heterogeneity of the disease presents a challenge: two patients with similar apnea–hypopnea indices (AHIs) may have vastly different symptom profiles, comorbidities, and long-term risks. Traditional diagnostic metrics, such as AHI, which measures the frequency of events per hour, often lack correlation with clinical outcomes like cardiovascular disease or excessive daytime sleepiness. A deeper understanding of pathophysiology and alternative emerging metrics is crucial for individualizing treatment, identifying high-risk phenotypes, and improving long-term care strategies.

In this chapter, we will explore the concept of hypoxic burden—a metric designed to quantify the frequency, depth, and duration of oxygen desaturations associated with sleep-disordered breathing (Fig. 19.1). We will examine the pathophysiological mechanisms by which intermittent hypoxemia during sleep contributes to systemic inflammation, oxidative stress, and sympathetic activation. Special attention will be given to how these processes influence the development and progression of pulmonary diseases, while also recognizing their impact on cardiovascular, neurocognitive, and metabolic diseases. By integrating this emerging evidence, we aim to provide a more nuanced understanding of OSA severity and its clinical implications.

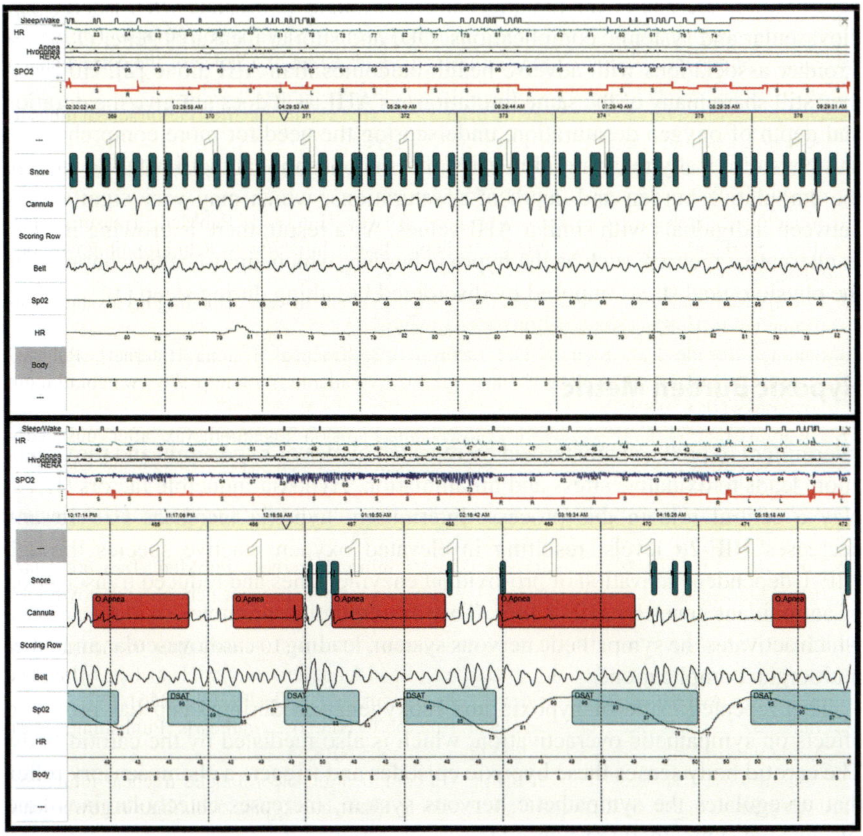

Fig. 19.1 Comparison of sleep tracings with and without hypoxic burden

Traditional Metrics of Obstructive Sleep Apnea

The severity of OSA has traditionally been quantified using the apnea–hypopnea index (AHI), which represents the number of apneas and hypopneas per hour of sleep. An AHI greater than 5 events per hour is the conventional diagnostic threshold for OSA, and the index is commonly used to categorize disease severity [11].

However, the AHI metric has several flaws. Based on the criteria of 5 events per hour as a diagnostic threshold for OSA, the HypnoLaus population study in Switzerland found that 83.8% of men and 60.8% of women aged 35–75 meet the diagnostic threshold, a prevalence that is inflated and likely does not represent people with clinically significant symptoms [12]. AHI also correlates poorly with clinical symptoms, sleep fragmentation, quality of life measures, and the extent of nocturnal oxygen desaturation.

To address some of these shortcomings, other conventional metrics, such as the oxygen desaturation index (ODI), are often used to assess intermittent hypoxemia, a hallmark physiological consequence of OSA [13]. Nocturnal oxygen desaturations are one of the key mechanisms thought to mediate OSA-related cardiovascular and systemic complications. ODI and similar measures generally show stronger associations with adverse health outcomes than AHI alone [2]. However, they still share many of the same limitations as AHI, as it does not give the duration and depth of oxygen desaturation, underscoring the need for more comprehensive and physiologically meaningful metrics. These conventional metrics fail to capture the cumulative burden and depth of desaturations, which may vary significantly between individuals with similar AHI values. As a result, there is growing interest in alternative metrics, such as the hypoxic burden, which aim to better characterize the physiological stress imposed by disordered breathing during sleep [14].

Hypoxic Burden Metric

Intermittent hypoxia, characterized by repeated cycles of hypoxemia and reoxygenation, leads to oxidative stress and inflammation. Hypoxia-inducible factors (HIFs) play a central role in this process. Intermittent hypoxia increases HIF-1α and decreases HIF-2α levels, resulting in elevated oxygen reactive species through HIF-1-dependent activation of pro-oxidant enzyme genes and reduced transcription of antioxidant genes by HIF-2 [15]. This dysregulation promotes oxidative stress, which activates the sympathetic nervous system, leading to cardiovascular and other multiorgan complications.

This repeated cycle of hypoxia and reoxygenation during sleep has profound effects on sympathetic overactivation, which is also mediated by the carotid body. The carotid body senses these hypoxic episodes and triggers a chemosensory reflex that upregulates the sympathetic nervous system, increases catecholamines, and sustains the sympathetic response [16].

The frequency, duration, and depth of apneas and hypopneas have more profound physiologic impacts and are better predictors of clinically significant adverse effects [17, 18]. Hypoxic burden is increasingly recognized as a valuable metric for assessing the severity and clinical impact of OSA (Fig. 19.1). Unlike the AHI, which primarily measures the frequency of respiratory events, hypoxic burden quantifies the cumulative area under the oxygen desaturation curve during sleep, capturing both the depth and duration of hypoxemic episodes [19]. Hypoxic burden at a threshold of 60% min/h. (i.e., 12 min of 5% desaturations every hour) is a strong predictor for cardiovascular morbidity and mortality (Fig. 19.2) [20]. As we discuss below, hypoxic burden is a strong predictor of clinically significant comorbid diseases related to OSA.

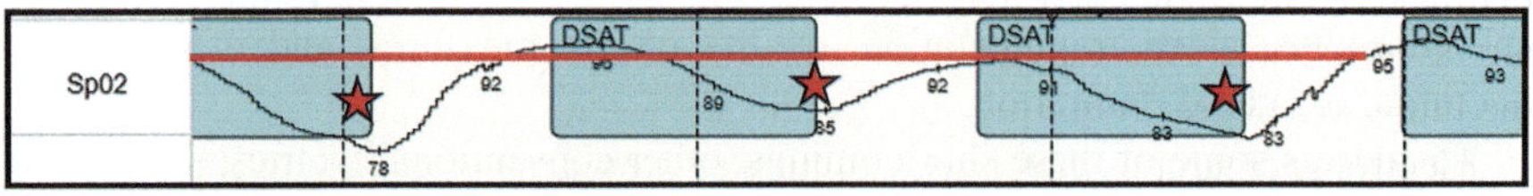

Fig. 19.2 Hypoxic burden measurement

The top panel shows stable respiratory parameters and oxygen saturation during sleep, indicating the absence of hypoxic burden.

The bottom panel demonstrates recurrent hypopneas with associated oxygen desaturations and fluctuations in respiratory flow, characteristic of sleep-disordered breathing with elevated hypoxic burden.

Hypoxic burden is measured by the area under the curve and expressed in units of %min/h (i.e., 60%min/h could represent 12 min of 5% desaturations every hour). This metric assesses the depth and duration of each desaturation.

Hypoxic Burden and Its Clinical Implications in Pulmonary Medicine

In chronic respiratory diseases, including chronic obstructive pulmonary disease (COPD), interstitial lung disease (ILD), and sleep-disordered breathing (SDB), a higher hypoxic burden has been consistently linked to adverse outcomes such as increased risk of pulmonary hypertension, right heart dysfunction, and mortality [21–23]. As described above, hypoxic burden captures both the depth and duration of oxygen desaturation events, offering a more comprehensive assessment of nocturnal hypoxemia than traditional indices such as the apnea–hypopnea index. Its growing clinical relevance highlights the need for pulmonologists to understand the clinical relevance and go beyond standard sleep study metrics when evaluating cardiopulmonary risk.

Chronic hypoxemia and intermittent hypoxemia are central pathophysiologic drivers of pulmonary vascular remodeling and pulmonary hypertension in these conditions. Recurrent episodes of hypoxia, whether sustained or intermittent, promote pulmonary vasoconstriction, vascular smooth muscle proliferation, and endothelial dysfunction [24]. In patients with sleep apnea, the PA pressures can progressively rise as the hypoxia worsens, and also correlate cyclically with apnea episodes. It has been demonstrated that these cyclic elevations of PA pressures can exceed 60 mmHg [25, 26]. Over time, these changes lead to elevated pulmonary arterial pressures and increased right ventricular afterload, contributing to right heart strain and failure. Recognition of these mechanisms is critical for timely intervention before irreversible vascular remodeling occurs.

In COPD, nocturnal hypoxemia is prevalent and plays a key role in the development of pulmonary hypertension and cardiovascular comorbidity [27]. The overlap syndrome of COPD and OSA further amplifies the hypoxic burden and its downstream effects. At a cellular level, hypoxic burden upregulates hypoxia-inducible factor 1-alpha (HIF-1α), which leads to a pro-inflammatory and pro-fibrotic signaling cascade via the EGFR/PI3K/AKT pathway [28, 29]. Thus, there is increased fibrocyte activation, migration, and airway fibrosis in these hypoxic settings. Protease balances, such as that of neutrophil elastase, are also disrupted and can cause endothelial damage and vascular dysfunction [30]. It leads to a higher risk of pulmonary hypertension, cardiovascular disease, increased frequency of COPD exacerbations and hospitalizations, as well as increased mortality [31]. Hypoxic burden also has a negative effect on skeletal muscle strength. It can lead to decreased respiratory muscle strength, forced vital capacity, and worsened dyspnea and functional limitations [32]. Identification of sleep disorders in patients with COPD is critical. Targeted therapies, including nocturnal oxygen supplementation and positive airway pressure, may help mitigate these risks in selected patients [31].

Obesity hypoventilation syndrome (OHS) represents another clinical context where hypoxic burden is particularly pronounced. Patients with OHS are characterized by a combination of obesity, sleep-disordered breathing, and daytime hypercapnia ($PaCO2 \geq 45$ mmHg) during wakefulness, occurring in the absence of alternative etiologies for hypoventilation. These patients have chronic hypercapnia and profound nocturnal hypoxemia, which are associated with insulin resistance, systemic inflammation, endothelial dysfunction, and heightened cardiometabolic risk [33]. In this population, there is a significant overlap (up to 90%) with OSA, as obesity is a major shared risk factor [34]. Hypoxic burden has been shown to independently predict adverse outcomes, including all-cause and cardiovascular mortality. The development and progression of pulmonary hypertension driven by chronic nocturnal hypoxemia may play a central role in the clinical deterioration of OHS [35]. Obesity hypoventilation syndrome (OHS) is associated with significantly higher in-hospital and post-discharge mortality compared to both eucapnic obese patients and those with obstructive sleep apnea (OSA) alone, especially in the context of acute-on-chronic hypercapnic respiratory failure and high hypoxic burden. Hospitalized patients with OHS experience increased rates of ICU admission, need for mechanical ventilation, longer length of stay, and higher healthcare costs, with in-hospital mortality rates reported up to 15% and 18-month post-discharge mortality as high as 23% [36]. The best treatment for OHS is extreme weight loss, but this can be difficult and take significant time. With significant overlap with OSA, early identification and initiation of positive airway pressure may improve long-term outcomes by reducing hypoxic burden [37].

Large population-based studies such as the Sleep Heart Health Study and the Osteoporotic Fractures in Men Study have demonstrated a graded relationship between hypoxic burden and mortality risk [21, 23]. Higher cumulative hypoxic exposure during sleep confers proportionally greater risk, underscoring the prognostic significance of this metric. These findings support incorporating hypoxic burden into both research and routine clinical assessment protocols.

For pulmonologists, incorporating hypoxic burden into clinical evaluation may enhance risk stratification and inform therapeutic decisions, especially in patients with coexisting cardiopulmonary or metabolic disease. As evidence continues to accumulate, hypoxic burden may become a pivotal marker in the management of chronic respiratory disorders. Its integration into future guidelines could ultimately improve patient-centered outcomes through more personalized care.

Multisystem Effects of Hypoxic Burden

In cardiovascular disease, hypoxic burden is independently associated with incident coronary artery disease, heart failure, atrial fibrillation, and other arrhythmias, even after adjusting for traditional sleep apnea metrics. These effects are mediated through sympathetic activation, oxidative stress, systemic inflammation, and endothelial dysfunction [38]. The Sleep Heart Health Study demonstrated that hypoxic burden, rather than event frequency alone, is a robust predictor of cardiovascular morbidity and mortality in community-based populations [23].

Beyond the cardiovascular system, chronic and intermittent hypoxemia have been implicated in the development and progression of chronic kidney disease, metabolic syndrome, including insulin resistance and dyslipidemia, and neurocognitive decline [39–42]. These associations are thought to arise from similar pathophysiologic mechanisms that disrupt homeostasis and contribute to long-term organ dysfunction.

While these systemic effects are increasingly recognized, the primary focus of this chapter is on the pulmonary consequences of hypoxic burden, as described above.

Diagnosis of OSA

The diagnosis of OSA centers on identifying characteristic sleep-disordered breathing events, with in-laboratory polysomnography (PSG) remaining as the diagnostic gold standard. PSG provides detailed physiologic data, including airflow, respiratory effort, oxygen saturation, EEG-defined sleep stages, and cardiac rhythm, thus allowing precise quantification of AHI and hypoxic burden. It is especially indicated in patients with excessive daytime sleepiness or high pretest probability, where its diagnostic yield and ability to characterize complex sleep-related pathology are highest [11].

For patients without significant comorbidities, home sleep apnea testing offers a practical alternative, measuring airflow, effort, and oximetry. However, PSG is preferred in those with overlapping conditions such as COPD, CHF, or neuromuscular disease, where simplified monitoring may underestimate disease severity or miss central events [11].

Screening tools like STOP-Bang, the Berlin Questionnaire, and the Epworth Sleepiness Scale may aid in triage but are not diagnostic. While useful in perioperative or primary care settings, definitive diagnosis and risk stratification require objective sleep testing to inform management decisions and assess comorbidity burden [43–45].

Management of OSA

The cornerstone of OSA management is continuous positive airway pressure (CPAP) as first-line therapy in fixed or auto-titrating modes [46]. CPAP acts as a pneumatic splint, keeping the upper airway open during sleep and thereby reducing the intermittent airway collapse, hypoxic burden, and the downstream effects of intermittent hypoxia, including oxidative stress and sympathetic overactivation [2]. Bi-level devices can be used in patients who cannot tolerate CPAP; however, there is no clear benefit of bi-level PPV [46]. For patients with OSA, OHS, and COPD with OSA overlap syndrome, the first-line management is CPAP therapy [47, 48].

Oxygen supplementation is not a treatment for OSA, but it can be considered for those who cannot tolerate PAP therapy and are having arrhythmias. Patients should be counseled that while nocturnal oxygen improves nocturnal hypoxemia, it does not significantly reduce blood pressure and cardiovascular risk [49]. In fact, oxygen therapy may potentially increase the duration of apnea–hypopnea events [50]. While oxygen therapy can be used as a bridge for those patients who cannot tolerate PAP therapy, patients should be referred for evaluation for oral appliances, upper airway stimulation therapy, and surgical options, as we discuss below.

Medical and behavioral interventions play a vital role in OSA management, especially among patients who are overweight or have metabolic comorbidities. Weight loss is one of the most impactful strategies; even modest reductions in body weight can significantly reduce the severity of OSA [51]. Intensive lifestyle programs, bariatric surgery, and newer pharmacotherapies such as glucagon-like peptide-1 (GLP-1) receptor agonists have shown promising results in promoting substantial and sustained weight loss. Emerging evidence supports the use of GLP-1 receptor agonists, such as liraglutide, semaglutide, and tirzepatide (GLP-1 and GIP co-agonist), for achieving clinically significant and sustained weight loss, which in turn is strongly associated with reductions in OSA severity, as measured by both AHI and hypoxic burden [52, 53]. Recent randomized controlled trials have shown that tirzepatide can reduce AHI by up to 29 events per hour (representing a 58.7% reduction from baseline), with nearly half of patients reaching AHI thresholds below which PAP therapy may no longer be indicated. These benefits occur independently of concurrent PAP use and are accompanied by improvements in blood pressure, systemic inflammation, and sleep-related quality of life [54]. GLP-1 receptor agonists do not replace PAP therapy as first-line treatment, but they are a powerful tool addressing obesity as a major underlying risk factor for OSA.

Additionally, behavioral modifications, including avoiding alcohol and sedative use, which relax upper airway muscles, and practicing positional sleeping to avoid supine-related airway collapse, can be especially beneficial in patients with mild to moderate OSA or positional OSA.

For patients who are intolerant of CPAP or require additional therapeutic options, oral appliances such as mandibular advancement devices mechanically reposition the lower jaw forward, thereby enlarging the upper airway space during sleep and reducing airway obstruction. These are most effective in mild to moderate OSA [55]. Surgical options may be appropriate for individuals with specific anatomic obstructions or who have failed conservative treatments. Modified uvulopalatopharyngoplasty can widen the oropharyngeal airway, and hypoglossal nerve stimulation offers benefits by activating upper airway dilator muscles during sleep [56, 57]. A comprehensive, individualized treatment plan that integrates PAP therapy, medical therapy, behavioral changes, and procedural interventions offers the best chance of improving sleep quality and reducing the long-term health consequences of OSA.

Conclusions

In conclusion, OSA is a highly prevalent disorder with far-reaching implications for systemic health. Emerging evidence highlights that hypoxic burden—a measure of the depth and duration of oxygen desaturations—offers a more clinically meaningful assessment of OSA severity than the traditional AHI metric. At the core of OSA's pathophysiologic impact lies the cycle of intermittent hypoxia, which triggers repeated sympathetic surges through mechanisms involving oxidative stress, systemic inflammation, and neurohumoral dysregulation. This cyclical sympathetic activation contributes to a cascade of effects across multiple organ systems, underscoring the importance of early recognition and targeted management of hypoxemia in sleep-disordered breathing. Understanding and quantifying hypoxic burden may help refine risk stratification and therapeutic decision-making. Effective diagnosis and management of OSA requires a combination of accurate, objective testing and a personalized, multidisciplinary treatment approach. Polysomnography remains the diagnostic gold standard, while a range of therapeutic options—including CPAP, lifestyle modifications, GLP1/GIP agonists, and surgical procedures—offer tailored strategies to reduce hypoxic burden and improve patient outcomes. Early identification and comprehensive care are essential to mitigating the systemic effects of OSA and enhancing overall health and quality of life.

References

1. Benjafield AV, Ayas NT, Eastwood PR, Heinzer R, Ip MSM, Morrell MJ, et al. Estimation of the global prevalence and burden of obstructive sleep apnoea: a literature-based analysis. Lancet Respir Med. 2019;7(8):687–98.
2. Veasey SC, Rosen IM. Obstructive sleep apnea in adults. N Engl J Med. 2019;380(15):1442–9.
3. Drager LF, Togeiro SM, Polotsky VY, Lorenzi-Filho G. Obstructive sleep apnea: a cardiometabolic risk in obesity and the metabolic syndrome. J Am Coll Cardiol. 2013;62(7):569–76.
4. Jehan S, Auguste E, Zizi F, Pandi-Perumal SR, Gupta R, Attarian H, et al. Obstructive sleep apnea: women's perspective. J Sleep Med Disord. 2016;3(6):1064.
5. Bayliss DA, Millhorn DE, Gallman EA, Cidlowski JA. Progesterone stimulates respiration through a central nervous system steroid receptor-mediated mechanism in cat. Proc Natl Acad Sci USA. 1987;84(21):7788–92.
6. Lin T-Y, Lin P-Y, Su T-P, Li C-T, Lin W-C, Chang W-H, et al. Risk of developing obstructive sleep apnea among women with polycystic ovarian syndrome: a nationwide longitudinal follow-up study. Sleep Med. 2017;36:165–9.

7. Turan O, Akinci B, Ikiz AO, Itil O, Oztura I, Ada E, et al. Airway and sleep disorders in patients with acromegaly. Clin Respir J. 2018;12(3):1003–10.
8. Ozcan KM, Selcuk A, Ozcan I, Ozdas T, Ozdogan F, Acar M, et al. Incidence of hypothyroidism and its correlation with polysomnography findings in obstructive sleep apnea. Eur Arch Otorrinolaringol. 2014;271(11):2937–41.
9. Dempsey JA, Veasey SC, Morgan BJ, O'Donnell CP. Pathophysiology of sleep apnea. Physiol Rev. 2010;90(1):47–112.
10. Simpson R, Oyekan AA, Ehsan Z, Ingram DG. Obstructive sleep apnea in patients with Down syndrome: current perspectives. Nat Sci Sleep. 2018;10:287–93.
11. Kapur VK, Auckley DH, Chowdhuri S, Kuhlmann DC, Mehra R, Ramar K, et al. Clinical practice guideline for diagnostic testing for adult obstructive sleep apnea: an American academy of sleep medicine clinical practice guideline. J Clin Sleep Med. 2017;13(3):479–504.
12. Heinzer R, Vat S, Marques-Vidal P, Marti-Soler H, Andries D, Tobback N, et al. Prevalence of sleep-disordered breathing in the general population: the HypnoLaus study. Lancet Respir Med. 2015;3(4):310–8.
13. Rashid NH, Zaghi S, Scapuccin M, Camacho M, Certal V, Capasso R. The value of oxygen desaturation index for diagnosing obstructive sleep apnea: a systematic review. Laryngoscope. 2021;131(2):440–7.
14. Parekh A. Hypoxic burden – definitions, pathophysiological concepts, methods of evaluation, and clinical relevance. Curr Opin Pulm Med. 2024;30(6):600–6.
15. Prabhakar NR, Peng Y-J, Nanduri J. Hypoxia-inducible factors and obstructive sleep apnea. J Clin Invest. 2020;130(10):5042–51.
16. Prabhakar NR, Peng Y-J, Nanduri J. Carotid body hypersensitivity in intermittent hypoxia and obstructive sleep apnoea. J Physiol Lond. 2023;601(24):5481–94.
17. Oksenberg A, Leppänen T. Duration of respiratory events in obstructive sleep apnea: In search of paradoxical results. Sleep Med Rev. 2023;68:101728.
18. Wu H, Zhan X, Zhao M, Wei Y. Mean apnea-hypopnea duration (but not apnea-hypopnea index) is associated with worse hypertension in patients with obstructive sleep apnea. Medicine (Baltimore). 2016;95(48):e5493.
19. Trzepizur W, Blanchard M, Ganem T, Balusson F, Feuilloy M, Girault J-M, et al. Sleep apnea-specific hypoxic burden, symptom subtypes, and risk of cardiovascular events and all-cause mortality. Am J Respir Crit Care Med. 2022;205(1):108–17.
20. Martinez-Garcia MA, Sánchez-de-la-Torre M, White DP, Azarbarzin A. Hypoxic burden in obstructive sleep apnea: present and future. Arch Bronconeumol. 2023;59(1):36–43.
21. Azarbarzin A, Sands SA, Stone KL, Taranto-Montemurro L, Messineo L, Terrill PI, et al. The hypoxic burden of sleep apnoea predicts cardiovascular disease-related mortality: the Osteoporotic Fractures in Men Study and the Sleep Heart Health Study. Eur Heart J. 2019;40(14):1149–57.
22. Punjabi NM, Caffo BS, Goodwin JL, Gottlieb DJ, Newman AB, O'Connor GT, et al. Sleep-disordered breathing and mortality: a prospective cohort study. PLoS Med. 2009;6(8):e1000132.
23. Redline S, Yenokyan G, Gottlieb DJ, Shahar E, O'Connor GT, Resnick HE, et al. Obstructive sleep apnea-hypopnea and incident stroke: the sleep heart health study. Am J Respir Crit Care Med. 2010;182(2):269–77.
24. Sylvester JT, Shimoda LA, Aaronson PI, Ward JPT. Hypoxic pulmonary vasoconstriction. Physiol Rev. 2012;92(1):367–520.
25. Tilkian AG, Guilleminault C, Schroeder JS, Lehrman KL, Simmons FB, Dement WC. Hemodynamics in sleep-induced apnea. Studies during wakefulness and sleep. Ann Intern Med. 1976;85(6):714–9.
26. Buda AJ, Schroeder JS, Guilleminault C. Abnormalities of pulmonary artery wedge pressures in sleep-induced apnea. Int J Cardiol. 1981;1(1):67–74.
27. Kent BD, Mitchell PD, McNicholas WT. Hypoxemia in patients with COPD: cause, effects, and disease progression. Int J Chron Obstruct Pulmon Dis. 2011;14(6):199–208.

28. Wang C-H, Lo C-Y, Huang H-Y, Wang T-Y, Weng C-M, Chen C-J, et al. Oxygen desaturation is associated with fibrocyte activation via epidermal growth factor receptor/hypoxia-inducible factor-1α axis in chronic obstructive pulmonary disease. Front Immunol. 2022;13:852713.
29. Zhang HX, Yang JJ, Zhang SA, Zhang SM, Wang JX, Xu ZY, et al. HIF-1α promotes inflammatory response of chronic obstructive pulmonary disease by activating EGFR/PI3K/AKT pathway. Eur Rev Med Pharmacol Sci. 2018;22(18):6077–84.
30. Lodge KM, Vassallo A, Liu B, Long M, Tong Z, Newby PR, et al. Hypoxia increases the potential for neutrophil-mediated endothelial damage in chronic obstructive pulmonary disease. Am J Respir Crit Care Med. 2022;205(8):903–16.
31. Marin JM, Soriano JB, Carrizo SJ, Boldova A, Celli BR. Outcomes in patients with chronic obstructive pulmonary disease and obstructive sleep apnea: the overlap syndrome. Am J Respir Crit Care Med. 2010;182(3):325–31.
32. Saglam M, Vardar-Yagli N, Savci S, Inal-Ince D, Calik-Kutukcu E, Arikan H, et al. Functional capacity, physical activity, and quality of life in hypoxemic patients with chronic obstructive pulmonary disease. Int J Chron Obstruct Pulmon Dis. 2015;10:423–8.
33. de Athayde RAB, de Oliveira Filho JRB, Lorenzi Filho G, Genta PR. Obesity hypoventilation syndrome: a current review. J Bras Pneumol. 2018;44(6):510–8.
34. Masa JF, Corral J, Alonso ML, Ordax E, Troncoso MF, Gonzalez M, et al. Efficacy of different treatment alternatives for obesity hypoventilation syndrome. pickwick study. Am J Respir Crit Care Med. 2015;192(1):86–95.
35. Castro-Añón O, Golpe R, Pérez-de-Llano LA, López González MJ, Escalona Velasquez EJ, Pérez Fernández R, et al. Haemodynamic effects of non-invasive ventilation in patients with obesity-hypoventilation syndrome. Respirology. 2012;17(8):1269–74.
36. Mokhlesi B, Masa JF, Afshar M, Almadana Pacheco V, Berlowitz DJ, Borel J-C, et al. The effect of hospital discharge with empiric noninvasive ventilation on mortality in hospitalized patients with obesity hypoventilation syndrome. An individual patient data meta-analysis. Ann Am Thorac Soc. 2020;17(5):627–37.
37. Masa JF, Pépin J-L, Borel J-C, Mokhlesi B, Murphy PB, Sánchez-Quiroga MÁ. Obesity hypoventilation syndrome. Eur Respir Rev. 2019;28:151.
38. Javaheri S, Barbe F, Campos-Rodriguez F, Dempsey JA, Khayat R, Javaheri S, et al. Sleep apnea: types, mechanisms, and clinical cardiovascular consequences. J Am Coll Cardiol. 2017;69(7):841–58.
39. Lin C-H, Lurie RC, Lyons OD. Sleep apnea and chronic kidney disease: a state-of-the-art review. Chest. 2020;157(3):673–85.
40. Gaines J, Vgontzas AN, Fernandez-Mendoza J, Bixler EO. Obstructive sleep apnea and the metabolic syndrome: the road to clinically-meaningful phenotyping, improved prognosis, and personalized treatment. Sleep Med Rev. 2018;42:211–9.
41. Kent BD, Grote L, Ryan S, Pépin J-L, Bonsignore MR, Tkacova R, et al. Diabetes mellitus prevalence and control in sleep-disordered breathing: the European Sleep Apnea Cohort (ESADA) study. Chest. 2014;146(4):982–90.
42. Wallace A, Bucks RS. Memory and obstructive sleep apnea: a meta-analysis. Sleep. 2013;36(2):203–20.
43. Chung F, Abdullah HR, Liao P. STOP-bang questionnaire: a practical approach to screen for obstructive sleep apnea. Chest. 2016;149(3):631–8.
44. Netzer NC, Stoohs RA, Netzer CM, Clark K, Strohl KP. Using the Berlin questionnaire to identify patients at risk for the sleep apnea syndrome. Ann Intern Med. 1999;131(7):485–91.
45. Johns MW. A new method for measuring daytime sleepiness: the Epworth sleepiness scale. Sleep. 1991;14(6):540–5.
46. Patil SP, Ayappa IA, Caples SM, Kimoff RJ, Patel SR, Harrod CG. Treatment of adult obstructive sleep apnea with positive airway pressure: an American academy of sleep medicine clinical practice guideline. J Clin Sleep Med. 2019;15(2):335–43.
47. Venkatesan P. GOLD COPD report: 2025 update. Lancet Respir Med. 2025;13(1):e7–8.

48. Srivali N, Thongprayoon C, Tangpanithandee S, Cheungpasitporn W, Won C. The use of continuous positive airway pressure in COPD-OSA overlap syndrome: a systematic review. Sleep Med. 2023;108:55–60.
49. Gottlieb DJ, Punjabi NM, Mehra R, Patel SR, Quan SF, Babineau DC, et al. CPAP versus oxygen in obstructive sleep apnea. N Engl J Med. 2014;370(24):2276–85.
50. Mehta V, Vasu TS, Phillips B, Chung F. Obstructive sleep apnea and oxygen therapy: a systematic review of the literature and meta-analysis. J Clin Sleep Med. 2013;9(3):271–9.
51. Kuna ST, Reboussin DM, Strotmeyer ES, Millman RP, Zammit G, Walkup MP, et al. Effects of weight loss on obstructive sleep apnea severity. Ten-year results of the sleep AHEAD study. Am J Respir Crit Care Med. 2021;203(2):221–9.
52. Yang R, Zhang L, Guo J, Wang N, Zhang Q, Qi Z, et al. Glucagon-like Peptide-1 receptor agonists for obstructive sleep apnea in patients with obesity and type 2 diabetes mellitus: a systematic review and meta-analysis. J Transl Med. 2025;23(1):389.
53. El-Solh AA, Gould E, Aibangbee K, Jimerson T, Hartling R. Current perspectives on the use of GLP-1 receptor agonists in obesity-related obstructive sleep apnea: a narrative review. Expert Opin Pharmacother. 2025;26(1):51–62.
54. Malhotra A, Grunstein RR, Fietze I, Weaver TE, Redline S, Azarbarzin A, et al. Tirzepatide for the treatment of obstructive sleep apnea and obesity. N Engl J Med. 2024;391(13):1193–205.
55. Marklund M, Verbraecken J, Randerath W. Non-CPAP therapies in obstructive sleep apnoea: mandibular advancement device therapy. Eur Respir J. 2012;39(5):1241–7.
56. MacKay S, Carney AS, Catcheside PG, Chai-Coetzer CL, Chia M, Cistulli PA, et al. Effect of multilevel upper airway surgery vs medical management on the apnea-hypopnea index and patient-reported daytime sleepiness among patients with moderate or severe obstructive sleep apnea: the SAMS randomized clinical trial. JAMA. 2020;324(12):1168–79.
57. Kim DH, Kim SW, Han JS, Kim G-J, Park JH, Basurrah MA, et al. Comparative effectiveness of hypoglossal nerve stimulation and alternative treatments for obstructive sleep apnea: a systematic review and meta-analysis. J Sleep Res. 2024;33(3):e14017.

Chronic Tracheostomy Tubes 20

Padmanabh Bhatt and Frances Mae West

History and Indications for Chronic Tracheostomy

Tracheostomy is a procedure in which a stoma is created between a patient's neck and trachea. The term is derived from the Greek phrase "I cut the trachea" [1]. Tracheostomies have been described in ancient history and were first mentioned in the Hindu Rig Veda, ca. 1000–2000 BC, and the Ebers Papyrus, ca. 1550 BC. The procedure was historically performed emergently to relieve airway obstruction from foreign bodies, with Homer reportedly performing a tracheostomy in the eighth century BC to relieve choking, and Alexander the Great doing the same with his sword to relieve a soldier choking on an animal bone.

Tracheostomies became rare over the next millennium, owing to being criticized as a barbaric procedure. The procedure re-emerged in the sixteenth century, again being used to treat upper airway obstruction from foreign bodies, tonsillar adenopathy, or quinsy. The first instance of a trocar being placed after a tracheostomy is from 1590 by Sanctorius, now a common practice in modern medicine. In early American medicine, one of the physicians caring for George Washington, who was thought to have died from acute epiglottitis, recommended the creation of a tracheostomy to relieve impending upper airway obstruction but was overruled by colleagues.

P. Bhatt · F. M. West (✉)
Allergy and Critical Care Medicine, Department of Pulmonary, Philadelphia, PA, USA
e-mail: frances.west@jefferson.edu

G. C. Kane et al. (eds.), *Oxygen*, https://doi.org/10.1007/978-3-032-18934-9_20

The polio epidemic revolutionized tracheostomies in the 1950s. With a large influx of patients presenting with respiratory failure due to neuromuscular weakness, in the absence of effective positive-pressure ventilators, patients were initially tracheostomized and subsequently bag ventilated for days by medical students—saving countless lives [2]. The development of effective and safe positive-pressure ventilators expanded the role of tracheostomy in subacute and chronic respiratory failure, allowing physicians to titrate the level of respiratory support in accordance with patients' recovery. In parallel was the development of intensive care units, where patients with severe respiratory impairment could be treated and monitored in a discrete unit. The development of the percutaneous tracheostomy, initially described in 1969 [3], has broadened the remit of tracheostomy creation from operating rooms to the bedside, and the procedure is now routinely performed by general surgeons, intensive care physicians, and pulmonologists in addition to ENT and thoracic surgeons. A separate chapter in this book explores the creation of a tracheostomy in the intensive care unit. For patients requiring long-term tracheostomy, the utilization of softer and lower-pressure cuffs has dramatically reduced the incidence of tracheal injuries, fistulae, and tissue necrosis.

In the modern age, indications for tracheostomy creation can be grouped into four main categories: ventilation and oxygenation, airway protection, airway obstruction, and pulmonary toilet or secretion management. In many patients, these indications overlap.

Patients with acute respiratory failure who undergo endotracheal intubation and cannot be liberated from mechanical ventilation are subsequently tracheostomized to help with ventilator weaning, engagement in physical therapy and rehabilitation, ability to speak, and overall improved quality of life compared to persistent endotracheal intubation.

This chapter will focus on the use of chronic tracheostomy tubes and give special consideration to how oxygen is delivered for patients who require it.

Anatomy of a Tracheostomy and Ventilatory Considerations

After the creation of a tracheal stoma, a tracheostomy is left in place to facilitate ventilation and prevent stomal closure. Oxygen therapy may be supplied directly to a tracheostomy tube or via an oxygen mask. Tracheostomies may have an inner and outer cannula. The outer cannula keeps the device in place and can be secured with sutures, a collar, or both, until a mature tract is formed. The inner cannula is designed to facilitate toileting and prevent tube obstruction; it may be disposable or reusable, with non-disposable types requiring regular cleaning before reuse. Tubes with inner and outer cannulas are termed dual cannula tubes, while those with only an outer cannula are termed single cannula tubes. While the inner cannula can help with toileting, it reduces the diameter of the airway through which a patient breathes, resulting in increased resistance. This is of special importance in spontaneously breathing patients, or those on ventilator weans, as this increase in resistance can be significant. There are several brands and types of tracheostomy tubes available in

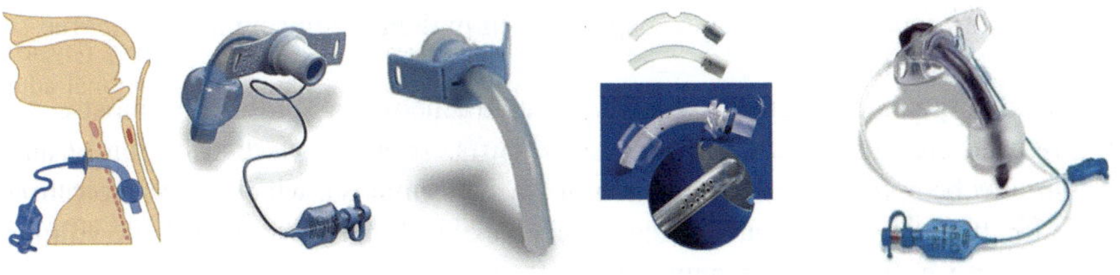

Fig. 20.1 From left to right: Appropriate positioning of a tracheostomy in the neck, a cuffed tracheostomy tube, an uncuffed tracheostomy tube, fenestrated tracheostomy tubes, a cuffed tracheostomy tube with subglottic suctioning apparatus

the market, and these variations may impact both ventilation and oxygenation. Figure 20.1 outlines the various tracheostomies that are commonly used.

The outer and inner diameters are listed on each type of tracheostomy tube, with the outer diameter (OD) referring to the size of the stoma created in the neck and the inner diameter (ID) referring to the size of the tube via which air passes. In addition, tracheostomy tubes come in different lengths, which can also affect resistance. These factors should be taken into consideration for patients weaning from tracheostomy. Nonetheless, work of breathing and resistance are reduced with tracheostomy tubes when compared to endotracheal tubes, a benefit that increases with higher tidal volumes and inspiratory flow rates [4]. This same study showed that patients who failed extubation had a higher work of breathing than when tracheostomized. This phenomenon is not solely explained by modest reductions in dead space ventilation and airway resistance. The authors hypothesize that the other benefits of tracheostomy such as improved secretion clearance and upper airway control contribute to the improved breathing pattern.

The majority of tracheostomy tubes are made of polyvinyl chloride (PVC), silicone, or polyurethane. While an in-depth review of these materials is outside the scope of this book, PVC is utilized because it is malleable and conforms with ease to patients' anatomy, while silicone can resist biofilm build-up and be cleaned with ease. Metal tubes are falling out of use due to cost, the lack of a cuff, and their rigid, nonconforming nature.

Tracheostomies can either be cuffed or cuffless. Patients receiving positive-pressure ventilation are usually managed with cuffed tracheostomy tubes, as the inflated cuff ensures that the volume of gas from the ventilator is delivered into the respiratory system rather than being allowed to escape into the upper airway, hence allowing effective ventilation. The cuff should be inflated with enough air to ensure apposition with the trachea, but not overinflated to prevent tracheal injury—the sequelae of which include tracheo-esophageal and tracheo-brachiocephalic artery fistulas, and tracheal stenosis. A cuff pressure of 20–30 cm H_2O is recommended to balance these indications, as the tracheal capillary perfusion pressure is approximately 25–35 mmHg (34–47 cm H_2O). Importantly, the cuff pressure should be checked as part of routine monitoring as it can change with movement and positioning. In patients with a sudden change in respiratory parameters and loss of ventilator volumes, cuff integrity should always be examined—cuff ruptures can evolve into a medical emergency, especially in patients requiring a high degree of ventilator support.

Broadly speaking, there are four types of tracheostomy cuffs. The most commonly used are high-volume, low-pressure cuffs. These allow distribution of cuff pressure to be spread over a large area of tracheal mucosa, which, with their thin-walled nature, prevent focal tracheal injury despite longer-term use. Low-volume low-pressure cuffs, as their name suggests, inflate with lower volumes but still maintain low pressures. Animal and preclinical studies suggest these cuffs may reduce mucosal injury compared to high-volume, low-pressure cuffs; however, this has not yet been investigated in humans [5]. Tight-to-shaft cuffs are designed to sit tightly with the tracheostomy tube when deflated, in order to minimize the tracheostomy diameter and make tube exchanges easy. This property also improves spontaneous ventilation with cuff deflation. These cuffs are generally inflated with sterile water, as they are gas-permeable. While not routinely used, foam cuffs are occasionally considered as an alternative in select cases. They do not require air or water to form a seal, but instead, the foam expands spontaneously to form a seal with the trachea. Foam cuffs are generally used for patients with irregular tracheostomies or those with a high risk of tracheal injury.

As patients are liberated from the ventilator, the tube can be changed to a cuffless one, which allows for speaking and reduces the risk of tracheal and mucosal injury. This allows air to pass from the respiratory system through the larynx into the upper airway, allowing speech. A deflated cuff increases the risk of gross aspiration, and given the lack of a tracheal seal, the tracheostomy may move or hinge along its axis at the stoma site, especially if weighed down with unsupported ventilator tubing. Patients may use a one-way Passy-Muir valve, which is placed at the proximal end of the tracheostomy to allow phonation. This allows air to enter the tracheostomy, but not exit, forcing it through the vocal cords. As a safety measure, the patient or caregivers must be able to remove the valve, as it can become occluded with secretions.

Some tracheostomy tubes have fenestrations on the outer curvature above the tracheostomy cuff. These allow phonation even with an inflated cuff, as some air escapes the fenestrations and goes through the vocal cords. Fenestrated tubes may also provide a lower-resistance route during exhalation, perhaps reducing the work of breathing. This can be important in patients with limited respiratory reserve. These tubes are occasionally used in the setting of gradual ventilator weaning and may improve quality of life by enhancing communication, but have their own risks, including the formation of granulation tissue at the site of fenestrations at the anterior trachea and concomitant tracheal narrowing [6]. In patients not requiring continuous mechanical ventilation, the benefits of these tubes can be achieved with uncuffed tracheostomy tubes or smaller tubes with deflated cuffs, with lower complication rates, so they are not used frequently in this population [7]. Further discussion of fenestrated tubes and their effect on speech is discussed later in this chapter.

Extra length tracheostomy (XLT) tubes are longer tracheostomy tubes and are defined either as proximal XLTs with a longer proximal segment or as distal XLTs with longer distal segments. The former are often used in obese individuals, those with excessive neck soft tissue, or large neck circumference. Distal XLTs are used in patients with distal tracheal obstruction or those with tracheomalacia. Imaging and bronchoscopy can identify patients with challenging tracheal and neck anatomy that may benefit from XLT tracheostomies. The concept of airway resistance must be considered when choosing a longer tracheostomy tube, and this is especially important in XLT tubes with small inner diameters, which further significantly increase airway resistance and thus work of breathing in spontaneously ventilating patients or those on ventilator weans. However, airway diameter has a much larger effect, to the fourth power, compared to length as described in Poiseuille's law:

$$R = \frac{8\eta L}{\pi r^4}$$

Where η is viscosity, a constant, L is the length of the tube, and r is the cross-sectional radius.

XLT tubes can cause complications related to tube positioning, with the distal tip placement leading to selective lung ventilation and atelectasis, or posterior wall contact causing granulation tissue formation, tracheal stenosis, tracheomalacia, or tracheal wall injury with rare fistula formation.

Delivery of Supplemental Oxygen in Patients with Tracheostomies

Many patients with a tracheostomy continue to require supplemental oxygen. In patients who continue to require positive-pressure ventilation, the fraction of inspired oxygen (FiO_2) can be adjusted on the ventilator. Positive end-expiratory pressure (PEEP) improves oxygenation by recruiting alveolar units, improving V/Q matching, and reducing atelectotrauma. Lastly, as previously discussed in this book, CO_2 clearance is key to maintaining a physiological alveolar partial pressure of oxygen (PAO_2) following Dalton's Law of Partial Pressures. Excessive CO_2 retention reduces PAO_2, which subsequently leads to hypoxemia. Physicians can ensure adequate ventilation through tracheostomies.

Once a patient is weaned off a ventilator, they may still require supplemental oxygen to maintain normoxemia. A tracheostomy cuff mask connected to a Venturi device can be used to titrate FiO_2. This provides high-flow oxygen delivery, which ensures adequate oxygen delivery to the respiratory tract at flow rates that prevent a feeling of air hunger, while also providing a small amount of PEEP. The FiO_2 is a rough guide as the tracheostomy isn't tightly connected to the tracheostomy cuff mask but rather operates on a blow-by principle. The actual FiO_2 delivered into the respiratory tract depends on the degree of room air admixture and the amount of inspiratory flow the patient generates. Heat and humidification are lost from bypassing the nasal cavity, and oropharynx can be added to prevent excessive drying of the respiratory epithelium and facilitate mucociliary clearance.

Heat moisture exchangers (HMEs) capture heat and moisture in a patient's exhaled breath in a humidification chamber and release it with the next inspired breath. When compared to heated humidified high-flow circuits, HMEs provide significantly less humidification to the airway and thus may not be ideal in patients with high secretion burden [8, 9]. While heated humidified high-flow oxygen therapy has been shown to provide improved oxygenation and positive airway expiratory pressures when delivered nasally, these effects are significantly reduced when delivered through a tracheostomy tube.

Sleep in Patients with Tracheostomies

Sleep is an important aspect of quality of life in patients with chronic respiratory failure requiring tracheostomies. Patients temporarily tracheostomized following surgery for head and neck cancer generally reported a negative experience with sleep, especially with associated noise [10]. The mode of nocturnal ventilation in patients who are able to tolerate increasing periods of spontaneous breathing has also been studied, with some evidence that low nocturnal pressure support may be superior to spontaneous breathing in terms of total sleep time [11]. Conversely, patients undergoing tracheostomy for obstructive sleep apnea demonstrate dramatic improvements in apnea–hypopnea index, nocturnal oxygenation, sleep-related mortality, and overall sleep architecture [12].

Ensuring adequate oxygenation during sleep is crucial to ensuring sleep quality, reducing morbidity, and the long-term development of pulmonary hypertension. An important aspect is preventing obstruction of the tube by secretions, which may entail regular tracheostomy care and suctioning. Provision of humidified, high-flow oxygen during sleep ensures adequate oxygen delivery, reduces secretions, and moistens the airway while also providing PEEP, which, in combination, prevents hypoxic events and optimizes mucociliary function. High-flow oxygen is safe to use through a tracheostomy cuff mask, and the FiO_2 should be adjusted to maintain $SpO_2 > 92\%$. As such, patients may initially require nocturnal pulse oximetry monitoring to ensure adequate oxygenation.

Patients with tracheostomies generally experience mild hypercapnia during sleep, similar to individuals without tracheostomies due to a degree of hypoventilation. However, in those receiving positive-pressure ventilation with deflated cuffs, additional volume loss during sleep can further contribute to elevated CO_2 levels [13]. Consequently, patients receiving mechanical ventilation may require increased inspiratory pressures during sleep to maintain adequate alveolar ventilation.

Tracheostomy Complications and Emergencies

Bleeding from the tracheostomy site is a common occurrence, and a small amount may be physiological after tracheostomy creation or after tracheostomy changes. Irritation of tracheal mucosa from the tracheostomy itself or suction catheters can also cause minor bleeding.

Tracheostomy tube displacement can result in an emergency, with complete tube displacement termed decannulation, and partial displacement called dislodgement. For patients on mechanical ventilation, the initial signs of tube displacement can be inability to deliver tidal volumes, subcutaneous emphysema and hypoxia. The fourth National Audit Project (NAP4) of the Royal College of Anesthetists and the Difficult Airway Society in the United Kingdom noted this complication in the largest registry of airway complications ever compiled. The authors reported that these patients were often not monitored with capnography, which led to delays in recognition of tube displacement, resulting in cardiac arrest in some cases. One of the major recommendations from these societies is that "*Capnography must be available at each bed space in the ICU and should be used continuously while patients are being mechanically ventilated*" [14].

Risk factors for tracheostomy tube displacement include loose tracheostomy ties, significant coughing, and excessive traction on the tracheostomy. Obese patients without XLT tracheostomy tubes may be at risk for dislodgement due to inadequate tube length. Inability to pass a suction catheter through the tube is suggestive of dislodgement. Tracheostomies that are under a week old have immature tracts, which are likely to close quickly in the setting of displacement. In patients who are tracheostomy-dependent, in this situation, endotracheal intubation is often necessary to protect the airway and ensure ventilation. Displacement of tracheostomy in the initial period is therefore a true medical emergency. In patients who have mature tracheostomies, i.e., over two weeks old, it is often possible to reinsert the tracheostomy through the existing stoma, and positioning may be confirmed by bronchoscopy. Other early complications of tracheostomy are discussed in a complementary chapter.

Tracheostomy tube obstruction can also lead to an emergency, especially in ventilator-dependent patients with an inflated cuff. Often, this obstruction is due to a build-up of secretions, either physiological or in the setting of respiratory infections. This highlights the importance of regular tracheostomy care, as well as heated humidified circuits, as previously discussed. In patients who have suspected tracheostomy obstruction, suctioning should be performed to restore lumen patency. The inner cannula can also be removed and cleaned or exchanged. In the setting of persistent obstruction or inability to pass a suction catheter, tube dislodgement should be considered. As previously discussed, mature tracheostomy tubes can be replaced relatively simply. Patients with fresh tracheostomies that are obstructed and refractory to suctioning and replacement of the inner cannula may need endotracheal intubation and interrogation of the tracheostomy in an operative setting.

Late complications of tracheostomy are those that occur after seven days. Tracheal stenosis is relatively common, occurring in up to 26% of patients [15]. Risk factors include insults leading to local tissue necrosis or granulation tissue formation, i.e., use of fenestrated tracheostomy tubes, cuff overinflation, and tracheal infections. The majority of tracheal stenoses are less than 50% of the tracheal diameter and are mostly asymptomatic. Most symptomatic stenoses can be treated with bronchoscopic dilatation [16].

Tracheomalacia is a known but uncommon late complication of tracheostomy, occurring in 2.6% of patients [17]. The etiology is destruction of tracheal cartilage leading to a loss of mechanical integrity. When symptomatic, a distal XLT can be used to bypass the area of tracheomalacia. Definitive treatments are similar to those of patients without tracheostomies, including airway stents.

Patients with tracheostomies are at increased risk of aspiration pneumonia due to secretions pooling above the cuff. Up to 50% of patients aspirate, and the majority of these are silent aspiration events [18]. Although cuff inflation may reduce the risk of macro-aspiration events, it does not reduce the risk of microaspiration. Thus, engaging with speech and language pathologists is a crucial aspect of these patients' care.

The formation of a tracheo-esophageal (TE) fistula is a rare complication, with an incidence rate of 3% [19]. This is caused by erosion of the posterior tracheal wall, leading to an anomalous connection with the esophagus. Risk factors are similar to those leading to a trachea-brachiocephalic artery fistula, including excessive cuff pressures, high airway pressures, and use of corticosteroids. Further, the presence of a nasogastric tube also increases the risk of fistulization. Signs of a TE fistula include suctioning of gastric contents or feeds from the respiratory tract, gastric distension, and volume loss if the patient is ventilator-dependent. As spontaneous closure of the defect is rare, and patients with chronic tracheostomies may not be candidates for complex surgery, conservative approaches include placement of a feeding jejunostomy and gastric decompression, or total parenteral nutrition [20].

Speech and Swallowing in Patients with Tracheostomies

Challenges with phonation are common in tracheostomized patients. Patients who are ventilator-dependent with inflated cuffs will largely not be able to phonate, unless fenestrated tubes are used. As patients wean from the ventilator, one-way speaking valves with deflated cuffs allow for a degree of phonation, provided patients are able to generate the necessary vital capacity to produce speech. Prolonged duration without speech can be challenging, hindering the ability to communicate—this highlights the importance of intensive speech therapy in tracheostomized patients [21].

Newer single-fenestrated tubes with smooth edges, such as the Blom tracheostomy tube, have been developed in an attempt to reduce granulation tissue formation. In a study of 30 non-ventilator-dependent patients requiring tracheostomy, there was no difference in oxygen saturation, respiratory rate, or heart rate at baseline or after speech in patients using a standard fenestrated or non-fenestrated inner cannula with a Passy-Muir speaking valve or a Blom tracheostomy tube [22]. Furthermore, there was no difference in the decibel level of speech between these groups. However, in mechanically ventilated patients, the Blom tracheostomy tube with a fully inflated tube cuff allowed for effective speech and verbal communication [23].

Patients' ability to manage secretions should be evaluated before trialing speaking valves, as buildup of secretions in the trachea and around the tracheostomy tube can hinder adequate exhalation and result in respiratory failure and hypoxia. Patients may require supplemental oxygen while trialing a speaking valve. This can be provided with a tracheostomy mask over the speaking valve, or through an oxygen delivery adaptor on some speaking valves. Humidification can also be added to this circuit. In patients with small-diameter tracheostomies, the majority of inspiratory flow may be through the upper airway, in which case supplemental oxygen can be delivered through a facemask or nasal cannula. Pulse oximetry is recommended initially during speech valve trials to ensure adequate oxygenation.

Dysphagia and difficulties with oral intake are common challenges in tracheostomized patients, and professional bodies advise formal swallow assessment with videofluoroscopic swallow study or fiberoptic endoscopic evaluation of swallowing prior to initiation of oral intake [24]. In particular, attempting oral intake with the cuff inflated can be challenging and further contribute to abnormal swallowing mechanics and dysphagia. Oral intake is generally considered safer in patients with capped tracheostomies and deflated cuffs. Unfortunately, some patients with severe dysphagia may be unable to resume oral feeding for a prolonged period [25].

Decannulation

Once the underlying condition prompting tracheostomy placement has improved, clinicians can begin evaluating the appropriate timing and strategy for tracheostomy decannulation. In order to do this, the patient must be able to tolerate spontaneous breathing around the clock while maintaining appropriate oxygenation, usually targeted at SpO_2 greater than 92%. If the tracheostomy was created for airway protection, the underlying neurological or muscular pathology must have improved such that the patient can keep their airway patent independently. The patient must also be able to manage and clear their own secretions, with minimal assistance with suctioning.

In some patients, especially those who have spent prolonged periods on mechanical ventilation or with significant sarcopenia, closer attention should be paid to the ability to spontaneously ventilate. Anatomical dead space increases with tracheostomy removal, as does overall airway resistance, and if patients do not have adequate respiratory muscle reserve to overcome this, CO_2 levels rise, which can subsequently lead to hypoxia.

Some patients may not be candidates for decannulation, especially those with permanent upper airway obstruction due to masses or surgery. Additionally, patients with devastating neurological injury may never recover to the extent that they can independently maintain their own airway.

Before decannulation is considered, patients' upper airways are assessed by encouraging phonation while occluding the proximal end of the tracheostomy tube with a deflated cuff. Normal phonation indicates no significant upper airway obstruction, while respiratory distress or stridor indicates obstruction that may need to be evaluated endoscopically or with imaging. Next, the presence of a strong and effective cough is assessed as a proxy for the ability to manage one's secretions.

Traditionally, once patients are deemed suitable for decannulation, their tracheostomy tubes are capped—physiologically simulating removal. The time for which the tubes are left capped is gradually increased to ensure patients will tolerate decannulation. An alternative approach involves downsizing the tracheostomy tube, which allows more air to enter through the upper airway and reduces the dependence on the tracheostomy for ventilation. Once a small enough tube is tolerated, the patient is decannulated. This approach allows the patient time to build the respiratory muscle strength to provide the entire tidal volume through the upper airway. Both these techniques have demonstrated high rates of decannulation success [26].

A critique of these approaches is that they are excessively conservative and unnecessarily delay decannulation. Moreover, some patients do not tolerate extended capping trials due to discomfort and pooling of secretions, but may nonetheless tolerate decannulation. Resultantly, novel protocols for decannulation based on suctioning frequency, as a marker of patients' ability to manage secretions, have been investigated and appear to lead to earlier decannulation, fewer pulmonary infections, and shorter hospital stays, without a difference in decannulation failure [27], supporting a more central role for secretion frequency in assessing for tracheostomy decannulation.

The utility of high-flow oxygen delivery has also been investigated in patients thought to be at high risk of weaning failure, with the hypothesis being that high-flow oxygen could improve neuro-ventilatory drive, reduce work of breathing, and improve ventilation, similar to the effects seen in patients receiving oxygen through high-flow nasal cannulas. However, a small study did not support this hypothesis, suggesting important differences between tracheostomy, high-flow oxygen, and high-flow nasal cannula [28]. Thus, the majority of patients with tracheostomies receive supplemental oxygen through either a tracheostomy collar or conventional low-flow oxygen. Indeed, evidence suggests that weaning with tracheostomy leads to a quicker ventilator wean compared to pressure support [29]. However, clinicians must ensure that these patients have adequate respiratory muscle function and can tolerate the relatively low-flow rates and FiO_2 that these techniques offer. Lastly, continuous positive airway pressure (CPAP) can also be used for ventilator weaning [30]—physiologically, these patients may oxygenate better than those on a tracheostomy collar or low-flow oxygen due to the PEEP supplied by the machine. However, this may limit patients from engaging with speech and language pathology and other rehabilitation activities.

In patients who are decannulated but have a high propensity to fail, tracheostomy plugs can be placed in the tracheostomy site to maintain its patency in case toileting or replacement of the tracheostomy tube is required.

Generally, mature tracheostomy tracts begin to close two days after decannulation and are fully closed by a week after decannulation. Patent tracts beyond 3–6 months are pathological and termed tracheocutaneous fistulas.

Tracheostomy Safety at Home

Adequate care of the tracheostomy is key to avoiding complications and preventing infections. Therefore, patients and caregivers must be appropriately educated prior to discharge about how to care for them, how to handle tracheostomy emergencies, and when to ask for help.

At a minimum, patients and caregivers should be able to demonstrate how to clean the stoma, exchange or clean the inner cannula, change the tracheostomy tube, and change tracheostomy ties [31].

In the event of displacement, the ability to advance a suction catheter to confirm location and replace the tracheostomy is key. It is advisable for patients to have the same size tracheostomy and one size smaller in case of emergencies.

Summary

The evolution of tracheostomy tubes and advances in mechanical ventilation have allowed patients to live chronically with tracheostomy tubes or to wean from mechanical ventilation following critical illness. Practitioners must be aware of how oxygenation and ventilation are affected by various tracheostomy tubes in concert with patients' individual characteristics or clinical conditions when selecting a tracheostomy tube and oxygen therapy. Awareness and monitoring of complications following tracheostomy are important to prevent clinical decompensation in the tracheostomized patients requiring mechanical ventilation in the hospital. Tracheostomy weaning must be monitored closely and in a manner that ensures the patient will tolerate decannulation. Patients living with chronic tracheostomies must be educated and demonstrated routine tracheostomy care to prevent complications.

Declarations

Competing Interests The author(s) has no competing interests to declare that are relevant to the content of this manuscript.

Ethics Approval The author(s) declares that this manuscript does not include primary research with human participants.

The author(s) declares that this manuscript does not include primary studies involving animals.

References

1. Davis KJ, Campbell RS, Johannigman JA, Valente JF, Branson RD. Changes in respiratory mechanics after tracheostomy. Arch Surg. 1999;134:59–62.
2. van Heurn LW, Goei R, de Ploeg I, Ramsay G, Brink PR. Late complications of percutaneous dilatational tracheotomy. Chest. 1996;110:1572–6.
3. Pryor L, Ward E, Cornwell P, O'Connor S, Chapman M. Patterns of return to oral intake and decannulation post-tracheostomy across clinical populations in an acute inpatient setting. Int J Lang Commun Disord. 2016;51:556–67.
4. Norwood S, Vallina VL, Short K, Saigusa M, Fernandez LG, McLarty JW. Incidence of tracheal stenosis and other late complications after percutaneous tracheostomy. Ann Surg. 2000;232:233–41.
5. Leder SB, Pauloski BR, Rademaker AW, Grammer T, Dikeman K, Kazandjian M, Mendes J, Logemann JA. Verbal communication for the ventilator-dependent patient requiring an inflated tracheotomy tube cuff: a prospective, multicenter study on the Blom tracheotomy tube with speech inner cannula. Head Neck. 2013;35:505–10.
6. Ke M, Wu X, Zeng J. The treatment strategy for tracheoesophageal fistula. J Thorac Dis. 2015;7:S389–97.
7. Stripoli T, Spadaro S, Di Mussi R, et al. High-flow oxygen therapy in tracheostomized patients at high risk of weaning failure. Ann Intensive Care. 2019;9:4.
8. Frost EA. Tracing the tracheostomy. Ann Otol Rhinol Laryngol. 1976;85:618–24.
9. Pandian V, Boisen SE, Mathews S, Cole T. Are fenestrated tracheostomy tubes still valuable? Am J Speech Lang Pathol. 2019;28:1019–28.
10. Camacho M, Certal V, Brietzke SE, Holty J-EC, Guilleminault C, Capasso R. Tracheostomy as treatment for adult obstructive sleep apnea: a systematic review and meta-analysis. Laryngoscope. 2014;124:803–11.
11. Freeman-Sanderson A, Togher L, Phipps P, Elkins M. A clinical audit of the management of patients with a tracheostomy in an Australian tertiary hospital intensive care unit: Focus on speech-language pathology. Int J Speech Lang Pathol. 2011;13:518–25.
12. Cook TM, Woodall N, Harper J, Benger J, Project FNA. Major complications of airway management in the UK: results of the Fourth National Audit Project of the Royal College of Anaesthetists and the Difficult Airway Society. Part 2: intensive care and emergency departments. Br J Anaesth. 2011;106:632–42.
13. Roche-Campo F, Thille AW, Drouot X, Galia F, Margarit L, Cordoba-Izquierdo A, Mancebo J, d'Ortho M-P, Brochard L. Comparison of sleep quality with mechanical versus spontaneous ventilation during weaning of critically III tracheostomized patients. Crit Care Med. 2013;41:1637–44.
14. Dieperink W, Aarts LPHJ, Rodgers MGG, Delwig H, Nijsten MWN. Boussignac continuous positive airway pressure for weaning with tracheostomy tubes. Respiration. 2008;75:427–31.
15. West JB. The physiological challenges of the 1952 Copenhagen poliomyelitis epidemic and a renaissance in clinical respiratory physiology. J Appl Physiol (1985). 2005;99:424–32.
16. Elpern EH, Scott MG, Petro L, Ries MH. Pulmonary aspiration in mechanically ventilated patients with tracheostomies. Chest. 1994;105:563–6.
17. Adam SI, Srinet P, Aronberg RM, Rosenberg G, Leder SB. Verbal communication with the Blom low profile and Passy-Muir one-way tracheotomy tube speaking valves. J Commun Disord. 2015;56:40–6.
18. Chikata Y, Oto J, Onodera M, Nishimura M. Humidification performance of humidifying devices for tracheostomized patients with spontaneous breathing: a bench study. Respir Care. 2013;58:1442–8.
19. Kuhn MA, Gillespie MB, Ishman SL, et al. Expert consensus statement: management of dysphagia in head and neck cancer patients. Otolaryngol Head Neck Surg. 2023;168:571–92.
20. Hernandez Martinez G, Rodriguez M-L, Vaquero M-C, et al. High-flow oxygen with capping or suctioning for tracheostomy decannulation. N Engl J Med. 2020;383:1009–17.

21. Nakanishi N, Oto J, Itagaki T, Nakataki E, Onodera M, Nishimura M. Humidification performance of passive and active humidification devices within a spontaneously breathing tracheostomized cohort. Respir Care. 2019;64:130–5.
22. Watt JW, Devine A. Does dead space ventilation always alleviate hypocapnia? Long-term ventilation with plain tracheostomy tubes. Anaesthesia. 1995;50:688–91.
23. Pandian V, Miller CR, Schiavi AJ, et al. Utilization of a standardized tracheostomy capping and decannulation protocol to improve patient safety. Laryngoscope. 2014;124:1794–800.
24. Jubran A, Grant BJB, Duffner LA, Collins EG, Lanuza DM, Hoffman LA, Tobin MJ. Effect of pressure support vs unassisted breathing through a tracheostomy collar on weaning duration in patients requiring prolonged mechanical ventilation: a randomized trial. JAMA. 2013;309:671–7.
25. Rogers SN, Russell L, Lowe D. Patients' experience of temporary tracheostomy after microvascular reconstruction for cancer of the head and neck. Br J Oral Maxillofac Surg. 2017;55:10–6.
26. Mitchell RB, Hussey HM, Setzen G, et al. Clinical consensus statement: tracheostomy care. Otolaryngol Head Neck Surg. 2013;148:6–20.
27. Pandian V, Boisen S, Mathews S, Brenner MJ. Speech and safety in tracheostomy patients receiving mechanical ventilation: a systematic review. Am J Crit Care. 2019;28:441–50.
28. Paraschiv M. Tracheoesophageal fistula—a complication of prolonged tracheal intubation. J Med Life. 2014;7:516–21.
29. Toy FJ, Weinstein JD. A percutaneous tracheostomy device. Surgery. 1969;65:384–9.
30. Berges AJ, Lina IA, Ospino R, Tsai H-W, Ding D, Izzi JM, Hillel AT. Impact of low-volume, low-pressure tracheostomy cuffs on acute mucosal injury in swine. Otolaryngol Head Neck Surg. 2022;167:716–24.
31. Shin B, Kim K, Jeong B-H, Eom JS, Song WJ, Kim H. Clinical implications of differentiating between types of post-tracheostomy tracheal stenosis. J Thorac Dis. 2017;9:4413–23.

Use of Oxygen at the End of Life

21

Margaret Kreher

Defining End of Life

Supplemental oxygen therapy is frequently requested and implemented in the hospital setting in response to hypoxemia and complaints of dyspnea [1]. The rationale behind supplemental oxygen use at the end of life is variable, including patient/family request, goal-directed use, and use for symptom relief [2]. The review of the palliative use of oxygen at the end of life begins with a fundamental understanding of the definition of end of life. End of life is the period during the trajectory of serious illness characterized by rapid physical decline occurring in the last days to weeks of life [3]. The rapidity of decline may occur at different rates depending upon the severity of underlying illnesses, acute insults, and progression and complications of the terminal disease and its treatments. End-of-life symptoms include pain, anxiety, and dyspnea, and are the most common symptoms experienced by patients in the last days to weeks of life. Dyspnea can be present in up to 30–90% of patients at the end of life, depending on diagnosis and complications [4].

Hypoxia Versus Dyspnea

Dyspnea is a sensory experience for a patient. Patients describe the sensation as not being able to take a deep breath, feeling short of breath, or feeling tight in the chest. The perception of dyspnea is the result of interactions between receptors within the CNS and between the CNS and peripheral receptors in the upper airways, lungs, and chest wall [5]. The interplay between physical, emotional, spiritual, and social distress affects the dyspnea experience. The complaint of dyspnea may or may not

M. Kreher (✉)
Division of Palliative Care, Department of Family Medicine, Thomas Jefferson University, Philadelphia, PA, USA
e-mail: margaret.kreher@jefferson.edu

G. C. Kane et al. (eds.), *Oxygen*, https://doi.org/10.1007/978-3-032-18934-9_21

be associated with hypoxia. Hypoxia is insufficient tissue oxygenation that results in abnormal metabolism [6]. Hypoxia is a measured parameter, and dyspnea is the sensation perceived by the patient. The presence of hypoxia at the end of life may or may not be associated with dyspnea. This is important as patients may not display distress despite hypoxemia at the very end of life, shortly before death.

Evaluation

General principles for evaluating patients with dyspnea and or hypoxia include careful history and physical examination. Identifying the cause of dyspnea and intervening when feasible are the first steps in treating dyspnea. Dyspnea can occur in the setting of hypoxemia, anxiety, panic, pleural effusion, pericardial effusion, fluid overload, pneumothorax, pain, increased intra-abdominal pressure, and other acute and chronic medical conditions. Easy to fix problems, such as technical problems with oxygen delivery, should be part of the initial assessment by the clinician. Standard tools for dyspnea measurement, such as the numeric rating scale (NRS) for patients who can communicate or the respiratory distress observation scale (RDOS) for patients who cannot communicate, are part of a standardized practice to assess the patient for respiratory distress [7]. NRS ratings above 4–5 and RDOS ratings above 3 are significant and in need of assessment and intervention.

History/Evidence

Oxygen supplementation at the end of life remains part of practice patterns for comfort measures [2]. As the evidence base for palliative interventions at the end of life expands, more information regarding how to best utilize oxygen at the end of life has become available.

For patients with severe hypoxic respiratory failure, oxygen supplementation is part of the treatment for dyspnea at the end of life. In patients with COPD and severe hypoxemia, $PaO2 \leq 55$ mm Hg at rest, oxygen supplementation improves dyspnea, survival, and functional status [8]. Supplemental oxygen in nonhypoxic or mildly hypoxic patients at the end of life provides no more relief of dyspnea than air flow alone [9]. For patients with severe lung disease, chronic dyspnea, and mild or no hypoxemia, supplemental oxygen may impact dyspnea during exercise but does not improve dyspnea overall or quality of life [10]. The technology of noninvasive forms of respiratory support for hospitalized patients with severe respiratory disease has advanced and become easier to access over time. It is important to develop an understanding of the role noninvasive forms of respiratory support play in addressing symptoms at the end of life. It has become more common to encounter hospitalized patients with lung disease or end-stage malignancy, most often involving the lung, who are on high-flow nasal cannula oxygen (HFNC) or noninvasive positive-pressure ventilation (NPPV) as part of a stabilization strategy for relief of hypoxemia and dyspnea [11].

Recommendations

Understanding where the patient is within the course of illness, specifically within the dying trajectory, is critical. Establishing prognosis is the first step in the management of end-of-life care. Communicating this information is also essential to the provision of such care. Effective communication is the basis for establishing priorities, care goals, and the extent of medical interventions. Knowing what goals of care are for a patient who is in the last days to weeks of life guides the evaluation and intervention(s) for dyspnea and/or hypoxemia. For example, a patient who is at the end of life may have goals for life prolongation to achieve specific patient/family milestones or may have cultural/religious beliefs that include life support as an accepted intervention at the end of life. Alternatively, a patient with knowledge of a prognosis of days to weeks may choose to have symptoms managed and forego life-supporting measures.

Patients at the end of life who are experiencing dyspnea benefit from providers determining the cause of dyspnea and treating dyspnea, dependent upon patient goals and feasibility of interventions. For the nonhypoxic or minimally hypoxic patient with dyspnea, airflow, relaxation techniques, opiates, and anxiolytics are all part of the care plan to relieve dyspnea. For patients with severe hypoxic respiratory failure whose PaO_2 is <55 mm Hg, oxygen supplementation may be a beneficial part of dyspnea treatment along with air flow, relaxation techniques, opiates, and anxiolytics. For the patient who is at the end of life, whose goals are symptom-focused and who has severe hypoxic respiratory failure with refractory dyspnea despite treatment, sedation titrated to an acceptable dyspnea level can be part of a care plan established through shared decision-making between clinicians and patients and their families [1].

Noninvasive respiratory support, such as noninvasive positive pressure (NPPV), high-flow nasal cannula (HFNC), or nasal cannula support, may be consistent with care goals in the last days to weeks of life. Noninvasive positive pressure ventilation (NPPV) can support patients with acute and chronic respiratory failure. This type of ventilation provides support for both the inspiratory and expiratory phases of respiration and is part of treatment plans for COPD, CHF, ALS, sleep apnea, and interstitial lung disease. Such support may provide relief from dyspnea and may prolong life. Discomfort may be associated with noninvasive respiratory support. The discomfort associated with noninvasive respiratory support should be part of the discussion of interventions. Noninvasive positive pressure (NPPV) masks and non-rebreather masks can feel claustrophobic to patients. Masks may impede a patient from eating and drinking. Nasal cannulas and high-flow nasal cannulas (HFNC) can be irritating to the nose depending on the flow. High-flow rates create noise for a patient wearing the cannula, which can add difficulty to communication with loved ones and caregivers. Patients who are in the last hours to days of life may no longer achieve the benefits of noninvasive respiratory support [12].

The use of NPPV in hypoxic respiratory failure as a means of dyspnea control at the end of life presents challenges. Patients are awake and may have goals in the short-term to prolong life. A portion of patients at the end of life find it helpful for dyspnea control [13]. Providing patient/family-centered anticipatory guidance is helpful as dying patients clinically change and the benefit, and tolerance of NPPV may change. Counsel regarding the uncertainty of duration of symptom relief, life prolongation, and/or prolongation of the dying process is part of shared decision-making between clinician and patient. If the patient remains symptomatic from dyspnea despite maximizing NPPV settings or is no longer alert because of the dying process, then NPPV is nonbeneficial. It is important to reassess patients frequently for physical signs of comfort or discomfort and to assess patients' satisfaction with dyspnea control [14]. Standards of care and frequent assessment by standardized tools assessing respiratory distress should be employed. If the patient feels claustrophobic, a small dose of benzodiazepine can alleviate anxiety. When NPPV is no longer part of goal-concordant care, opioids and benzodiazepines are part of the treatment to decrease dyspnea and anxiety. Because NPPV provides pressure support, its discontinuation is similar to removing ventilatory support at the very end of life. Titration of medications with opiates as the mainstay for dyspnea control and benzodiazepines for anxiety is part of the standard of care for patients dying with respiratory failure and dyspnea.

The other form of noninvasive respiratory support utilized for hypoxic patients at the end of life is HFNC. HFNC can present barriers to hospital discharge. Frequently, the oxygen flow rates exceed what is possible to support in the home or inpatient hospice units. Patients and families sometimes do not perceive HFNC treatment as an intensive form of care and are surprised that it cannot be provided in the home. Discussion of care goals in this setting would include discussion of titration of HFNC, adjustment of medications to achieve satisfactory dyspnea control, and establishing a flow rate compatible with discharge to a home setting or an inpatient hospice unit setting.

The dependence upon HFNC for dyspnea control may preclude a safe discharge home at the end of life. In this situation, a careful assessment of patient care goals and needs, as well as respiratory needs help determine if a patient would desire titration of HFNC to room air to avoid prolonging the dying process, as may occur with the continuation of supplemental oxygen. Careful attention to psychosocial, spiritual, and physical needs is necessary, no matter the decision. Anxiety and fear are highly prevalent in awake patients when discussing the tapering of noninvasive respiratory support. Patient-centered education addressing concerns about the withdrawal process can help ease anxiety. Medication management in this setting is determined by patient preference, symptom burden, and clinical judgment. Adequate symptom control is necessary prior to the taper of HFNC. A published case series suggests a protocol of reducing FiO_2 and liter flow rate by 25% at 10-min intervals with bolus opiate or anxiolytic, depending on symptoms. If the patient becomes dyspneic or uncomfortable, weaning stops until the provided medication has an effect and the patient is comfortable [15].

Conclusion

Care of the patient with dyspnea and/or hypoxia who is seriously ill should include good prognostication as to whether a patient is within the last days to weeks of life, followed by communication of the prognosis to the patient and family. Supportive counsel is essential, as are establishing goals for care. Evaluate and treat dyspnea in terms of the goals of care. Oxygen as a treatment for dyspnea may have a limited role in those patients who are not hypoxic or who are minimally hypoxic. In those situations, airflow may be just as beneficial for the treatment of dyspnea. Opioids remain the mainstay for dyspnea, which is refractory to treatment of underlying causes. Anxiolytics and relaxation techniques have a role dependent upon symptoms. HFNC and NPPV are commonly part of the support for patients with hypoxia and dyspnea at the end of life. Goal-directed care includes discussion of what is to come in terms of benefits, achieving goals, and prolongation of living and/or dying. For patients, the decisions at the end of life are not an "all or none" phenomenon. Patients with dyspnea and hypoxemia often choose NPPV, HFNC, or nasal cannula oxygen if it meets their goals and assists with symptom control. Goals change over time as illness progresses, and decisions are based on symptoms and the complex interplay of emotions and relationships. Periodically reassessing the efficacy of interventions in relieving symptoms and achieving goals is part of the care plan for seriously ill patients at the end of life [16]. There remains much to learn regarding the treatment of hypoxic/dyspneic patients at the end of life, given the evolving technology of noninvasive oxygen therapies and the heterogeneity of severely ill patients and the unique clinical, cultural, spiritual, and social scenarios each patient presents.

Declarations

Competing Interests The author has no competing interests to declare that are relevant to the content of this manuscript.

Ethics Approval The author declares that this manuscript does not include primary research with human participants.

The author declares that this manuscript does not include primary studies involving animals.

References

1. Kamal AH, Maguire JM, Wheeler JL, Currow DC, Abernethy AP. Dyspnea review for the palliative care professional: treatment goals and therapeutic options. J Palliat Med. 2012;15:106–14. https://doi.org/10.1089/jpm.2011.0110.7.
2. Quinn-Lee L, Weggel J, Moch SD. Use of oxygen at the end of life: attitudes, beliefs and practices in Wisconsin. WMJ. 2018;117(1):7–12.
3. Hui D, Nooruddin Z, Didwaniya N, et al. Concepts and definitions for "Actively Dying," "End of Life," "Terminally Ill," "Terminal Care": systematic review. JPSM. 2014;1:77–89. https://doi.org/10.1016/j.jpainsymman.2013.02.021.

4. Spinazzola G, Ferrone G, Michi T, et al. Focus on the role of non-invasive respiratory support (NRS) during palliative care in patients with life limiting respiratory disease. J Clin Med. 2024;13:5165. https://doi.org/10.3390/jcm131751165.
5. Hashmi MF, Modi P, Basit, et al. Dyspnea. (Updated 2023 Feb 19). In: StatPearls (Internet). Treasure Island (Fl): StatPearls Publishing; 2025 Jan-. Available from: https://www.ncbi.nlm.nih.gov/books/NBK499965.
6. Bhutta BS, Alghoula F, Berim I. Hypoxia. (updated 2024 Mar 4). In: StatPearls (Internet). Treasure Is (Fl): StatPearls Publishing; 2025 Jan-, Available from: https://www.ncbi.nlm.nih.gov/books/NBK482316/.
7. Zhuang Q, Yang GM, Neo S, Cheung YB. Validity, reliability, and diagnostic accuracy of the respiratory distress observation scale for assessment of dyspnea in adult palliative care patients. J Pain Symptom Manag. 2019;57(2):304–10.
8. Guyatt GH, McKim DA, Austin P, et al. Appropriateness of domiciliary oxygen delivery. Chest. 2000;118:1303–8.
9. Abernathy AP, McDonald CF, Frith PA, et al. Effect of palliative oxygen versus room air in relief of breathlessness in patients with refractory dyspnoea: a double-blind, randomized controlled trial. Lancet. 2010;376:784–93.
10. Long-term oxygen Treatment Trial Group. A randomized trial of long-term oxygen for COPD with moderate desaturation. N Engl J Med. 2016;375:1617–27.
11. Sullivan DR, Kim H, Gozalo PL, et al. Trends in noninvasive and invasive mechanical ventilation among Medicare beneficiaries at the end of life. JAMA Intern Med. 2021;181(1):93–102.
12. Campbell ML, Yarandi H, Dove-Meadows E. Oxygen is nonbeneficial for most patients who are near death. JPSM. 2013;45(3):517–23.
13. Curtis JR, Cook DJ, Sinuff T, Society of Critical Care Medicine Palliative Noninvasive Positive Ventilation Task Force, et al. Noninvasive positive pressure ventilation in critical and palliative care settings: understanding the goals of therapy. Crit Care Med. 2007;35(3):932–9.
14. Nava S, Ferrer M, Esquinas A, et al. Palliative use of noninvasive ventilation in end-of-life patients with solid tumors: a randomized feasibility trial. Lancet Oncol. 2013;14(3):219–27.
15. Brackett H, Forman A, et al. Compassionate removal of heated high-flow nasal cannula for end of life: case series and protocol development. J Hosp Palliat Nurs. 2021;23(4):360–6.
16. Jennerich AL. An approach to caring for patients and family of patients dying in the ICU. Chest. 2024;166(1):127–35.

Part IV

Acute Respiratory Failure

Basic Principles of Mechanical Ventilation

22

Christopher O'Hara and Urvashi Vaid

History of Oxygen and Mechanical Ventilation

Respiratory disease and respiratory failure have plagued humanity throughout our existence. There is surviving documentation as far back as 400 BCE from texts such as the *Hippocratic Corpus*, in which symptoms such as shortness of breath, blue skin discoloration, and labored breathing are described. They recognized that the disease was most severe when patients were expectorating sputum and even described complications such as empyema [1]. Despite the impressive depth of their observations, there was still a gap in their understanding of anatomy, physiology, and pathophysiology; they believed that the lungs cooled the heart or that they provided a life-giving spirit, and attributed illness to humoral theory [2].

It was not until centuries later that the understanding of respiratory illness started to evolve. There were major advances both in the understanding of the human body and the elements needed to support life. In the sixteenth century, the anatomist Andreas Vesalius began to better understand the anatomy of the thoracic cavity, even using bellows to inflate animal lungs [1]. In the eighteenth century, a new gas was discovered independently by Joseph Priestley and Carl Scheele, namely what we know now as oxygen (called "fire air" by Scheele) [3]. It was noted that it supported combustion better than ambient air, and Priestley observed that this newly isolated gas allowed candles to burn brighter and

C. O'Hara
Northwestern Medicine Regional Medical Group – McHenry Hospital, McHenry, IL, USA
e-mail: Christopher.ohara@nm.org

U. Vaid (✉)
The Korman Respiratory Institute and the Division of Pulmonary, Allergy and Critical Care, The Department of Medicine at the Sidney Kimmel Medical College of Thomas Jefferson University, Philadelphia, PA, USA
e-mail: Urvashi.Vaid@jefferson.edu

G. C. Kane et al. (eds.), *Oxygen*, https://doi.org/10.1007/978-3-032-18934-9_22

improved the energy and lifespan of a mouse. Antoine Lavoisier conducted further combustion experiments with this substance, leading him to the conclusion that air is a mixture of two gases, "azote" (nitrogen in English) and "vital air," which he later called oxygen. This work debunked the prior theory of combustion, Phlogiston, which believed that all flammable material contained a material called phlogiston, which was released during combustion and laid the foundation for our understanding of cellular respiration and oxygen's role in respiratory failure and death [3]. Previous chapters at the beginning of the book describe the discovery of oxygen in greater detail.

Despite continued advancement in the understanding of respiratory physiology and failure, there were scant treatment options available until the twentieth century. The polio epidemic necessitated innovation. While polio is a motor neuron disease, and not a respiratory pathogen, in severe cases, it can cause diaphragmatic paralysis and death. Children were most prone to diaphragm failure. It was a harrowing disease to witness; James L. Wilson, a resident physician at Harvard at the time, wrote the following "Of all the experiences that the physician must undergo, none can be more distressing than to watch respiratory paralysis in a child ill with poliomyelitis... Using with increasing vigor every available accessory muscle of neck, shoulder and chin, silent, wasting no breath for speech, wide-eyed and frightened, conscious almost to the last breath" [4]. Their lungs were unaffected, but they were unable to breathe.

At the time, there was no sustainable treatment for respiratory failure until Philip Drinker and Louis Shaw developed the "Drinker Respirator" in 1929, colloquially known as the "iron lung." The iron lung was a 2-meter-long metal tank enclosing the thorax, sealing the neck with rubber collars and leaving the head to atmospheric pressure. It utilized air pumps and bellows to create negative pressure around the thorax, allowing for inspiration. While this was a major advancement, the iron lung had a narrow indication; it was a life-sustaining treatment option for neuromuscular weakness, but it did not augment oxygenation [5]. The Drinker respirator provided ventilatory support.

Interestingly, the transition from negative-pressure ventilation to positive-pressure ventilation was also sparked by a poliovirus epidemic. In 1952, there was another polio epidemic in Copenhagen. Dr. Bjorn Ibsen (an Anesthesiologist) promoted tracheostomy and positive-pressure ventilation, then delivered by hand-bag ventilation, and mortality dropped from 87% to approximately 40%. At the epidemic's worst, 70 patients were being manually ventilated, often by medical students, 1500 of whom provided 165,000 total hours of care. This experience not only catalyzed the development of modern positive-pressure ventilators but also laid the foundation for modern intensive care units [5].

By the 1960s and 1970s, indications for mechanical ventilators had expanded to treat not only neuromuscular failure but also respiratory failure of all causes. Today, invasive mechanical ventilation is a critical intervention in the treatment of hypoxemic respiratory failure and reflects thousands of years of incremental advancement in our understanding of physics, chemistry, biology, and disease. Noninvasive ventilation for acute respiratory failure is covered in other chapters.

Respiratory Physiology

To understand the role of mechanical ventilation in hypoxemic respiratory failure, respiratory anatomy and physiology must first be reviewed. The two main functions of the lungs are the delivery of oxygen and the elimination of carbon dioxide from the bloodstream. While they appear to be simple concepts, they produce a tremendous physiologic challenge. As a result, the lung can appear to be a simple organ on its surface, but microscopically is extremely complex, and its essential functions are intrinsically related to its structure.

Oxygen arrives in the bloodstream from the atmosphere. After the brainstem signals the diaphragm to contract, air flows through the mouth or nares into the upper airway, travels past the vocal cords, and into the trachea. There, the airway branches into the left and right mainstem bronchi. The airways continue to branch through 23 generations, eventually leading to the terminal bronchioles and alveoli where gas exchange occurs [6]. There are approximately 400 million alveoli, which are microscopic sacs at the end of the airway, classically described as individual units, arranged like a "cluster of grapes," but in fact they are interconnected, and air can communicate between individual alveoli via small gaps called Pores of Kohn [7]. Alveoli are composed of three types of cells—type I pneumocytes, type II pneumocytes, and alveolar macrophages. Type I pneumocytes are epithelial cells that surround the alveoli and cover approximately 95% of the alveolar surface area [6]. Type II pneumocytes produce a substance called surfactant, a combination of protein and phospholipids coating the inner surface of the alveoli, which helps prevent alveolar collapse (atelectasis) [6]. The wall of the alveolus is extremely thin and shares a basement membrane with the pulmonary capillary endothelium [6]. The pulmonary capillaries surround the alveoli like a sheet, separated only by a thin layer of interstitial fluid, and have a diameter just wide enough to allow passage of a single layer of red blood cells [6]. The extremely close relationship between the alveoli and pulmonary capillaries allows for extremely efficient gas exchange between the lungs and the blood. Oxygen is transferred from the lungs to the blood via passive diffusion, driven by the concentration gradient between oxygen in the alveoli and oxygen in the deoxygenated blood [6].

Matching ventilation (the volume of air the lungs move) and perfusion (the volume of blood delivered to the lungs) is a central concept in determining oxygenation. This concept is called the ventilation/perfusion (V/Q) ratio. Ideally, the V/Q ratio would be 1, meaning all oxygen inhaled would be transferred into the blood [8]. However, even in healthy lungs, the V/Q ratio is approximately 0.8 [9]. This is due to regional differences in ventilation and perfusion. Both ventilation and perfusion are greatest at the lung bases; perfusion increases more than ventilation in the bases in the upright lung, lowering the ratio at the base of the lung. Ventilation is greatest at the base of the lungs simply due to their larger volume at the bases and the fact that pleural pressure is less negative at the bases in the upright lung, allowing for a greater change in alveolar volume with every breath as the alveoli start out smaller at end expiration [8]. Dr. West described how perfusion to the lungs is related to gravity and three pressures: pulmonary alveolar pressure, pulmonary artery pressure, and pulmonary venous pressure. Gravity acts to increase the pressure in the pulmonary artery and veins, while alveolar pressure remains relatively constant [9]. These pressure differences divide the lung into three "zones." Zone 1 is at the lung apex, where the pressure of the distended alveoli is greater than both pulmonary artery pressure and venous pressure, leading to a relative decrease in perfusion compared to ventilation, resulting in a $V/Q > 1$. In the middle of the lung, pulmonary artery pressure is greater than alveolar pressure, allowing for better matching of ventilation and perfusion. Zone 3 is at the base of the lungs, where both pulmonary artery and venous pressure are greater than alveolar pressure, leading to $V/Q < 1$ [10].

After oxygen is taken up into the blood, it is delivered to the tissues. It undergoes passive diffusion from the systemic capillaries into the tissue and the cells, and finally into the mitochondria. Fascinatingly, the partial pressure of oxygen in the mitochondria is an order of magnitude lower than when it started in the atmosphere, typically 1–3 mmHg [11]. However, in many disease states, oxygen uptake is impacted, leading to hypoxemia (low blood oxygen content) and eventually hypoxia (low tissue oxygen content). There are five different mechanisms of hypoxemia [10]:

1. Low inspired oxygen content.
2. Hypoventilation.
3. Diffusion limitation.
4. Shunt.
5. V/Q mismatch.

Before diving into the mechanisms of hypoxemia, it is important to review the alveolar gas equation (see below). This formula is used to estimate the partial pressure of oxygen in the alveoli [10].

The alveolar gas equation is as follows:

$$PaO_2 = FiO_2 \times \left(P_{atmos} - PH_2O\right) - \left(\frac{PaCO_2}{Q}\right)$$

Where PaO_2 is the partial pressure of alveolar oxygen.

FiO_2 is the fraction of inspired oxygen (21% while breathing ambient air).
Patmos is the atmospheric pressure (760 at sea level).
PH_2O is the vapor pressure at the alveoli (47 mmHg at body temperature).
$PaCO_2$ is the partial pressure of carbon dioxide in the blood.
Q is the respiratory quotient, the ratio of carbon dioxide produced to oxygen consumed (this varies with diet, but is assumed to be 0.8).

If numbers are plugged in, assuming values 0.21*(760–47)-40/0.8, the resulting PaO_2 is 99.73 mmHg.

Low Inspired Oxygen Content

This commonly occurs at altitude and can be easily understood with the alveolar gas equation. At altitude, while the FiO_2 of the oxygen in the air is the same as sea level (21%), the atmospheric pressure is lower. Let's use the extreme example of Mount Everest, where at the summit, the atmospheric pressure is only 235 mmHg. If 235 mmHg is plugged into the alveolar gas equation (rather than 760 mmHg at sea level), the resulting PaO_2 is −10.5 mmHg. This is physiologically impossible to sustain and results in an increase in minute ventilation and a low partial pressure of arterial carbon dioxide. This lowering of the CO_2 allows an increase in the partial pressure of oxygen in the blood. This will be further elaborated in detail in the Chapter "Ascent into Thin Air: How Oxygen Is Reduced at Elevation Due To Barometric Pressure" [10].

Hypoventilation

While one might assume hypoventilation causes hypoxemia due to inadequate oxygen uptake into the lungs, this is not actually the case. First, it is important to clarify what is meant by ventilation: it refers to the volume of air moving into the lungs; therefore, hypoventilation is inadequate air movement for the body's demands. Ventilation is primarily driven by the body's pH; increasing blood CO_2 will lower the blood's pH, triggering an increase in ventilation to help compensate. With these concepts in mind, the alveolar gas equation can explain how hypoventilation causes hypoxemia. If the partial pressure of CO_2 is doubled from 40 to 80 mmHg (as would occur if ventilation were half of what the body demanded), the equation then looks like this: 0.21*(760–47)–80/0.8, resulting in a PaO_2 of 49.73 mmHg (how PaO_2 affects oxygen delivery will be discussed later) [10].

Diffusion Limitation

As discussed before, oxygen traverses through the extremely thin respiratory membrane or alveolar–capillary interface) from the lungs into the bloodstream. Gases can be either diffusion-limited or perfusion-limited. Diffusion limitation implies that the rate of gas transfer across the membrane is limited by the properties of the membrane, while perfusion-limited gases diffuse very readily through the membrane, so gas transfer is limited by the volume of blood delivered per unit time, i.e., the more blood that flows through the circuit, the more gas is transferred. In normal circumstances, oxygen transfer is perfusion-limited. However, various pathologic conditions can cause it to be diffusion-limited, such as pulmonary edema and interstitial lung disease, in which the alveolar–capillary membrane is thickened, or in high-output heart failure, in which blood is moving so rapidly that there is inadequate time for oxygen to fully equilibrate [10].

Shunt

This refers to the passage of blood from the right side of the heart to the left side of the heart without participating in gas exchange. This results in deoxygenated blood mixing with oxygenated blood, which leads to decreased arterial oxygen content and hypoxemia. Shunts can either be intrapulmonary (such as pneumonia, acute atelectasis, or atrialvenous [AV] malformations) or intracardiac (patent foramen ovale [PFO] or atrial or ventricular septal defects [ASD or VSD]). These classically present as refractory hypoxemia. In other words, hypoxemia that does not respond to increasing inspired oxygen content.

Ventilation/Perfusion (V/Q) Mismatch

V/Q is the most frequent cause of hypoxemia and exists as a spectrum. One extreme, lack of ventilation, was discussed under shunt, but at the opposite end of the spectrum is dead space. Dead space refers to areas of the lung that are ventilated but do not have any blood flow. Even in healthy humans, there is a proportion of physiologic dead space, with gas exchange only possible at the level of the respiratory bronchioles (which immediately precede the terminal bronchioles). There is about 150 mL of physiologic dead space in a healthy human. Various pathologies can cause pathologic dead space, such as pulmonary embolism. In V/Q mismatch, the delicate balance of ventilation and perfusion is disrupted, either by relative decreases in ventilation for the amount of perfusion or decreases in perfusion for the amount of ventilation.

These five mechanisms are fundamental concepts to help understand alterations in oxygenation, but clinically, they rarely exist in isolation.

There is an important distinction between hypoxemia and hypoxia, though these terms often are used interchangeably. Hypoxemia is inadequate partial pressure of oxygen in the blood, while hypoxia is inadequate partial pressure of oxygen in the tissues (leading to anaerobic metabolism). While hypoxia is most often caused by hypoxemia, it is important to understand that the vast majority of oxygen delivered to tissues is not dissolved in the blood serum; it is carried by hemoglobin. This can be quantified by the following equation [12]:

$$\mathrm{CaO_2} = \left(\mathrm{Hb} \times 1.36 \times \mathrm{SaO_2}\right) + \left(0.0031 \times \mathrm{PaO_2}\right)$$

Where CaO_2 is the arterial oxygen content.

Hb is the hemoglobin concentration (in g/dL).
1.36 is the milliliters of oxygen bound per gram of hemoglobin
SaO_2 is the arterial oxygen saturation.
0.0031 is the solubility coefficient of oxygen in serum
PaO_2 is the partial pressure of oxygen in the blood.

When plugging in normal values, the equation yields: 15*1.36*1 + 0.0031*100, which simplifies to 20.4 ml/dL (oxygen carried by hemoglobin) + 0.31 ml/dL (oxygen carried in the serum), indicating that 98.5% of oxygen is delivered to the tissue by hemoglobin. Hemoglobin pathologies can also lead to hypoxia even with a completely intact oxygen diffusion mechanism into the bloodstream (examples: severe anemia or carbon monoxide poisoning).

Basics of Mechanical Ventilation

Mechanical ventilation is a life support modality used to augment oxygenation, ventilation, or both in patients who are unable to do so on their own. It is important to keep in mind that it is not a treatment modality; rather, it keeps the patient alive and gas exchange and acid-base status as close to normal, while treating the underlying condition. The most common indications for mechanical ventilation are general anesthesia, hypoxemic respiratory failure, hypercapnic respiratory failure (perhaps better described as ventilatory failure), increased ventilatory demand, and airway protection [13]. Table 22.1 outlines some of the common pathologies that require mechanical ventilation for these indications.

The journey of oxygen from the atmosphere to the mitochondria was discussed previously in this book, but prior to its arrival in the lungs, a discussion of how oxygen arrives at the lungs in mechanically ventilated patients is required. At most centers, there is onsite storage of liquid oxygen, which is transported to the patient's room, and 100% oxygen is delivered to the ventilator at high pressure (typically 50 PSI). It then travels through a pressure regulator, which reduces the input pressure, and then goes into a blender, which mixes oxygen and room air to achieve the set FiO_2; it is then warmed and humidified. The ventilator is connected to a dual-limb circuit, with an inspiratory limb and an expiratory limb, which is attached to the endotracheal tube (or tracheostomy tube). Once inspiration has completed, during exhalation, air is passively expired through the expiratory limb.

Table 22.1 Examples of pathologies and the indication for mechanical ventilation required to support the patient

Indication	Example
Hypoxemic respiratory failure	Pneumonia, ARDS
Hypercapnic respiratory failure (ventilatory failure)	COPD exacerbation, severe asthma exacerbation, acute on chronic obesity hypoventilation syndrome
Airway protection	Severe altered mental status, anaphylaxis
Increased ventilatory demand	Severe metabolic acidosis
Pre-procedure	General anesthesia

Ventilator Settings and Respiratory Mechanics

Mechanical ventilation assists in ventilation and oxygenation. Ventilation focuses on the movement of air and the removal of CO_2 (thus predominantly adjusting the minute ventilation for a patient by manipulating volume and/or flow). Oxygenation is adjusted by increasing the FiO_2 and mean airway pressure, thus increasing the driving force of oxygen across the alveolar–capillary interface. Modern mechanical ventilation delivers breaths using positive pressure.

One might ask: How does the ventilator know when to start and end a breath? There are three characteristics of a breath, denoted by three variables. The first variable is the trigger (what causes the ventilator to initiate a breath). There are two different types of triggers, or two different ways the ventilator knows when to deliver a breath: time trigger, where the ventilator will deliver a breath based on the set respiratory rate (for example, if the rate were set at 12 breaths per minute, the ventilator would deliver a breath every 5 seconds), and patient-triggered, where the patient's respiratory effort will trigger the delivery of a breath. Now that the breath is initiated, the ventilator needs to decide how long and in what mode it delivers the breath. This brings us to the next variable, which is the limit. The limit is typically either pressure, where the maximum allowed inspiratory pressure is set, or flow, where the ventilator delivers the breath at a set flow rate. The last variable is the cycle, which is the setting the ventilator uses to end inspiration and transition to exhalation. Exhalation is a passive process in mechanical ventilation, and expiratory flow will vary depending on the disease pathology until either the patient reaches their resting lung volume or the next breath is triggered [13]. Figure 22.1 graphically depicts the breath characteristics of a ventilator breath.

All these variables must be programmed into the ventilator. The nuances of ventilator management are outside the scope of this text, but the basics will be reviewed. First, the mode of ventilation must be selected. This controls how breaths are triggered. The two most important are "assist control" (AC) and "support" modes. In assist control, the ventilator will provide both patient-triggered breaths and time-triggered breaths. There are two main subsets of AC, which are volume control (AC/VC) and pressure control (AC/PC). In both modes, respiratory rate (RR), positive end-expiratory pressure (PEEP), and fraction of inspired oxygen (FiO_2) are set. AC/

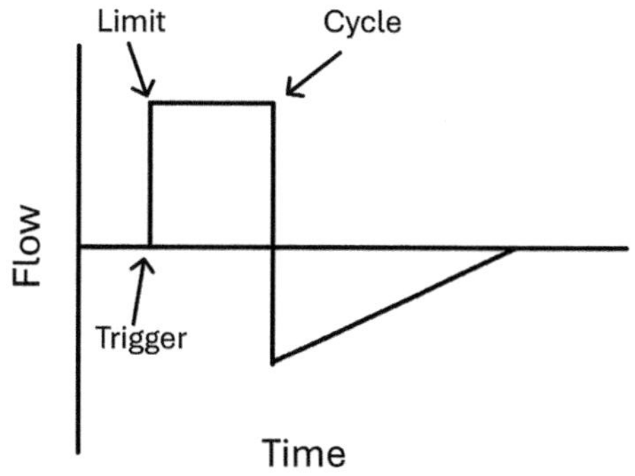

Fig. 22.1 Ventilator flow/time square waveform demonstrating trigger/limit/cycle. Once the breath is triggered, flow increases until it hits the limit (in this case, flow), and cycles off when the preset volume is delivered

VC is a "patient/time triggered, flow limited, volume cycled" mode. In this mode, RR, tidal volume (VT), PEEP, FiO_2, and inspiratory flow are set. The breath is triggered, the ventilator delivers air at a certain flow rate until the preset tidal volume is reached, then the vent cycles off and transitions to exhalation. Flow can be delivered either at a constant flow rate (square waveform) or by degrading over time (ramp waveform). In the square waveform, the breath is typically shorter, which may be beneficial for patients requiring a high respiratory rate or who have bronchospasm, but a degrading flow better mimics natural breathing and is more comfortable for patients. Of particular importance is the volume set for the tidal volume. A patient's tidal volume is dependent physiologically on their height and gender, and based on numerous landmark studies, it is now recommended to set the initial VT between 6 ml/Kg and 10 ml/Kg of ideal body weight. More on this in the chapters on acute respiratory distress syndrome (ARDS) and proning [13].

AC/PC is similar, but these breaths are "patient/time triggered, pressure limited, and time cycled." The main settings are RR, inspiratory pressure (which is additive to PEEP), inspiratory time, PEEP, and FiO_2. In AC/PC, the breath is triggered, air is delivered at the set pressure for a set time, after which the ventilator cycles to exhalation [13].

The other most common mode of ventilation is the support mode, where all breaths are patient-triggered. While both pressure support ventilation (PSV) and volume support modes exist, volume support is almost never used in practice. PSV is a "patient triggered, pressure limited, flow cycled" mode. In pressure support, there is no set respiratory rate (because all breaths are patient-triggered). Instead, one sets an inspiratory pressure (additive to PEEP, like in PCV), FiO_2, PEEP, and flow threshold. This is a flow-cycled breath. You might recall that in normal respiratory physiology, inspiratory flow is highest at the beginning of the breath, and slows throughout inspiration until it stops, after which expiration begins. PSV takes advantage of this and will cycle the breath (turn off) when flow reaches a certain percentage of peak flow (i.e., 25% of the maximal flow). The patient initiates a breath, and air is delivered at a set pressure until the flow degrades a set percentage, at which time the ventilator cycles to exhalation. PSV allows the patient the most control (they control the respiratory rate, volume, inspiratory time, and inspiratory flow) and is the best-tolerated mode of ventilation. There are drawbacks—there is no backup rate, so care must be taken to avoid medications that contribute to respiratory depression and to monitor for hypoventilation [13]. Table 22.2 summarizes the breath characteristics by ventilator mode.

There are many other modes of ventilation, but these are the three most used. The different modes of ventilation have their advantages and disadvantages; however, in

Table 22.2 Breath characteristics by common ventilator modes

Ventilator mode	Trigger	Limit	Cycle
Assist control—volume	Patient/time	Flow	Volume
Assist control—pressure	Patient/time	Pressure	Time
Pressure support	Patient	Pressure	Flow

all modes, patients need to be carefully monitored to see how they respond to the programmed settings. In volume control, inspiratory pressures are monitored, and conversely, in pressure control, tidal volumes and minute ventilation are monitored. The resulting pressure (in volume control) or volume (in pressure control) is related to the patient's respiratory mechanics, which comprises airway resistance and lung compliance. Acute changes in pressure or volume (depending on the mode) can suggest changes in the clinical condition and may require changes to ventilator settings [13].

Airway resistance plays an important role in respiratory mechanics, as one can imagine how a patient with an acute attack of asthma appears clinically—wheezy and in marked respiratory distress as they struggle to exhale every breath. Airway resistance is the opposition of airflow within the airways and is inversely and exponentially proportional to airway caliber: the smaller the airway, the higher the resistance to flow [14]. The equation below defines this relationship.

$$R = \frac{8l\eta}{\pi r^4}$$

Where R is resistance

l is the length of the circuit
η is the fluid viscosity
r is the radius

Airway resistance can increase acutely in airway disease (like asthma and COPD), intubations with small-diameter endotracheal tubes, secretions or kinks blocking the tube, or when the patient bites the endotracheal tube [13].

Compliance, another important concept in ventilation, is the change in volume over change in pressure, or the amount of pressure required to achieve a certain volume. Measured compliance is an interplay of numerous factors: chest wall pressure, abdominal pressure, and lung compliance. A stiff, low-compliance respiratory system can be due to diseases such as acute respiratory distress syndrome (ARDS), interstitial lung disease (ILD), pulmonary edema, abdominal compartment syndrome, or obesity. Conversely, patients with emphysema have higher compliance due to destruction of lung parenchyma and decreased elastic recoil [13].

The maximal inspiratory pressure measured on the ventilator comprises both resistive pressures and compliance pressures, and it is vital to monitor both to best identify changes in respiratory mechanics. These pressures can be measured using a ventilator maneuver called an inspiratory hold. When performing an inspiratory hold, the ventilator will deliver a full breath, then "hold" or stop all flow at the end of inspiration. The resulting pressure (known as the plateau pressure or P_{Plat}) is the measured pressure in the absence of flow, removing resistance pressures from the equation. Using a plateau pressure, both resistance and compliance can be calculated while in volume-control settings with a square waveform. First, obtain a plateau pressure with an inspiratory hold. To measure compliance, use the tidal volume and divide that by the driving pressure (defined as P_{Plat} – PEEP) [14]. The equation below defines the relationship between compliance, tidal volume, and airway pressures.

$$C = \frac{V_T}{\left(P_{\text{Plat}} - \text{PEEP}\right)}$$

Where C is compliance

V_T is tidal volume
P_{Plat} is plateau pressure
PEEP is positive end-expiratory pressure

To calculate airway resistance, use the peak inspiratory pressure, subtract the plateau pressure, and divide this by the inspiratory flow. Take care to note the units for this: flow on the ventilator is reported in L/min, whereas resistance is reported in cmH_20/L/sec, so it may be necessary to convert from L/min to L/sec. This is a useful exercise while caring for mechanically ventilated patients because although changes in tidal volume and flow will change the resulting inspiratory pressures, resistance, and compliance should remain the same. Tracking resistance and compliance better enables the quantification of changes in the patient's respiratory mechanics and clinical condition and allows a response to them as needed [13].

The equation for resistance is as follows:

$$R = \frac{P_{\text{Peak}} - P_{\text{Plat}}}{\dot{V}}$$

Where R is resistance

P_{Peak} is peak airway pressure
P_{Plat} is plateau pressure
$\dot{V}$ is inspiratory flow

How to Modulate Oxygenation in Mechanically Ventilated Patients

One of the most common indications for mechanical ventilation is acute hypoxemic respiratory failure, and there are various strategies that can be used to modulate the delivery and uptake of oxygen in mechanically ventilated patients. The primary and simplest way is adjusting FiO_2 to achieve the patient's oxygenation goals. This can be titrated from 21% to 100%. Another common way to modulate oxygenation is "PEEP titration." PEEP can augment oxygenation via alveolar recruitment. Atelectasis (collapse of alveoli and/or lung units) is a common complication in mechanically ventilated patients; lying supine in bed can cause the dependent areas of the lung to shrink and collapse, leading to shunt physiology. PEEP helps prevent this by applying a distending force to these alveoli even during expiration and reducing the shunt. PEEP is commonly, and somewhat incorrectly, thought of as the only pressure to assist with alveolar recruitment, when in actuality, the mean airway pressure is the main driver of oxygenation. Mean airway pressure is the average pressure in the airway over an entire respiratory cycle and is composed of both pressures during inspiration and expiration (PEEP). Ultimately, mean airway pressure affects multiple properties that improve oxygenation, including diffusion gradient, gas compression, and increasing the surface area for gas exchange. It is calculated by taking the inspiratory pressure multiplied by inspiratory time, adding it to PEEP multiplied by expiratory time, divided by total time [13]. The equation for mean airway pressure is as follows:

$$\overline{\mathrm{Paw}} = \frac{(T_I \times \mathrm{PIP}) + (T_E \times \mathrm{PEEP})}{T_{\mathrm{Tot}}}$$

Where $\mathrm{P}\overline{\mathrm{aw}}$ is the mean airway pressure
T_I is inspiratory time
PIP is positive inspiratory pressure
T_E is expiratory time
PEEP is positive end-expiratory pressure.
T_{Tot} is total inspiratory time

There are numerous other strategies that can be used to help augment oxygenation in critically ill patients, usually reserved for patients with severe disease and refractory hypoxemia. Several chapters in this book are dedicated to describing these in detail.

Prone positioning, where the patients are turned from their backs to their stomachs (usually for 16 hours a day), is one strategy. This works by assisting in V/Q matching. As mentioned earlier, patients who are mechanically ventilated will develop some degree of atelectasis in the dependent portions of the lung, but in ARDS, this process is particularly prominent, and the other portions of the lung cannot maintain oxygenation. By placing the patient in the prone position, recruitment of the previously atelectatic dependent lung will increase the V and match Q better. Please refer to the chapters on prone positioning for more details (Chaps. 28, 29).

Neuromuscular blockade is another common strategy for augmenting oxygenation. This does not directly improve gas transfer or lung injury; instead, it is hypothesized to decrease oxygen consumption throughout the body. While oxygen is typically perfusion-dependent, numerous diseases can cause it to become diffusion-limited. Neuromuscular blockade can help combat this by increasing the saturation of deoxygenated blood, so less time is required for equilibration of alveolar oxygen and blood oxygen [15].

Inhaled pulmonary vasodilators (such as epoprostenol or nitric oxide) are another strategy. While they have been proven to help with oxygenation, there is no proven mortality benefit with their use. Inhaled pulmonary vasodilators work by improving

V/Q matching. The drug is delivered only to well-ventilated portions of the lung and acts locally to vasodilate and increase blood flow to these portions, leading to an improvement in oxygenation. Conversely, usage of intravenous pulmonary vasodilators could have the opposite effect, by promoting blood flow to poorly ventilated areas of the lung and worsening V/Q matching. In addition, if diffusion is poor and blood flow is accelerated through the lung, there is less time for oxygen diffusion across the membrane into hemoglobin. Intravenous vasodilators can also worsen hypotension, so if there is a decision to initiate these, patients must be closely monitored while on these agents [15].

Monitoring

It is important to closely monitor the oxygenation status of patients receiving mechanical ventilation, especially those with hypoxemic respiratory failure. The simplest way to monitor these patients is with peripheral oxygen saturation, though this measurement can become unreliable in severe illness due to malperfusion of the extremities, and is less accurate in patients with darker skin tones. Arterial blood gases are another strategy; most will only report a partial pressure of oxygen, though with co-oximetry, saturation can be directly measured as well.

In patients with ARDS, there are other tools used to help trend oxygenation and the severity of lung injury. P/F ratio is the most common one used in adults with ARDS. This uses the partial pressure of oxygen and divides it by FiO_2 (fraction, not percentage). A P/F ratio between 200 and 300 is considered mild ARDS, between 100 and 200 is moderate, and <100 is severe ARDS. However, this requires an arterial blood draw, so recent recommendations include the S/F ratio as a surrogate for this measurement. This uses the peripheral oxygen saturation divided by FiO_2. Please refer to the chapters on ARDS for further details [16].

The oxygenation index is another monitoring tool, though it is more frequently used in pediatric literature. It is calculated by taking the mean airway pressure, multiplying it by FiO_2 (as a percentage), and dividing by PaO_2. In the neonatal literature, severity is graded as 15 or less for mild, 16–25 for moderate, 26–40 for severe, and greater than 40 for severe. This is a superior tool for monitoring lung injury as it incorporates mean airway pressure, which, as discussed before, can augment oxygenation independent of FiO_2 [14].

Oxygen Goals and Toxicity

Scientists have long studied what the appropriate oxygenation target is in critically ill patients. One might think "more is better," and plan to target a SpO_2 of 100% in all patients; however, oxygen itself can be harmful to patients.

Oxygen toxicity can occur with hyperoxia via the production of reactive oxygen species (ROS). Oxygen is responsible for one of the early mass extinctions of life, allowing for the emergence of organisms that were able to neutralize its toxic effects and later use it for energy. Endogenous antioxidants are present in all humans, but a high partial pressure of oxygen can overcome these defenses and lead to injury. This is seen in stable patients with ILD undergoing surgery and can be seen in ARDS as well, and excessive oxygen administration has been shown to be an independent risk factor for mortality in critically ill patients [17].

There have been numerous large randomized controlled trials attempting to identify the ideal oxygen goal in adult critically ill patients. While the methods differ slightly, they compare lower oxygen targets with higher oxygenation targets. There was no difference found between these groups, suggesting that lower oxygen targets are safe and can help avoid the risks associated with hyperoxia [7, 18, 19]. A pediatric study comparing lower and higher oxygenation targets did support a lower oxygenation target of SpO_2 88–92% when it came to the outcome of duration of organ support or death [20].

Conclusions

Modern understanding of the role of oxygen and mechanical ventilation took centuries, requiring incremental advancements in anatomy, physiology, chemistry, and physics. Today, mechanical ventilation is one of the cornerstones of critical care medicine, serving as a life-sustaining measure in respiratory failure.

Ventilators are sophisticated machines, and ventilator management requires an understanding of pulmonary physiology, mechanisms of hypoxemia, ventilator modes, respiratory mechanics, and strategies to augment oxygenation in refractory hypoxemia.

Declarations

Competing Interests The author(s) have no competing interests to declare that are relevant to the content of this manuscript.

Ethics Approval The author(s) declare that this manuscript does not include primary research with human participants.

The author(s) declare that this manuscript does not include primary studies involving animals.

References

1. Slutsky AS. History of mechanical ventilation. From vesalius to ventilator-induced lung injury. Am J Respir Crit Care Med. 2015;191(10):1106–15. https://doi.org/10.1164/rccm.201503-0421PP. PMID: 25844759.
2. Lutz PL. Chapter 4/The age of Plato and Aristotle. In: The rise of experimental biology. Totowa: Humana Press Inc; 2002. p. 30.
3. West JB. Carl Wilhelm Scheele, the discoverer of oxygen, and a very productive chemist. Am J Physiol Lung Cell Mol Physiol. 2014;307(11):L811–6. https://doi.org/10.1152/ajplung.00223.2014. Epub 2014 Oct 3. PMID: 25281638.

4. Wilson JL. Respiratory failure in poliomyelitis: treatment with the drinker respirator. Am J Dis Child. 1932;43(6):1433–1454. oi:https://doi.org/10.1001/archpedi.1932.01950070002001.
5. Stefanakis G, Nyktari V, Papaioannou A, Askitopoulou H. Hippocratic concepts of acute and urgent respiratory diseases still relevant to contemporary medical thinking and practice: a scoping review. BMC Pulm Med. 2020;20(1):165. https://doi.org/10.1186/s12890-020-01193-9. PMID: 32522288; PMCID: PMC7288510.
6. Hsia CC, Hyde DM, Weibel ER. Lung Structure and the Intrinsic Challenges of Gas Exchange. Compr Physiol. 2016;6(2):827–95. https://doi.org/10.1002/cphy.c150028. PMID: 27065169; PMCID: PMC5026132.
7. Semler MW, Casey JD, Lloyd BD, Hastings PG, Hays MA, Stollings JL, Buell KG, Brems JH, Qian ET, Seitz KP, Wang L, Lindsell CJ, Freundlich RE, Wanderer JP, Han JH, Bernard GR, Self WH, Rice TW, PILOT Investigators and the Pragmatic Critical Care Research Group. Oxygen-saturation targets for critically ill adults receiving mechanical ventilation. N Engl J Med. 2022;387(19):1759–69. https://doi.org/10.1056/NEJMoa2208415. Epub 2022 Oct 24. PMID: 36278971; PMCID: PMC9724830.
8. Powers KA, Dhamoon AS. Physiology, pulmonary ventilation and perfusion. [Updated 2023 Jan 23]. In: StatPearls [Internet]. Treasure Island (FL): StatPearls Publishing; 2025 Jan-. Available from: https://www.ncbi.nlm.nih.gov/books/NBK539907/
9. Petersson J, Glenny RW. Gas exchange and ventilation-perfusion relationships in the lung. Eur Respir J. 2014;44(4):1023–41. https://doi.org/10.1183/09031936.00037014. Epub 2014 Jul 25. PMID: 25063240.
10. Gertler R. Respiratory mechanics. Anesthesiol Clin. 2021;39(3):415–40. https://doi.org/10.1016/j.anclin.2021.04.003. PMID: 34392877; PMCID: PMC8360707.
11. Bassingthwaighte JB, Raymond GM, Dash RK, Beard DA, Nolan M. The pathway for oxygen: tutorial modelling on oxygen transport from air to mitochondrion: the pathway for oxygen. Adv Exp Med Biol. 2016;876:103–10. https://doi.org/10.1007/978-1-4939-3023-4_13. PMID: 26782201; PMCID: PMC4828238.
12. TreacherDF,LeachRM.Oxygentransport-1.Basicprinciples.BMJ.1998;317(7168):1302–1306. https://doi.org/10.1136/bmj.317.7168.1302. PMID: 9804723; PMCID: PMC1114207.
13. Tobin MJ. Principles and practice of mechanical ventilation. 3rd ed. McGraw-Hill; 2012.
14. Shen H, Qu D, Na W, Liu S, Huang S, Hui Y. Comparison of the OI and PaO2 /FiO2 score in evaluating PARDS requiring mechanical ventilation. Pediatr Pulmonol. 2021;56(5):1182–8. https://doi.org/10.1002/ppul.25194. Epub 2020 Dec 14. PMID: 33289279.
15. Pipeling MR, Fan E. Therapies for refractory hypoxemia in acute respiratory distress syndrome. JAMA. 2010;304(22):2521–7. https://doi.org/10.1001/jama.2010.1752. PMID: 21139113.
16. Bilan N, Dastranji A, Ghalehgolab Behbahani A. Comparison of the spo2/fio2 ratio and the pao2/fio2 ratio in patients with acute lung injury or acute respiratory distress syndrome. J Cardiovasc Thorac Res. 2015;7(1):28–31. https://doi.org/10.15171/jcvtr.2014.06. Epub 2015 Mar 29. PMID: 25859313; PMCID: PMC4378672.
17. Alva R, Mirza M, Baiton A, Lazuran L, Samokysh L, Bobinski A, Cowan C, Jaimon A, Obioru D, Al Makhoul T, Stuart JA. Oxygen toxicity: cellular mechanisms in normobaric hyperoxia. Cell Biol Toxicol. 2023;39(1):111–43. https://doi.org/10.1007/s10565-022-09773-7. Epub 2022 Sep 16. PMID: 36112262; PMCID: PMC9483325.
18. ICU-ROX Investigators and the Australian and New Zealand Intensive Care Society Clinical Trials Group, Mackle D, Bellomo R, Bailey M, Beasley R, Deane A, Eastwood G, Finfer S, Freebairn R, King V, Linke N, Litton E, McArthur C, McGuinness S, Panwar R, Young P, ICU-ROX Investigators the Australian and New Zealand Intensive Care Society Clinical Trials Group. Conservative oxygen therapy during mechanical ventilation in the ICU. N Engl J Med. 2020;382(11):989–98. https://doi.org/10.1056/NEJMoa1903297. Epub 2019 Oct 14. PMID: 31613432.
19. Martin DS, Gould DW, Shahid T, Doidge JC, Cowden A, Sadique Z, Camsooksai J, Charles WN, Davey M, Francis-Johnson A, Garrett RM, Grocott MPW, Jones J, Lampro L, Mackle DM, O'Driscoll BR, Richards-Belle A, Rostron AJ, Szakmány T, Warren A, Young PJ, Rowan KM, Harrison DA, Mouncey PR, UK-ROX Investigators. Conservative oxygen therapy in

mechanically ventilated critically ill adult patients: the UK-ROX Randomized Clinical Trial. JAMA. 2025:e259663. https://doi.org/10.1001/jama.2025.9663. Epub ahead of print. PMID: 40501321; PMCID: PMC12163715.

20. Peters MJ, Gould DW, Ray S, Thomas K, et al. Conservative versus liberal oxygenation targets in critically ill children (Oxy-PICU): a UK multicentre, open, parallel-group, randomised clinical trial. Lancet. 2024;403(10424):355–64. https://doi.org/10.1016/S0140-6736(23)01968-2. ISSN 0140-6736. https://www.sciencedirect.com/science/article/pii/S0140673623019682

Artificial Airways

23

Shourjo Chakravorty and Michael Baram

Introduction

This chapter describes the mechanical properties of endotracheal tubes (ETT) and tracheostomy tubes. There is also a brief discussion about the complications of these tubes. The complications are discussed in further detail in other chapters.

Endotracheal Tube

Fundamentals of the Endotracheal Tube

The basic function of the endotracheal tube (ETT) is to provide an artificial airway that can provide gas exchange by way of oxygenation and ventilation. The ETT was first utilized in the early 1900s, and in its most basic form, is a tube that goes through the vocal cords and into the trachea [1]. The tube also serves as mechanical protection for the lungs from aspiration of blood and gastric contents, which can cause an inflammatory response (chemical pneumonitis) [2]. The ETT can be utilized in many settings, including prehospital, operating room, emergency room, and intensive care unit. In the operating room, the ETT is used to secure the airway and facilitate mechanical ventilation while patients are under general anesthesia. Other situations for which patients are intubated include hypoxic respiratory failure due to low oxygen levels, hypercapnic respiratory failure due to high carbon dioxide levels, hemodynamic instability and shock in critically ill patients, metabolic

S. Chakravorty · M. Baram (✉)
The Korman Respiratory Institute and the Division of Pulmonary, Allergy and Critical Care, The Department of Medicine at the Sidney Kimmel Medical College of Thomas Jefferson University, Philadelphia, PA, USA
e-mail: Michael.Baram@jefferson.edu

G. C. Kane et al. (eds.), *Oxygen*, https://doi.org/10.1007/978-3-032-18934-9_23

instability with metabolic acidemia, airway protection for those with anaphylaxis or significant encephalopathy resulting in altered mental status, and finally to bypass an airway obstruction [3].

The History of the Endotracheal Tube

The concept of artificial airways can be traced back to ancient times when Hippocrates first described tracheal intubation in humans [4]. Many centuries later, in 1543, Vesalius placed a reed into the trachea of a pig to treat a pneumothorax [5]. In 1754, Benjamin Pugh performed the first endotracheal intubation to resuscitate a neonate with a coiled wire covered by leather [6]. Major advances in ETTs occurred in the early 1840s, in conjunction with the development of the first anesthetics. Historically, postoperative pneumonia and aspiration of gastric contents were a frequent problem after surgical procedures. In 1869, Trendelenburg designed the first inflatable cuff, which created a seal to prevent aspiration during anesthesia [7]. In 1893, Eisenmenger introduced the idea of an external pilot balloon [8]. Rubber tubes were used in the early 1900s; however, they were thought to be too hard and cause excessive bleeding. As polymer technology advanced, a disposable polyvinyl chloride tube was introduced in 1968 [2]. Time and science have made the walls of the ETT thinner to allow larger inner diameters to improve airflow. Although disposable for humans, these tubes are durable and often reused between animals in the veterinary community.

Parts of the Endotracheal Tube

Below is an example of a typical ETT (Fig. 23.1).

A typical adult ETT is made of transparent polyvinyl chloride and is 33 cm (about 1.1 ft) long and comes in many different diameters [2]. The curvature of the ETT conforms to the shape of the airway when the head is in a neutral position. Markings along the tube length denote the distance in centimeters from the tip. This allows personnel to track the depth of the tube after placement. There is a radiopaque continuous strip embedded in the length of the tube, which allows the distal tip to be identified on a chest radiograph, another technique for confirming proper positioning of the tube [9]. The tip of the tube is slanted, with the bevel facing left. In most cases, the ETT is introduced on the right side of the standard left-handed laryngoscope. The left slanted bevel allows better visualization of the area in front of the tube and allows for easier passage through the vocal cords. Opposite the bevel, there is an additional side hole called the Murphy eye. Its purpose is to allow passage of gas and thus ventilation should the tip of the tube become obstructed with mucus or if the ETT is lodged in the right mainstem bronchus [10]. The Murphy eye allows ventilation of the left lung. All tubes have a standard adapter that allows a variety of respiratory or anesthesia equipment to be attached to the tube. Basic connectors are 15 mm (about 0.6 in) and 22 mm (about 0.9 in) in size. The

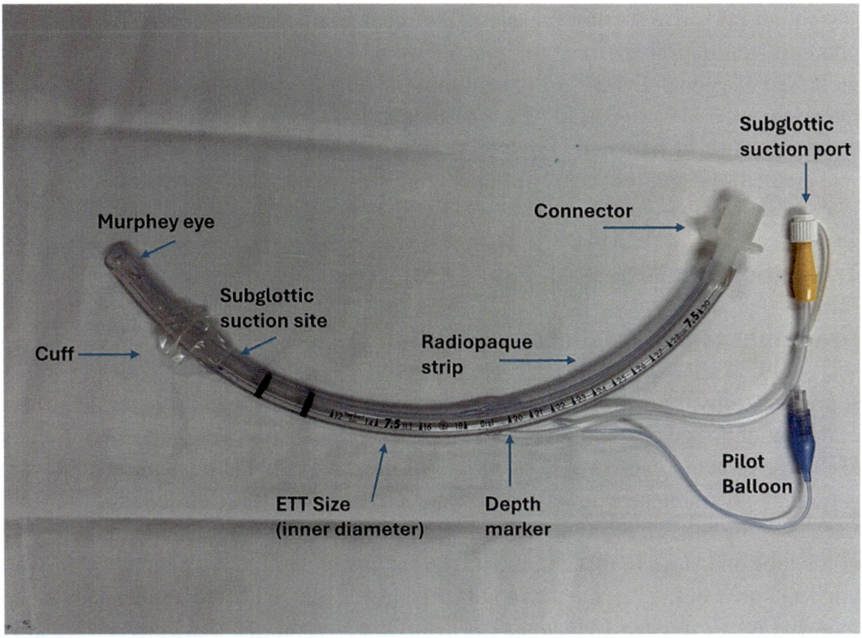

Fig. 23.1 Anatomy of an ETT

connector allows the ETT to be connected to airway equipment such as a bag mask, which can be used for manual ventilation or to a mechanical ventilator. The air-filled cuff is an important feature of the ETT in adults. Importantly, pediatric tubes are typically not cuffed [11]. The cuff allows for a positive-pressure seal and protects the lower airways from upper airway secretions. In children, the cricoid ring is sufficiently narrow to form a seal by itself, though many argue that cuffed tubes should be more available in the pediatric population [11]. The pilot balloon is connected to the cuff through a narrow lumen. The pilot balloon's integrity acts as a surrogate for the cuff pressure. If the pilot balloon is flaccid, the cuff is likely to be as well. To reduce the risk of overinflation pressure injury, there are specific devices to measure cuff pressures. A subglottic suction port allows for the aspiration of secretions that are collected above the cuff. Suctioning above the cuff decreases the risk of infection and aspiration, though it can cause mucosal trauma [12]. The nomenclature by which tubes are referred to is related to their inner diameter. If a large enough tube is not chosen, too much air will leak around the cuff and impair ventilation to the patient. Typically, an 8.0 or 8.5 for adult men and 7.5 to 8.0 for adult women is an optimal choice [13].

There is a common misconception about the role of the ETT cuff. The cuff can act to reduce aspiration risk; however, there can still be downward seepage of pharyngeal contents around the cuff that can cause inflammatory and infectious complications in the lungs. It would be more accurate to say that the cuff does not stop gastric content aspiration but can act to slow how often aspiration occurs. The more significant role of the cuff is to create a seal around the ETT to maintain a closed system and positive airway pressure. This seal in the airway allows for positive-pressure ventilation to increase mean airway pressure, which in turn leads to increased oxygen delivery during inspiration. During exhalation, positive end-expiratory pressure, (PEEP or EPAP), can be applied to avoid atelectasis, which is a common cause of hypoxemia due to ventilation–perfusion mismatch. Without the seal created by an appropriately inflated cuff, this would not be possible.

Tracheostomy Tubes

Fundamentals of Tracheostomy Tubes

A tracheostomy is an artificial opening through a stoma made in the anterior surface of the patient's neck extending into the trachea. Tracheostomy tubes are used for gas exchange in acute and chronic respiratory failure, to provide a patent a stable airway, and to help manage airway secretions, similar to the functions of an ETT. Most tracheostomy tubes have an inner and outer cannula. The outer cannula is the body of the tube and stays in place in the trachea and is secured to the patient's skin with tracheostomy ties. The inner cannula fits inside the outer cannula and can be removed for purposes of cleaning the inspissated secretions that collect over time [14]. Similar to the ETT, tracheostomy tubes are labeled based on inner diameter. Tracheostomy tubes can be cuffed or uncuffed. When a tracheostomy tube has an inflatable balloon around the outer cannula, it is called a cuffed tracheostomy. When the cuff is "up," or inflated, it allows for a closed system where air is prevented from escaping around the tube. If the cuff is "down" or deflated, air can flow out during expiration via the tracheostomy tube *and* around the tube and up through the larynx, facilitating the use of the vocal cords and thus allowing vocalization. Patients who need an airway but do not necessarily need the ventilator can be managed with a cuffless tracheostomy, where air can move around and also through the tube. When patients are clinically improving, their tracheostomy tubes are often "downsized" (reduced in diameter) and eventually are changed to a cuffless tube when they no longer need ventilatory support. In some cases, a fenestrated tracheostomy is used. These tubes have openings at the bend of the outer or inner cannula, which improves the passage of air into the upper airway, helping patients with speech and sensation

Table 23.1 Comparisons of tracheostomy tubes: uncuffed versus cuffed

Uncuffed tubes	Cuffed tubes
Larger internal diameter	Allows use of lower gas flow
Lower resistance to flow	Reduces risk of aspiration
Mitigates the increase in the work of breathing	Avoids multiple laryngoscopies and intubations
Allows easy suctioning	Reduces air pollution/debris from above the ventilator circuit
Avoids trauma to the subglottic region	Improves ventilation and end tidal CO_2 monitoring

Modified for Lewith et al. [15]

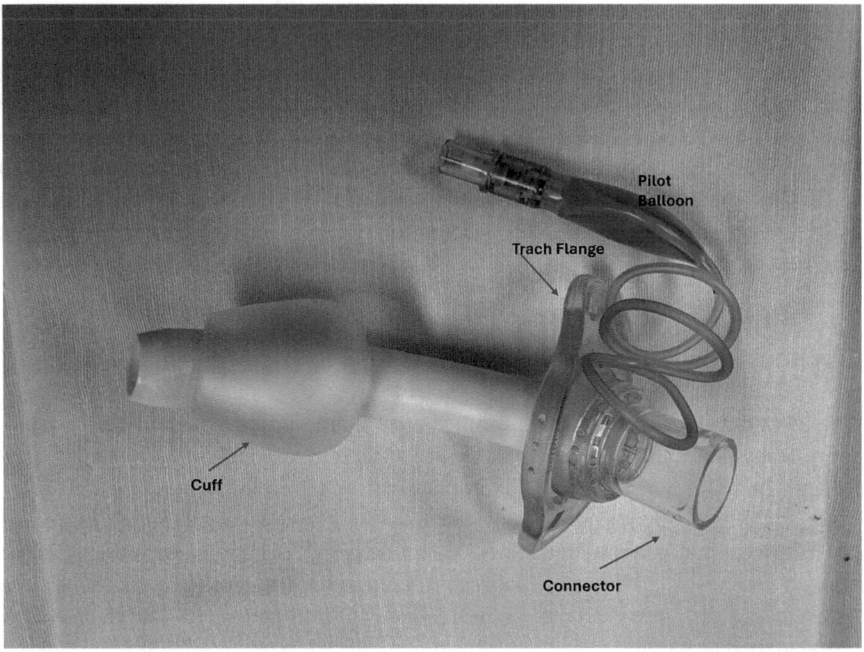

Fig. 23.2 Anatomy of a tracheostomy tube

[15] (Table 23.1). The flange helps secure the device to the neck. Figure 23.2 provides a visual example of a cuffed tracheostomy tube with important parts labeled.

A tracheostomy tube is not simply "a tube in the neck." There is much more to consider regarding the pulmonary physiology that involves a tracheostomy tube. This "tube in the neck" shortens the airway by bypassing the nasopharynx and pharynx, which in turn reduces the work of breathing and dead space. This change in anatomy has a profound effect on physiology, specifically by improving gas exchange and reducing the work for carbon dioxide clearance. For the "pink puffer" with severe emphysema, even this 10% reduction in work of breathing can have a major effect on the feeling of dyspnea by reducing oxygen consumption demand. This work of breathing directly affects calorie wasting, as significant energy is wasted during periods of increased work of breathing. This is one of the reasons those with severe emphysema often develop pulmonary cachexia [16].

A specific and often underutilized form of tracheostomy is transtracheal oxygen (TTO) therapy, which functions as an ultra-skinny tracheostomy that assists in oxygenation by increasing the fraction of inspired oxygen (FiO_2) in the trachea. This location maximizes the trachea as an oxygen reservoir and reduces dead space ventilation. Benefits of TTO also include improved patient compliance with oxygen therapy due to less nasal irritation, and it is thought to be more comfortable [17]. Practically speaking, patients find TTO to be more cosmetically appealing, as the tubing can be hidden under their clothing. As TTO improves oxygen at lower flow rates, patients can increase exercise tolerance. By insufflating supplemental oxygen near the carina, the anatomic dead space decreases, thus improving alveolar ventilation. Over time, patients can be away from home longer with decreased oxygen flow rates, which improves quality of life. Though TTO has numerous physiologic and practical benefits, it is underutilized by physicians due to complications related to the procedural placement of the TTO catheter and complications related to TTO itself. These include the formation of large mucous balls resulting in partial tracheal obstruction, posterior tracheal wall ulceration, and the formation of a granulation tumor at the insertion site [18].

Tracheostomy Cuffs

The advantages of the cuff/balloon in the ETT are similar with cuffed tracheostomy tubes. The balloon is essential in providing increased oxygenation in a closed system, but comes with risks. It is imperative for clinicians to monitor cuff pressures to reduce tracheal mucosal ischemia from high cuff pressures. Increased pressure can cause decreased blood flow and local ischemia. To mitigate these risks, a variety of cuffs are available and include high-volume low-pressure cuffs (most common), low-volume high-pressure cuffs, foam-filled cuffs, or newer taper-shaped cuffs.

A high-volume low-pressure (HVLP) tracheostomy cuff is designed to create a seal against the tracheal wall using a larger volume of air at a lower pressure than other cuff designs [19]. These cuffs are specifically meant to minimize pressure-related damage to the trachea while still providing an effective seal. HVLP cuffs have a larger surface area of contact with the tracheal wall. They can achieve a seal at lower pressures, which reduces the risk of tracheal damage like fistulation, stenosis, and ulceration. Even when deflated, HVLP cuffs occupy more space in the trachea than low-volume low-pressure (LVHP) cuffs, which can sometimes cause issues with ventilatory weaning, or with speaking valve use.

Low-volume low-pressure (LVLP) cuffs are used in endotracheal tubes and tracheostomy tubes to reduce the risk of tracheal injury. These are less commonly used than HVLP cuffs. They use lower inflation volumes and pressure to try to minimize damage to the tracheal wall. LVLP cuffs can create better seals with less volume and pressure. Studies have suggested that LVLP cuffs may help reduce the risk of aspiration. They have smaller internal volumes than HVLP [20].

Foam-filled cuffs are primarily used to help manage persistent cuff leaks and reduce tracheal wall damage, especially in those with existing wall damage. The foam expands to conform to the trachea shape, creating a seal at lower cuff pressures than the air-filled cuffs. They require special care and attention as they are self-inflating in nature and are at risk for deflation and unintentional removal [21].

Taper-shaped cuffs are designed to improve tracheal seal and to reduce aspirations compared to traditional cylindrical cuffs. Their tapered design creates a smaller contact area with the trachea, potentially minimizing pressure points and improving the seal against leaks. They also tend to be more comfortable for patients and have been associated with reduced dysphonia and postoperative throat pain. Oxygenation is not impacted by the choice of the type of cuff applied [22]. Table 23.1 outlines the comparison of tracheostomy tubes, cuffed versus uncuffed.

Sizing of Tracheostomy Tubes

An "XLT" refers to an extended-length tracheostomy tube. There are two main types of "XLT": a proximal XLT, which is for patients who are obese and/or have thick neck circumference, and a distal XLT, which is used for patients with long trachea or tracheal obstructions such as stenosis or malacia [23]. A proximal XLT has a portion of the canula that is longer proximal to the stoma (higher in the airway), whereas a distal XLT has a portion of the canula that is longer distal to the stoma (lower in the airway). In a proximal XLT tube, the added distance is from the flange to the bend to accommodate the increased girth of the neck. In a distal XLT tube, the added length is distal to the bend of the tracheostomy tube to accommodate the cuff sitting closer to the carina. This longer tube may be required to accommodate larger patients, airway obstruction, or to help provide support for tracheomalacia.

Patients undergoing mechanical ventilation in critical care units often have undergone a computed tomography (CT) scan of the chest for various indications. These scans can be used to measure the amount of pretracheal soft tissue, which may help practitioners recognize which patients would benefit from an XLT. CT imaging allows for noninvasive anatomical measurements [24]. Using imaging can help with procedural planning and improve the fit of the tracheostomy tubes.

Specialty Tubes

An armored endotracheal tube is a type of tube with a reinforced metal coil embedded within its wall. This reinforcement makes the tube more resistant to kinking, compression, laceration, and/or obstruction. These features are particularly useful in situations where the airway is prone to bending, obstruction, or compression, for example, during head and neck surgeries, or in patients with difficult upper airway anatomy [25].

A double-lumen tube is an endotracheal tube designed to isolate the lungs anatomically and physiologically. These special tubes are used to provide independent ventilation to one lung. Single-lung ventilation, or lung isolation, is the mechanical and functional separation of the two lungs to allow for the selective ventilation of only one lung [26]. The other lung that is not being ventilated passively deflates or is displaced by the surgeon to facilitate surgical exposure for noncardiac operations in the chest, such as thoracic, esophageal, aortic, and spine procedures.

Antiseptic-impregnated tubes have been used to prevent complications such as ventilator-related pneumonia (VAP) in patients requiring prolonged mechanical ventilation. Tubes impregnated with chlorhexidine and violet crystal have shown some preliminary evidence that they could reduce VAP incidence. Use of Noble metal alloy-coated tubes (gold, silver, palladium) has resulted in a delayed onset of VAP and showed decreased utilization of antibiotics in ventilated patients. Lastly, silver sulfadiazine-coated tubes have been shown to prevent bacterial colonization on the surface of the tube, and this compound can be applied to help prevent infection in patients with long-standing tracheostomies [27].

Supraglottic Airway Devices

Supraglottic airway devices, such as a laryngeal mask airway (LMA), are adjunct airway devices that can be used to deliver oxygen and ventilate patients [28]. These devices sit above the vocal cords in the pharynx, rather than being inserted into the trachea like an ETT or tracheostomy. An LMA is a tube with an elliptical cuff that is inserted into the hypopharynx, creating a seal around the laryngeal inlet (Fig. 23.3). One important consideration of using this device is oxygen leakage, or the potential for oxygen to leak around the supraglottic airway seal, especially during spontaneous ventilation, though leakage tends to be less common with the use of an LMA. The first supraglottic airways were used in the 1980s, where they were

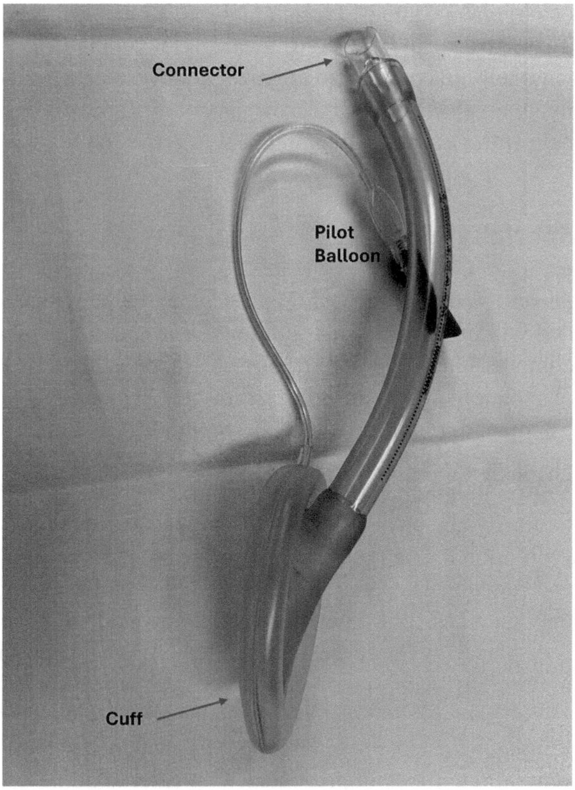

Fig. 23.3 Anatomy of an LMA

primarily deployed in the operating room. Since then, their use has become more widespread, including in the field settings with emergency services, the intensive care unit, and the emergency department. The LMA is a suitable alternative to bag-mask ventilation to reduce the risk of gastric inflation, thus lowering the risk of aspiration, though it is far less protective than an endotracheal tube [29]. LMAs are an effective method of ventilation and should be utilized unless they are ineffective in patients requiring prolonged mask ventilation. The I-Gel is another supraglottic device that is easy to use and widely available in many medical settings and emergency situations. The I-Gel devices are unique in that they have a pre-shaped non-inflatable cuff. They are made from a gel-like substance, which may be easier to insert because there is no cuff to inflate. The I-Gel also allows insertion of standard endotracheal tubes [30]. These devices can be used for all ages.

Pediatric Endotracheal Tubes

Pediatric ETTs differ from adult ETTs in size and cuff design. Pediatric airways are smaller and shorter in diameter, as the narrowest part of the airway is at the cricoid cartilage, unlike in adults, where the vocal cords are the narrowest point. The tongue is larger, and the larynx is more anterior in children [31]. Historically, uncuffed ETTs were favored due to concern about tracheal injury and pressure necrosis, but cuffed tubes are now more common except in neonates [32]. The cuffed ETT maintains positive airway pressure to improve oxygenation. Modern cuffed ETTs are designed with lower pressure and larger volumes of cuffs to mitigate the risk of mucosal injury. These cuffs help create seals and prevent air leaks in the typically more cylindrical pediatric airway. While the choice of tube size is always important, it can have even more consequences for pediatrics. If a very small ETT is inserted for example, there is a risk of inadequate ventilation and decreased reliability of end tidal carbon dioxide monitoring. There is also a risk of oxygen leakage (as stated previously), anesthetic gas leakage, aspiration, and high airway pressures. If an overly large ETT is placed, serious complications can include airway damage, ulceration, scar, ischemia, post-intubation croup, and in severe cases subglottic stenosis [33].

Nasopharyngeal Airways

A nasopharyngeal airway (NPA) device or "nasal trumpet" is a hollow plastic or soft rubber tube that can improve oxygenation and ventilation in cases where bag-valve-mask ventilation is ineffective or a subglottic airway device is not available [34]. NPAs are inserted into the nose and placed through the posterior pharynx, clearing the airway by displacing the posterior tongue and soft palate. NPAs do not typically cause patients to gag. Thus, this device is recommended over an oropharyngeal airway in patients with an intact gag reflex. NPAs are helpful when a patient's mouth is difficult to open or access, as in cases of trismus or angioedema. NPAs serve as adjuncts for ventilation and oxygenation. They are often used only as a temporizing measure before obtaining a more secure airway via intubation or until the patient can breathe independently [35]. Nevertheless, NPAs are valuable tools for quickly establishing and maintaining a patent airway, especially during emergencies. NPAs are easily sized by measuring the distance from the nose to the tragus of the ear. The ease of measuring, inserting, and suctioning makes it a reliable airway adjunct.

Complications

Endotracheal Tube Complications

Complication rates are hard to report due to the varying indications for intubation. Another chapter covers the procedure of intubation (Chap. 24). Some mechanical complications related to having an endotracheal tube in place include local irritation of the throat and vocal cords. The injury may be as simple as irritation or a hoarse voice, or it may be more severe, like tracheal injury or potentially life-threatening laryngeal edema. Endotracheal tubes that are in place for more than two weeks may result in granulomas, tracheal stenosis, or even tracheomalacia. The incidence of these injuries is often related to the duration of intubation.

Early Complications of Tracheostomy

There are inherent risks in placing a tracheostomy tube. Immediate complications include airway irritation and bleeding, pneumothorax, which may induce subcutaneous emphysema, injury to the recurrent laryngeal nerve, and infection. A small amount of bleeding is expected during a tracheostomy procedure, usually from superficial vessels. Severe bleeding should undergo bronchoscopy. Bleeding may also occur in the setting of airway trauma due to frequent or improper suctioning [36]. A collapsed lung, or pneumothorax, occurs when air accumulates in the pleural space. The development of a partial or complete pneumothorax has been reported to be up to 17% in patients undergoing tracheostomy placement [37]. Current dilatational techniques have lower risks. Patients with chronic obstructive pulmonary disease are at higher risk due to intrinsic air-trapping, which causes their chest to be barrel-shaped, causing the apex of the lung to be much higher in the chest cavity. Subcutaneous emphysema is the result of air or gas escaping under the skin. It can develop rapidly and may be the first clinical sign of pneumothorax. It can result from trauma during the tracheotomy procedure or tracheal intubation. The most common sign is swelling around the neck and chest pain. Other signs and symptoms include a tender sore throat, an aching neck, difficulty in swallowing, breathlessness, wheezing, and distension. Subcutaneous emphysema has a characteristic crackling feel when palpating the skin, which is termed subcutaneous crepitus [38].

Injury to the recurrent laryngeal nerve is a known early complication of tracheostomy. Patients may become hoarse (if able to phonate), develop dysphagia, aspiration, and vocal cord paralysis. The risk is higher during cases in which the tracheostomy tube is not maintained at midline and has become significantly misplaced. Tracheostomy tubes can be obstructed by blood or mucus, and this can be a life-threatening event if not managed properly. Patency of the airway is maintained with humidification, good hygiene, cleaning of the inner cannula, and proper suctioning of the airway. Utilizing double cannula tubes decreases the risk of mucus plugging because the inner cannula can be removed for cleaning while the outer cannula maintains patency of the tract [39].

Late Complications of Tracheostomy

Late complications of tracheostomy procedures include tracheal stenosis, tracheomalacia, and the development of tracheoesophageal fistula. Tracheal stenosis is a narrowing of the trachea, which can develop from prolonged intubation and can lead to pressure injury and scarring due to high cuff pressures. Tracheal stenosis develops at the stoma site or at the level of the cuff. When stenosis occurs at the stoma site, it is usually due to bacterial infection and chondritis. Even a tracheal tube fenestration can cause local irritation as it rubs across the lining of the trachea. Diligent tracheostomy care includes appropriate downsizing of the tube and providing cuffless tracheostomy when able, which can decrease the risk of tracheal stenosis. Diagnosis of this complication is often delayed. It may present as an increased cough or difficulty clearing secretions. If the individual is on mechanical ventilation, the presentation may be difficult in weaning with intermittent high peak airway pressures [40]. Tracheomalacia is the weakening of the tracheal wall, often due to wall trauma, which can develop after recurrent infections and overinflation of the cuff. Signs and symptoms of tracheomalacia include shortness of breath, hoarse voice, chronic cough, difficulty swallowing, recurring respiratory tract infections, and, during mechanical ventilation, there is often the presence of a cuff leak or the need to overinflate the cuff to maintain tidal volumes and minute ventilation. If tracheomalacia is suspected, bronchoscopy or a dynamic CT scan of the trachea can reveal excessive expiratory collapse of the trachea [41]. A tracheoesophageal fistula (TE-F) is a rare complication of tracheostomy placement, occurring in less than 1% of cases. A TE-F is a connection between the trachea and the esophagus, which can develop in patients with injury to the posterior wall of the trachea. Patients typically present with copious secretions and recurrent aspirations of secretions, food, and/or liquids, which can lead to life-threatening pulmonary complications. For patients receiving tube feeds, there should be a high suspicion of TE-F if tube feedings are noted in the tracheostomy tube or around the stoma. The diagnosis of tracheoesophageal fistula is made by high-resolution CT scan, contrast esophagram, or endoscopy [42].

Conclusion

Endotracheal tubes and tracheostomy tubes are crucial for providing oxygenation and ventilation, especially in emergency and critical care settings, and in the operating room. They deliver oxygen and inhaled gases directly to the lungs while protecting the airway from aspiration. The cuff in the airway allows for positive-pressure ventilation creating a closed circuit to increase the mean airway pressure, which in turn leads to increased oxygen delivery during inspiration. The cuff allows for positive-pressure ventilation and positive end-expiratory pressure and thus aids oxygenation. Tracheostomy tubes are placed in patients who require a longer or permanent airway and can offer similar physiologic benefits for oxygenation and ventilation, and can deliver positive pressure when the cuff is inflated. Airway adjuncts such as an LMA or a nasal trumpet are also important to consider, depending on the clinical situation. Although they can be considered simple airway tubes, there is a very significant science and history underpinning the evolution of these medical devices.

Declarations

Competing Interests The authors have no competing interests to declare that are relevant to the content of this manuscript.

Ethics Approval The authors declare that this manuscript does not include primary research with human participants.

The authors declare that this manuscript does not include primary studies involving animals.

References

1. Szmuk P, Ezri T, Evron S, Roth Y, Katz J. A brief history of tracheostomy and tracheal intubation, from the bronze age to the space age. Intensive Care Med. 2007;34(2):222–8.
2. Haas CF, Eakin RM, Konkle MA, Blank R. Endotracheal Tubes: old and NewDiscussion. Respir Care [Internet]. 2014;59(6):933–955. Available from: http://rc.rcjournal.com/content/59/6/933.
3. Shebl E, Burns B. Respiratory failure in adults [Internet]. National Library of Medicine: StatPearls Publishing; 2023. Available from: https://www.ncbi.nlm.nih.gov/books/NBK526127/
4. Tsoucalas G, Sgantzos M, Androutsos G. Hippocrates, principles on abdominal surgery in ancient Greece during the fifth century BC. Surg Innov. 2016;23(2):212–3.
5. Pratt LW, Ferlito A, Rinaldo A. Tracheotomy: historical review. Laryngoscope. 2008;118(9):1597–606.
6. O'Donnell CPF, Gibson AT, Davis PG. Pinching, electrocution, ravens' beaks, and positive pressure ventilation: a brief history of neonatal resuscitation. Arch Dis Child Fetal Neonatal Ed [Internet]. 2006;91(5): F): F369–F373. Available from: https://pubmed.ncbi.nlm.nih.gov/16923936/
7. Fallatah SM, Al-metwalli RR, Alghamdi TM. Endotracheal tube cuff pressure: an overlooked risk. Anaesth Pain Intensive Care. 2021;25(1).
8. Bryant J, Werner J, Moss E, Tobias JD. Can the Intracuff pressure be estimated by palpation of the pilot balloon? ICU Dir. 2013;4(4):170–2.

9. Khan A, Al-Jahdali H, Al-Ghanem S, Gouda A. Reading chest radiographs in the critically ill (part I): Normal chest radiographic appearance, instrumentation and complications from instrumentation. Ann Thoracic Med. 2009;4(2):75.
10. Anaesthesia in. Tracheal tubes, tracheostomy tubes and airways – clinical tree [Internet]. Clinical Tree 2023 [cited 2025 Jul 1]. Available from: https://clinicalpub.com/tracheal-tubes-tracheostomy-tubes-and-airways/
11. Shah A, Carlisle JB. Cuffed tracheal tubes: guilty now proven innocent. Anaesthesia. 2019;74(9):1186–90.
12. de Souza CR, Santana VTS. Impact of supra-cuff suction on ventilator-associated pneumonia prevention. Rev Bras Ter Intensiva [Internet] 2012;24(4):401–406. Available from: https://www.ncbi.nlm.nih.gov/pmc/articles/PMC4031821/.
13. Ahmed RA, Boyer TJ. Endotracheal tube (ET) [Internet]. PubMed. Treasure Island (FL): StatPearls Publishing; 2023. Available from: https://www.ncbi.nlm.nih.gov/books/NBK539747/
14. Hess DR, Altobelli NP. Tracheostomy Tubes. Respir Care [Internet]. 2014;59(6):956–973. Available from: http://rc.rcjournal.com/content/59/6/956.
15. Lewith H, Athanassoglou V. Update on management of tracheostomy. BJA Educ [Internet] 2019;19(11):370–376. Available from: https://www.bjaed.org/article/S2058-5349(19)30125-8/fulltext.
16. Sanders KJC, Kneppers AEM, van de Bool C, Langen RCJ, Schols AMWJ. Cachexia in chronic obstructive pulmonary disease: new insights and therapeutic perspective [Internet]. U.S. National Library of Medicine; 2016 [cited 2025 Jul 31]. Available from: https://pmc.ncbi.nlm.nih.gov/articles/PMC4799856/
17. Christopher KL, Spofford BT, Brannin PK, Petty TL. Transtracheal oxygen therapy for refractory hypoxemia. JAMA [Internet] 1986;256(4):494–497. Available from: https://pubmed.ncbi.nlm.nih.gov/3723742/.
18. Siddiqui F, Campbell S, Ie S, Biscardi F, Rubio E. Three decades of transtracheal oxygen therapy: a review of the associated complications with an illustrative case presentation. Lung India [Internet] 2017 [cited 2023 Aug 18];34(5):448–448. Available from: https://www.ncbi.nlm.nih.gov/pmc/articles/PMC5592757/#:~:text=Transtracheal%20oxygen%20therapy%20is%20a
19. Berges AJ, Lina IA, Ospino R, Tsai HW, Ding D, Izzi JM, et al. Impact of low-volume, low-pressure tracheostomy cuffs on acute mucosal injury in swine. Otolaryngol Head Neck Surg [Internet] 2022 Oct;167(4):716–724. Available from: https://pubmed.ncbi.nlm.nih.gov/35998065/
20. Young PJ, Pakeerathan S, Blunt MC, Subramanya S. A low-volume, low-pressure tracheal tube cuff reduces pulmonary aspiration*. Crit Care Med. 2006;34(3):632–9.
21. Rajendram R, Barker G. Self-expanding foam-filled tracheostomy tube cuffs and the management of airway emergencies. Anaesthesia. 2013;68(4):436–7.
22. Huang WM, Huang XA, Du YP, Li LX, Wu FF, Hong SQ, et al. Tapered cuff versus conventional cuff for ventilator-associated pneumonia in ventilated patients: a meta-analysis of randomized controlled trials. Can Respir J. 2019;2019:1–7.
23. Bathula SS, Srikantha L, Patrick T, Stern NA. Immediate postoperative complications in adult tracheostomy. Cureus. 2020;12(12):e12228.
24. Corbett M, Hughes I, O'Shea J, Davey MG, Savage J, Hughes J, et al. X-ray and CT scan based prediction of best fit tracheostomy tube—a pilot study. Diagnostics. 2020;10(8):506.
25. Vijayakumar V, Ganesamoorthi A. Armored endotracheal tube: concerns in intensive care unit. Indian J Crit Care Med. 2017;21(1):60–1.
26. Bora V, Kritzmire SM, Arthur ME. Double Lumen Endobronchial Tubes [Internet]. PubMed. Treasure Island (FL): StatPearls Publishing; 2020. Available from: https://www.ncbi.nlm.nih.gov/books/NBK535366/ 1.
27. Gasparetto J, Bressianini Jurkonis L, Ramos Dantas L, Hansen Suss P, Francisco Tuon F. Low-cost antiseptic-impregnated tracheostomy tube for the prevention of ventilator-associated pneumonia caused by multidrug-resistant bacteria: in vitro and pilot study in humans. Rev

Argent Microbiol [Internet] 2024;56(4):359–363. Available from: https://pubmed.ncbi.nlm.nih.gov/39068088.

28. Simon LV, Torp KD. Laryngeal mask Airway [Internet]. Nih.gov. StatPearls Publishing; 2019. Available from: https://www.ncbi.nlm.nih.gov/books/NBK482184/
29. De Rosa S, Messina A, Sorbello M, Rigobello A, Colombo D, Piccolo A, Bonaldi E, Gennaro P, Urukalo V, Pellizzari A, Bonato R, Carboni SC. Laryngeal mask Airway supreme vs. the Spritztube tracheal cannula in anaesthetised adult patients: a randomised controlled trial. Eur J Anaesthesiol. 2019;36(12):955–62. [PubMed]
30. Sabuncu U, Kusderci HS, Oterkus M, Abdullayev R, Demir A, Uludag O, Ozdas S, Goksu M. AuraGain and i-Gel laryngeal masks in general anesthesia for laparoscopic cholecystectomy. Performance characteristics and effects on hemodynamics. Saudi Med J. 2018;39(11):1082–9.
31. Park S, Shin SW, Kim HJ, Byeon GJ, Yoon JU, Kim EJ, et al. Choice of the correct size of endotracheal tube in pediatric patients. Anesth Pain Med. 2022;17(4):352.
32. Dariya V, Moresco L, Bruschettini M, Brion LP. Cuffed versus uncuffed endotracheal tubes for neonates. Cochrane Database Syst Rev 2022;2022(1).
33. Weber T, Salvi N, Orliaguet G, Wolf A. Cuffed vs non-cuffed endotracheal tubes for pediatric anesthesia. Paediatr Anaesth. 2009;19:46–54.
34. Atanelov Z, Rebstock SE. Nasopharyngeal Airway [Internet]. PubMed. Treasure Island (FL): StatPearls Publishing; 2024. Available from: https://www.ncbi.nlm.nih.gov/books/NBK513220/
35. Roberts K, Whalley H, Bleetman A. The nasopharyngeal airway: dispelling myths and establishing the facts. Emerg Med J. 2005;22(6):394–6.
36. Santiago-Rosado LM, Sigmon DF, Lewison CS. Tracheal Trauma [Internet]. PubMed. Treasure Island (FL): StatPearls Publishing; 2020. Available from: https://www.ncbi.nlm.nih.gov/books/NBK500015/
37. Kwon MA, Cho C, Park JH. Life-threatening tension pneumothorax after unsuccessful tracheostomy tube exchange in a trauma patient – a case report. Anesthesia Pain Med. 2020;15(1):124–8.
38. Alshoubi A, Mathew A. Subcutaneous emphysema following open tracheostomy during tracheostomy mask ventilation. Am J Case Rep. 2022:23.
39. Culp JM, Patel G. Recurrent laryngeal nerve injury [Internet]. PubMed. Treasure Island (FL): StatPearls Publishing; 2021. Available from: https://www.ncbi.nlm.nih.gov/books/NBK560832/
40. Sarper A, Ayten A, Eser I, Ozbudak O, Demircan A. Tracheal stenosis after tracheostomy or intubation: review with special regard to cause and management. Tex Heart Inst J [Internet] ;32(2):154. Available from: https://pmc.ncbi.nlm.nih.gov/articles/PMC1163461/
41. Yang D, Cascella M. Tracheomalacia [Internet]. Nih.gov. StatPearls Publishing; 2021. Available from: https://www.ncbi.nlm.nih.gov/books/NBK553191/.
42. Paraschiv M. Tracheoesophageal fistula – a complication of prolonged tracheal intubation. J Med Life [Internet] 2025;7(4):516. Available from: https://pmc.ncbi.nlm.nih.gov/articles/PMC4316129/

Assuring Oxygenation During Emergency Endotracheal Intubation in the ICU

24

Saikou Saidy and Frances Mae West

Introduction

Endotracheal intubation is a critical intervention frequently employed in intensive care to manage patients with respiratory failure. This procedure entails the insertion of an endotracheal tube via the oropharynx or nasal passage, through the vocal cords, and into the trachea. Indications for intubation include the patient's inability to sustain effective ventilation, maintain adequate oxygenation, control pulmonary secretions, or secure the airway against the risk of aspiration into the airway. It is common for patients to receive supplementary oxygen therapy prior to intubation. Following the administration of sedative or neuromuscular blocking agents, there is an absence of spontaneous ventilation, rendering the patient reliant on the oxygen reservoir within the functional residual capacity (FRC). Consequently, preoxygenation and apneic oxygenation, which involve the administration of high fraction of inspired oxygen (FiO_2) to maximize the patient's oxygen saturation levels before and after induction, are crucial to maintain adequate oxygenation during the apneic period of the intubation process. Select patients with severe oxygenation, ventilation, metabolic, or physiologic deficits may benefit from an awake or minimally sedated intubation strategy. This chapter delves into the methodologies, techniques, and critical considerations requisite for ensuring optimal oxygenation during intubation from the vantage point of an intensivist. This chapter is organized into the following sections: understanding the physiology and rationale for preoxygenation, pre-intubation assessment preoxygenation, and intubation technique.

S. Saidy · F. M. West (✉)
The Korman Respiratory Institute and the Division of Pulmonary, Allergy, and Critical Care, The Department of Medicine at the Sidney Kimmel Medical College of Thomas Jefferson University, Philadelphia, PA, USA
e-mail: Frances.West@jefferson.edu

G. C. Kane et al. (eds.), *Oxygen*, https://doi.org/10.1007/978-3-032-18934-9_24

Understanding the Physiology and Rationale for Preoxygenation

The primary aim of preoxygenation is to maximize the oxygen concentration in the functional residual capacity (FRC), thereby creating a buffer that can support the body's oxygen needs during the period of apnea that occurs during intubation [1, 2].

When inhaling ambient air, the gas composition within the functional residual capacity (FRC) of the lungs is approximately 13–14% oxygen (O_2), 78–80% nitrogen (N_2), and 5–6% carbon dioxide (CO_2). This composition results from alveolar O_2 uptake and the production of CO_2, while N_2 remains largely unaffected due to its inert characteristics [3, 4]. Conversely, during preoxygenation with 100% fraction of inspired oxygen (FiO_2), the nitrogen within the pulmonary alveoli is displaced with oxygen. This process sometimes refers to denitrogenating, a term used interchangeably with reoxygenation. Consequently, the FRC gaseous mixture adjusts to approximately 85–90% oxygen, less than 5% nitrogen, and 5–6% carbon dioxide. [5, 6]

The extent of oxygenation of the functional residual capacity during the preoxygenation process is measured by the end-tidal oxygen (EtO_2), which refers to the oxygen concentration assessed in the exhaled breath at the end of expiration. It is measured using a gas analyzer and closely mirrors the alveolar oxygen fraction [2, 7, 8].

The target end-tidal oxygen value during preoxygenation is ≥90%, which takes about 3–5 minutes of breathing 100% oxygen in healthy adults. This value correlates with an optimal extension of safe apnea time during airway management. However, EtO_2 levels between 85% and 90% are permissible in practice, especially in emergency situations [2, 7, 8]. Moderate illness reduces apnea time significantly, with normal nonobese adults maintaining SpO_2 > 90% for 8 minutes to approximately 5 minutes for a moderately ill adult [9] (Fig. 24.1).

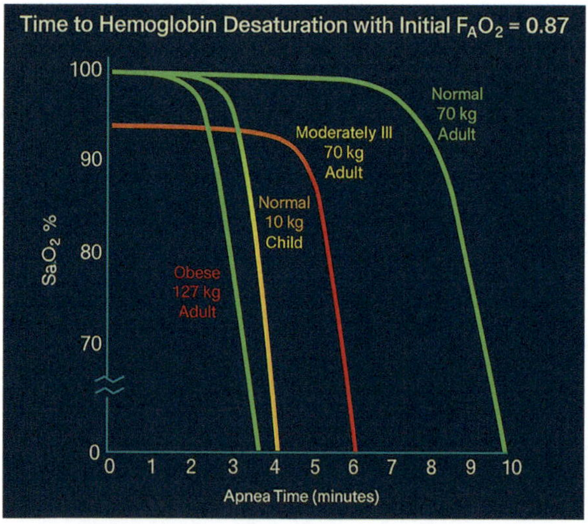

Fig. 24.1 SaO_2 versus time of apnea for various types of patients [9]. (Adapted from Benumof et al. [9])

The most prevalent indication for intubation in the medical intensive care unit (ICU) is respiratory failure, accounting for over 50% of all intubations. Patients with respiratory pathology exhibit reduced functional capacity, shunt physiology, and hypoxemia, which impedes the ability of high-concentration oxygen to effectively denitrogenate the functional residual capacity (FRC) and replace alveolar nitrogen with oxygen during preoxygenation. These physiologic challenges make it difficult to achieve a targeted end-tidal oxygen concentration of 90% and leave patients vulnerable to rapid desaturation during apnea [10, 11]. This high end-tidal oxygen content protects the patient from hypoxemia and hypoxia.

Effective preoxygenation and monitoring of end-tidal oxygen (EtO_2) are especially important in the critical care setting [10]. Given the special challenges in preoxygenating critically ill patients, the Society of Critical Care Medicine (SCCM) recommends employing advanced preoxygenation techniques, which include the use of positive end-expiratory pressure (PEEP) or a high-flow nasal cannula (HFNC) for optimized pre- and apneic oxygenation [1, 10, 12]. Both of these techniques improve the oxygen delivery by positive pressure to recruit atelectatic lung and improve oxygen diffusion.

Pre-intubation Assessment

Critically ill patients are at an increased risk for difficult preoxygenation, rapid desaturation, and subsequent hemodynamic collapse during intubation. This makes a thorough pre-intubation assessment very crucial for these patients. Such an evaluation should include an assessment of patients for anatomical or physiological factors that may cause difficulty with the intubation process. This allows intensivists to make modifications in the intubation process to minimize risk. In the next few paragraphs, the components of pre-intubation assessment are explored. The concept of anatomically and physiologically difficult airways is reviewed, and alternative options are discussed that can be utilized to minimize risk in patients with an anticipated difficult airway [10, 13, 14].

The American Society of Anesthesiologists (ASA) defines a difficult airway as any scenario where there is anticipated or unanticipated difficulty or failure in any airway management steps, including face-mask ventilation, laryngoscopy, ventilation using a supraglottic airway, tracheal intubation, extubation, and invasive airway access. Factors contributing to a difficult airway can be anatomical or physiological [15].

Anatomically Difficult Airway

An anatomically challenging airway is characterized as one in which the structural or physical attributes of the patient's airway anatomy are expected to complicate airway management for a skilled practitioner. These challenges include any anatomical considerations that may contribute to challenges associated with face-mask ventilation, supraglottic airway placement, laryngoscopy, tracheal intubation, or front-of-neck access [15–17]. The assessment of the patient's airway complexities is performed using established risk evaluation instruments such as the Mallampati score and the MACOCHA score [17, 18]. The Mallampati score is employed to categorize oropharyngeal visibility with the mouth in an open position, graded from I to IV, wherein grades III or IV indicate limited visibility of oropharyngeal structures and are associated with an increased likelihood of difficult intubation. Although this score is widely utilized, it has limitations in critical care settings, as it serves primarily as an anatomical predictor and possesses moderate sensitivity and specificity, along with a low negative predictive value, rendering it insufficient for reliably excluding the possibility of difficult intubation [17, 18].

To address the complexities inherent in evaluating challenging airways in the intensive care unit (ICU), the MACOCHA score, a more advanced assessment tool, has been validated for use with ICU patients. This score comprises seven critical variables: a Mallampati classification of III or IV, the presence of obstructive sleep apnea syndrome, restricted cervical spine mobility, limited oral aperture (less than 3 cm), coma status, severe hypoxemia (oxygen saturation levels below 80%), and whether the individual performing the intubation is not an anesthesiologist. The MACOCHA score is interpreted by summing the points for each risk factor present; a score of 3 or higher should prompt preparation for a potentially difficult airway and consideration of additional support or advanced airway techniques [19, 20]. The score has demonstrated superior predictive accuracy, sensitivity, and specificity, along with an impressive negative predictive value of 98% for identifying difficult intubation scenarios among critically ill patients [19, 20].

Physiologically Difficult Airway

A physiologically difficult airway is characterized by underlying physiological abnormalities that increase the risk of severe complications during intubation. ICU patients with respiratory failure, severe hypoxemia, severe metabolic acidosis, acute right ventricular failure, intracranial hypertension, hypotension, or shock requiring emergency intubation represent patients who would be considered a difficult physiological airway.

Although comprehensive data quantifying the exact prevalence of physiologically difficult airways in the intensive care unit (ICU) is limited, it is reasonable to conclude that a significant portion of ICU patients exhibit physiological abnormalities that elevate the risk of life-threatening complications during intubation [15, 21, 22]. Diagnoses such as pneumonia, heart failure, and acute respiratory distress syndrome (ARDS) cause alveolar filling and contribute to poor oxygen diffusion, other diagnoses of pulmonary embolism and atelectasis affecting ventilation/perfusion (V/Q) mismatch, creating scenarios of hypoxemia.

There is no validated scoring system designed to evaluate physiologically difficult airways, and as discussed, the MACOCHA score predominantly addresses anatomical and operator-related factors, incorporating only a few components of physiological risk. Consequently, the assessment of a physiologically difficult airway largely depends on the experience and clinical judgment of the intensivist [13, 19, 20, 22] (Table 24.1).

Evaluation of Rapid Desaturation Risk Factors

Intensivists should conduct an exhaustive pre-intubation analysis to identify patients predisposed to rapid desaturation. Key risk groups include individuals with acute respiratory distress syndrome (ARDS), chronic pulmonary pathology, or compromised cardiac function. Identifying these factors is essential for taking preemptive measures like ensuring adequate preoxygenation and implementing a reliable apneic oxygenation technique. An alternative yet often overlooked method of awake intubation can be used to minimize the risk of apneic desaturation [14, 16, 23].

Monitoring Oxygen Levels During Intubation in the ICU

Continuous monitoring of arterial oxygen saturation (SpO_2) via pulse oximetry is the standard methodology for tracking oxygen levels during endotracheal intubation in the intensive care unit (ICU). Pulse oximetry provides a real-time, continuous assessment of arterial hemoglobin saturation. It is imperative that the SpO_2 alarm thresholds on monitoring systems are configured to trigger alerts at saturation levels below the targeted 92% to ensure patient safety. Within the ICU environment, it is advisable to adjust the alarm volume to a higher setting and position the monitor display for unobstructed visibility by the healthcare team to facilitate prompt responsiveness. However, it must be recognized that the accuracy of the pulse oximeter can be affected by several factors, such as skin pigmentation, perfusion index, hypotension, and motion. Advanced monitoring technologies like the Oxygen Reserve Index (ORI), which uses multiwavelength pulse co-oximetry designed to provide an early warning of impending hypoxemia in patients with moderate

Table 24.1 Anatomical and physiological predictors of difficulty with airway

Anatomical predictors	Physiological predictors
Limited head and neck extension Limited mouth opening (Mallampati class III or IV) Obesity and increased neck circumference Limited mandibular protrusion and a short thyromental distance Operator inexperience with direct laryngoscopy Obstructing or distorting lesions in the upper airway	Hemodynamic instability (shock, hypovolemia, or right ventricular failure) Reduced functional residual capacity (FRC) or increased oxygen consumption (due to obesity, sepsis, or pregnancy) Severe hypoxia and rapid desaturation Large minute ventilation (patients compensating for metabolic acidosis) Full stomach increases the risk of aspiration

Adapted from Heidegger [16]

hyperoxia (PaO_2 100–200 mm Hg), offer potential advantages by providing an earlier indication of potential desaturation events [26]. However, the adoption and utility of such indices are still under evaluation and have not reached a standardized protocol across clinical settings [10, 24–26].

Preoxygenation and Apneic Oxygenation Techniques During Intubation

Noninvasive Ventilation (NIV)

This technique delivers 100% oxygen by using positive pressure applied via a tight-fitting mask. It is particularly beneficial for patients experiencing acute hypoxic respiratory failure, as it reduces the risk of oxygen desaturation more effectively than high-flow nasal cannula and other conventional oxygen therapies. The Society of Critical Care Medicine endorses the use of NIV for preoxygenation in patients with severe hypoxemia, characterized by a partial pressure of oxygen/fraction of inspired oxygen (PaO_2/FiO_2) ratio of less than 150 mm Hg [10, 27–29].

The advantages of NIV include the provision of pressure support and positive end-expiratory pressure (PEEP), which facilitate alveolar recruitment and enhance alveolar oxygenation. It is important to note that logistical complexity and time required to initiate NIV may preclude its use in the most urgent intubations. Other drawbacks include patient discomfort or intolerance and the risk of aspiration. Clinical trials have shown that a window of 3–5 minutes is adequate for optimal preoxygenation without delaying definitive airway management [27, 31, 32].

Contraindications to the use of NIV for preoxygenation in the ICU include the following: poor mental status (Glasgow Coma Scale <8), substantial facial injury, active vomiting, recent airway or esophageal surgery, severe hemodynamic instability, or cardiac arrest [10, 18].

High-Flow Nasal Oxygen (HFNC)

This method administers high-flow rates (typically ranging from 40 to 60 L/min) of heated and humidified oxygen, with a fraction of inspired oxygen (FiO_2) up to 100%. The Society of Critical Care Medicine recommends the use of HFNC in scenarios where laryngoscopy is anticipated to be challenging [10, 12, 30]. Since high-flow oxygen provides oxygen even during apneas due to Brownian motion, it adds some physiologic reserve. Consequently, HFNC is suitable for preoxygenation and also supports apneic oxygenation during laryngoscopy and any subsequent intubation attempts [11, 30, 31].

Disadvantages include requiring specialized equipment and higher oxygen consumption. It is inferior to NIV in patients with severe respiratory hypoxemia (PaO_2/

$FiO_2 < 150$). There are no absolute contraindications to the use of HFNC except for severe facial injury that makes fitting of the nasal canula impossible.

A study enrolling 322 patients with acute hypoxemic respiratory failure from 28 ICUs failed to show a difference in post-intubation hypoxemia, suggesting non-inferiority of one method over the other [32].

Bag-Valve-Mask (BVM) Ventilation

BVM ventilation facilitates the administration of high fraction of inspired oxygen (FiO_2) via a self-inflating bag attached to a face mask, with optional positive end-expiratory pressure (PEEP). Optimal oxygenation efficiency with BVM necessitates proper technique in its application [33].

A two-hand mask seal technique incorporating head-tilt and chin-lift or jaw-thrust maneuvers is recommended for optimal ventilation. The two-hand seal method demonstrates superior sealing efficacy compared to the single-hand technique and should be prioritized when an additional operator is present [16, 33].

The oxygen flow rate should be no less than 15 liters per minute, and ventilation should be delivered at a frequency of 10 breaths per minute (equivalent to one breath every 6 seconds). To prevent gastric air entry, a minimal tidal volume should be delivered to achieve a visible chest rise [33].

Although BVM continues to represent the standard care modality for oxygenation and ventilation during cardiopulmonary resuscitation (CPR), its application in preoxygenation and apneic oxygenation remains subject to ongoing debate. Despite its efficacy in maintaining adequate oxygenation, BVM usage carries inherent risks such as gastric insufflation and subsequent aspiration [10, 34].

The Society of Critical Care Medicine's 2023 guidelines advocate for advanced preoxygenation methods, utilizing high-flow nasal oxygen (HFNO) and noninvasive ventilation (NIV), rather than BVM, for patients experiencing acute hypoxemic respiratory failure. Consequently, BVM should be preferentially employed for patients requiring intubation for indications other than respiratory failure and who present with normal functional residual capacity (FRC).

Non-Rebreather Mask (NRM)

A non-rebreather mask works by delivering a high concentration of oxygen without positive pressure. It consists of a face mask connected to a reservoir bag and one-way valves that allow patients to inhale oxygen from both the reservoir bag and the mask, preventing exhaled air from entering the reservoir bag. The NRM has the advantage of simplicity and the ability to deliver high inspired oxygen concentrations without the need for a skilled operator. However, its main drawback is the lack of PEEP and the fact that the actual delivered FiO_2 can be variable and often lower than expected [12, 35, 36].

Combination Techniques

ICU patients, especially those with acute respiratory failure, are more difficult to preoxygenate and are at increased risk of rapid desaturation during apnea. This makes the use of noninvasive ventilation (NIV) for preoxygenation and simultaneously or sequentially using HFNC to provide continuous oxygen flow during the apneic phase, further reducing the risk of desaturation [37].

Intubation Techniques in the ICU

The next section will explore different techniques for endotracheal intubation in the ICU and describe how the technique, medication selection, and timing can affect oxygenation and ventilation in critically ill patients.

Rapid Sequence Intubation

Rapid sequence intubation (RSI) is a technique used to rapidly secure the airway in patients who are at risk of aspiration or require immediate airway management. It involves the sequential administration of a potent sedative (induction agent) followed immediately by a rapid-onset neuromuscular blocking agent and subsequent laryngoscopy within 30–60 seconds after administration of the medications. As the paralytics are taking effect, BVM can be utilized to reduce the risks of hypoxemia if aspiration is considered low risk. This process facilitates endotracheal intubation under optimal conditions, minimizing the risk of aspiration [10, 38, 39].

RSI is the most widely used intubation technique in the intensive care unit (ICU) accounting for 62.2% of intubations due to its benefits in providing rapid airway protection, particularly in patients at high risk for aspiration. It is associated with improved success rates on the first intubation attempt, which is crucial for minimizing complications that can arise from multiple attempts [11].

Performing RSI in the ICU requires careful patient selection, thorough pre-intubation optimization, and skilled personnel to mitigate the risk of complications like severe hypoxemia, hypotension, and cardiovascular collapse. It is also important to note that neuromuscular blockers also carry risks of anaphylaxis, prolonged paralysis, and metabolic disturbances. Although widely used, there is limited data on direct patient-centered outcome data comparing RSI with alternative intubation strategies in the ICU. Therefore, in high-risk patients, alternative techniques such as delayed sequence intubation or awake intubation may be considered. These methods can offer safer airway management in scenarios where traditional RSI may present increased risks [11, 38].

Delayed Sequence Intubation

Delayed sequence intubation (DSI), also known as medication-assisted preoxygenation, is a technique utilized in the intubation of patients who are agitated, delirious, or otherwise unable to tolerate standard preoxygenation methods. In this approach, a sedative is administered to induce sedation while maintaining airway reflexes and spontaneous respiration, therefore allowing for effective preoxygenation. Once adequate preoxygenation is achieved, a neuromuscular blocking agent is administered, allowing intubation to proceed similarly to rapid sequence intubation (RSI) [10, 40, 41].

DSI is particularly advantageous for patients at risk of critical desaturation who are unable to cooperate with conventional preoxygenation techniques. Observational studies have indicated that DSI can significantly enhance oxygen saturation prior to intubation in high-risk, agitated patients, without introducing major complications [10, 42].

In delayed sequence intubation, the use of neuromuscular blockade can be avoided. This technique involves administering ketamine to achieve dissociation or a hypnotic agent such as propofol [43, 44]. Randomized trials have indicated that this approach can provide suitable intubating conditions without the need for neuromuscular blockade. However, it presents a higher risk of difficult intubation and airway discomfort compared to using neuromuscular blockade. According to the Society of Critical Care Medicine, intubation without neuromuscular blockade may lead to inferior intubating conditions and increased complications. Therefore, it should be reserved for high-risk situations where the use of neuromuscular blockade is contraindicated or not practical [10, 45, 46].

Awake Intubation

While awake intubations negate the need for RSI drugs, they are sometimes described using direct laryngoscopy and with the patient in a semi-recumbent position. An awake fiberoptic intubation, or bronchoscopic intubation, is a less commonly used technique to manage critical airways [29]. The fourth National Audit Project (NAP4) of the Royal College of Anesthetists and the Difficult Airway Society in the United Kingdom is the largest registry of airway complications ever compiled. The report concludes that awake fiberoptic intubation (AFOI) is underutilized, which may lead to a decrease in trained personnel, thereby perpetuating its infrequent use. While AFOI is largely considered for anatomic difficult airways, the physiologically difficult airway is another underrecognized clinical situation where AFOI may be indicated to prevent respiratory or cardiovascular collapse [47]. The predictors of anatomic and physiologically difficult airways are outlined in Table 24.1 [16, 48]. AFOI or awake bronchoscopic intubation with a video bronchoscope offers a significant advantage over an eye-piece bronchoscope, which only allows the operator to visualize the larynx and participate in the procedure. High-definition video monitors are now available from both reusable and disposable bronchoscope manufacturers, the latter being an affordable option present in modern-day ICUs [49]. The optimal patient position is sitting upright to prevent position-related reductions in FRC (Fig. 24.2). The patient can be oxygenated with either continuous nasal NIVV or HFNC throughout the intubation process [50–52]. This procedure requires a cooperative patient, and a clinical situation that affords some time to perform appropriate topical anesthesia includes atomization of 200 mg 4% lidocaine to the tonsillar pillars and laryngeal structures, as well as 5% lidocaine ointment on a standard Berman oral airway to anesthetize the distal soft palate. A 9 or 10 cm intubating airway (Williams) is used to facilitate intubation of the trachea with the laryngoscope, and the ETT is then passed over the bronchoscope into the trachea [50]. Patients receive minimal or no moderate sedation.

In a single-center retrospective study of 219 emergency intubations over 1 year in a medical ICU, patients intubated with an awake bronchoscopic technique had a higher first pass rate of intubation compared to direct or video laryngoscopic techniques (96% vs. 78%; $P = 0.003$) and higher FiO_2 requirement (0.73 ± 0.27 vs. 0.63 ± 0.30; $P = 0.044$) [53]. There was no difference in hypoxemic events between the groups; however, it is notable that the patients chosen for AFOI had higher BMI (28.4 vs. 25.9; $P = 0.027$) and a higher FiO_2 requirement (0.73 ± 0.27 vs. 0.63 ± 0.30; $P = 0.044$) prior to intubation. This method has also been shown to be effective in patients experiencing acute right heart failure and pulmonary hypertension [54].

While this method of endotracheal intubation remains underutilized due to the attainment or maintenance of skill, medical ICUs employing dual-trained pulmonologists and intensivists may be uniquely positioned to consider this technique for management of the difficult physiological airway, given their experience with diagnostic bronchoscopy.

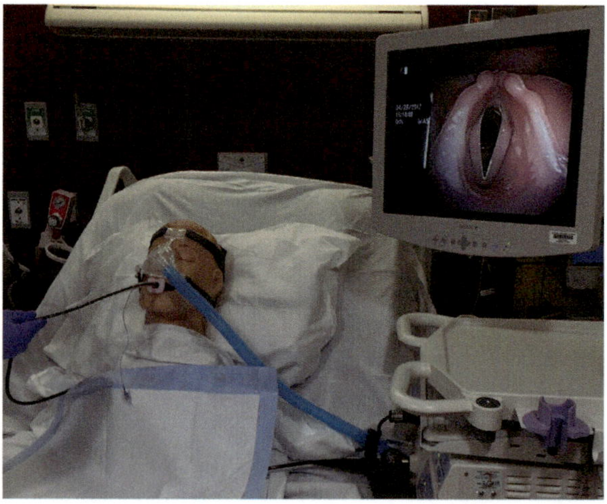

Fig. 24.2 Awake bronchoscopic intubation in the ICU. This simulated patient is seated upright and being oxygenated with nasal noninvasive ventilation throughout the procedure. The airway is visualized on a video monitor so that all practitioners can visualize the procedure and assist if needed

Conclusion

Ensuring optimal oxygenation during intubation in the intensive care setting requires a multifaceted understanding of physiology and practical techniques. This entails a comprehensive assessment of the patient's unique anatomical and physiological challenges. Mastery of preoxygenation strategies and proficiency in various intubation techniques—such as rapid sequence intubation, delayed sequence intubation, and awake bronchoscopic intubation—are crucial. These techniques must be tailored to each patient's specific needs and potential risks to ensure a safe and effective procedure. By combining thorough pre-intubation assessments with the strategic application of both conventional and alternative intubation techniques, risks can be mitigated with optimization of preoxygenation, ultimately enhancing the likelihood of successful intubation and improved patient outcomes in this high-stakes environment.

References

1. Tanoubi I, Drolet P, Donati F. Optimizing preoxygenation in adults. Can J Anaesth. 2009;56(6):449–66.
2. Nimmagadda U, Salem MR, Crystal GJ. Preoxygenation: physiologic basis, benefits, and potential risks. Anesth Analg. 2017;124(2):507–17.
3. Williams EM, Hamilton RM, Sutton L, Viale JP, Hahn CE. Alveolar and dead space volume measured by oscillations of inspired oxygen in awake adults. Am J Respir Crit Care Med. 1997;156(6):1834–9.
4. Sapoval B, Kang M-Y, Dinh-Xuan AT. Modeling of gas exchange in the lungs. Compr Physiol. 2020;11(1):1289–314.
5. Samain E, Farah E, Delefosse D, Marty J. End-tidal oxygraphy during pre-oxygenation in patients with severe diffuse emphysema. Anaesthesia. 2000;55(9):841–6.
6. Nimmagadda U, Salem MR, Joseph NJ, Lopez G, Megally M, Lang DJ, et al. Efficacy of preoxygenation with tidal volume breathing. Comparison of breathing systems. Anesthesiology. 2000;93(3):693–8.
7. Nimmagadda U, Chiravuri SD, Salem MR, Joseph NJ, Wafai Y, Crystal GJ, et al. Preoxygenation with tidal volume and deep breathing techniques: the impact of duration of breathing and fresh gas flow. Anesth Analg. 2001;92(5):1337–41.
8. Caputo ND, Oliver M, West JR, Hackett R, Sakles JC. Use of end tidal oxygen monitoring to assess preoxygenation during rapid sequence intubation in the emergency department. Ann Emerg Med. 2019;74(3):410–5.
9. Benumof JL, Dagg R, Benumof R. Critical hemoglobin desaturation will occur before return to an unparalyzed state following 1 mg/kg intravenous succinylcholine. Anesthesiology. 1997;87(4):979–82.
10. Acquisto NM, Mosier JM, Bittner EA, Patanwala AE, Hirsch KG, Hargwood P, et al. Society of critical care medicine clinical practice guidelines for rapid sequence intubation in the critically ill adult patient. Crit Care Med. 2023;51(10):1411–30.
11. Russotto V, Myatra SN, Laffey JG, Tassistro E, Antolini L, Bauer P, et al. Intubation practices and adverse Peri-intubation events in critically ill patients from 29 countries. JAMA. 2021;325(12):1164–72.
12. Bailly A, Ricard J-D, Le Thuaut A, Helms J, Kamel T, Mercier E, et al. Compared efficacy of four preoxygenation methods for intubation in the ICU: retrospective analysis of Mcgrath mac videolaryngoscope versus macintosh laryngoscope (MACMAN) trial data. Crit Care Med. 2019;47(4):e340–8.

13. Karamchandani K, Nasa P, Jarzebowski M, Brewster DJ, De Jong A, Bauer PR, et al. Tracheal intubation in critically ill adults with a physiologically difficult airway. An international Delphi study. Intensive Care Med. 2024;50(10):1563–79.
14. De Jong A, Myatra SN, Roca O, Jaber S. How to improve intubation in the intensive care unit. Update on knowledge and devices. Intensive Care Med. 2022;48(10):1287–98.
15. Apfelbaum JL, Hagberg CA, Connis RT, Abdelmalak BB, Agarkar M, Dutton RP, et al. 2022 american society of anesthesiologists practice guidelines for management of the difficult airway. Anesthesiology. 2022;136(1):31–81.
16. Heidegger T. Management of the difficult airway. N Engl J Med. 2021;384(19):1836–47.
17. Detsky ME, Jivraj N, Adhikari NK, Friedrich JO, Pinto R, Simel DL, et al. Will this patient be difficult to intubate?: the rational clinical examination systematic review. JAMA. 2019;321(5):493–503.
18. Roth D, Pace NL, Lee A, Hovhannisyan K, Warenits A-M, Arrich J, et al. Airway physical examination tests for detection of difficult airway management in apparently normal adult patients. Cochrane Database Syst Rev. 2018;5(5):CD008874.
19. De Jong A, Molinari N, Terzi N, Mongardon N, Arnal J-M, Guitton C, et al. Early identification of patients at risk for difficult intubation in the intensive care unit: development and validation of the MACOCHA score in a multicenter cohort study. Am J Respir Crit Care Med. 2013;187(8):832–9.
20. Luedike P, Totzeck M, Rammos C, Kindgen-Milles D, Kelm M, Rassaf T. The MACOCHA score is feasible to predict intubation failure of nonanesthesiologist intensive care unit trainees. J Crit Care. 2015;30(5):876–80.
21. Myatra SN, Divatia JV, Brewster DJ. The physiologically difficult airway: an emerging concept. Curr Opin Anaesthesiol. 2022;35(2):115–21.
22. Hickey AJ, Cummings MJ, Short B, Brodie D, Panzer O, Madahar P, et al. Approach to the physiologically challenging endotracheal intubation in the intensive care unit. Respir Care. 2023;68(10):1438–48.
23. Mosier JM, Sakles JC, Law JA, Brown CA, Brindley PG. Tracheal intubation in the critically Ill. Where we came from and where we should go. Am J Respir Crit Care Med. 2020;201(7):775–88.
24. Saidy S, Iqbal A, Baig SH. Pulse oximetry discrepancies and occult hypoxemia in ICU patients: predictors and clinical outcomes. J Intensive Care Med. 2025:8850666251351594.
25. Semler MW, Casey JD, Lloyd BD, Hastings PG, Hays MA, Stollings JL, et al. Oxygen-saturation targets for critically ill adults receiving mechanical ventilation. N Engl J Med. 2022;387(19):1759–69.
26. Hille H, Le Thuaut A, Asfar P, Quelven Q, Mercier E, Le Meur A, et al. Impact of non-invasive oxygen reserve index versus standard SpO2 monitoring on peripheral oxygen saturation during endotracheal intubation in the intensive care unit: protocol for the randomized controlled trial NESOI2. PLoS One. 2024;19(9):e0307723.
27. Gibbs KW, Semler MW, Driver BE, Seitz KP, Stempek SB, Taylor C, et al. Noninvasive ventilation for Preoxygenation during emergency intubation. N Engl J Med. 2024;390(23):2165–77.
28. Munshi L, Mancebo J, Brochard LJ. Noninvasive respiratory support for adults with acute respiratory failure. N Engl J Med. 2022;387(18):1688–98.
29. Barjaktarevic I, Esquinas AM, West FM, Albores J, Berlin D. Noninvasive ventilation in difficult endotracheal intubation: systematic and review analysis. Anaesthesiol Intensive Ther. 2017;49(4):294–302.
30. Guitton C, Ehrmann S, Volteau C, Colin G, Maamar A, Jean-Michel V, et al. Nasal high-flow preoxygenation for endotracheal intubation in the critically ill patient: a randomized clinical trial. Intensive Care Med. 2019;45(4):447–58.
31. Jaber S, Monnin M, Girard M, Conseil M, Cisse M, Carr J, et al. Apnoeic oxygenation via high-flow nasal cannula oxygen combined with non-invasive ventilation preoxygenation for intubation in hypoxaemic patients in the intensive care unit: the single-centre, blinded, randomised controlled OPTINIV trial. Intensive Care Med. 2016;42(12):1877–87.

32. Frat J-P, Ricard J-D, Quenot J-P, Pichon N, Demoule A, Forel J-M, et al. Non-invasive ventilation versus high-flow nasal cannula oxygen therapy with apnoeic oxygenation for preoxygenation before intubation of patients with acute hypoxaemic respiratory failure: a randomised, multicentre, open-label trial. Lancet Respir Med. 2019;7(4):303–12.
33. Casey JD, Janz DR, Russell DW, Vonderhaar DJ, Joffe AM, Dischert KM, et al. Bag-mask ventilation during tracheal intubation of critically ill adults. N Engl J Med. 2019;380(9):811–21.
34. Panchal AR, Bartos JA, Cabañas JG, Donnino MW, Drennan IR, Hirsch KG, et al. Part 3: adult basic and advanced life support: 2020 american heart association guidelines for cardiopulmonary resuscitation and emergency cardiovascular care. Circulation. 2020;142(16_suppl_2):S366–468.
35. Coudroy R, Frat J-P, Girault C, Thille AW. Reliability of methods to estimate the fraction of inspired oxygen in patients with acute respiratory failure breathing through non-rebreather reservoir bag oxygen mask. Thorax. 2020;75(9):805–7.
36. Sorg ME, Chatburn RL. Oxygen delivery with an open oxygen mask and other conventional masks: a simulation-based study. Respir Care. 2022;67(3):316–21.
37. Binks MJ, Holyoak RS, Melhuish TM, Vlok R, Hodge A, Ryan T, et al. Apnoeic oxygenation during intubation in the intensive care unit: a systematic review and meta-analysis. Heart Lung. 2017;46(6):452–7.
38. Stollings JL, Diedrich DA, Oyen LJ, Brown DR. Rapid-sequence intubation: a review of the process and considerations when choosing medications. Ann Pharmacother. 2014;48(1):62–76.
39. Sorbello M, Paternò DS, Zdravkovic I, La Via L. Pharmacological approach to rapid sequence induction/intubation: a contemporary perspective. Curr Opin Anaesthesiol. 2025;38(4):369–74.
40. Weingart SD, Trueger NS, Wong N, Scofi J, Singh N, Rudolph SS. Delayed sequence intubation: a prospective observational study. Ann Emerg Med. 2015;65(4):349–55.
41. Weingart SD. Preoxygenation, reoxygenation, and delayed sequence intubation in the emergency department. J Emerg Med. 2011;40(6):661–7.
42. Fotopoulou G, Theocharis S, Vasileiou I, Kouskouni E, Xanthos T. Management of the airway without the use of neuromuscular blocking agents: the use of remifentanil. Fundam Clin Pharmacol. 2012;26(1):72–85.
43. Grillot N, Lebuffe G, Huet O, Lasocki S, Pichon X, Oudot M, et al. Effect of remifentanil vs neuromuscular blockers during rapid sequence intubation on successful intubation without major complications among patients at risk of aspiration: a randomized clinical trial. JAMA. 2023;329(1):28–38.
44. Koenig SJ, Lakticova V, Narasimhan M, Doelken P, Mayo PH. Safety of propofol as an induction agent for urgent endotracheal intubation in the medical intensive care unit. J Intensive Care Med. 2015;30(8):499–504.
45. Lundstrøm LH, Duez CHV, Nørskov AK, Rosenstock CV, Thomsen JL, Møller AM, et al. Effects of avoidance or use of neuromuscular blocking agents on outcomes in tracheal intubation: a Cochrane systematic review. Br J Anaesth. 2018;120(6):1381–93.
46. Lundstrøm LH, Duez CH, Nørskov AK, Rosenstock CV, Thomsen JL, Møller AM, et al. Avoidance versus use of neuromuscular blocking agents for improving conditions during tracheal intubation or direct laryngoscopy in adults and adolescents. Cochrane Database Syst Rev. 2017;5(5):CD009237.
47. Cook TM, Woodall N, Frerk C, Fourth National Audit Project. Major complications of airway management in the UK: results of the Fourth National Audit Project of the Royal College of Anaesthetists and the Difficult Airway Society. Part 1: anaesthesia. Br J Anaesth. 2011;106(5):617–31.
48. Myatra SN, Divatia JV, Brewster DJ. The physiologically difficult airway: an emerging concept. Curr Opin Anaesthesiol. 2022;35(2):115–21. https://doi.org/10.1097/ACO.0000000000001102. PMID: 35165233.
49. Russotto V, Myatra SN, Laffey JG, INTUBE Study Investigators, et al. Intubation practices and adverse peri-intubation events in critically ill patients from 29 countries. JAMA. 2021;325:1164–72.

50. Barjaktarevic I, Berlin D. Bronchoscopic intubation during continuous nasal positive pressure ventilation in the treatment of hypoxemic respiratory failure. J Intensive Care Med. 2015;30(3):161–6. https://doi.org/10.1177/0885066613510680. Epub 2013 Nov 15. PMID: 24243561.
51. Berlin D, Singh I, Barjaktarevic I, Friedman O. A technique for Bronchoscopic intubation during high-flow nasal cannula oxygen therapy. J Intensive Care Med. 2016;31(3):213–5. https://doi.org/10.1177/0885066615582020. Epub 2015 Apr 23. PMID: 25911299.
52. Badiger S, John M, Fearnley RA, Ahmad I. Optimizing oxygenation and intubation conditions during awake fibre-optic intubation using a high-flow nasal oxygen-delivery system. Br J Anaesth. 2015;115(4):629–32. https://doi.org/10.1093/bja/aev262. Epub 2015 Aug 7. PMID: 26253608.
53. Ma KC, Chung A, Aronson KI, Krishnan JK, Barjaktarevic IZ, Berlin DA, Schenck EJ. Bronchoscopic intubation is an effective airway strategy in critically ill patients. J Crit Care. 2017;38:92–6. https://doi.org/10.1016/j.jcrc.2016.10.022. Epub 2016 Nov 4. PMID: 27875775.
54. Johannes J, Berlin DA, Patel P, Schenck EJ, West FM, Saggar R, Barjaktarevic IZ. A technique of awake Bronchoscopic endotracheal intubation for respiratory failure in patients with right heart failure and pulmonary hypertension. Crit Care Med. 2017;45(9):e980–4. https://doi.org/10.1097/CCM.0000000000002586. PMID: 28682836.

Complications of Mechanical Ventilation 25

Padmanabh Bhatt and Michael Baram

Introduction

The mechanical ventilator, although an extraordinary invention that has saved countless lives, comes with the risk of significant complications. It is well understood that ventilators do not correct the underlying lung pathology but rather provide oxygen and assist in carbon dioxide (CO_2) removal to allow oxygen-dependent metabolism to occur. In the setting of pathological stress that requires mechanical ventilation, the body still needs to continue to use oxygen to convert glucose into energy through aerobic respiration. Loss of efficient oxygen delivery can increase the work of breathing. There is constant tension between increasing blood oxygen delivery and damage caused by the ventilator. This chapter will discuss some of the main risk factors and causes of ventilator-induced lung injury (VILI) while providing suggestions about how these can be mitigated.

The Traumas

Barotrauma

Barotrauma is an injury to the lung caused by excessive airway pressure, and by extension, transalveolar or transpulmonary pressures. In physiological

P. Bhatt · M. Baram (✉)
The Korman Respiratory Institute and the Division of Pulmonary, Allergy and Critical Care, The Department of Medicine at the Sidney Kimmel Medical College of Thomas Jefferson University, Philadelphia, PA, USA
e-mail: Michael.baram@jefferson.edu

G. C. Kane et al. (eds.), *Oxygen*, https://doi.org/10.1007/978-3-032-18934-9_25

circumstances, humans breathe with negative-pressure ventilation—the diaphragm and external intercostal muscles contract, increasing intrathoracic volume, thereby reducing intrathoracic pressure, leading to inspiration. Normal expiration is mostly a passive process, although intercostal and abdominal muscles can contract to allow forced expiration. Mechanical ventilation inverts this. The ventilator forces air under positive pressure during inhalation, while exhalation remains a mostly passive process driven by chest wall and lung compliance. The pressure distributed to the lungs by the ventilator is not uniform. The airways within the lungs are not fluid pipes. Due to the tapering nature of the airways, flow is time dependent, which means that inflamed, narrow distal airways will see less pressure than relatively normal regions. As healthier airways and lung units cause less airflow resistance, they receive more gas and oxygen from the ventilator. However, these excessive volumes can become deleterious. This differential in flow/pressure is the root cause of ventilator-induced lung injury. Ultimately, the microscopic endpoint of barotrauma is the rupture of alveoli, leading to extra-alveolar air accumulation. The macroscopic and clinically relevant manifestations are pneumothorax, pneumomediastinum, and subcutaneous emphysema. These can be dramatic, and in extreme circumstances, lead to tension physiology. Knowledge and avoidance of barotrauma is crucial.

The incidence of barotrauma with modern lung-protective ventilation strategies is likely under 10% [1]. The etiology of respiratory failure necessitating mechanical ventilation certainly plays a role in barotrauma, with both restrictive processes like interstitial lung disease, pneumonia, and acute respiratory distress syndrome (ARDS) and obstructive pathologies like asthma and chronic obstructive airways disease being involved. This is likely due to reduced lung compliance in the former pathologies, where similar tidal volumes lead to higher airway pressures resulting in barotrauma. Conversely, progressive dynamic hyperinflation in obstructive pathologies results in barotrauma.

A major cause of barotrauma is high airway pressures, with plateau pressures (Pplat) being key. The plateau pressure is reflective of the pressure experienced by the small airways and alveoli at the end of inspiration. Although there are no values of Pplat where barotrauma definitely does or does not occur, there is generally a higher incidence of barotrauma with Pplat higher than 35 cm H_2O. Thus, every effort should be made to target a Pplat under this value, or more cautiously, 30 cm H_2O. The concept of stress is important here. It refers to and is related to transpulmonary pressure—the distending pressures seen by alveoli, which is the difference between the alveolar and pleural pressures per unit area. Excessive stress causes barotrauma.

In ARDS, only a small fraction of relatively healthy alveoli perform the ventilatory workload of the lungs. This is the "baby lung" concept of the disorder, whereby the functional lung volume in an adult with ARDS may be closer to a child, or in severe forms of the disorder, a baby. This baby lung receives the majority of tidal volume, and therefore the stress experienced by this functioning lung volume may be higher than what is observed globally. Preventing VILI in the baby lung is crucial as it is the functional component of the respiratory system. Lastly, a word about positive end expiratory pressure (PEEP) and baby lung. The right amount of PEEP can increase the functional residual capacity, and thus, increase the size of baby lung—thereby allowing healthier lung to participate in gas exchange, while also reducing the stress experienced by each alveolar unit. However, excessive PEEP can contribute to barotrauma. This original concept of the baby lung described by Gattinoni et al. has now been modified to the "sponge lung." [2] The "baby lung" was thought of as a distinct anatomical part of the lung—the only part participating in gas exchange in the lung affected by ARDS. Now, with the advent of CT scans and prone positioning, it is known that the part of the lung that is affected by ARDS is fluid and can move. The lungs are like a sponge with fluid and inflammation that are gravitationally dependent and can move anatomically based on the position of the patient. More on proning in later chapters.

Neuromuscular blockade (NMB) has been studied in critically ill ventilated patients, with some indications that in the right patients, it can reduce the risk of barotrauma. [3, 4] NMB can be particularly useful in patients with dynamic hyperinflation-induced barotrauma, as it allows for complete control of the respiratory cycle and takes away the patient's native respiratory drive. However, the risks of NMB—critical illness myopathy and neuropathy, among others—must be balanced with the benefits.

The development of barotrauma likely portends a worse prognosis, is associated with higher mortality, longer ICU stays, and longer duration of mechanical ventilation. Large bronchopleural fistulae are also associated with higher mortality [5]. The caveat with the above studies is that the patients experiencing barotrauma likely had poorer lung compliance and worse disease to start off with, and thus, while barotrauma is not a direct cause of death, it may serve as a marker for more severe illness.

Atelectotrauma

The concept of atelectotrauma comes from animal models of mechanical ventilation, whereby the cyclic opening and closing of alveoli create sheer forces that damage neighboring non-atelectatic alveoli [6]. These interactions cause activation of alveolar macrophages and release of mitochondrial alarmins, which ultimately lead to the local release of pro-inflammatory cytokines [7]. Subsequent neutrophil infiltration causes a vicious cycle of inflammation, ultimately leading to increased alveolar–capillary permeability, which further reduces the number of functioning alveolar units and worsens gas exchange.

How to minimize atelectotrauma, especially in a world of low tidal volume ventilation? Adequate PEEP is crucial to mitigate the serial opening and closing of alveolar units. PEEP keeps alveolar units open throughout the respiratory cycle and thus reduces the risk of atelectotrauma. Secondly, providing as low an FiO_2 as possible is key, as oxygen readily crosses the alveolar–capillary membrane into the bloodstream while nitrogen, the most abundant gas in the atmosphere, is mostly in equilibrium with dissolved nitrogen in the blood. Thus, high FiO_2 washes out alveolar nitrogen, and as the alveolar oxygen crosses into the bloodstream, absorptive atelectasis ensues.

In the normal lung, surfactant acts to reduce surface tension in the alveoli, thus preventing them from collapsing at the end of expiration. While surfactant administration has been shown to reduce leukocyte infiltration, pro-inflammatory cytokines, and lower surface tension in preclinical models of VILI, human data do not support its use [8].

Biotrauma

Biotrauma describes the effect of inflammatory humoral mediators that cause VILI, and in some cases, multiorgan dysfunction. Biotrauma is seen with excessive alveolar inflation pressures, excessive alveolar volumes, and with atelectotrauma, but is separate from the mechanical concepts discussed previously.

Preclinical data suggest that overventilation with high tidal volumes or excessive pressures results in the release of TNF-α, IL-6, IL-1β, and macrophage inflammatory peptide 2 [9]. These are pro-inflammatory cytokines which in turn cause leukocyte chemotaxis and further contribute to local inflammation. Indeed, early studies in human subjects illustrated that patients receiving lung-protective ventilation, with low tidal volumes and higher PEEP, compared to traditional ventilation methods with higher tidal volumes and lower PEEP, had lower levels of the above pro-inflammatory cytokines locally in the lung and in the systemic circulation [10]. Further, biotrauma can happen quickly, with elevated pro-inflammatory cytokines seen in both the systemic circulation and in the lung within an hour of subjecting patients to traditional ventilation methods [11].

Reducing biotrauma is key as elevated levels of TNF-α, IL-6, and IL-8 in patients with acute lung injury are associated with multiorgan failure and mortality [12, 13].

Other Considerations

Hyperoxia and Its Risks

Normal SpO_2 and PaO_2 in healthy individuals are greater than 95% and 75 mmHg, respectively. Additionally, oxyhemoglobin comprises the majority of the blood's oxygen-carrying capacity, and thus, the higher the SpO_2, the more oxygen is carried in the blood. Further, in critically ill patients, especially those with septic shock and ARDS, tissue oxygen extraction is impaired due to microcirculatory and mitochondrial dysfunction, and thus a higher oxygen delivery (DO_2) may be required to match tissue oxygen consumption (VO_2). Lastly, a higher oxygen target possibly protects against the risk of hypoxia. The combination of the above led to the historic dogma of aiming for hyperoxia in critically ill and mechanically ventilated patients, with SpO_2 and PaO_2 targets of >96% and > 100 mmHg, respectively.

However, it is now known that hyperoxia carries significant risks and more conservative targets of oxygenation are likely safer.

Hyperoxia and Barotrauma

Common teaching is that manipulating PEEP and FiO_2 impacts oxygenation. In the previous discussion, the importance of the "right amount of PEEP" was highlighted, and how both under- and over-utilizing PEEP could contribute to barotrauma. Indeed, one can imagine a setting where an overzealous clinician exposes a patient to high amounts of PEEP in order to strive for ever higher SpO_2 and PaO_2 targets, but in the process exposes the patient to barotrauma.

The concept of mean airway pressure is also relevant. Apart from PEEP and FiO_2, higher mean airway pressures improve oxygenation, primarily by recruiting more alveolar units, increasing functional residual capacity (FRC), and improving V/Q matching. This is achieved by increasing the time spent in inspiration and by maneuvers to increase inspiratory airway pressures (MIP). However, excessive airway pressures can result in barotrauma.

Hyperoxia and Atelectotrauma

Hyperoxia causes washout of nitrogen from alveoli, and as oxygen is readily absorbed in the blood, the result can be alveolar collapse/atelectasis. As discussed previously, recurrent alveolar opening and closing result in atelectotrauma. Patients with poor regional ventilation, like those with chronic obstructive pulmonary disease (COPD), significant mucous plugging, or with airway foreign bodies, are particularly at risk, as once the pre-existing oxygen diffuses into the blood, the affected alveoli receive minimal ventilation to keep them open.

Patients with surfactant abnormalities, which can be seen with ARDS, are also at risk for recurrent atelectotrauma.

Lastly, patients who have a high VO_2 (utilization of oxygen), i.e., those with fever, hyperthyroidism, and sepsis, have a faster rate of alveolar O_2 extraction and are therefore at higher risk of atelectotrauma.

Hyperoxia, Biotrauma, and Reactive Oxygen Species

Cellular injury from oxygen toxicity is primarily caused by the formation of reactive oxygen species (ROS). Injury-causing ROS include the superoxide anion, hydroxyl radical, and hydrogen peroxide. The initial data for cellular injury from reactive oxygen species came from mouse models with mutations in various superoxide dismutase genes, which are key in breaking down ROS to prevent cellular injury. Mice with these mutations would die shortly after birth and showed significant mitochondrial injury.

On a cellular level, ROS-mediated cellular damage involves both apoptosis and necrosis and affects both endothelial and epithelial cells. While the higher the FiO_2, the greater the risk of ROS-induced biotrauma. An FiO_2 above 0.6 increases the risk of lung injury. Overall, the time required to develop biotrauma is inversely related to the FiO_2, with higher levels causing damage even within 24 hours. However, even short periods of moderate hyperoxia, 28%, result in the detection of inflammatory and oxidative stress-mediated damage as measured in expired breath condensate [14].

The Mechanical Ventilator Irony

Despite the above-mentioned risks inherent to ventilators, respect needs to be given to the simplicity of moving oxygen into the lungs. Other chapters review the safety and potential benefit of permissive hypercapnia, but there is a limit to how low oxygen levels can drop. Dr. West elegantly showed that elite athletes can tolerate hypoxemia with PaO_2 in the 30 mmHg while climbing mountains. Human bodies are clearly very efficient in oxygen utilization [15]. Most hospitalized patients cannot tolerate this degree of hypoxemia. Instead, a PaO_2 of 70 mmHg is targeted. The same pressures that damage lungs are what drive up arterial partial pressures of oxygen. The mean airway pressure, or area under the pressure–time curve, is reflective of the PaO_2 being driven into the lung and blood. Thus, to increase oxygenation, clinicians must maximize the area under the pressure–time curve, without increasing peak and plateau pressures. Utilizing strategies of improving V/Q matching, vasodilator use, and optimizing air flow without causing alveolar distension represent the art of oxygen delivery in the setting of critical illness [16]. There are times when oxygen saturation above 92% cannot be achieved. In this less-than-ideal scenario, permitting mild hypoxemia may be better than increasing ventilator settings which can worsen lung injury. In this age of medicine, Extracorporeal Membrane Oxygenation (ECMO) is an alternative means to provide oxygen without the risks of ventilators [17]. However, ECMO carries its own risks. More on this in later chapters.

Effects of Mechanical Ventilation on Other Organ Systems

Cardiovascular

Intrathoracic Pressures and Hemodynamics

The heart shares the thorax with the lungs and is therefore directly affected by changes in intrathoracic pressure caused by mechanical ventilation. The degree to which intrathoracic pressure is transmitted through the lungs and onto the heart and great vessels depends on both lung and chest wall compliance. In scenarios with low lung compliance and/or high chest wall compliance, pressure changes from mechanical ventilation are either absorbed by the lungs themselves, in the former case, or transmitted through the chest wall in the latter case. Such scenarios include pneumonia, ARDS, and sternotomy. In these situations, the heart and great vessels are relatively shielded from the pressure changes associated with mechanical ventilation. The converse is also true, in conditions with high lung compliance, like emphysema, or low chest wall compliance, the heart and great vessels are more exposed to changes in intrathoracic pressures.

Hypotension is a common complication of mechanical ventilation and is seen in over 40% of patients initiated on mechanical ventilation [18]. There are several etiologies for this. Firstly, increased intrathoracic pressures are transmitted to the right atrium, which reduces the pressure gradient with peripheral or systemic circulation. Increased intrathoracic pressures lead to reduced right-sided preload. This, in turn, reduces cardiac output and contributes to hypotension.

Another effect of increased intrathoracic pressure is an increase in right ventricular afterload, both macroscopically and microscopically, due to compression of small pulmonary vessels by distended alveoli. The combination of reduced RV preload with increased afterload can put significant strain on the more compliant but weaker RV, further reducing cardiac output. It is notable that patients with preexisting right heart disease, pulmonary hypertension, cardiomyopathies, and inferior myocardial infarctions can suffer catastrophic cardiovascular collapse with mechanical ventilation, especially with liberal use of vasodilating sedating medications.

The effects of mechanical ventilation on the left heart are not as significant but can also be consequential. The increased RV afterload can lead to septal bulging to the left, leading to reduced LV preload, which may be exacerbated by the reduction in RV cardiac output. Conversely, mechanical ventilation reduces transmural pressures across the LV, leading to a reduction in LV afterload, which might be beneficial depending on the clinical picture. Thus, overall, the LV sees a reduction in both preload and afterload.

The effects of positive-pressure ventilation, as described above, can be beneficial to certain patient populations. Mechanical ventilation can be helpful in patients with heart failure exacerbations, as the reduction in preload and LV afterload can help optimize electromechanical coupling.

Patients with respiratory failure have elevated energy requirements driven by the high work of breathing. This, in turn, increases myocardial energy demands. The initiation of mechanical ventilation can reduce myocardial energy demands, which may be beneficial in critically ill patients or those with myocardial infarction or LV failure.

Lastly, a word about coronary perfusion in mechanical ventilation. Increased intrathoracic pressures reduce coronary perfusion pressure, especially if providing high airway pressures or PEEP. However, this may be balanced by the reduction in myocardial energy/oxygen demands as discussed above.

Overall, one could simplistically state that mechanical ventilation is a friend of the LV but a foe of the RV.

A Note on the Effects of Sedatives on Hemodynamics

Analgesia and sedation are crucial in mechanically ventilated patients to manage the pain, delirium, anxiety, and distress associated with critical illness. Unfortunately, the majority of agents used for analgosedation have an adverse cardiovascular risk profile.

Most analgosedatives used in the ICU cause vasodilation. This is especially true for propofol and dexmedetomidine. Propofol causes vasodilation and venodilation, while also blunting sympathetic outflow that further reduces vascular tone. Additionally, propofol has a direct negative inotropic effect. Dexmedetomidine is an alpha 2 agonist, developed to act centrally and has anxiolytic and weak analgesic properties. It is known to cause both hypotension and hypertension, depending on the balance of effect on central alpha 2a or peripheral alpha 2b receptors, respectively. In the majority of cases, the central alpha 2a effect is stronger, leading to vasodilation and hypotension.

Benzodiazepines (BZDs) were historically used with much greater frequency in the ICU, but their use has reduced due to a higher incidence of delirium compared to propofol and dexmedetomidine, and the concern for oversedation. Lastly, there is also a risk of a paradoxical reaction to BZDs, presenting with increased agitation and hostile behavior, which worsens with escalating doses.

Neurologic

Mechanical ventilation can cause a number of neurological adverse effects, including increases in intracranial pressure (ICP), sleep dysfunction, among others, which will be detailed in this section.

Raised Intracranial Pressure

Mechanical ventilation can increase ICP through a number of mechanisms, although the main driver is the elevation in central venous pressure from increased intrathoracic pressures, reducing the pressure gradient that facilitates cerebral venous drainage. This is seen particularly with high PEEP and airway pressures. Poorly compliant lungs or reduced lung recruitment further contribute to elevated central venous pressures. Mechanical ventilation leading to elevated ICP is particularly problematic in patients with CNS pathologies that raise ICP—intracranial space-occupying lesions, hemorrhage, or in situations with loss of endogenous ICP autoregulation.

In mechanically ventilated patients where hypercarbia is an intentional or unintentional ventilation strategy, the ensuing cerebral vasodilation can further increase intracranial pressure.

It is important to note that the primary focus in neurointensive care is on cerebral perfusion pressure (CPP), rather than ICP on its own. The following simple equation outlines the relationship between the two:

$$\text{CPP} = \text{MAP} - \text{ICP}$$

Where MAP is the mean arterial pressure.

As previously discussed, mechanical ventilation can result in hypotension, thus reducing CPP.

In summary, ICP and CPP must be monitored in patients with any brain pathology that lends itself to raised ICPs undergoing mechanical ventilation.

Disordered Sleep

Unfortunately, disordered sleep is common in mechanically ventilated patients. Assessing sleep in critically ill patients is challenging, as there is a dearth of tools to quantify the amount and quality of sleep patients get. However, polysomnography studies demonstrate reduced total sleep time and marked reductions in rapid eye movement (REM) sleep in the critically ill [19, 20].

These changes are likely multifactorial, but related to anxiety, pain, and delirium associated with critical illness, and discomfort associated with mechanical ventilation. Some experts advise allowing patients to "rest" on assist control ventilation overnight rather than pressure support; there is limited evidence supporting this. Further, significant sleep disturbance due to loud sounds and patient care likely also contributes. Abnormal sleep also contributes to ICU delirium and persists in most patients after discharge.

Clearly, improving sleep quality is important in critically ill and mechanically ventilated patients. Melatonin is currently recommended by professional societies to reduce the risk of delirium, likely by optimizing sleep quality.

Direct Ventilator Injury

Myopathy

Ventilator-induced diaphragmatic dysfunction (VIDD) is relatively common, affecting up to 65% of patients at the time of their first spontaneous breathing trial, and can be seen within the first day of mechanical ventilation [21]. Further, the longer the duration of mechanical ventilation, the greater the risk and severity of developing VIDD. This puts patients and clinicians in a challenging scenario, as respiratory muscle fatigue is a common indication for initiation of mechanical ventilation, but the treatment is associated with worsening of the underlying disorder.

The etiology of VIDD is multifactorial, but involves a combination of oxidative stress, mitochondrial dysfunction, and diaphragmatic proteolysis. The diaphragm is particularly susceptible to atrophy from disuse, compared to peripheral muscles, although critical illness myopathy and peripheral neuropathy do share some pathological markers with VIDD. In addition to proteolysis, peripheral muscle weakness is characterized by downregulation of myofibrillar proteins and loss of myosin filaments.

The primary insults causing VIDD are likely muscle disuse, especially with the use of controlled mechanical ventilation. In addition to the diaphragm, other respiratory muscles can also atrophy. This can be independent of VIDD and does not necessarily correlate with it. Peripheral myopathy and neuropathy are caused by a multitude of factors, including the use of systemic corticosteroids, NMB, hyperglycemia, prolonged immobilization, and systemic inflammatory response. Steroids, interestingly, do not seem to be directly implicated in the development of VIDD.

Diagnosing VIDD presents challenges, as several components of diaphragmatic muscle testing used in non-intubated patients cannot be applied to patients receiving mechanical ventilation. Often, the first sign of VIDD is difficulty weaning and liberating patients from the ventilator. In general, testing is delayed while the underlying pathology that necessitated initiation of mechanical ventilation is considered resolved. The sniff maneuver with ultrasonographic visualization of the diaphragm and negative inspiratory effort testing can be performed at the bedside. More advanced studies, such as transdiaphragmatic pressure measurement and diaphragmatic electromyography, may also be available at specialist centers.

Clearly, both VIDD and critical illness myopathy and neuropathy are clinically significant. Both increase the risk of in-hospital and long-term mortality, duration of mechanical ventilation, ICU length of stay, and the need for tracheostomy for slower and prolonged ventilator weaning.

The treatment and prevention of VIDD is an evolving field. It is hypothesized that avoiding excessive ventilator support, i.e., allowing about 60–80% spontaneous breathing effort, may reduce the incidence of VIDD. However, this must be balanced against patient self-inflicted lung injury (PSILI) incurred through patient-ventilator dyssynchrony, resulting in barotrauma and volutrauma. Additionally, excessive work of breathing can also cause diaphragmatic injury. Similarly, avoidance of NMB and deep sedation is more likely to reduce both the risk of VIDD and critical illness myopathy [22]. Strict glucose control has been shown to reduce the risk of developing myopathy [23]. Lastly, there are emerging studies testing the utility of phrenic nerve stimulation and diaphragmatic rehabilitation in patients requiring prolonged mechanical ventilation, although these are still in their nascency and require further corroboration before they can enter routine clinical care.

Loss of Cough and Mucociliary Clearance

The etiology of reduced mucociliary clearance in mechanically ventilated patients is likely multifactorial but involves the physical barrier of the endotracheal tube disrupting the mucociliary escalator, gas under positive pressure forcing secretions more distally, and the drying of airway secretions due to inhalation of dry gas. Moreover, critical illness myopathy and VIDD weaken the cough reflex, further impairing mucociliary clearance and increasing the risk of ventilator-associated pneumonia, atelectasis, and mucous plugging.

A marker of mucociliary clearance is bronchial mucous transport velocity. Indeed, patients with lower velocities, i.e., poorer mucociliary clearance, have a higher incidence of pneumonia and secretion retention [24].

Both non-pharmacologic and pharmacological techniques have been studied to improve mucociliary clearance and cough in mechanically ventilated patients. Non-pharmacological techniques include the use of a cough-assist mechanical insufflation-exsufflation device and are associated with higher ventilator liberation success, although the quality of data is low [25]. Societal bodies encourage the use of chest physiotherapy and PEEP in order to augment mucociliary clearance and reduce the risk of ventilator-associated pneumonias [26]. Pharmacologic therapies include the use of N-acetylcysteine to break down mucin polymers, hypertonic saline to increase the water content of mucous, therefore, making it easier to mobilize. However, neither of these techniques has demonstrated encouraging clinical data in non-cystic fibrosis patients.

Ventilator-Associated Pneumonia

Ventilator-associated pneumonia (VAP) is defined as a diagnosis of pneumonia in a patient who has required mechanical ventilation for greater than 48 hours. The prevalence of VAP is around 10%, with estimates varying depending on the definition applied and the population studied. Among the factors that make VAP challenging to treat are higher rates of resistant organisms compared to community-acquired pneumonias, with studies reporting greater than 60% of VAPs attributed to drug-resistant organisms. These organisms include *Pseudomonas, Klebsiella, Acinetobacter*, and *Staphylococcus aureus*.

VAP prevention is challenging, as the most common etiology of VAP is a micro-aspiration event. Limiting the time a patient is intubated is critical in preventing VAP, and thus regular sedation holidays, avoiding excessive sedation, avoiding NMB use where possible, and daily spontaneous breathing trials are all important. Measures aimed at preventing micro- and macro-aspiration are also key. These include elevating the head of the bed and intermittent subglottic suction. Regular oral care and toothbrushing are vital, as it prevents oropharyngeal colonization of pathogenic organisms [27].

Early initiation of enteral feeding has been linked to reduced infectious complications in mechanically ventilated patients, with a possible signal favoring post-pyloric over gastric feeding to reduce aspiration rates. Lastly, early mobilization and exercise programs have been shown to reduce VAP rates, possibly by reducing the duration of mechanical ventilation [28].

Lowering the Risk of Ventilator-Induced Lung Injury

A significant component of ventilator-induced lung injury results from trying to achieve "normal" oxygen levels. In this section, measures clinicians can take to reduce the risk of VILI will be discussed.

Settle for Less

As previously discussed, traditional oxygen saturations of >97% did not portend better outcomes compared with lower saturation targets, and patients likely suffered lung injury in their pursuit. Similarly, in the majority of critically ill medical patients, some hypercarbia is probably safe, with professional societies allowing pH values as low as 7.15 to offer lung-protective ventilation. Is it possible to aim for even lower oxygen targets to provide ultra-lung-protective ventilation? It is known from physiologic data that mountaineers can function and carry out complex tasks and make detailed plans despite significant hypoxia. Individuals at elevations of 5500 m above sea level have an SpO_2 in the 75–85% range, and indeed, mountaineers on Mount Everest have SpO_2s in the 55–65% range with PaO_2 values around 25 mmHg [15].

While at high altitude, acclimatization plays a pivotal role in the ability to adapt to the low partial pressure of O_2. It results in a rightward shift of the oxygen dissociation curve, and mountaineers ostensibly have minimal issues with tissue oxygen consumption, both of which do not hold true in critically ill patients. However, further studies are required to identify a safer lower oxygen target in the critically ill population.

Targeted Temperature Management

The practice of targeted temperature management has been shown to reduce systemic oxygen demand and induce an anti-inflammatory state. In animal experiments, individuals with VILI due to high tidal volume ventilation subjected to mild or moderate hypothermia showed a reduction in the mediators of biotrauma and histopathological improvement [29]. Given the reduction in systemic oxygen demand in hypothermic individuals, it is possible that they may require lower oxygen targets, reducing the risk of VILI.

There is no evidence currently supporting the use of hypothermia in humans with respiratory failure; however, trials are ongoing [30].

Neuromuscular Blockade

Patients with respiratory failure, and particularly ARDS, have a high minute ventilation and a sensation of dyspnea. This results in the potential for patient-ventilator dyssynchrony and P-SILI. Studies with animals in ARDS suggest that the activity of abdominal muscles while undergoing mechanical ventilation can cause lung injury, and paralyzing those abdominal muscles is associated with lower levels of inflammatory mediators and less histopathological lung damage [31].

Further, one can reasonably assume that paralyzed muscles require less oxygen to function. Thus, it may be possible to offer a lower oxygen saturation target for such patients.

However, the use of NMB must be weighed against its risks as previously discussed. Partial paralysis could be a consideration that may allow many of the benefits of full NMB but with fewer side effects. Further work is required to study the clinical impact of NMB use in preventing VILI.

Improving V/Q Matching

Physiologically, humans have an imbalance between ventilation and perfusion of lung units. In a healthy individual in the upright position, there is an excess of ventilation in the apical lung zones, with concomitant excess of perfusion in the lower lung zones. This V/Q mismatch is further worsened in disease. For example, in ARDS, alveolar units in some parts of the lung are flooded with inflammatory fluid, increasing the shunt, whereas other, more normal alveolar units may be overinflated, increasing dead space. The heterogeneity of the injured lung exacerbates V/Q mismatch.

Improving V/Q matching by opening previously atelectatic areas of lung through optimizing PEEP, recruitment maneuvers, or positioning allows more lung units to be ventilated, reducing the risk of localized barotrauma in the uninjured or "baby" lung. It also reduces the formation of stress concentrators, which further limits stress and strain in healthy lungs. A key evidence-based intervention to improve V/Q matching by recruiting atelectatic alveolar units is prone positioning, which is discussed elsewhere in this book.

Another benefit of improved V/Q matching is improved gas exchange, improving hypoxia and reducing hypercarbia. Thus, clinicians may be able to reduce FiO_2 to safer levels, mitigating hyperoxia. An improvement in CO_2 clearance facilitates low tidal volume lung-protective ventilation.

Inhaled pulmonary vasodilators have been shown to improve P/F ratios and V/Q matching in patients with heterogeneous infiltrates leading to respiratory failure. These therapies are delivered to ventilated alveolar units and thereafter come into contact with nearby blood vessels and cause vasodilation, leading to improved perfusion to the ventilated lung units. Several inhaled pulmonary vasodilators are available, including epoprostenol and nitric oxide. Although theoretically beneficial, these medications usually only have a transient effect and thus are only recommended as acute, rescue therapies. Indeed, several studies have failed to show a mortality benefit with the use of these agents. The risks involved with using pulmonary vasodilators include paradoxical worsening of V/Q matching, especially in patients with COPD, as it prevents hypoxic vasoconstriction; worsening pulmonary edema, especially in patients with left heart disease; and acute kidney injury.

Conclusion

This chapter highlights the challenges of using mechanical ventilators in the critically ill. Although they provide life-supporting oxygen, they can cause life-threatening damage in the same breath. There continues to be evolution in ventilatory strategies and efforts to mitigate the damage they can cause. Much of the recent research revolves around VILI and traumas described in this chapter. The overarching goal is to minimize the time spent on ventilators. Even with the best protocols, we will always have to contend with this double-edged sword of mechanical ventilatory support and the harm that it can do. The art of medicine lies in achieving this delicate balance of aiming to reduce complications while maximizing benefits.

References

1. Anzueto A, Frutos-Vivar F, Esteban A, Alía I, Brochard L, Stewart T, Benito S, Tobin MJ, Elizalde J, Palizas F, David CM, Pimentel J, González M, Soto L, D'Empaire G, Pelosi P. Incidence, risk factors and outcome of barotrauma in mechanically ventilated patients. Intensive Care Med. 2004;30(4):612–9. https://doi.org/10.1007/s00134-004-2187-7. Epub 2004 Feb 28. PMID: 14991090.
2. Gattinoni L, Pesenti A. The concept of "baby lung". Intensive Care Med. 2005;31(6):776–84. https://doi.org/10.1007/s00134-005-2627-z. Epub 2005 Apr 6. PMID: 15812622.
3. Alhazzani W, Alshahrani M, Jaeschke R, Forel JM, Papazian L, Sevransky J, Meade MO. Neuromuscular blocking agents in acute respiratory distress syndrome: a systematic review and meta-analysis of randomized controlled trials. Crit Care. 2013;17(2):R43. https://doi.org/10.1186/cc12557. PMID: 23497608; PMCID: PMC3672502.
4. Papazian L, Forel JM, Gacouin A, Penot-Ragon C, Perrin G, Loundou A, Jaber S, Arnal JM, Perez D, Seghboyan JM, Constantin JM, Courant P, Lefrant JY, Guérin C, Prat G, Morange S, Roch A, ACURASYS Study Investigators. Neuromuscular blockers in early acute respiratory distress syndrome. N Engl J Med. 2010;363(12):1107–16. https://doi.org/10.1056/NEJMoa1005372. PMID: 20843245.
5. Pierson DJ, Horton CA, Bates PW. Persistent bronchopleural air leak during mechanical ventilation. A review of 39 cases. Chest. 1986;90(3):321–3. https://doi.org/10.1378/chest.90.3.321. PMID: 3743142.
6. Retamal J, Bergamini BC, Carvalho AR, Bozza FA, Borzone G, Borges JB, Larsson A, Hedenstierna G, Bugedo G, Bruhn A. Non-lobar atelectasis generates inflammation and structural alveolar injury in the surrounding healthy tissue during mechanical ventilation. Crit Care. 2014;18(5):505. https://doi.org/10.1186/s13054-014-0505-1. PMID: 25200702; PMCID: PMC4172813.
7. Wu J, Yan Z, Schwartz DE, Yu J, Malik AB, Hu G. Activation of NLRP3 inflammasome in alveolar macrophages contributes to mechanical stretch-induced lung inflammation and injury. J Immunol. 2013;190(7):3590–9. https://doi.org/10.4049/jimmunol.1200860. Epub 2013 Feb 22. PMID: 23436933; PMCID: PMC3608749.
8. Willson DF, Truwit JD, Conaway MR, Traul CS, Egan EE. The adult Calfactant in acute respiratory distress syndrome trial. Chest. 2015;148(2):356–64. https://doi.org/10.1378/chest.14-1139. PMID: 25855884.
9. Tremblay L, Valenza F, Ribeiro SP, Li J, Slutsky AS. Injurious ventilatory strategies increase cytokines and c-fos m-RNA expression in an isolated rat lung model. J Clin Invest. 1997;99(5):944–52. https://doi.org/10.1172/JCI119259. PMID: 9062352; PMCID: PMC507902.

10. Ranieri VM, Suter PM, Tortorella C, De Tullio R, Dayer JM, Brienza A, Bruno F, Slutsky AS. Effect of mechanical ventilation on inflammatory mediators in patients with acute respiratory distress syndrome: a randomized controlled trial. JAMA. 1999;282(1):54–61. https://doi.org/10.1001/jama.282.1.54. PMID: 10404912.
11. Stüber F, Wrigge H, Schroeder S, Wetegrove S, Zinserling J, Hoeft A, Putensen C. Kinetic and reversibility of mechanical ventilation-associated pulmonary and systemic inflammatory response in patients with acute lung injury. Intensive Care Med. 2002;28(7):834–41. https://doi.org/10.1007/s00134-002-1321-7. Epub 2002 Jun 15. PMID: 12122519.
12. Parsons PE, Eisner MD, Thompson BT, Matthay MA, Ancukiewicz M, Bernard GR, Wheeler AP, NHLBI Acute Respiratory Distress Syndrome Clinical Trials Network. Lower tidal volume ventilation and plasma cytokine markers of inflammation in patients with acute lung injury. Crit Care Med. 2005;33(1):1–6. https://doi.org/10.1097/01.ccm.0000149854.61192.dc. discussion 230–2. PMID: 15644641.
13. Parsons PE, Matthay MA, Ware LB, Eisner MD, National Heart, Lung, Blood Institute Acute Respiratory Distress Syndrome Clinical Trials Network. Elevated plasma levels of soluble TNF receptors are associated with morbidity and mortality in patients with acute lung injury. Am J Physiol Lung Cell Mol Physiol. 2005;288(3):L426–31. https://doi.org/10.1152/ajplung.00302.2004. Epub 2004 Oct 29. PMID: 15516488.
14. Carpagnano GE, Kharitonov SA, Foschino-Barbaro MP, Resta O, Gramiccioni E, Barnes PJ. Supplementary oxygen in healthy subjects and those with COPD increases oxidative stress and airway inflammation. Thorax. 2004;59(12):1016–9. https://doi.org/10.1136/thx.2003.020768. PMID: 15563698; PMCID: PMC1746910.
15. Grocott MP, Martin DS, Levett DZ, McMorrow R, Windsor J, Montgomery HE, Caudwell Xtreme Everest Research Group. Arterial blood gases and oxygen content in climbers on Mount Everest. N Engl J Med. 2009;360(2):140–9. https://doi.org/10.1056/NEJMoa0801581. PMID: 19129527.
16. Awsare B, Herman J, Baram M. Management strategies for severe respiratory failure: as extracorporeal membrane oxygenation is being considered. Crit Care Clin. 2017;33(4):795–811. https://doi.org/10.1016/j.ccc.2017.06.003. Epub 2017 Jul 29. PMID: 28887928.
17. Gupta E, Awsare B, Hirose H, Cavarocchi N, Baram M. Don't drive blind: driving pressure to optimize ventilator management in ECMO. Lung. 2020;198(5):785–92. https://doi.org/10.1007/s00408-020-00381-y. Epub 2020 Jul 23. Erratum in: Lung. 2020 Oct;198(5):793. doi:10.1007/s00408-020-00385-8. Hiroshi, Hitoshi [corrected to Hirose, Hitoshi]. PMID: 32705400; PMCID: PMC7377310.
18. Russotto V, Myatra SN, Laffey JG, Tassistro E, Antolini L, Bauer P, Lascarrou JB, Szuldrzynski K, Camporota L, Pelosi P, Sorbello M, Higgs A, Greif R, Putensen C, Agvald-Öhman C, Chalkias A, Bokums K, Brewster D, Rossi E, Fumagalli R, Pesenti A, Foti G, Bellani G, INTUBE Study Investigators. Intubation practices and adverse peri-intubation events in critically ill patients from 29 countries. JAMA. 2021;325(12):1164–72. https://doi.org/10.1001/jama.2021.1727. Erratum in: JAMA. 2021 Jun 22;325(24):2507. doi:10.1001/jama.2021.9012. PMID: 33755076; PMCID: PMC7988368.
19. Cooper AB, Thornley KS, Young GB, Slutsky AS, Stewart TE, Hanly PJ. Sleep in critically ill patients requiring mechanical ventilation. Chest. 2000;117(3):809–18. https://doi.org/10.1378/chest.117.3.809. Erratum in: Chest 2001 Mar;119(3):993. PMID: 10713011.
20. Elliott R, McKinley S, Cistulli P, Fien M. Characterisation of sleep in intensive care using 24-hour polysomnography: an observational study. Crit Care. 2013;17(2):R46. doi:https://doi.org/10.1186/cc12565. PMID: 23506782; PMCID: PMC3733429.
21. Dres M, Dubé BP, Mayaux J, Delemazure J, Reuter D, Brochard L, Similowski T, Demoule A. Coexistence and impact of limb muscle and diaphragm weakness at time of liberation from mechanical ventilation in medical intensive care unit patients. Am J Respir Crit Care Med. 2017;195(1):57–66. https://doi.org/10.1164/rccm.201602-0367OC. PMID: 27310484.
22. Peñuelas O, Keough E, López-Rodríguez L, Carriedo D, Gonçalves G, Barreiro E, Lorente JÁ. Ventilator-induced diaphragm dysfunction: translational mechanisms lead to therapeuti-

cal alternatives in the critically ill. Intensive Care Med Exp. 2019;7(Suppl 1):48. https://doi.org/10.1186/s40635-019-0259-9. PMID: 31346802; PMCID: PMC6658639.
23. Callahan LA, Supinski GS. Hyperglycemia-induced diaphragm weakness is mediated by oxidative stress. Crit Care. 2014;18:R88. https://doi.org/10.1186/cc13855.
24. Konrad F, Schreiber T, Brecht-Kraus D, Georgieff M. Mucociliary transport in ICU patients. Chest. 1994;105(1):237–41. https://doi.org/10.1378/chest.105.1.237. PMID: 8275739.
25. Rose L, Adhikari NK, Leasa D, Fergusson DA, McKim D. Cough augmentation techniques for extubation or weaning critically ill patients from mechanical ventilation. Cochrane Database Syst Rev. 2017;1(1):CD011833. https://doi.org/10.1002/14651858.CD011833.pub2. PMID: 28075489; PMCID: PMC6353102.
26. Cork G, Wade C, Gordon A, Vaughan-France A, Palmer A, Walker K, Jones U. Airway clearance techniques for the intubated adult: a scoping review. ACPRC Issue 2022 J. 2022;54(3):120–39.
27. Zhao T, Wu X, Zhang Q, Li C, Worthington HV, Hua F. Oral hygiene care for critically ill patients to prevent ventilator-associated pneumonia. Cochrane Database Syst Rev. 2020;12:Art. No.:CD008367. https://doi.org/10.1002/14651858.CD008367.pub4.
28. Qi W, Murphy TE, Doyle MM, Ferrante LE. Association between daily average of mobility achieved during physical therapy sessions and hospital-acquired or ventilator-associated pneumonia among critically ill patients. J Intensive Care Med. 2023;38(5):418–24. https://doi.org/10.1177/08850666221133318. Epub 2022 Oct 22. PMID: 36278257; PMCID: PMC10065937.
29. Aslami H, Kuipers MT, Beurskens CJ, Roelofs JJ, Schultz MJ, Juffermans NP. Mild hypothermia reduces ventilator-induced lung injury, irrespective of reducing respiratory rate. Transl Res. 2012;159(2):110–7. https://doi.org/10.1016/j.trsl.2011.10.005. Epub 2011 Nov 10. PMID: 22243795.
30. Shanholtz CB, Terrin ML, Harrington T, Chan C, Warren W, Walter R, Armstrong F, Marshall J, Scheraga R, Duggal A, Formanek P, Baram M, Afshar M, Marchetti N, Singla S, Reilly J, Knox D, Puri N, Chung K, Brown CH, Hasday JD. Design and rationale of the CHILL phase II trial of hypothermia and neuromuscular blockade for acute respiratory distress syndrome. Contemp Clin Trials Commun. 2023;33:101155. https://doi.org/10.1016/j.conctc.2023.101155. Epub 2023 May 18. PMID: 37228902; PMCID: PMC10191700.
31. Zhang X, Wu W, Zhu Y, Jiang Y, Du J, Chen R. Abdominal muscle activity during mechanical ventilation increases lung injury in severe acute respiratory distress syndrome. PLoS One. 2016;11(1):e0145694. https://doi.org/10.1371/journal.pone.0145694. Erratum in: PLoS One 2016 Feb 09;11(2):e0149325. doi:10.1371/journal.pone.0149325. PMID: 26745868; PMCID: PMC4712828.

Treatment of Pneumothorax: Role for Oxygen

26

Tyler R. Grenda

The approach to ideal management of pneumothorax, particularly spontaneous pneumothorax, has been a point of debate for decades. Descriptions of pneumothorax and early management date back centuries [1]. Several approaches have been proposed over the course of time to accelerate the resolution of the pneumothorax. A case report from 1947 describes the successful use of inhaled 100% supplemental oxygen over the course of 10 days in a patient presenting with spontaneous pneumothorax [2]. The author suggested future controlled trials based on this case report. This report added to the armamentarium for treatment, for what was described at that time as "benign, idiopathic, spontaneous pneumothorax." As further evidence of the burden of this problem, the author described in 1943 that there were approximately 873 Army hospital admissions in the United States for this diagnosis, with a common treatment approach of "bed rest and mild sedation" [2]. Furthermore, the average hospitalization in this patient cohort was 40 days. Other contemporary approaches described included injection of an "irritant solution" into the pleural space, aspiration of the pleural cavity, and lavage of the pleural cavity with 100% oxygen to "hasten" resolution of the pneumothorax [2]. Figure 26.1 depicts a relatively small pneumothorax (left lung, anteriorly) on a CT scan that might prompt the treating physicians to consider observation with consideration for supplemental oxygen as management.

The Australian trial published in 2020 did establish several important findings to guide the management of patients who present with moderate-to-large spontaneous pneumothoraces that do not require immediate chest tube placement or intervention on clinical grounds. The trial, however, did not provide substantial guidance on the appropriate use of oxygen, as all patients in the conservative management group

T. R. Grenda (✉)
Division of Thoracic Surgery, The Department of Surgery at the Sidney Kimmel Medical College of Thomas Jefferson University, Philadelphia, PA, USA
e-mail: tyler.grenda@jefferson.edu

G. C. Kane et al. (eds.), *Oxygen*, https://doi.org/10.1007/978-3-032-18934-9_26

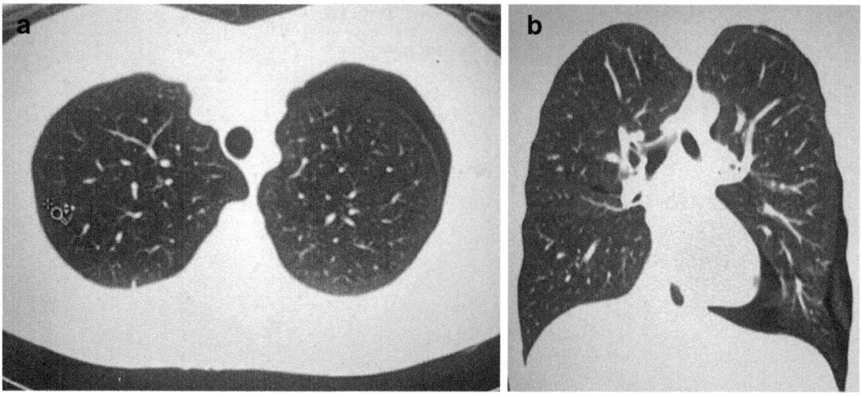

Fig. 26.1 (**a**, **b**) Demonstration of a small pneumothorax (featured above in a cross section (panel **a**) of a chest CT in the left lung anteriorly and in a coronal view (panel **b**)) in a patient presenting with shortness of breath and chest pain without a history of underlying lung disease

received oxygen if the O_2 saturation was less than 92%. This multicenter randomized trial focused on younger patients, aged 40–50 years, who would most typically be presenting with a spontaneous pneumothorax, comparing an intervention arm with a conservative treatment arm, which focused principally on observation prior to discharge and follow-up. It would be important to note that 25 of the 162 randomized patients in the conservative arm crossed over to an intervention based upon a prespecified protocol and worsening of their pneumothorax and/or clinical status. In addition, 23% of patients in the observation group and 15% of patients in the intervention group were lost to follow-up. However, 129 of 131 patients (98.5%) in the interventional group achieved re-expansion, whereas 118 of 125 patients (94.5%) in the conservative group achieved expansion within 8 weeks. While the study was not statistically significant in terms of the primary outcome comparing the two strategies, the significance of this study was that it challenged the previous dogma that an interventional approach was best for moderate-to-large pneumothoraces based upon the study criteria [3].

Outside of the clinical realm, laboratory studies have attempted to evaluate the role of inhaled oxygen and the resolution of experimental pneumothoraces in animal models [4, 5]. This body of work suggests a role for inhaled supplemental oxygen in the resolution of pneumothorax. Some studies in animal models have attempted to explain the role of supplemental oxygen in spontaneous pneumothorax through the "nitrogen washout theory" [6]. Since nitrogen is poorly absorbed into tissue, the idea is to replace the nitrogen-rich pneumothorax with 100% oxygen that may leak from the lung parenchyma. The oxygen that moves into the pleural space can be absorbed by adjacent tissue, thereby allowing the pleural spaces to normalize. An alternate physiological hypothesis is that the increased gradient between air and the pneumothorax (composed of approximately 79% nitrogen and 21% oxygen), and gas in the lung, which has a higher concentration of oxygen, exists for patients who are on supplemental O2. As a result, there is a gradient of movement of air between the pneumothorax space and the lung, favoring reabsorption. These explanations have attempted to bridge the gap between what was observed in animal studies and findings observed in clinical investigations.

Previous, non-randomized studies established the role for conservative management of spontaneous pneumothorax [7]. Subsequent efforts to demonstrate the specific efficacy of supplemental oxygen therapy have mainly focused on the primary spontaneous pneumothorax population [7]. However, there have been limited data on the utility of supplemental oxygen in non-hypoxemic patients with spontaneous pneumothorax [8]. Previous small institutional studies demonstrated increased absorption of pneumothorax in patients presenting with spontaneous pneumothorax receiving inhaled concentrated supplemental oxygen [8–10]. Additional efforts have focused on establishing treatment guidelines and identifying patients who may be managed with observation and supplemental oxygen, particularly in the primary spontaneous pneumothorax population [11, 12]. However, there was a paucity of high-quality, randomized evidence comparing conservative interventions for the management of primary spontaneous pneumothorax [13]. In addition, there is heterogeneity in patient populations, study design, and the application of supplemental oxygen among studies, highlighting the need for well-designed randomized trials. Subsequent randomized studies have provided some data surrounding the role of conservative management versus chest tube placement in moderate-to-large primary spontaneous pneumothorax, but have not clearly defined the efficacy of supplemental oxygen [13].

It is important to recognize that specific clinical scenarios may require immediate procedural intervention for management, rather than initial conservative management, such as a large pneumothorax with concern for a tension pneumothorax. Figure 26.2 demonstrates a large right pneumothorax that requires a chest tube placement. In this context, patients may require decompression of the pleural space

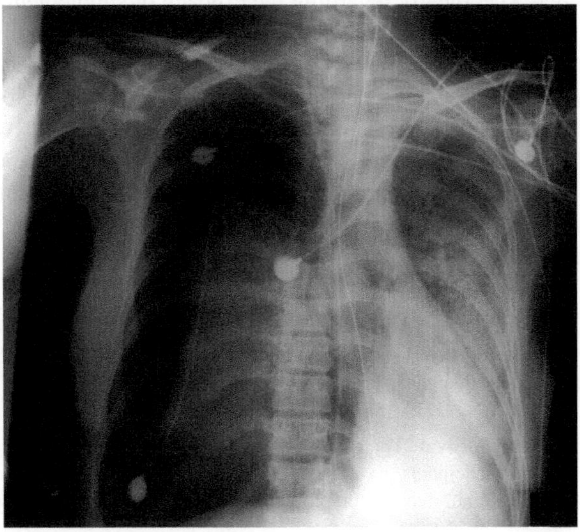

Fig. 26.2 A large right pneumothorax (panel **a**) and following right chest tube placement (panel **b**). The role of oxygen use in this clinical scenario is simply supportive and not intended to alter the pathophysiology

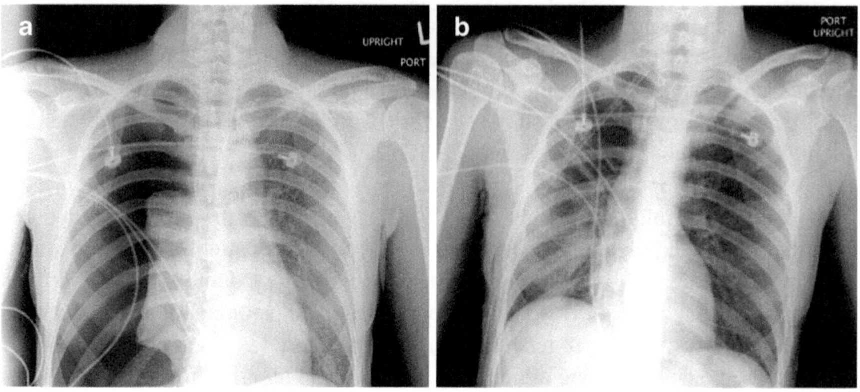

Fig. 26.3 (**a**, **b**) On the left is a chest X-ray demonstrating a right pneumothorax. On the right is the same patient after placement of the chest tube with re-expansion of the right lung and the return of the mediastinal structures to a more midline position

with chest tube placement or initial needle decompression followed by a chest tube in select clinical situations. Furthermore, patients with recurrent, large, and/or symptomatic pneumothoraces may need consideration for chest tube placement or other interventions. While oxygen may not play a role as the primary intervention in episodes of tension pneumothorax, it is important to highlight that oxygen may play a secondary role in patient management. Figure 26.3a, b demonstrates a large pneumothorax and the impact of placing a thoracostomy tube for management of the right pneumothorax.

Currently, there is some data to support the use of supplemental oxygen in the management of spontaneous pneumothorax, particularly primary spontaneous pneumothorax. However, evidence from well-designed, randomized trials is limited, specifically regarding the efficacy of supplemental oxygen in primary spontaneous pneumothorax in the absence of hypoxia. While non-randomized evidence may support the role of oxygen, more data are needed in this area. Future randomized studies are needed to identify patients with primary spontaneous pneumothorax who are most likely to benefit from supplemental oxygen and avoid subsequent procedural interventions. In addition, identifying metrics for ideal oxygen titration to optimize pneumothorax resolution will be important to further evaluate this role. Overall, oxygen will remain a key aspect of managing pneumothorax.

Declarations

Competing Interests The author has no competing interests to declare that are relevant to the content of this manuscript.

Ethics Approval The author declares that this manuscript does not include primary research with human participants.

The author declares that this manuscript does not include primary studies involving animals.

References

1. Kaya SO, Karatepe M, Tok T, Onem G, Dursunoglu N, Goksin I. Were pneumothorax and its management known in 15th-century anatolia? Tex Heart Inst J. 2009;36(2):152–3.
2. Press E. Oxygen inhalation in the treatment of spontaneous pneumothorax. Ann Intern Med. 1947;27(1):135–7.
3. Brown SGA, Ball EL, Perrin K, Asha SE, Braithwaite I, Egerton-Warburton D, Jones PG, Keijzers G, Kinnear FB, Kwan BCH, Lam KV, Lee YCG, Nowitz M, Read CA, Simpson G, Smith JA, Summers QA, Weatherall M, Beasley R. PSP investigators. conservative versus interventional treatment for spontaneous pneumothorax. N Engl J Med. 2020;382(5):405–15. https://doi.org/10.1056/NEJMoa1910775. PMID: 31995686.
4. England GJ, Hill RC, Timberlake GA, et al. Resolution of experimental pneumothorax in rabbits by graded oxygen therapy. J Trauma. 1998;45(2):333–4.
5. Hill RC, DeCarlo DP Jr, Hill JF, Beamer KC, Hill ML, Timberlake GA. Resolution of experimental pneumothorax in rabbits by oxygen therapy. Ann Thorac Surg. 1995;59(4):825–7. discussion 827–828.
6. Grasmuk-Siegl E, Valipour A. "Nitrogen wash-out" in non-Hypoxaemic patients with spontaneous pneumothorax: a narrative review. J Clin Med. 2023;12(13):4300.
7. Stradling P, Poole G. Conservative management of spontaneous pneumothorax. Thorax. 1966;21(2):145–9.
8. Park CB, Moon MH, Jeon HW, et al. Does oxygen therapy increase the resolution rate of primary spontaneous pneumothorax? J Thorac Dis. 2017;9(12):5239–43.
9. Northfield TC. Oxygen therapy for spontaneous pneumothorax. Br Med J. 1971;4(5779):86–8.
10. Chadha TS, Cohn MA. Noninvasive treatment of pneumothorax with oxygen inhalation. Respiration. 1983;44(2):147–52.
11. Baumann MH, Noppen M. Pneumothorax. Respirology. 2004;9(2):157–64.
12. Baumann MH, Strange C, Heffner JE, et al. Management of spontaneous pneumothorax: an American College of Chest Physicians Delphi Consensus Statement. Chest. 2001;119(2):590–602.
13. Ashby M, Haug G, Mulcahy P, Ogden KJ, Jensen O, Walters JA. Conservative versus interventional management for primary spontaneous pneumothorax in adults. Cochrane Database Syst Rev. 2014;2014(12):Cd010565.
14. Brown SGA, Ball EL, Perrin K, et al. Conservative versus interventional treatment for spontaneous pneumothorax. N Engl J Med. 2020;382(5):405–15.

Respiratory Failure in Pneumonia and ARDS

27

Lauren McDonnell and Michael Baram

Introduction

Pneumonia and acute respiratory distress syndrome (ARDS) are two leading causes of respiratory failure and, as such, are common diagnoses made in the ICU [1, 2]. Both cause increased work of breathing as well as hypoxemia. The two clinical diagnoses can be difficult to differentiate from each other and are often seen concurrently, as pneumonia is both a leading cause and a common complication of ARDS [3, 4]. To add confusion to this topic, pneumonia is a disease, while ARDS is a syndrome. This chapter will explain the nuances of each and their effect on oxygen delivery in a host, as well as management strategies [5, 6]. Since pneumonia is the most common precipitator of ARDS, pneumonia will be reviewed first, followed by ARDS. Despite improving care for these ill patients, there remains an underrecognition of ARDS.

L. McDonnell
The Korman Respiratory Institute and the Division of Pulmonary and Critical Care, Thomas Jefferson University, Philadelphia, PA, USA

M. Baram (✉)
The Korman Respiratory Institute and the Division of Pulmonary, Allergy and Critical Care, The Department of Medicine at the Sidney Kimmel Medical College of Thomas Jefferson University, Philadelphia, PA, USA
e-mail: Michael.baram@jefferson.edu

G. C. Kane et al. (eds.), *Oxygen*, https://doi.org/10.1007/978-3-032-18934-9_27

Pneumonia

An infection of the lower respiratory tract, pneumonia occurs when there is an accumulation of microbes within the alveoli. The root of the pathologic findings of mucus production and alveolar filling is an inflammatory response to the invasion of microbes, resulting in the migration of white cells to the lungs and the release of cytokines. These cytokines affect oxygen diffusion and V/Q matching. These microbes are most commonly viral or bacterial in origin. Less prevalent in the US, mycobacteria are a common cause worldwide, with fungal and parasitic etiologies as the least common and typically found in immunosuppressed hosts [5, 7, 8]. Bacterial pneumonia is typically further differentiated into community-acquired pneumonia (CAP), hospital-acquired pneumonia (HAP), or ventilator-acquired pneumonia (VAP). Testing, treatment, and/or supportive care remain highly effective treatments, while vaccinations have helped reduce the severity of pneumonia infections across different populations.

Etiologies and Pathophysiology

The etiology of pneumonia is dependent on the host and their exposures. In the US, the most identified typical strains of community-acquired pneumonia are *Streptococcus pneumoniae* and *Haemophilus influenzae,* while the most identified atypical strains are Legionella and Mycoplasma. Common viral etiologies historically have included rhinovirus, RSV, and influenza; however, in recent years, SARS-CoV-2 has been most prevalent and has had a major impact on the healthcare system and management of pneumonia [7, 9]. Immunocompromised hosts may be more predisposed to fungal infections such as Histoplasma, Blastomyces, and Coccidioides based on regional locations. Hospital-acquired and ventilator-associated organisms include *E. coli*, *Pseudomonas*, *Enterobacter*, and *Staphylococcus aureus* [9].

As will become evident in the next section, pneumonia differs from ARDS in that the alveolar–capillary membrane remains intact, and the host response is typically confined to the affected alveolar spaces. Inflammation also plays a large role in both; however, in pneumonia, proteins responding to epithelial and endothelial injury disrupt the homeostasis of a host's microbiome and allow for overgrowth of bacteria. Release of inflammatory mediators creates an alveolar–capillary leak that causes exudative congestion and often results in a positive feedback loop that continues to propagate inflammation and bacterial growth. Certain bacteria promote inflammation and interfere with the vasoconstriction of impaired alveoli, leading to shunt [8, 9]. This alveolar filling process and shunting all contribute to the hypoxemia seen with pneumonia. The large physiologic reserve that healthy lungs provide protects patients from needing oxygen supplementation. However, patients with low reserves or an overwhelming inflammatory response are at a higher risk of requiring oxygen support. Hence, increasing oxygen needs are often a trigger for hospitalization. When looking at pneumonia severity scores, the need for oxygen is a heavily weighted component of the calculation.

Clinical Findings and Diagnosis

Patients with pneumonia exhibit a high alveolar–arterial (Aa) gradient as the obstructed alveoli limit the amount of oxygen able to diffuse across the membrane [10]. An inflammation-induced capillary leak results in hypoxemia, decreased compliance, increased secretions, and increased respiratory drive that can result in dyspnea, tachypnea, and pleuritic chest pain [5, 8]. This leak also results in radiographic infiltrates, while circulating inflammatory mediators often cause fever [8]. Pain, dyspnea, hypoxia, and fever are also likely to result in tachycardia. A typical immune response results in leukocytosis. In later decompensated stages or in immunocompromised patients, patients may have encephalopathy, hypothermia, or hypotension. In non-immunocompromised hosts, there is usually a correlation between the degree of infiltrates and the degree of hypoxia; CT scans of the lungs have a better correlation to the degree of hypoxemia than chest radiographs. Viral symptoms may differ slightly in the physical exam and may be less remarkable compared with the level of debility. A rash may also be present.

While no pathogen is identified in the majority of bacterial pneumonia cases, sputum and blood culture sampling, as well as urine antigen testing for Legionella and pneumococcus, are still recommended for patients with severe disease [7, 11–13]. Once a diagnosis of exclusion, viral etiologies are now frequently identifiable by PCR via nasopharyngeal or oropharyngeal swabs, so viral testing should be done if disease is present in the community [14]. It may be difficult to rule out concurrent or superimposed bacterial pneumonia in patients with viral pneumonia [7, 12].

Management

Management of pneumonia depends on the type of pneumonia but largely focuses on early recognition of the disease and its causative organisms, providing anti-infective agents where available, supporting respiratory status, and avoiding further injury, such as ventilator-induced lung injury or development of ARDS. As the focus of this chapter is respiratory failure in pneumonia, it will discuss inpatient management of patients requiring oxygen support. To prevent progression of injury, early recognition and treatment of pneumonia is key. Prompt measures to dampen the immune disturbance provoked by pneumonia can play a role in avoiding the development of ARDS [11]. Steroid use remains a highly controversial topic.

Community-Acquired Pneumonia

Early recognition is essential and focuses on testing for pathogens and timely, appropriate, empiric antibiotic therapy for suspected bacterial pneumonia [11, 12]. Empiric antibiotic selection should be targeted at the most likely pathogens and take into account prior infection history [7, 12]. For example, drug-resistant pneumococci should be considered in those older than 65, patients who have taken antibiotics in the prior 3 months, or those with chronic medical conditions and/or immunosuppression. Pseudomonas pneumonia is more common in patients who are malnourished, have bronchiectasis, or are on steroids or antibiotic therapy for longer than a week in the prior month. In nonintensive care settings, fluoroquinolones or beta-lactam and macrolide are sufficient empiric therapy for CAP, unless Pseudomonas or MRSA is suspected. In these cases, an antipseudomonal beta-lactam should be chosen along with an antipseudomonal fluoroquinolone, and vancomycin should be added if MRSA is suspected. For those in the ICU, combination therapy with a beta-lactam, macrolide or respiratory fluoroquinolone, and vancomycin or linezolid is advised unless other risk factors are present. Historically, 5–7 days of therapy was considered sufficient; some guidelines recommend as little as 3 days, assuming good clinical response [13]. This duration needs to be extended in patients with delayed response or in pseudomonal, MRSA, or Legionella pneumonia [14, 15]. These recommendations are for empiric therapy only. In an age of growing antibiotic resistance, narrowing antibiotics when additional favorable data becomes available is critical. Other medications, such as inhalers and mucolytics, should be used in selective cases and only if they provide symptomatic relief.

Corticosteroids in CAP

The recent CAPE-COD trial demonstrated that hydrocortisone may have a mortality benefit in severe CAP [16]. Patients received intravenous hydrocortisone 200 mg daily for 4 or 7 days, depending on clinical status, then tapered for an additional 8–14 days [16]. With the fine line for distinction between pneumonia and ARDS, many of these study patients did have ARDS by definition.

Hospital-Acquired/Ventilator-Associated Pneumonia (HAP/VAP)

The core principles for treating hospital-acquired pneumonia—early recognition, sampling, and empiric antibiotics with a de-escalation plan—remain similar to the management of CAP. However, multidrug-resistant organisms are more common and atypical organisms less so, so this must be considered when choosing the initial antibiotic therapy program. As patients with endotracheal or tracheal tubes may have developed colonization, it is important to correlate a positive sample with clinical signs and symptoms of pneumonia. Utilizing early samples prior to colonization of ETT has been correlated with a reduction in antibiotic use. Treatment should be guided by the local hospital antibiogram but should ensure that agents are active against *Staphylococcus aureus*, *Pseudomonas* species, and Gram-negative bacilli. MRSA coverage (vancomycin or linezolid) should be added to patients at risk for resistance, as MRSA is common; otherwise, MSSA coverage should suffice. Initial Gram-negative coverage should be broad-spectrum, typically piperacillin-tazobactam, cefepime, or levofloxacin. If patients have risk factors for gram-negative resistance, a second gram-negative agent from a different class (typically an aminoglycoside or fluoroquinolone) should be added until susceptibilities become available [8, 17]. The importance of de-escalation cannot be overstated. Stopping or narrowing the antibiotic strategy is important to reducing drug resistance and drug side effects.

Viral Pneumonia

Management of viral pneumonia largely consists of supportive care, but some antiviral therapies can have a major impact on outcomes. This includes oxygen delivery, ensuring adequate hydration and maximizing rest to decrease oxygen demand. Certain viruses do have therapies approved for use. These include oseltamivir/peramivir/zanamivir for influenza and ribavirin for RSV, parainfluenza, and adenovirus [14]. While earlier trials showed no benefit (and possibly even harm) in using steroids for viral pneumonias, more recent data have supported the use of dexamethasone in SARS-CoV-2 infections [7]. Vaccinations are a highly effective way to prevent or reduce the severity of an infection.

Oxygen Therapy

Oxygen therapy in pneumonia can be provided in a number of ways: nasal cannula, facemasks, high-flow nasal cannula (HFNC), noninvasive positive pressure (NIPPV), and mechanical ventilation. Nasal cannulas and facemasks are used in milder diseases, while HFNC, NIPPV, and mechanical ventilation are used in more severe cases. Due to the invasiveness of the final option, along with the increased potential for ventilator-induced lung injury, mechanical ventilation should be a last resort. HFNC delivers a higher, adjustable flow of oxygen (up to 100 L/min, depending on the device) via a larger-bore nasal cannula. This flow can provide relief of dyspnea and a small amount of positive end-expiratory pressure (PEEP) (proportional to flow) that may improve gas exchange in the lower airways by recruiting atelectatic alveoli. At lower levels of flow (35–45 L), HFNC may also improve hypoxemia and dyspnea, inspiratory effort, and minute ventilation by clearing CO_2 from the upper airways and minimizing anatomical dead space. To keep mucociliary function intact and assist in secretion clearance while minimizing damage to the mucosa, heated, humidified air should be used. Noninvasive positive pressure ventilation (NIPPV) is a second type of noninvasive strategy. Typically delivered via nasal, oronasal, or full-face mask, as well as a helmet, NIPPV allows for spontaneous breathing with pressure assistance in both the inspiratory and expiratory phases. NIPPV used with only continuous positive airway pressure mode (CPAP) is most helpful for hypoxic respiratory failure. In this mode, the machine delivers a continuous amount of pressure, allowing for the application of PEEP. This PEEP assists with oxygenation by recruiting alveoli and improving intrapulmonary shunts. Patients with a component of hypercapnic respiratory failure or significant work of breathing benefit from a bilevel mode, setting both inspiratory pressure and expiratory pressure. The inspiratory pressure increases tidal volume, allowing for improved ventilation and CO_2 clearance, while the end-expiratory pressure improves oxygenation as discussed above. Inspiratory pressure is also helpful in off-loading the work of breathing and may improve a patient's distress. In patients who are unable to tolerate NIPPV or who fail to respond, invasive mechanical ventilation is required [18]. In this case, principles of lung-protective ventilation (6 cc/kg of IBW) should be utilized to prevent VILI, and FiO_2 and PEEP should be titrated to patient response, keeping in mind the principles discussed previously. As pneumonia is the leading pulmonary cause of ARDS, it is important to be vigilant and monitor for progression of lung injury.

The role of oxygen in pneumonia is multifactorial. The most intuitive reason is that oxygen helps overcome hypoxemia by improving the simple diffusion gradient in the lung. The improved oxygenation improves organ function by allowing oxidative phosphorylation to occur. If there is an inadequate oxygen supply, the body can revert to anaerobic metabolism, which creates lactic acidosis, which then increases the work of breathing. Furthermore, some patients with mild hypoxemia, or sometimes no measurable hypoxemia, feel anxious. It is a sensation that can improve with minimal oxygen supplementation.

ARDS

ARDS is a broad syndrome with multiple causes that is often unpredictable in its response to therapy [5]. This classification as a syndrome—a group of signs and symptoms that tend to accompany each other and that lack a clear cause or treatment course—inherently complicates recognition and management. There are many studies that show that in 40% of cases, clinicians have delayed recognizing that a patient has met criteria for an ARDS diagnosis [19].

From Dr. Thomas Petty's definition of adult respiratory distress syndrome to the current physiologic concept of oxygen deficiency, at its core, ARDS is a clinical syndrome characterized by inflammation and noncardiogenic pulmonary edema, resulting in hypoxia [4–6, 20]. While no confirmatory test currently exists, the Berlin criteria, established in 2012, have long been the standard for clinical diagnosis, but recently underwent revision at a consensus conference in 2023 [20, 21]. The original Berlin criteria specified that to meet criteria for ARDS, the following must be present:

- Occurrence within 1 week of a known clinical insult.
- Bilateral opacities not fully explained by pleural effusions, lobar/lung collapse, or opacities, cardiac failure, or fluid overload.
- A PaO_2/FiO_2 (P/F) ratio less than or equal to 300 on PEEP or CPAP of five or more cm H_2O [21].

The new definition proposed in 2023 built upon the existing definition, but added the following:

Table 27.1 Characteristics and outcomes of ARDS

ARDS severity from 2023 Berlin criteria	P/F ratio	S/F ratio	Mortality (%)
Mild ARDS	200–300 mm Hg	235–315	27
Moderate ARDS	100–200 mm Hg	123–235	32
Severe ARDS	<100 mm Hg	123	45

Adopted from: ARDS Definition Task Force [21]

- High-flow nasal oxygen with a minimum flow rate of ⩾30 L/min may be used when calculating the P/F ratio.
- Pulse oximetry may be used to identify hypoxemia when a blood gas is not available: SpO_2:FiO_2 ⩽ 315 (if oxygen saturation as measured by pulse oximetry is ⩽97%).
- Ultrasound may be used as an imaging modality to evaluate for bilateral opacities, especially in resource-limited areas.
- In resource-limited settings, positive end-expiratory pressure, oxygen flow rate, or specific respiratory support devices are not required [20].

Refinement of the definitions has helped correlate the severity of the disease with outcomes (Table 27.1). Oxygenation scores in the form of P/F and S/F ratios are the key indices to follow. These definitions help with prognostication, decisions on treatment plans, and help standardize research. The severity of the disease is based on oxygen needs, highlighting the impairment of gas exchange through the alveoli. Imaging, compliance, and cause are less predictive of outcomes.

Etiologies and Pathophysiology

A key component in ARDS is the concept of a precipitating event. As the definition states, ARDS must occur within 1 week of a clinical insult. Types of insults are divided into two categories: pulmonary (direct) and extrapulmonary (indirect). A pulmonary insult is one in which there is a direct injury to the lung that results in local inflammation, such as pneumonia, inhalation, or aspiration. An extrapulmonary trigger occurs as a result of systemic conditions causing systemic inflammation, such as sepsis, pancreatitis, drug toxicity, trauma, burns, or transfusion-related injury [4, 5, 7].

In both pulmonary and extrapulmonary categories of insult, ARDS is a result of dysregulation of a host's injury response pathways, leading to excessive inflammation and disruption of the alveolar–capillary membrane. In a normal lung, gas exchange occurs at the alveolar–capillary membrane. This membrane is composed of thin layers of alveolar and capillary endothelial cells that form tight junctions to keep fluid from filling the alveolar space. Damage to the epithelial layers of the membrane activates proinflammatory and procoagulant pathways, increasing the permeability of intercellular junctions. This injury allows for alveolar flooding of protein-rich fluid and white blood cells, leading to shunting and ventilation/perfusion (V/Q) mismatch. Typically, oxygen transport is more impaired than CO_2 removal. Surfactant is also deactivated, leading to decreased compliance and atelectasis. This, in turn, causes an inconsistent alveolar response, with some alveoli fully inflating while others do not. Activation of the procoagulant pathways leads to microvascular thrombus formation, resulting in an increase in dead space and impaired gas exchange, further hampering oxygenation. These thrombi can also lead to pulmonary hypertension and right ventricular dysfunction, while the interaction of platelets and neutrophils forms fibrous complexes and hyaline membranes, further resulting in lung injury [4, 5, 7, 22].

Part of the inflammatory issue can be a robust SIRS response or an inability to turn off the inflammatory cascade. This lack of ability to return to normal could be seen during the recent COVID pandemic, where relatively mild primary infection symptoms could progress to severe ARDS. In addition, children had multisystem inflammatory syndrome (MIS-C), which was quantified with rising inflammatory markers out of proportion to their viral burden. Please see Chap. 34 on the ARDS tincture of time chapter, where the recovery process is discussed.

Diagnosis and Clinical Findings in ARDS

Unfortunately, no diagnostic test exists for ARDS, so the clinician must be vigilant for patients meeting the criteria discussed above. As the name indicates, ARDS is a syndrome that makes unique diagnostic testing very difficult. Any patient with worsening hypoxemia should have developing ARDS on the differential. Since oxygen has a narrow gradient for diffusion, monitoring the alveolar–arterial (AA) gradient and P/F ratio can be helpful in screening for ARDS as well as for assessing resolution. When the alveolar–capillary membrane is impaired with shunt physiology or V/Q mismatch is present, as in ARDS, the AA gradient will be high [10]. Other clinical findings are also explained by the pathophysiology described above. The bilateral pulmonary edema seen on imaging is a result of alveolar filling and is manifested clinically by increased work of breathing and worsening of hypoxemia. The resultant shunt and V/Q mismatch cause severe hypoxemia. Increased dead space results in hypercarbia and high minute ventilation. Pulmonary hypertension and right ventricle (RV) dysfunction may result in an enlarged RV or dilated IVC on TTE and can cause right heart failure. Patients are at risk for superimposed infections, as a healthy alveolar–capillary membrane releases antibacterial proteins, which help protect against pathogen entry in healthy areas of the lung. This protection is lost once this barrier is disrupted [5]. Poor lung compliance is manifested as high peak airway and plateau pressures on the ventilator.

Management of ARDS

Ventilator Management

Despite advances in recent years, ARDS remains a difficult syndrome to treat and carries a high mortality rate. While a few techniques, such as lung-protective ventilation (low tidal volume, low plateau pressure, and low driving pressure) and proning, have been shown to have a mortality benefit, management of ARDS focuses mainly on addressing the cause, supporting the patient through the acute injury, while avoiding further harm. To this end, one main goal of ARDS management is a lung-protective strategy that focuses on avoiding ventilator-induced lung injury. (Please see Chap. 25.) This approach is based on the inconsistent alveolar inflation that occurs—some alveoli inflate completely while others do not inflate at all, causing the effective ventilation area of the lung to be significantly reduced. This phenomenon has led some to coin the term "baby lung" [22]. Typical ventilation strategies in this situation are likely to lead to strain and high transpulmonary pressures that can eventually result in volutrauma and barotrauma and worsening of the lung injury. This can perpetuate a cyclical pattern of harm by further disrupting the endothelial barrier and causing further inflammation, thus continuing the ongoing lung damage. Because of this, a primary goal in ARDS management is to avoid alveolar overdistension and minimize transpulmonary pressure. This lung-protective approach is supported by data from the original ARMA trial, which showed a mortality benefit with lower tidal volumes—4–6 cc/kg as opposed to 12 cc/kg and a plateau pressure less than 30 cmH_2O [23, 24]. It should be noted that ideal body weight should be used when calculating the appropriate tidal volume target. Another component of lung-protective ventilation is the concept of driving pressure. This is defined as the ratio between tidal volume and pulmonary compliance and is calculated by subtracting PEEP from the plateau pressure. Driving pressures under 14 cm H_2O correlate with better outcomes. As the formula suggests, this can be attempted by lowering tidal volume and optimizing positive end-expiratory pressure (PEEP) [24].

In targeting lower tidal volumes, the practitioner must allow for permissive hypercapnia. Although a safe level of acidosis has not been established, it is generally thought allowable to tolerate a pH down to 7.2, assuming the patient suffers no ill hemodynamic effects [22]. It is also important to note that low tidal volume ventilation is usually poorly tolerated by awake patients, resulting in ventilator asynchrony. As this can also have deleterious effects, it is important to try to minimize asynchrony. In many cases, sedatives and analgesics will be necessary. Occasionally, paralytic agents may need to be added, but when doing so, adequate sedation must be assured. Some patients may tolerate pressure control ventilation better than volume control. While a meta-analysis showed no difference in mortality or oxygenation when comparing the two modes, it must be noted that pressure control ventilation sacrifices the practitioner's ability to control tidal volumes [25].

Table 27.2 Comparing two PEEP strategies, high versus low

FiO_2 on vent	0.3	0.4	0.4	0.5	0.5	0.6	0.7	0.7	0.8	0.9	0.9	0.9	1
Low peep	5		8		10			12	14			16	18
High peep	5	8					14		14		16	18	18–24

Adopted from multiple Refs. [22, 24, 26]

Strategies such as PEEP optimization and prone positioning aim to improve oxygenation. Higher PEEP strategies have been shown to be beneficial in ARDS by recruiting collapsed alveoli and creating a larger surface for gas exchange, improving hypoxemia [6, 22, 24, 26]. Too much PEEP, however, can be detrimental by causing alveolar overdistension, so patients must be monitored for PEEP responsiveness. This is typically done by incrementally increasing PEEP and monitoring for improved compliance, typically by calculating driving pressures (Table 27.2). Once driving pressure starts to increase or oxygenation suffers, PEEP titration should cease [26]. Higher PEEP may also result in hypotension, as venous return to the heart is decreased as intrathoracic pressure increases. Recruitment maneuvers, performed by implementing very high PEEP for a short period of time, are no longer recommended as they provide only a temporary benefit at the risk of decreased venous return and alveolar overdistension/barotrauma [22, 26].

Adjunctive Management

Prone positioning is discussed at length elsewhere in this book, but has been shown to be beneficial in ARDS by increasing lung recruitment and improving V/Q mismatch, as volume and distension are more evenly distributed throughout the lung [6, 22, 24, 26].

Additional strategies that have been shown to have a benefit in ARDS are conservative fluid strategies, neuromuscular blockade, glucocorticoids, inhaled vasodilators, and ECMO. Conservative fluid strategies aim to avoid pulmonary edema and subsequent capillary leak, which can worsen V/Q mismatch and pulmonary venous pressures. Conservative fluid approaches have been shown to improve ventilator-free and ICU-free days [22, 24, 26]. Early neuromuscular blockade (NMB) has had mixed results in trials but may be helpful in patients with ventilator asynchrony or strong respiratory effort by decreasing ventilator synchrony and improving compliance. NMB may also decrease inflammation. Patients who do require paralysis should be heavily sedated to avoid consciousness while paralyzed. Paralytics should be weaned as soon as possible, as patients incur a risk of increased muscle loss, pressure injuries, and VTE [22, 24, 26]. Glucocorticoids, in theory, could help dampen the inflammatory response of patients with ARDS. Their use remains controversial in ARDS management, as there have been mixed outcomes in trials, and they are not without side effects (immunosuppression, hyperglycemia, myopathy), but certain phenotypes may benefit, especially if administered early in the course [4, 22, 26]. Inhaled vasodilators have been shown to improve oxygenation, but do not affect mortality. By dilating pulmonary blood vessels, blood flow is redirected from a poorly ventilated lung to an adequately ventilated lung, thus improving V/Q mismatch. While not routinely recommended, they may be helpful as a bridge or salvage therapy in patients with refractory hypoxemia [4, 22, 26]. ECMO can support ultraprotective ventilation by essentially providing the lungs with oxygenated blood. In addition, ECMO may be helpful in lowering stress delivered to the lungs, thereby avoiding VILI. Complications include bleeding and neurological complications (ICH, stroke, and seizures), so ECMO should be considered in patients with few comorbidities, who are early in their course (less than 7 days on mechanical ventilation) and have refractory hypoxemia and acidosis [4, 22, 24, 26].

One of the many challenges of managing ARDS patients is that there are interventions that have been shown to improve oxygenation, but they fail to change morbidity and mortality rates. For example, inhaled NO improves oxygenation saturation but has not been proven to improve mortality.

Conclusion

It is often clinically hard to distinguish when pneumonia becomes ARDS. Clinicians should always be vigilant in inpatient assessment and care and try to reduce risk. Oxygen, antibiotics, ventilator pressures, and other medications should be assessed at every interaction. Increases in oxygen needs indicate a change in status, so this is an important data point to track. Conversely, as the pathology of pneumonia and ARDS improves, the oxygen requirements improve as well. The evolution to find a solution to ARDS has increased the understanding of lung physiology. Continued research into preventing, treating, supporting, and curing patients with ARDS has provided iterative advances in our management strategies for affected patients.

Declarations

Competing Interests The authors have no competing interests to declare that are relevant to the content of this manuscript.

Ethics Approval The authors declare that this manuscript does not include primary research with human participants.

The authors declare that this manuscript does not include primary studies involving animals.

References

1. Mirabile VS, Shebl E, Sankari A, Bracken B. Respiratory failure in adults. In: StatPearls [Internet]. Florida: Treasure Island: StatPearls Publishing; 2025. Available from: https://www.ncbi.nlm.nih.gov/books/NBK526127/.
2. NIH. Respiratory failure – causes and risk factors | NHLBI, NIH [Internet]. www.nhlbi.nih.gov. 2022. Available from: https://www.nhlbi.nih.gov/health/respiratory-failure/causes.

3. Luyt CE, Bouadma L, Morris AC, Dhanani JA, Kollef M, Lipman J, et al. Pulmonary infections complicating ARDS. Intensive Care Med. 2020;46(12):2168–83. https://doi.org/10.1007/s00134-020-06292-z.
4. Meyer NJ, Gattinoni L, Calfee CS. Acute respiratory distress syndrome. Lancet. 2021;398(10300):622–37. https://doi.org/10.1016/S0140-6736(21)00439-6.
5. Bos LDJ, Ware LB. Acute respiratory distress syndrome: causes, pathophysiology, and phenotypes. Lancet. 2022;400(10358):1145–56. https://doi.org/10.1016/S0140-6736(22)01485-4.
6. Gorman EA, O'Kane CM, McAuley DF. Acute respiratory distress syndrome in adults: diagnosis, outcomes, long-term sequelae, and management. Lancet. 2022;400(10358):1157–70. https://doi.org/10.1016/S0140-6736(22)01439-8.
7. Long ME, Mallampalli RK, Horowitz JC. Pathogenesis of pneumonia and acute lung injury. Clin Sci. 2022;136(10):747–69. https://doi.org/10.1042/CS20210879.
8. Mandell LA, Niederman MS. Pneumonia. In: Longo D, Fauci A, Kasper D, Hauser S, Jameson J, Loscalzo J, Holland S, Langford C, editors. [Internet]. Harrison's principles of internal medicine. 22nd ed. McGraw Hill; 2026. https://accesspharmacy.mhmedical.com/content.aspx?bookid=3541&sectionid=294613915.
9. Jain V, Vashisht R, Yilmaz G, Bhardwaj A. Pneumonia pathology. In: StatPearls [Internet]. Florida: Treasure Island: StatPearls Publishing; 2025. Available from: https://www.ncbi.nlm.nih.gov/books/NBK526116/.
10. Hantzidiamantis PJ, Amaro E. Physiology, alveolar to arterial oxygen gradient. In: StatPearls [Internet]. Florida: Treasure Island: StatPearls Publishing; 2025. Available from: https://www.ncbi.nlm.nih.gov/books/NBK545153/.
11. Lee KY. Pneumonia, acute respiratory distress syndrome, and early immune-modulator therapy. Int J Mol Sci. 2017;18(2):388. https://doi.org/10.3390/ijms18020388.
12. Metlay JP, Waterer GW, Long AC, Anzueto A, Brozek J, Crothers K, et al. Diagnosis and treatment of adults with community-acquired pneumonia. An official clinical practice guideline of the American Thoracic Society and Infectious Diseases Society of America. Am J Respir Crit Care Med. 2019;200(7):e45–67. https://doi.org/10.1164/rccm.201908-1581ST. PMID: 31573350; PMCID: PMC6812437.
13. IDSA. CAP Clinical pathway. [Internet]. Available from: https://www.idsociety.org/globalassets/idsa/practice-guidelines/community-acquired-pneumonia-in-adults/cap-clinical-pathway-final-online.pdf.
14. Freeman AM, Leigh JTR. Viral pneumonia. In: StatPearls [Internet]. Florida: Treasure Island: StatPearls Publishing; 2025. Available from: https://www.ncbi.nlm.nih.gov/books/NBK513286/.
15. Regunath H, Oba Y. Community-acquired pneumonia. In: StatPearls [Internet]. Florida: Treasure Island: StatPearls Publishing; 2025. Available from: https://www.ncbi.nlm.nih.gov/books/NBK430749/.
16. Dequin PF, Meziani F, Quenot JP, Kamel T, Ricard JD, CRICS-TriGGERSep Network, et al. Hydrocortisone in severe community-acquired pneumonia. N Engl J Med. 2023;388(21):1931–41. https://doi.org/10.1056/NEJMoa2215145.
17. Kalil AC, Metersky ML, Klompas M, Muscedere J, Sweeney DA, Palmer LB, et al. Management of adults with hospital-acquired and ventilator-associated pneumonia: 2016 clinical practice guidelines by the Infectious Diseases Society of America and the American Thoracic Society. Clin Infect Dis. 2016;63(5):e61–e111. https://doi.org/10.1093/cid/ciw353.
18. Cutuli SL, Grieco DL, Menga LS, De Pascale G, Antonelli M. Noninvasive ventilation and high-flow oxygen therapy for severe community-acquired pneumonia. Curr Opin Infect Dis. 2021;34(2):142–50. https://doi.org/10.1097/QCO.0000000000000715. PMID: 33470666; PMCID: PMC9698117.
19. Bellani G, Laffey JG, Pham T, Fan E, Brochard L, Esteban A, et al. Epidemiology, patterns of care, and mortality for patients with acute respiratory distress syndrome in intensive care units in 50 countries. JAMA. 2016;315(8):788–800. https://doi.org/10.1001/jama.2016.0291.

20. Matthay MA, Arabi Y, Arroliga AC, Bernard G, Bersten AD, Brochard LJ, et al. A new global definition of acute respiratory distress syndrome. Am J Respir Crit Care Med. 2024;209(1):37–47. https://doi.org/10.1164/rccm.202303-0558WS.
21. ARDS Definition Task Force. Acute respiratory distress syndrome: the Berlin Definition. JAMA. 2012;307(23):2526–33. https://doi.org/10.1001/jama.2012.5669.
22. Banavasi H, Nguyen P, Osman H, Soubani AO. Management of ARDS – what works and what does not. Am J Med Sci. 2021;362(1):13–23. https://doi.org/10.1016/j.amjms.2020.12.019.
23. Acute Respiratory Distress Syndrome Network, Brower RG, Matthay MA, Morris A, Schoenfeld D, Thompson BT, Wheeler A. Ventilation with lower tidal volumes as compared with traditional tidal volumes for acute lung injury and the acute respiratory distress syndrome. N Engl J Med. 2000;342(18):1301–8. https://doi.org/10.1056/NEJM200005043421801. PMID: 10793162.
24. Liaqat A, Mason M, Foster BJ, Kulkarni S, Barlas A, Farooq AM, et al. Evidence-based mechanical ventilatory strategies in ARDS. J Clin Med. 2022;11(2):319. https://doi.org/10.3390/jcm11020319.
25. Chacko B, Peter JV, Tharyan P, John G, Jeyaseelan L. Pressure-controlled versus volume-controlled ventilation for acute respiratory failure due to acute lung injury (ALI) or acute respiratory distress syndrome (ARDS). Cochrane Database Syst Rev. 2015;2017(6):1–48.
26. Grotberg JC, Reynolds D, Kraft BD. Management of severe acute respiratory distress syndrome: a primer. Crit Care. 2023;27:289. https://doi.org/10.1186/s13054-023-04572-w.

Prone Positioning: Turning Hypoxia Around

28

Daniel Kramer and Robert Hilton

Introduction

Prone positioning has emerged as a critical intervention in the management of acute respiratory distress syndrome (ARDS) and severe hypoxemic respiratory failure. Though its physiologic underpinnings were first noted in the 1970s through observational studies and early radiologic investigations, it would take decades of research to fully elucidate the mechanisms by which prone positioning improves gas exchange, reduces ventilation–perfusion mismatch, and mitigates ventilator-induced lung injury. The practice gained renewed attention during the COVID-19 pandemic, when its benefits were leveraged at an unprecedented scale in both intubated and non-intubated patients. Despite clear evidence demonstrating improved oxygenation and, in select populations, reduced mortality, the adoption of prone positioning remains inconsistent across institutions. This chapter explores the history, physiologic rationale, and clinical evidence behind prone positioning, highlighting its evolution from an observed instinct to a lifesaving intervention in modern critical care.

D. Kramer (✉) · R. Hilton
The Korman Respiratory Institute and the Division of Pulmonary, Allergy and Critical Care, The Department of Medicine at the Sidney Kimmel Medical College of Thomas Jefferson University, Philadelphia, PA, USA
e-mail: Daniel.kramer@jefferson.edu; Robert.hilton@jefferson.edu

G. C. Kane et al. (eds.), *Oxygen*, https://doi.org/10.1007/978-3-032-18934-9_28

History Behind Prone Positioning

The modern understanding of the benefits of prone breathing began with the fortuitous observation of children with cystic fibrosis. In 1974 Dr. Robert Mellins observed that patients with advanced lung disease due to cystic fibrosis would position themselves on hands and knees, which he noted to be a natural instinct to improve ventilation [1]. Interestingly, around the same time, a study was performed utilizing radiologic techniques to study diaphragmatic movement in healthy subjects under general anesthesia, both during spontaneous breathing and passive ventilation while paralyzed. This idea was generated from the observation of impaired gas exchange in passively ventilated patients in the supine position. While it was understood that mechanical ventilation reduced the functional residual capacity (FRC) of patients, this was not felt to be sufficient to fully explain the observed physiologic changes. They found that, while in the supine position during spontaneous breathing on the ventilator, the dependent portion of the diaphragm had the greatest displacement. However, when the patient was paralyzed and passively ventilated, there was a cephalad shift of the end-expiratory position of the diaphragm, disproportionately disadvantaging the dependent portions. Most importantly, passive excursion of the diaphragm was least in the dependent portion, a finding that was not corrected by increasing positive end-expiratory pressure (PEEP) or tidal volumes [2]. This was corroborated clinically by the observation that prone positioning improved oxygenation in patients with acute hypoxemic respiratory failure, with a mean increase in PaO_2 of 69 mmHg when flipped from the supine to the prone position [3].

While studies would follow that would confirm this finding, it would take decades until prone positioning was found to meaningfully affect clinical outcomes in patients with acute respiratory distress syndrome (ARDS). In an article reviewing the modern understanding of prone positioning, Gattinoni et al. observed the long, slow progression of interest from the 1970s until 2020, at which point we saw an explosion of publications on the topic of prone position and ventilation. This explosion coincided with the outbreak of the COVID-19 pandemic, when the influx of severe respiratory disease led physicians to seek out all noninvasive mechanisms to improve respiratory function.

Physiologic Principles of Prone Positioning

Several physiologic and anatomic principles underlie the benefits of prone positioning in patients with acute respiratory failure. First and foremost, the understanding of transpulmonary pressure is essential to appreciate the benefits of prone positioning. Defined as the difference between alveolar pressure and pleural pressure, transpulmonary pressure represents a gradient of pressure from the alveolar side of the pulmonary-capillary membrane, through the lung parenchyma, and out into the pleural space. Typically, the distending pressure in the alveolus, along with a negative pressure within the pleural cavity, allows for the lung to maintain a baseline of recruited lung with normal breathing. This gradient is critical in maintaining alveolar stability, particularly during the static phase at end-exhalation. A sufficiently positive transpulmonary pressure supports alveolar inflation, whereas lower values predispose to alveolar collapse. In the supine position, pleural pressure becomes progressively less negative from the ventral to dorsal regions of the lung. This gradient results in lower transpulmonary pressures and correspondingly reduced alveolar volumes in the dorsocaudal lung regions. These dependent areas are further disadvantaged by gravitational forces and the anatomical phenomenon known as shape mismatch, wherein the dorsal lung is further compressed by gravity, and the ventral lung distends to fit the shape of the thoracic cavity [4]. This effect is also compounded by the differential effect of intra-abdominal pressures in the supine position, with a vertical gradient of increasing abdominal pressure forces on the thorax from ventral to dorsal in the supine position. This further increases pleural pressures, particularly in the dependent portions of the lungs. It is quite the conundrum that pleural pressure becomes less negative and abdominal pressure more positive along the vertical column moving toward the dependent part of the lung. This leads to a significant risk for atelectasis in these crucial areas of the lungs. This can be further compounded by morbid obesity, ascites, abdominal sepsis, abdominal trauma, and other etiologies known to further increase intra-abdominal pressure. Furthermore, there is a compressive effect of the heart on these dependent regions of the lung, which further compounds the issue.

In both the supine and prone positions, perfusion is highest in the dorsal lung [5]. While incompletely understood, this finding can be at least partially attributed to the higher proportion of vasculature in the dorsal lung, leading to an increased capacitance for blood flow. When a significant proportion of pulmonary perfusion is directed toward these collapsed dorsocaudal units, it can lead to significant ventilation–perfusion (V/Q) mismatch. This effect is magnified when the lung is acutely compromised in any process affecting the interstitium and/or alveoli, and when severe enough, it can lead to shunt physiology.

Transpulmonary pressure also plays a crucial role in lung physiology during active inhalation. Pleural pressures become increasingly negative during active inhalation, while alveolar pressure decreases only slightly, resulting in a net positive increase in transpulmonary pressure [6]. This ultimately results in the expansion of, as well as gas entry into, the alveoli. This effect is not evenly distributed throughout the lungs and is highly dependent on patient positioning and compressive forces on the respiratory system from the abdomen and chest wall.

To best appreciate the effects of transpulmonary pressure changes during the inspiratory phase and how prone positioning is beneficial, it is important to understand the change in respiratory system mechanics when individuals go from spontaneous breathing to more passive breathing during invasive mechanical ventilation. In spontaneously breathing individuals, the diaphragm is the dominant muscular force of inspiration. When the diaphragm is strong without compromise, its downward contraction and significant displacement during the inhalation phase allow for a favorable increase in the transpulmonary gradient, with its effect felt most in the dorsocaudal regions of the lungs, where the change in transpulmonary pressures is greatest. This ultimately allows for the greater ventilation observed in the most dependent lung regions. However, during passive mechanical ventilation and neuromuscular paralysis, the diaphragm becomes inactive, permitting intra-abdominal pressure to exert deleterious effects on transpulmonary pressures, via increased pleural pressures, on alveolar recruitment and ventilation. In the absence of active diaphragmatic contraction, insufflated gas is preferentially distributed to the ventral, nondependent regions of the lung. This can be attributed to the greater compliance and mobility of the ventral chest wall compared to the dorsal chest wall in the supine position. Moreover, the lack of diaphragmatic activity permits unopposed compressive forces from the heart and abdominal contents. These factors collectively promote atelectasis, particularly in the highly perfused dorsocaudal regions of the lung. This, again, is further exacerbated in the setting of acute lung pathology and conditions that raise intra-abdominal pressures. This physiology also raises concern for repeat alveolar collapse and reopening during mechanical ventilation, putting the patient at risk for atelectotrauma and ventilator-induced lung injury (VILI), both associated with increased morbidity and mortality. While these physiologic effects are clearly magnified in a ventilated patient with ARDS, physiologic studies demonstrate that even in healthy, spontaneously breathing subjects, transpulmonary pressures are more homogenously distributed in the prone position [7].

Prone positioning counteracts these effects by redistributing gravitational forces, improving shape matching between the lungs and thoracic cavity, and offloading the crucial dorsocaudal portions of the lungs from the pressures exerted by the abdomen and the heart. In the prone position, the greater mass of dorsal lung tissue is distributed more evenly along the broader, horizontally oriented dorsal chest wall. Elevated intra-abdominal pressures and the gravitational force of the heart are redistributed anteriorly, relieving compressive forces on the dorsocaudal lung regions. As a result, transpulmonary pressures are more evenly distributed across the lung, leading to improved recruitment of dorsal alveolar units and enhanced ventilation–perfusion (V/Q) matching. While the ventral lung becomes dependent in the prone position, it comprises a smaller proportion of total lung mass and receives relatively less perfusion. Therefore, any loss in ventilation in these anterior regions has a comparatively minor effect on global gas exchange. Importantly, these benefits are maintained and likely most crucial in passively ventilated patients, particularly with acute lung pathology.

In addition to the above benefits on the respiratory system, there are potential cardiac benefits of prone positioning, particularly with the right ventricle that is vulnerable to the negative effects of acute lung injury and hypoxic vasoconstriction. In a disease state such as ARDS, a failing right ventricle likely signifies an increased risk for mortality. However, it can also cause clinicians to overestimate the severity of lung injury based on the severity of hypoxemia. This can occur due to a low cardiac output state, causing a reduction in mixed venous O_2 passing through the diseased lung with impaired gas exchange. In addition, in some patients, this may be compounded by the opening of a patent foramen ovale via increased right-sided cardiac pressures, causing further shunting [8]. Therefore, improving right ventricular function can be essential in a subgroup of patients with respiratory failure with combined right ventricular failure. Prone positioning enhances ventilation–perfusion (V/Q) matching and oxygenation while reducing regions of both atelectasis and hyperinflation, which can otherwise compress the pulmonary vasculature. These changes contribute to a reduction in pulmonary vascular resistance (PVR), thereby decreasing right ventricular afterload. In addition, the physiologic benefits of prone positioning may justify a reduction in PEEP, further reducing right ventricular afterload [8]. These physiologic advantages have been corroborated by studies demonstrating that prone positioning can decrease PVR, decrease right ventricle size, improve right ventricular function, and reverse shunting through a patent foramen ovale [9, 10]. It is important to recognize that the cardiac benefits of prone positioning are not consistently demonstrated across all patients, as evidenced by current studies. This variability highlights the need for a comprehensive assessment of cardiac function both prior to and following the application of this intervention.

Prone Positioning in ARDS and Severe COVID-19

It can take a state of critical hypoxemia to appreciate all the mechanisms by which prone positioning augments our breathing. This is where the close relationship between ARDS and the understanding of proning begins. ARDS is typically characterized by diffuse pulmonary edema, dense consolidations of dependent lung, diffuse alveolar damage, and progressive fibrosis, all resulting in severe hypoxemia caused by diffusion deficit, shunting, and general V/Q mismatch (Fig. 28.1). These physiologic derangements are only magnified in the supine position based on the principles discussed in the prior section of this chapter. For this reason, there has been a long-standing interest in the utilization of prone positioning in ARDS as a low-cost, noninvasive strategy to mitigate both morbidity and mortality.

In the early 2000s, several studies explored the use of prone positioning in ARDS. Landmark trials by Gattinoni et al. in 2001, Mancebo et al. in 2006, and Taccone et al. in 2009 confirmed the previously suspected improvement in oxygenation, but failed to establish a mortality benefit [11–13]. Subsequent analysis of these studies suggested limitations due to insufficient proning duration, less severe hypoxemia, and variable lung protective ventilation strategies. It was felt, however, that if there is a reliable improvement in oxygenation and lung recruitment, there was strong potential for clinical benefit if the correct patient population and implementation could be identified.

The benefit of the prone position would finally materialize in the landmark PROSEVA trial published in 2013, which would successfully shift the broader management of ARDS to favor early proning [14]. Emphasizing timely and prolonged prone positioning, Guerin and colleagues randomized 466 patients to their study, over 100 more than the second largest proning study to date. Patients were enrolled within 48 h of meeting criteria for severe ARDS diagnosis with a PaO_2:FiO_2 ratio less than 150. The patients randomized to the intervention group were then committed to 16 h in the prone position per day. Proning would continue until they demonstrated clinical improvement, which was clearly defined in the trial design, or until

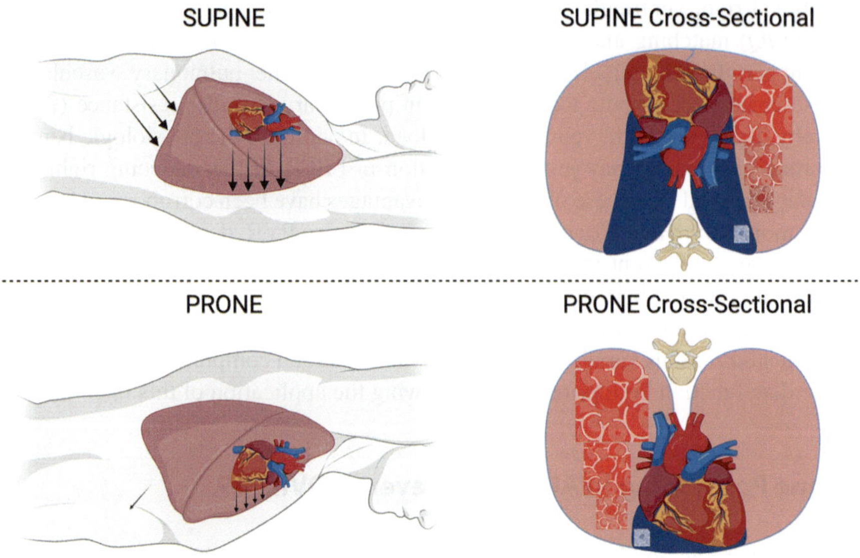

Fig. 28.1 These illustrations show the advantage of the prone position on oxygenation. The upper two pictures show the compression of the lungs by the heart and the abdominal contents, causing atelectasis, which worsens V/Q matching. The lower figures show the advantage of releasing the pressure. The two right-sided cross-section images show the dark blue shapes that represent compressed lung. The larger, redder alveoli represent the improved expansion and oxygenation in the unweighted body surface, both due to the gravitational effects of layering and from the compression by the heart. (Figure by Eliot Baram created in https://BioRender.com)

there was clinical decline prohibiting further proning, such as hemodynamic instability. The study would go on to demonstrate that patients who were proned had an absolute reduction in mortality of 16.8% at 28 days, and that benefit would sustain at 90 days—indicating one of the most significant reductions in mortality for ARDS since its first clinical description in 1967. Following PROSEVA, multiple meta-analyses would support the belief that prone positioning not only improved oxygenation but also, in the right patients under appropriate management, could improve mortality [15–17].

Since the publication of PROSEVA and supportive analyses, society guidelines have followed. The 2017 ATS/ESICM/SCCM guidelines strongly recommend proning for patients with PaO_2:FiO_2 ratios below 150 [18]. Guidelines from La Société de Réanimation de Langue Française (SRLF), the French society for critical care, recommend proning as the first line for patients with severe ARDS, as well [19]. With these guidelines in place, however, the uptake of proning for ARDS remained limited in the years after PROSEVA. Before 2020, proning rates hovered around 16.2% despite the described mortality benefits [20]. The limited uptake of this intervention was believed to be limited by the lack of routine familiarity, the lack of required staffing, and possibly a lack of institutional knowledge or experience. It was found that many hospitals lacked formal protocols, and staff were often unfamiliar with the logistics of safely proning patients.

Things changed dramatically in the ensuing COVID-19 pandemic of 2020. As critically ill patients with severe hypoxemic respiratory failure filled intensive care units across the world, hospitals were forced to look for strategies that could be implemented quickly and broadly to improve oxygenation. Hospitals from Wuhan to Milan to New York City began employing proning teams designated to facilitate the maneuver on as many ventilated patients as possible. Teams were frequently redeployed from operating rooms or physical therapy groups, whose services were underutilized. Proning utilization surged to over half of all severe ARDS patients, more than doubling previous rates [21]. What was once a somewhat niche intervention became a more routine practice, a striking example of how a global crisis can transform bedside care in real time.

Due to high volumes of patients with hypoxemic respiratory failure due to COVID-19, the proning strategy was expanded to non-intubated patients. Studies such as Cappo et al. (2020) and Elharrar et al. (2020) demonstrated that awake proning was both feasible and could improve oxygenation in patients with respiratory failure [22–24]. Evidence remains limited as to whether proning can prevent intubation or improve mortality, as the predictors of progression to respiratory failure remain innumerable [25].

The shift was so remarkable that it captured public attention beyond the walls of the ICU. The New York Times ran stories describing how nurses, respiratory therapists, and physicians worked in teams to rotate patients onto their stomachs in makeshift ICUs. The Atlantic highlighted how proning had become a "go-to" maneuver in overwhelmed hospitals, with caregivers in places like New York City describing it as a simple, decades-old technique that was suddenly saving lives. Reports from NPR and other outlets described how awake patients in emergency departments and hospital wards were being asked to lie on their stomachs as a first-line effort to stave off intubation—a practice that, prior to COVID-19, was almost unheard of outside of critical care units.

Unfortunately, as the COVID crisis has come to a close, with hospitals optimizing efficiency, the volume of staff available has dwindled, and proning rates have decreased substantially. In 2022, proning frequency dropped to 27.5% for severe ARDS, a near 50% drop from 2021 [21]. While it was above the mark from Tathum et al.'s estimates in 2019, this decline is discouraging. An intervention that represents an absolute risk reduction of 16–17% in mortality equates to a number needed to treat only seven patients. This exceeds the mortality benefit of statins in heart disease, antihypertensives in secondary stroke prevention, and coronary bypass surgery in coronary artery disease. This should remind us, providers and patients alike, that we must remain vigilant and committed to best practices. We can look to Aristotle for guidance, acknowledging "We are what we repeatedly do. Excellence, then, is not an act, but a habit"—as shared by Will Durant, summarizing Aristotle.

Conclusion

Prone positioning, once an observational curiosity, has evolved into an important strategy in the care of patients with severe hypoxemic respiratory failure, particularly for severe ARDS. Its physiologic benefits—ranging from improved ventilation–perfusion matching to reduced ventilator-induced lung injury and right ventricular strain—are supported by decades of research and reinforced by robust clinical trials like PROSEVA. Despite clear evidence of improved outcomes, including a substantial mortality benefit, its utilization remains inconsistent. The COVID-19 pandemic reaffirmed the value of proning as both a potentially lifesaving and scalable intervention, yet its underuse in the post-pandemic era underscores the challenges of sustaining evidence-based practices. As clinicians, our responsibility is to embed such proven strategies into routine care—not as a crisis response but as a habitual standard rooted in both science and clinical excellence.

Declarations

Competing Interests The authors have no competing interests to declare that are relevant to the content of this manuscript.

Ethics Approval The authors declare that this manuscript does not include primary research with human participants.

The authors declare that this manuscript does not include primary studies involving animals.

References

1. Mellins RB. Pulmonary physiotherapy in the pediatric age group. Am Rev Respir Dis. 1974;110(6 Pt 2):137–42.
2. Froese AB, Bryan AC. Effects of anesthesia and paralysis on diaphragmatic mechanics in man. Anesthesiology. 1974;41(3):242–55.
3. Douglas WW, Rehder K, Beynen FM, Sessler AD, Marsh HM. Improved oxygenation in patients with acute respiratory failure: the prone position. Am Rev Respir Dis. 1977;115(4):559–66.
4. Gattinoni L, Taccone P, Carlesso E, Marini JJ. Prone position in acute respiratory distress syndrome. Rationale, indications, and limits. Am J Respir Crit Care Med. 2013;188(11):1286–93.
5. Scholten EL, Beitler JR, Prisk GK, Malhotra A. Treatment of ARDS with prone positioning. Chest. 2017;151(1):215–24.
6. Neupane K, Jamil RT. Physiology, transpulmonary pressure. In: StatPearls. Treasure Island (FL): StatPearls Publishing; 2025.
7. Tawhai MH, Nash MP, Lin C-L, Hoffman EA. Supine and prone differences in regional lung density and pleural pressure gradients in the human lung with constant shape. J Appl Physiol. 2009;107(3):912–20.

8. Vieillard-Baron A, Boissier F, Pesenti A. Hemodynamic impact of prone position. Let's protect the lung and its circulation to improve prognosis. Intensive Care Med. 2023;49(6):692–4.
9. Vieillard-Baron A, Charron C, Caille V, Belliard G, Page B, Jardin F. Prone positioning unloads the right ventricle in severe ARDS. Chest. 2007;132(5):1440–6.
10. Mekontso Dessap A, Boissier F, Charron C, Bégot E, Repessé X, Legras A, et al. Acute cor pulmonale during protective ventilation for acute respiratory distress syndrome: prevalence, predictors, and clinical impact. Intensive Care Med. 2016;42(5):862–70.
11. Gattinoni L, Tognoni G, Pesenti A, Taccone P, Mascheroni D, Labarta V, et al. Effect of prone positioning on the survival of patients with acute respiratory failure. N Engl J Med. 2001;345(8):568–73.
12. Mancebo J, Fernández R, Blanch L, Rialp G, Gordo F, Ferrer M, et al. A multicenter trial of prolonged prone ventilation in severe acute respiratory distress syndrome. Am J Respir Crit Care Med. 2006;173(11):1233–9.
13. Taccone P, Pesenti A, Latini R, Polli F, Vagginelli F, Mietto C, et al. Prone positioning in patients with moderate and severe acute respiratory distress syndrome: a randomized controlled trial. JAMA. 2009;302(18):1977–84.
14. Guérin C. Prone positioning acute respiratory distress syndrome patients. Ann Transl Med. 2017;5(14):289.
15. Sud S, Friedrich JO, Adhikari NKJ, Taccone P, Mancebo J, Polli F, et al. Effect of prone positioning during mechanical ventilation on mortality among patients with acute respiratory distress syndrome: a systematic review and meta-analysis. CMAJ. 2014;186(10):E381–90.
16. Lee JM, Bae W, Lee YJ, Cho Y-J. The efficacy and safety of prone positional ventilation in acute respiratory distress syndrome: updated study-level meta-analysis of 11 randomized controlled trials. Crit Care Med. 2014;42(5):1252–62.
17. Beitler JR, Shaefi S, Montesi SB, Devlin A, Loring SH, Talmor D, et al. Prone positioning reduces mortality from acute respiratory distress syndrome in the low tidal volume era: a meta-analysis. Intensive Care Med. 2014;40(3):332–41.
18. Fan E, Del Sorbo L, Goligher EC, Hodgson CL, Munshi L, Walkey AJ, et al. An Official American Thoracic Society/European Society of Intensive Care Medicine/Society of Critical Care Medicine clinical practice guideline: mechanical ventilation in adult patients with acute respiratory distress syndrome. Am J Respir Crit Care Med. 2017;195(9):1253–63.
19. Papazian L, Aubron C, Brochard L, Chiche J-D, Combes A, Dreyfuss D, et al. Formal guidelines: management of acute respiratory distress syndrome. Ann Intensive Care. 2019;9(1):69.
20. Tatham KC, Ferguson ND, Zhou Q, Hand L, Austin P, Taneja R, et al. Evolution of practice patterns in the management of acute respiratory distress syndrome: a secondary analysis of two successive randomized controlled trials. J Crit Care. 2021;65:274–81.
21. Hochberg CH, Psoter KJ, Eakin MN, Hager DN. Declining use of prone positioning after high initial uptake in COVID-19 adult respiratory distress syndrome. Crit Care Med. 2023;51(11):1547–51.
22. Coppo A, Bellani G, Winterton D, Di Pierro M, Soria A, Faverio P, et al. Feasibility and physiological effects of prone positioning in non-intubated patients with acute respiratory failure due to COVID-19 (PRON-COVID): a prospective cohort study. Lancet Respir Med. 2020;8(8):765–74.
23. Elharrar X, Trigui Y, Dols A-M, Touchon F, Martinez S, Prud'homme E, et al. Use of prone positioning in nonintubated patients with COVID-19 and hypoxemic acute respiratory failure. JAMA. 2020;323(22):2336–8.
24. Weatherald J, Solverson K, Zuege DJ, Loroff N, Fiest KM, Parhar KKS. Awake prone positioning for COVID-19 hypoxemic respiratory failure: a rapid review. J Crit Care. 2021;61:63–70.
25. Marini JJ, Gattinoni L. Management of COVID-19 respiratory distress. JAMA. 2020;323(22):2329–30.

Complications of Prone Positioning

29

Christina J. Carrero and Urvashi Vaid

Introduction

Prone positioning is the deliberate placement of a patient lying face down for an extended period of time and has recently become the cornerstone intervention in the management of severe hypoxia, specifically in patients with ARDS. The evidence-based physiologic benefits include increased homogeneous distribution of transpulmonary pressure throughout lung tissue and improved ventilation-perfusion (V/Q) matching, thereby allowing for better oxygenation [1, 2]. Because of these well-documented advantages, prone positioning has been adopted worldwide throughout intensive care units (ICUs). Most recently, there has been an increase in the use of prone positioning during the COVID-19 pandemic, when healthcare providers relied on this intervention in both intubated and non-intubated patients to improve oxygenation and P_aO2/F_iO2 (P/F) ratios. The previous chapter dives deep into the history, physiologic advantages, and clinical uses of prone positioning. This chapter will delve into the complications of prone positioning.

In the 1970s, Charles Bryan was one of the first providers to use prone positioning to improve ventilation to the dorsal regions of the lung [3]. Later in 1986, two separate studies published reports describing the anatomy of ARDS as seen on CT imaging, demonstrating that lung densities were not homogeneously distributed throughout the lung parenchyma but primarily in dependent regions of the lung [3].

C. J. Carrero
Thomas Jefferson University Hospital, Philadelphia, PA, USA
e-mail: Christina.Carrero@jefferson.edu

U. Vaid (✉)
The Korman Respiratory Institute and the Division of Pulmonary, Allergy and Critical Care, The Department of Medicine at the Sidney Kimmel Medical College of Thomas Jefferson University, Philadelphia, PA, USA
e-mail: Urvashi.Vaid@jefferson.edu

G. C. Kane et al. (eds.), *Oxygen*, https://doi.org/10.1007/978-3-032-18934-9_29

The first randomized study that showed improved oxygenation and reduced mortality with early prone positioning in moderate-to-severe ARDS was the PROSEVA trial published in 2013 [4]. The physiologic rationale behind its effectiveness is rooted in a combination of anatomical, gravitational, and mechanical factors that influence lung function [3, 5].

Patients with hypoxic respiratory failure often have collapsed alveoli and dense consolidations, particularly in the posterior dependent lung regions, due to inflammation, edema, increased lung weight, and overall gravitational pull affecting dependent lungs the most [5]. In the supine position, the pressure exerted by the heart and mediastinal structures on the lungs worsens the collapse of lung parenchyma, compressing the posterior (dorsal) regions of the lungs [3, 5, 6]. These dorsal areas are more perfused due to gravity-dependent blood flow. This discrepancy leads to a ventilation-perfusion (V/Q) mismatch, where the well-perfused dorsal lung regions receive insufficient ventilation, and the less perfused anterior (ventral) regions receive excessive ventilation. The result is inefficient gas exchange and decreased arterial oxygenation. When a patient is turned into the prone position, the effects of gravity on the lungs are redistributed. Although perfusion remains relatively gravity-dependent, blood flow still favors the dorsal regions, while ventilation improves significantly in these same regions. This change occurs because the prone position reduces the compression on the dorsal lung tissue, opening the collapsed or consolidated lung tissue and alveoli (lung/alveolar recruitment). Consequently, ventilation and perfusion become better matched, which enhances the efficiency of oxygen exchange.

The scope of complications from prone positioning varies from minor skin pressure injuries to catastrophic end-organ failure. Some of these complications can become immediately apparent as a transient worsening of oxygenation, as the patient's cardiopulmonary system adjusts to the change in position. Proning a patient can result in endotracheal tube compression and difficulty with ventilation or cause facial edema from the gravitational shift in edema. Other complications occur slowly over time and can go unnoticed if not frequently monitored. Patients with multiple comorbidities, frailty, obesity, and poor nutritional status are all at higher risk of complications [7]. Keeping this in mind, prone positioning poses logistical barriers in patient care while the intervention is in action, such as monitoring the patient's status, securing medical devices (i.e., the endotracheal tube), and maintaining hygiene [8]. Mechanical pressure on dependent body parts, limited access to the ventral surface during physical exams, and changes to the patient's hemodynamics can all contribute to various complications while in the prone position [9].

Understanding these complications is vital for effective planning by healthcare providers to mitigate as much risk as possible to the patient while trying to provide the highest quality of care. It requires a coordinated effort from multidisciplinary providers to ensure patient safety. There are risks associated with moving to the prone position, remaining prone for 12–16 h and then returning to the supine position [4, 8]. Safely implementing prone positioning is patient-specific and heavily relies on proper technique, appropriate supportive materials, and continuous monitoring and reassessment [10]. Throughout this chapter, the complications of prone positioning will be discussed along with practical approaches to reduce complications.

Complications of Prone Positioning

Worsening of V/Q Matching and Timing of Initiation of the Prone Position

In an observational sub-study from November 2019 to March 2020, electrical impedance tomography (EIT) was used bedside as a noninvasive monitoring tool for ventilation and perfusion distribution. The summary of this observational study showed that patients in the prone position had a change in ventilation distribution to the dorsal lung regions and an increase in homogenization of gas and perfusion patterns, leading to improved V/Q matching [11]. Despite improved V/Q matching, multiple studies have shown that perfusion to the dorsal lung regions remains greater than to the ventral lung regions, despite positioning and gravitational forces. This explains a potential complication observed, namely, a lack of improvement in V/Q matching transiently post-proning. The perfusion of poorly ventilated lung zones (shunt) and the ventilation of poorly perfused lung zones (dead space) are the main causes of V/Q mismatch and arterial hypoxemia, and we know that the severity of hypoxemia determines the severity of ARDS and the patient's clinical outcome [3, 5, 9]. In comparing the timing of prone positioning initiated for early versus late (persistent) ARDS, prone positioning was found to increase the pulmonary shunt with no improvement in oxygenation in patients with persistent or late ARDS [12]. If prone positioning does not improve V/Q mismatch, what interventions could be used instead? An alternative therapy may be considered in patients with unilateral consolidations or atelectasis. By placing such patients in the lateral recumbent position with the "good" or less affected lung in the dependent position, oxygenation can be optimized while minimizing shunt and V/Q mismatch. Although the lateral position does not supersede prone positioning, it can offer patients redistribution of blood flow from the affected to the unaffected lung, reducing shunt and improving gas exchange [7, 10].

Hemodynamic Complications

Patients requiring mechanical ventilation very seldom present without any other comorbidities contributing to their overall clinical outcome. Some common coexisting conditions seen in patients with acute respiratory failure are diabetes, chronic kidney disease, coronary artery disease, COPD/emphysema, liver disease, and cancer [7]. Any time a patient is placed in the prone position, perfusion is not only altered within the lung, but also to other vital organs as well. Lying on the ventral portion of the body can shift organs and vessels, causing compression and increased compartment pressure. Despite using lung protective ventilation, increasing the PEEP in the presence of inflamed lung parenchyma can cause an increase in intrathoracic pressure. This increase in pressure, in addition to the abdomen compressed against the hospital bed in the prone position, may impede blood flow through the inferior vena cava and back to the heart. As thoracic and/or abdominal pressure rises, venous return declines, directly affecting preload, stroke volume, and cardiac output, placing patients at risk of hypoperfusion of vital organs. Decreased venous return directly correlates with hypoperfusion, leading to acute kidney injury, bowel ischemia or ileus, and delirium [8, 13]. If prone positioning is inevitable, it is imperative to closely monitor a patient's volume status with the goal of keeping them euvolemic, as per guidelines for the management of ARDS.

Moreover, cardiac arrhythmias can be triggered by the hemodynamic consequences of prone positioning, primarily hypoperfusion and hypoxemia. As described above, decreased venous return can lead to a decrease in cardiac output and hypoperfusion of the myocardium. In patients at risk, this lower cardiac output can induce cardiac ischemia. Cardiac output can be reduced by 24% [13]. This specifically can lead to myocardial stress and ischemic/stress-related arrhythmias like atrial fibrillation/flutter. Close attention to the positioning of ECG leads is important, especially in prolonged proning with EKGs obtained from leads placed posteriorly [14]. Other organ ischemia leading to injury, such as acute kidney injury, can lead to electrolyte imbalances, which play a direct role in cardiac contractility. If electrolytes are not promptly monitored and repleted, the patient can be at risk for both atrial and ventricular arrhythmias and torsades de pointes. Key monitoring points when it comes to cardiac arrhythmias include continuous cardiac monitoring, thorough pre-prone positioning assessment with baseline ECG, and frequent volume status and electrolyte monitoring with repletion as needed. Of course, hemodynamic changes can precipitate neurologic complications such as increased intracranial pressure and long-term sequelae of CNS hypoxia and delirium.

Airway Complications

Complications directly related to mechanical ventilation and airway management are endotracheal tube dislodgement or extubation and difficulties with secretion management. The logistics of proning a patient, despite a multidisciplinary team involved, may lead to the risk of the ETT sliding in too deep or out of position, or completely out of the patient's airway [10, 15]. Adequate sedation, analgesia, and, if needed, neuromuscular blockade (NMB) can help minimize this risk, therefore preventing ETT dislodgement. It is key that, regardless of the technique used (manual proning or a rotation bed), team members participating in the process have designated roles and responsibilities. If staffing permits, the respiratory therapist should control the airway and the patient's head throughout the entire turn, marking the position (in cm) of the ETT placement before and after prone positioning. In addition, prone positioning can promote increased sinus drainage, leading to increased secretions specifically from the nose and mouth. This can be managed with frequent suctioning and oral hygiene, placing the patient in a slight reverse Trendelenburg position to minimize pooling of secretions around the face and head and minimizing facial edema.

Chest X-rays are frequently required when patients are in acute respiratory failure to correlate clinical progress to radiologic progress, monitor for complications of mechanical ventilation like barotrauma, and determine accurate placement of lines, tubes, and catheters. Recent literature suggests that X-rays performed in the prone position can be reliable for assessing these factors [16]. Since patients are prone for 12–16 h, it might be prudent to plan to obtain routine imaging when the patient is in the supine position.

Aspiration risk has not been shown to be increased in the prone position, and the recommendations remain to continue enteral feeding for patients unless they show signs of intolerance to feeds.

Skin, Soft Tissue, and Musculoskeletal Complications

When patients remain in the prone position for 12–16 h, fluid shifts occur, resulting in facial swelling. Specifically related to proning, the patient's eyes, nose, mouth, and ears can all be pressed against a pillow or bed, increasing the risk of pressure-related injuries [17, 18]. If the patient is receiving NMB, it is important to remember to place a small transparent dressing or tape over the patient's eyes to protect from possible corneal abrasions or infection, given the lack of a functional corneal reflex while sedated or paralyzed. A way to prevent the other head and neck complications is frequent head rotation with the assistance of respiratory therapy, moving the ETT from one side of the mouth to the other as the head rotates from side to side. This is recommended every 2 h if possible. Care must be taken, though, to avoid excessive neck movement, as it can rarely lead to alteration of blood flow and/or injury to the carotid and vertebral arteries. It may even rarely lead to cervical spinal injuries [19].

Like frequent head rotation to prevent eye, ear, and nose complications, arm, leg, and neck range of motion activities help keep joints mobile and reduce the risk of atrophy long-term. Careful neck rotation is provided when the rotation of the ETT and head is complete. Arms can be rotated within the same interval and are usually referred to as "swimming" with one arm placed above the head and the other at the patient's side. Additionally, all critically ill patients are at risk for acute skin failure and pressure-related injuries. Just like in the supine position, prone positioning poses specific risk areas for skin breakdown, such as the ears, face, nose/mouth, shoulders, knees, and feet. By applying protective dressings to bony prominences prior to prone positioning, the team can help prevent skin breakdown from pressure or medical devices [10, 18].

Upper limb peripheral nerve palsies are not uncommon, given the long duration that patients are placed in this position. One meta-analysis estimated the incidence to be 13% [19] and found brachial plexus injuries to be the most frequent. The

Table 29.1 Organ system-based summary of the complications of prone positioning of patients in acute hypoxic respiratory failure, with contraindications listed

Head, ear, nose, throat	Face/nose/ear pressure injuries Ocular: increased ocular pressure Corneal abrasions Face/tongue/lip edema Endotracheal tube occlusion/kinking
Neurologic	Increased intracranial pressure (ICP) Cognitive impairment (prolonged hypoxia) Delirium/agitation (prolonged sedation)
Cardiovascular	Decreased venous return ➔ hypotension Cardiac arrhythmias (Ectopy, A-Fib, VT) Increased RV strain Exacerbate heart failure or pulmonary hypertension
Respiratory	Transient worsening of V/Q mismatch Barotrauma ➔ Pneumothorax Poor secretion management/clearance Endotracheal tube dislodgment
Gastrointestinal/genitourinary	Delayed gastric emptying Aspiration Hepatic congestion Acute kidney injury
Musculoskeletal	Muscle atrophy (immobility and neuromuscular blockade use) Joint strain/dislocations/spinal or peripheral nerve injury (swimming of arms, neck adjustments)
Absolute contraindications	Refractory increased ICP Unstable cervical, thoracic, lumbar spine; pelvic, skull, or facial fractures
Relative contraindications/ precautions	Open chest/unstable chest wall Bronchopleural fistula Open abdomen or abdominal distension Use of a bifurcated endotracheal tube (severe hemoptysis)

heterogeneity of the studies included and the complexity of the patients made it difficult to pinpoint the exact risk factors or incidence, but this is a potential complication that needs monitoring. Table 29.1 provides a summary of the system-based complications that may arise because of proning.

Conclusion

While prone positioning is a powerful therapeutic intervention specifically in patients with acute respiratory distress syndrome (ARDS) and acute hypoxic respiratory failure, this intervention can have significant adverse consequences. Although it improves oxygenation by enhancing alveolar recruitment and optimizing ventilation-perfusion matching, prone positioning introduces complex complications involving both the cardiac and pulmonary systems that require diligent monitoring. Hypoxia and hypoperfusion can lead to hemodynamic collapse, specifically due to decreased venous return, leading to hypotension, reduced cardiac output, multi-organ hypoperfusion, and cardiac arrhythmias. These effects are further amplified in patients with preexisting cardiac dysfunction, where the added stress on the heart and systemic circulation can precipitate life-threatening shock and end-organ damage. Musculoskeletal complications, facial and airway edema, pressure injuries, and technical challenges related to positioning, monitoring, and accessing the patient can also play a role in complicating the management of patients in the prone position.

In essence, when indicated, prone positioning should be the standard of care, given its mortality benefit in patients with moderate-to-severe ARDS. The caveat being that the use of prone positioning must be evaluated on a case-by-case basis, balancing its benefits against the potential for significant complications. Table 29.1 (below) outlines the complications by organ system. Successful implementation hinges on the availability of an experienced healthcare team, careful patient selection, pre-proning optimization, and ongoing reassessment. In the absence of an experienced team for carrying out the proning process, proning might be avoided, or transfer to an experienced facility could be explored. With meticulous attention to detail, the complications of prone positioning can often be mitigated, allowing clinicians to harness its lifesaving potential while minimizing harm.

Declarations

Competing Interests The authors have no competing interests to declare that are relevant to the content of this manuscript.

Ethics Approval The authors declare that this manuscript does not include primary research with human participants.

The authors declare that this manuscript does not include primary studies involving animals.

References

1. Guérin C, Li J, Grasselli G. Prone positioning. Intensive Care Med. 2024;50(6):968–70.
2. Slobod D, Damia A, Leali M, Spinelli E, Mauri T. Pathophysiology and clinical meaning of ventilation-perfusion mismatch in the acute respiratory distress syndrome. Biology. 2022;12(1):67.
3. Gattinoni L, Brusatori S, D'Albo R, Maj R, Velati M, Zinnato C, et al. Prone position: how understanding and clinical application of a technique progress with time. Anesthesiol Perioper Sci. 2023;1(1):3.
4. Guérin C, Reignier J, Richard JC, Beuret P, Gacouin A, Boulain T, et al. Prone positioning in severe acute respiratory distress syndrome. N Engl J Med. 2013;368(23):2159–68.
5. Rampon GL, Simpson SQ, Agrawal R. Prone positioning for acute hypoxemic respiratory failure and ARDS: a review. Chest. 2023;163(2):332–40.
6. Yang S, Sun Q, Yuan X, Wang J, Wang H, Hu W, et al. Effect of prone position on ventilation-perfusion matching in patients with moderate to severe ARDS with different clinical phenotypes. Respir Res. 2025;26(1):70.

7. Messerole E, Peine P, Wittkopp S, Marini JJ, Albert RK. The pragmatics of prone positioning. Am J Respir Crit Care Med. 2002;165(10):1359–63.
8. Papazian L, Munshi L, Guérin C. Prone position in mechanically ventilated patients. Intensive Care Med. 2022;48(8):1062–5.
9. Scholten EL, Beitler JR, Prisk GK, Malhotra A. Treatment of ARDS with prone positioning. Chest. 2017;151(1):215–24.
10. Dirkes S, Dickinson S, Havey R, O'brien D. Prone positioning: is it safe and effective? Crit Care Nurs Q. 2012;35(1):64–75.
11. Bachmann M, Basoalto R, Díaz O, Bruhn A, Bugedo G, Retamal J. Prone position improves ventilation-perfusion mismatch in patients with severe acute respiratory distress syndrome. Med Intensiva. 2023;47(3):175.
12. Yuan X, Zhao Z, Chao Y, Chen D, Chen H, Zhang R, et al. Effects of early versus delayed application of prone position on ventilation–perfusion mismatch in patients with acute respiratory distress syndrome: a prospective observational study. Crit Care. 2023;27(1):462.
13. Edgcombe H, Carter K, Yarrow S. Anaesthesia in the prone position. Br J Anaesth. 2008;100(2):165–83. https://doi.org/10.1093/bja/aem380. ISSN 0007-0912.
14. Nguyen HH, Trohman RG, Huang HD. Influence of prone positioning on electrocardiogram in a patient with COVID-19. JAMA Intern Med. 2020;180(11):1521–3.
15. Binda F, Galazzi A, Marelli F, Gambazza S, Villa L, Vinci E, et al. Complications of prone positioning in patients with COVID-19: a cross-sectional study. Intensive Crit Care Nurs. 2021;67:103088.
16. Lazarus MS, Hossain R, Villasana GM, Herring AA, Ye K, Jeudy J, Levsky JM, White CS, Haramati LB. Prone chest radiographs: distinguishing features and identification of support devices. Lung. 2022;200(4):441–5. https://doi.org/10.1007/s00408-022-00545-y. Epub 2022 Jun 16. PMID: 35708780; PMCID: PMC9201801.
17. DePasse JM, Palumbo MA, Haque M, Eberson CP, Daniels AH. Complications associated with prone positioning in elective spinal surgery. World J Orthop. 2015;6(3):351.
18. Girard R, Baboi L, Ayzac L, Richard JC, Guérin C, Proseva Trial Group. The impact of patient positioning on pressure ulcers in patients with severe ARDS: results from a multicenter randomized controlled trial on prone positioning. Intensive Care Med. 2014;40:397–403.
19. Binda F, Gambazza S, Marelli F, Rossi V, Lusignani M, Grasselli G. Upper limb peripheral nerve injuries in patients with ARDS requiring prone positioning: a systematic review with proportion meta-analysis. Intensive Crit Care Nurs. 2024;85:103766. https://doi.org/10.1016/j.iccn.2024.103766. ISSN 0964-3397. https://www.sciencedirect.com/science/article/pii/S0964339724001514.

ECMO and Its Contribution to Lung Recovery

30

Douglas R. Adams and Michael Baram

Introduction

This chapter will give a brief overview of the history of ECMO, review patient screening, basic ECMO physiology, ECMO care strategy, and the future of extracorporeal CO_2 removal ($ECCO_2R$). This chapter is intended to be a review. There are textbooks dedicated to just this topic [1, 2]. Since the goal of this textbook is to focus on oxygen, venous-venous (V-V) oxygenation will be the thrust, but venous arterial (V-A) will be discussed as well, since it provides oxygenated blood to the body but also provides cardiac support for a failed heart. The earliest roots of extracorporeal therapy were first pioneered at Jefferson University by Dr. Gibbon for cardiac surgery. In the current version of ECMO for bedside use, credit goes to Dr. Robert Bartlett.

History of ECMO

It is hard to separate the topics of cardiopulmonary bypass machines from current-day ECMO devices. Over the years, there has been evolving technology, a better understanding of heart-lung physiology, and improvements in supportive medicine such as sedation, ventilators, anticoagulation, etc. Credit is given to Dr. John Heysham Gibbon for creating the first heart-lung machine. Early in his career, he

D. R. Adams
Department of Anesthesiology and Perioperative Medicine, Sidney Kimmel Medical College of Thomas Jefferson University, Philadelphia, PA, USA

M. Baram (✉)
The Korman Respiratory Institute and the Division of Pulmonary, Allergy, and Critical Care, The Department of Medicine at the Sidney Kimmel Medical College of Thomas Jefferson University, Philadelphia, PA, USA
e-mail: Michael.baram@jefferson.edu

G. C. Kane et al. (eds.), *Oxygen*, https://doi.org/10.1007/978-3-032-18934-9_30

cared for a young patient who succumbed to a pulmonary embolism. Using a concept from the late 1800s when German scientists bubbled oxygen into blood to convert hypoxic blood to oxygen-rich blood, he created a mechanism of oxygenating blood outside of the body (extracorporeal oxygenation) using screens [3]. Dr. Gibbon and his wife, Mary Gibbon, are credited with being the first to operationalize extracorporeal oxygenation. The first successful cardiopulmonary bypass surgery occurred in 1953. Despite the survival of some patients, there were a few deaths that resulted in Dr. Gibbon turning to Mayo Clinic (Rochester, Minnesota) to improve the technology. His vision allowed the idea of using technology to oxygenate blood spring from the laboratory to clinical practice.

Over time, the technology improved, and the oxygenation process caused less strain on the red cells, resulting in less hemolysis. The evolution of modern ECMO came decades later. The cardiac surgeons in the operating room improved the process of cardiac surgery by using more efficient membrane oxygenators. The current principle of longer-term support outside of the operating room is the differentiation between bypass and ECMO. The first adult ECMO survivor was reported in the *New England Journal of Medicine* in 1972 by Dr. J. Donald Hill [4]. This frequently referenced article shows a patient hidden behind a room full of equipment. The patient was a young male survivor of a motor vehicle accident who developed acute respiratory distress syndrome (ARDS) and severe hypoxic respiratory failure. Esperanza Pineda (Esperanza, translated from Spanish, is hope) was the first neonatal ECMO survivor in 1975 [5]. Imagine getting informed consent for a novel therapy, which still had high mortality. Dr. Robert Bartlett and Esperanza continued a friendship for decades to come.

After these two landmark, well-referenced cases, there were several clinical trials that shed doubt on the clinical benefits of ECMO. The Zapol study in 1979 was a nine-site multicenter randomized trial studying severe ARDS [6]. Although this study did not show a survival benefit from ECMO support, the importance of this paper highlights the importance of patient selection and patient management on ECMO. In retrospect, these patients already had over a week of ARDS, and despite being provided with lung support, the patients were left on high ventilator settings and very high doses of anticoagulation. The next large, randomized study in 1994 did not show much better results [7]. In the Morris study, it was a single, inexperienced site that tried to focus on high ventilator settings to provide oxygenation and used ECMO to provide carbon dioxide removal ($ECCO_2R$) [7]. The ventilator remained on high positive end expiratory pressure (PEEP of 20 cm H_2O) and peak pressure in the mid-to-high 40s and 50s cm H_2O. This historic paper also failed to show survival benefits. Both studies were important to highlight the need for improved technology, better ECMO protocols, and improved medical management for the critically ill.

The next critical paper on ECMO came from England, with its highly structured and organized health care system affecting results. The CESAR trial, with the lead author being Giles Peek, randomized patients to centralization for ARDS and potential ECMO care versus no transfer to ARDS treatment centers [8]. Those randomized to centralized centers had access to ECMO if they required it versus no ECMO in peripheral hospitals (hub and spoke design). Eighteen percent of the patients randomized to centralized and potential ECMO care did not require ECMO. But with the intention-to-treat analysis, survival was 63% in transfer to ECMO centers versus 47% non-ECMO centers ($p = 0.03$). The difference between this 2009 study and studies from the previous decades was improvement in the oxygenator membranes, improved centrifugal pump heads, and a better understanding of rescue ventilator settings.

Another controversial study supporting ECMO was the EOLIA paper published in the *New England Journal of Medicine* in 2018 [9]. This multicenter randomized controlled study was stopped early since it was unlikely to achieve the predefined goal of a 20% mortality ARDS reduction. This ambitious goal was targeted to increase survival of severe ARDS from 40% to 60%. The results showed a 65% versus 54% survival in favor of the ECMO arm. The p-value was 0.09, not statistically significant, due to the overall lower mortality in both arms. The statistics did not result in a positive study, but that was due to the power analysis driving the 20% reduction in mortality. But most interesting was that the crossover arm still had a 57% mortality, suggesting early ECMO confers a benefit over late ECMO [9]. There was little doubt that ECMO improved oxygenation, but there were still doubters with regard to the overall survival benefit of ECMO.

It is intentional that specific inclusion and exclusion criteria were not referenced above. These details continue to be reassessed and refined. The nuanced use of ECMO continues to evolve with each patient. ECMO technology and training are becoming safer and more accessible. Smaller circuits have been created that have lower blood flow, which provide an effective tool for CO_2 removal with only a mild oxygenation effect. This technology is referred to as extracorporeal CO_2 removal ($ECCO_2R$). This technology helps reduce serum CO_2, thereby lowering minute ventilation requirements to allow a ventilator strategy that focuses on oxygenation rather than ventilation [10]. This technology has been applied to chronic obstructive pulmonary disease (COPD) with mixed results, but the technology continues to evolve. With steps forward, the safety and effectiveness of ECMO and $ECCO_2R$ continue to be better understood.

There were many retrospective studies that looked at unique populations. The results vary, but the recent COVID-19 pandemic has validated ECMO as a therapy to support the sickest patients. Networks were developed to coordinate the most effective deployment of this resource. Most clinicians recognized that in the appropriate setting, ECMO offers patients an opportunity to recover from respiratory failure. Part of the art of ECMO care is patient selection in addition to patient management.

Patient Selection

Outcomes of ECMO therapy are tied directly to patient selection. Not only must the patient have the physiologic reserve to survive, but there must also be a path to recovery or transplant. The lungs have tremendous potential to heal after injury. Early physiologic testing showed that lungs heal for a year after ARDS. This is demonstrated in CT images (see Figs. 30.1, 30.2, and 30.3). Newer experience with cystic fibrosis medication shows that decades of lung damage can heal and improve

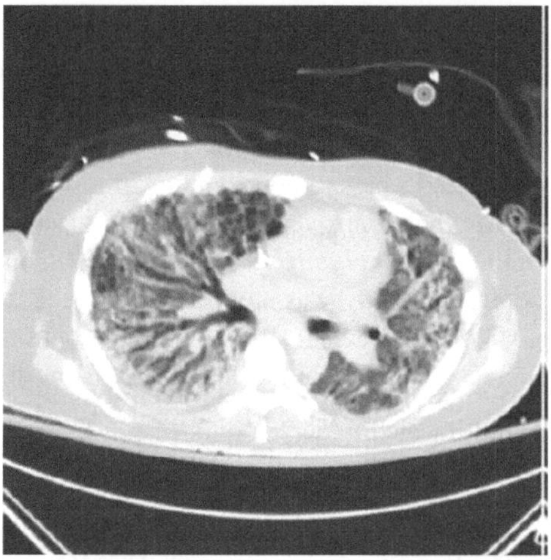

Fig. 30.1 ARDS with traction bronchiectasis—this image was collected during the worst ARDS period

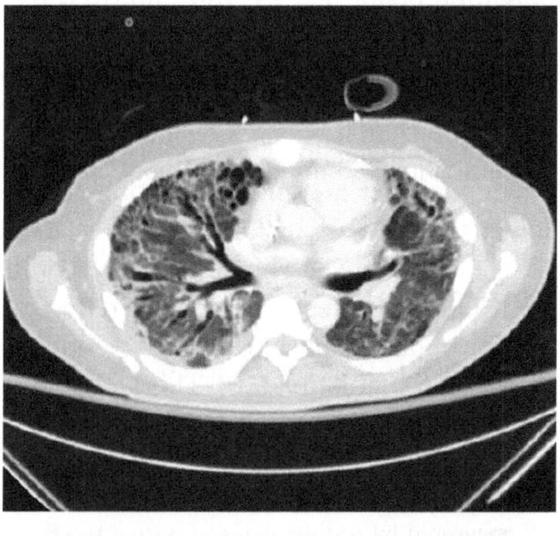

Fig. 30.2 Three months later, with improved inflammation

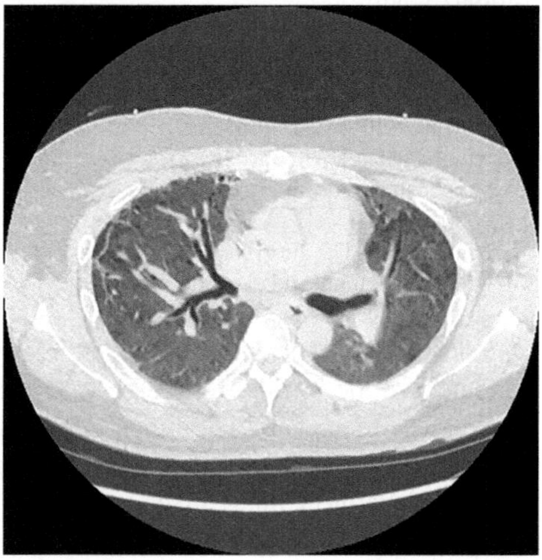

Fig. 30.3 Improved architecture 6 months later

for years after the insult is resolved [11]. The healing potential of lungs remains an area of important basic and clinical research. The central premise is that if patients can survive severe respiratory failure, they have a good chance of recovery.

For patient selection, it is very important to consider the three V-V ECMO strategies. Type 1 is to help recover from an acute illness. Type 2 is a bridge to transplant. Type 3 is a bridge to decision-making (i.e., trying to determine a diagnosis and if a transplant is an option). The focus of this chapter will be on Type 1, since the bridge to transplant depends on regional transplant practice. A bridge to decision-making is a nebulous area as clinicians try to make decisions about diagnostic and transplant options.

Premorbid Conditions and Scoring Systems

Even outside the technical aspect of decision-making about ECMO cannulation, there are many decisions about who should be cannulated. This field is evolving. Recognizing that ECMO is a tool to deliver oxygen for the short term, there must be a strategy on how the ECMO run will allow the underlying issue to resolve. Will the patient have enough healing potential that they will no longer need ECMO because the lungs will heal, or will the patient require a lung transplant, which is a limited resource? As a pulmonologist, medical history can help predict the trajectory. Chronic lung disease does not fare well on ECMO unless it is a bridge to transplant. Typically, by the time a patient with pulmonary fibrosis requires mechanical or ECMO support, the scarring in the parenchyma prevents healing. Patients with high oxygen needs prior to acute decompensation often have limited recovery reserve. Parenchymal scarring affects the lungs' ability to absorb oxygen but also causes a loss of the repair mechanisms. Although not an absolute contraindication, special thought needs to be given to patients on chronic oxygen. The ECMO community has been transitioning away from absolute contraindications to more relative contraindications. For example, there are some 70-year-old patients who have more physiologic reserve than those who are 50. But a history of CVA or intracranial hemorrhage also portends a risk of stroke and poor recovery potential, even if the patient is young.

The greatest component of ECMO decision-making is the trajectory of oxygen requirements. If the patient has been on high-pressure ventilator support with high oxygen content, this can help define survival odds. It is well understood that the high driving pressures from the ventilator convey a high mortality risk. It is unclear if the high ventilator pressure solely damages the lung or if it reflects the degree of lung injury. Either way, scoring systems often use days on a ventilator as a decision point.

There are a number of scoring systems that can be used to start the conversation about who should go on ECMO. They are by no means definitive. The RESP Score is one of the validated scores for V-V ECMO [12]. The major components are discrete medical points (Table 30.1). This tool and others are not perfect, but they do help frame the issues and collect pertinent data.

Table 30.1 Components of RESP score

Age
Immunocompromised state
Duration on vent
Peak vent pressure >42 ccmH_2O
Etiology of ARDS
CNS dysfunction
Infections other than pneumonia
Paralytics
NO use
Bicarbonate use
$PaCO_2$ is over 75 mmgHG

Another key component for patient selection is not just what data is collected, but how decision-making occurs. These are frequent high stakes decision—from a life and death perspective, cost of care, labor intensity, and use of limited/finite resources. In a similar manner to Pulmonary Emboli Response Teams (PERT), shared decision-making improves decision-making and encourages a more proactive response [13]. In the event that ECMO is declined as a viable option, shared decision-making reduces the moral burden. This model is used in many centers across the world.

Equipment

At its most basic, and what would satisfy the reader's knowledge for this book, an ECMO circuit contains a drainage or inflow cannula, a pump motor, an artificial lung, and a return or outflow cannula (Fig. 30.4). There are other accessory components of connections, heat exchangers, flow probes, and control devices, but these components will not be discussed since they are out of the scope of this oxygen textbook. It is important to recognize that maintaining core body temperature does improve oxygen delivery and offloading of oxygen to organs. Monitoring devices can provide insight into oxygen content, but even a gross visualization of the tubing can show the oxygen-depleted drainage cannulas then being oxygenated and returning to the body oxygen-rich (Fig. 30.5).

To understand the circuit, there must be consensus on certain nomenclature. The Extracorporeal Life Support Organization (ELSO) created a task force that ultimately penned the ELSO Maastricht Treaty that serves as the primary authority on ECMO nomenclature [14]. There are many fine details within the Maastricht Treaty; however, most of it is not necessary to discuss in this chapter. There are some highlights worth mentioning, though. The key to orienting communication on ECMO cannulation is the use of a hyphen (−). What comes prior to the hyphen is located between the patient and the motor pump, and that which comes after the hyphen is between the pump and the patient. A simple example would be V-A ECMO. The "V" prior to the hyphen means that there is a cannula within the patient's venous system that is serving as the drainage or inflow limb into the pump. The "A" after

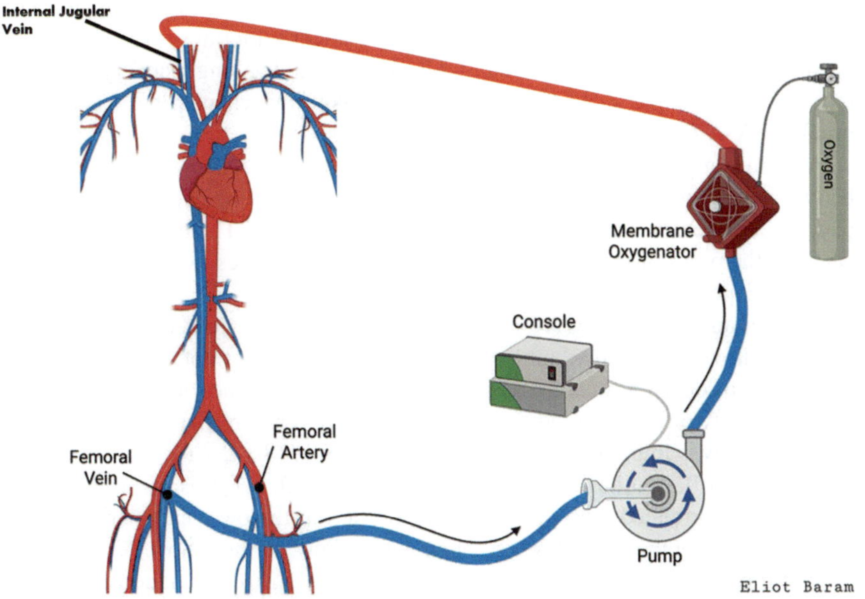

Fig. 30.4 A standard V-V ECMO with the drainage cannula in the right femoral vein with the oxygen-rich blood returning to the right Internal jugular vein. Notice this configuration is pulling oxygen-depleted blood from the venous side and returning oxygen-rich blood closer to the heart so the lungs can be supported. Image created by Eliot Baram in https://BioRender.com

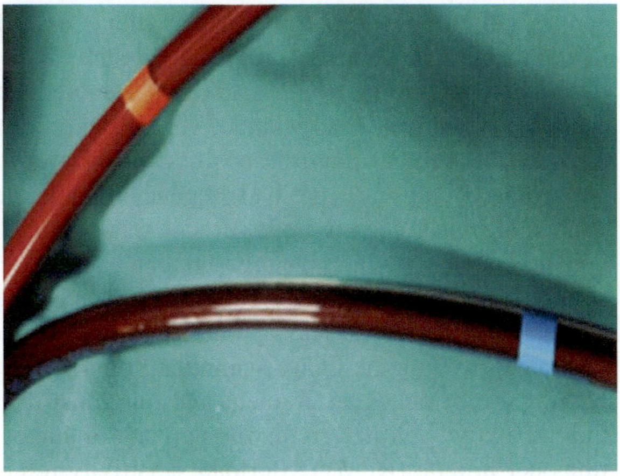

Fig. 30.5 Red tape—postmembrane blood, blue tape—premembrane blood

the hyphen denotes that the blood leaving the pump (and therefore the oxygenator) as the return or outflow limb is flowing into the patient's arterial system. As this is a book on oxygen, and the focus is on ECMO's role in aiding lung recovery, emphasis will be on the simple V-V ECMO circuit throughout this chapter, but it will touch briefly on V-A ECMO as well.

A more complex example would be something like VV-AV in which there would be two venous inflow cannulas to the pump system and two outflow limbs to the patient—one return via a vein and the other via an artery. There is even a significance to the order of the letters, but this complexity becomes extensive and is outside the scope of this chapter.

The cannulas themselves are variable in length, diameter, number and location of inflow/outflow ports, and whether they are heparin-coated or not. The most important aspect of decision-making regarding a cannula for an individual patient is the diameter (or two times the radius), often denoted by French (Fr) size. The Hagen-Poiseuille Law is imperative here: $Q = (\Delta P \times \pi \times R^4) / (8 \times L \times \mu)$.

The Hagen-Poiseuille Law importantly states that flow (Q) is most affected by and directly correlated with radius (R) due to the fourth power exponent. One can deduce, then, that the larger French cannula will allow for more flow. A practitioner must still optimize cannula size to the patient's body surface area, considering the size of their vasculature, however. This law highlights the importance of using ultrasound to maximize cannula size without causing vessel obstruction. Most cannula manufacturers report cannula size in French, which is equal to three times the outer circumference in millimeters (mm).

The most common type of pump motor used in ECMO circuits is the centrifugal pump. In some pediatric centers, roller pumps are used in neonates, but in adults, they only have a historical context. The important factors regarding centrifugal pumps are the pressure gradients as well as the flow dynamics. As the motor spins, it generates negative pressure on the drainage side of the patient or the portion prior to the hyphen in the nomenclature. The negative pressure pulls the (usually) deoxygenated, venous blood out of the body. The pressure after the centrifugal pump is positive as it flows back into the patient. These centrifugal pumps are preload dependent and afterload sensitive. Since the venous side has negative pressure, if there is not enough preload within the venous system, the negative pressure can cause "suck down" of the walls of the vessel. This can be visually seen as chatter in the ECMO cannulas (https://edecmo.org/chatter-causes-ivc-trauma/) [15]. Once the vessel walls become "sucked down" on the ECMO cannula, flow will decrease through the circuit as blood can no longer be drained, and one must troubleshoot how best to treat this—usually by either giving the patient volume or lowering the circuit's rotations per minute (RPM). Afterload sensitivity refers to the pressure the return flow is pushing against. This is most concerning for V-A ECMO. Imagine a patient initially going on ECMO, typically rather sick with a low systemic vascular resistance (SVR). As patients recover, their SVR does as well, increasing relatively. The set RPMs on the ECMO circuit are now attempting to flow against a higher level of resistance, usually resulting in a lower flow speed (say dropping from four liters per minute [lpm] to three lpm). Based on the patient's body surface area (BSA), three lpm of flow may not be adequate for perfusion, and again adjustments may have to be made—either lowering the SVR pharmacologically or increasing the RPMs to increase flow.

The last, yet most critical component worth exploring is the membrane oxygenator. It is for all intents and purposes the "lung" of the ECMO circuit. It can serve three main purposes for the patient: carbon dioxide (CO_2) removal, oxygen (O_2) delivery, and heat exchange. Most artificial lungs in use today utilize polymethyl pentene hollow fibers. These fibers allow for a longer lifespan compared to earlier models while still able to meet the metabolic demands of patients [16]. The ideal membrane lung allows for maximum gas exchange with minimal resistance to flow. They achieve this by having a large surface area, just like the actual human lung.

Sweep gas is an oxygen-air mixture delivered to the circuit. Adjusting the sweep rate, also defined in liters per minute, determines the degree of CO_2 removal from the patient. It is effectively the minute ventilation of the ECMO circuit. Sweep gas can be considered the same as alveolar ventilation on the ventilator. Initially, when a patient is placed on ECMO, a rule of thumb is to set the sweep gas flow rate equal to, or sometimes half of, the flow rate. Arterial blood gases can be sampled, and the sweep gas flow rate can then be adjusted by the equation: $\text{Sweep}_{\text{new}} = \text{sweep}_{\text{current}} \times (pCO_2/\text{desired } pCO_2)$ [17]. As an example, a sweep gas rate of 4 lpm can be considered equivalent to 4 lpm of minute ventilation. If the sweep gas rate were to be reduced all the way to zero, there would be no gas flow through the membrane lung. Blood would still flow through the membrane lung, but there would be no gas exchange occurring (this is done prior to removing a patient from V-V ECMO during the weaning process).

Sweep works via counter-current exchange. The oxygen-air mixed gas is delivered traveling in the opposite direction of blood flow, interfaces with the oxygen-poor blood at the membrane, allowing oxygen to diffuse from the gas to the blood. At the same time, the CO_2 is diffusing down a gradient from high concentration in the blood to low concentration in the gas for its removal. Ironically, most clinicians consider ECMO for oxygenation issues, but it is far more effective in removing CO_2. There are risks for rapid correction of hypercapnia.

A practitioner can assess the performance of an oxygenator by checking "pre" and "post" blood gases, analogous to venous blood gases and arterial blood gases, respectively. Oxygenators come with a sample port just before and after the oxygenator. This pre-oxygenator blood gas can be considered equivalent to a central venous blood gas, in which you would expect a relatively low pO_2 and relatively higher pCO_2. The post-oxygenator gas should see a marginal drop in pCO_2 and a drastic increase in pO_2. If there is not a drastic rise in pO_2, or if the absolute number is less than 300 mmHg, it may be a hint at inefficiency of the oxygenator. This is most likely due to clot buildup or fibrin deposition in the oxygenator. This reduction in oxygen diffusion is typically a sign that the oxygenator in the circuit needs to be exchanged.

How ECMO Helps: A Focus on Oxygen

As aerobic organisms, our metabolism is most linked to oxygen consumption and can be measured with the oxygen consumed every minute, VO_2. At rest, an adult's metabolism rate is approximately 120 cc/min/m^2 [17]. This rate is variable, increasing with activity, fevering, drugs, or decreasing with sedation, paralysis, or cooling. The amount of oxygen that is delivered to tissues is denoted by DO_2. This normally occurs by O_2 absorption in the lungs and delivery to tissues via the capillaries. Approximately 20–25% of oxygen is consumed per cardiac cycle. Hence, a "normal" central venous gas saturation is approximately 75–80%. ECMO helps in oxygen delivery, but at a cellular level, it does not improve oxygen consumption if there is mitochondrial dysfunction.

Maintaining a certain DO_2 to VO_2 ratio is imperative for patients to maintain normal aerobic metabolism. The amount of oxygen in the blood is best described with the oxygen content equation:

$$\mathrm{CaO_2} = \left(\mathrm{SaO_2} \times \mathrm{Hgb} \times 1.34\right) + \left(\mathrm{PaO_2} \times 0.003\right)$$

CaO_2, oxygen content; SaO_2, oxygen saturation; Hgb, hemoglobin; PaO_2, arterial partial pressure oxygen

As shown, the oxygen bound to hemoglobin is drastically more important than the oxygen dissolved in blood. Anemia can radically affect the oxygen content and, thus, delivery. Delivery itself depends on the patient's cardiac output:

$$\mathrm{DO_2} = \mathrm{CaO_2} \times \mathrm{CO} \times 10$$

DO_2, oxygen delivery; CaO_2, oxygen content; CO, cardiac output

Normal delivery of oxygen is 600 cc/min/m^{2,} which is approximately five times what is consumed. This 5:1 ratio of oxygen delivery to consumption is an important ratio to maintain. As oxygenation becomes increasingly impaired by disease states, with a relative inability to maintain cardiac output, the 5:1 ratio decreases until aerobic metabolism becomes anaerobic, leading to lactic acid byproduct buildup.

As cardiopulmonary disease progresses, the patient becomes relatively hypoxic and hypercapnic. Hypoxic pulmonary vasoconstriction, while having a role in shunting blood flow to functional alveoli, does place stress on the right ventricle (RV) [18]. As pulmonary disease progresses, increasing in severity to acute respiratory distress syndrome (ARDS), these effects become more pronounced. That is, until a patient is placed on a mechanical ventilator, when oxygenation and ventilation may be partially restored. Mechanical ventilator helps to correct the effects of hypoxia and hypercapnia on pulmonary vascular resistance (PVR), which stresses the right ventricle but induces its own stressors on the RV. Mechanical ventilation will induce a change in both the preload and afterload of the RV [19]. If, however, ARDS is severe enough, mechanical ventilation may not be sufficient to correct hypoxia and hypercapnia. In addition, the stress of mechanical ventilation may be injurious to the lungs and prevent recovery.

Enter V-V ECMO. ECMO will be extremely efficient in managing a patient's hypoxia and hypercapnia, thereby reducing the afterload stress for the RV. Depending on cannulation strategy and flow, there is also the possibility of a reduction of RV preload as the drainage cannula applies negative pressure throughout the vena cava [20].

As V-V ECMO is now managing the patient's gas exchange, the patient becomes less reliant on mechanical ventilation. Lung rest, or so-called ultra-low volume lung rest, strategies can now be utilized to allow the lung to heal with less theoretical risk from mechanical ventilation and barotrauma. Although there is debate on the best strategy for ventilator settings, ELSO recommendations are for the following goals: Inspiratory plateau pressure <25 cm H_2O, PEEP >10 cm H_2O, RR 4–15 breaths/min, with an FiO_2 as low as possible to maintain saturations [21].

Veno-Arterial ECMO and Differential Hypoxia

The cardiac and pulmonary systems are intimately entwined with one another. Although cardiogenic shock, cardiopulmonary arrest, or other indications for veno-arterial ECMO (V-A ECMO) are often not specifically due to hypoxia, it is still a support modality worth mentioning in a book on oxygen.

Veno-arterial ECMO is primarily a cardiac support modality. Just as in V-V ECMO, there is a venous drainage component, which then proceeds through the motor and oxygenator prior to returning to the patient. Unlike V-V ECMO, however, the return outflow limb infuses into the patient's arterial system as opposed to the venous system. This is important in several ways. Most importantly, you are now entirely bypassing the cardiopulmonary system. Unlike V-V ECMO, you are no longer reliant on cardiac output for oxygen delivery. So, while this system is primarily for cardiac support, lung rest can also be achieved if there is concomitant pulmonary disease, as the ECMO oxygenator is still providing oxygenation and ventilation support.

The arterialized blood flows retrograde through the arterial system if the patient is cannulated peripherally. The oxygenated blood enters via the femoral artery, flowing up past the abdominal aortic arterial branches, pressurizing the left subclavian, left carotid, and innominate vessels prior to settling in the aortic root to distribute through the coronaries. The recovering heart is tasked with ejecting blood against this retrograde flow.

As alluded to, there are an array of reasons why a patient may end up on V-A ECMO, many of which are without pulmonary disease or hypoxia. A short, partial list of these would be cardiogenic shock, massive pulmonary embolism with hemodynamic changes, and cardiac arrest. While lung pathology and hypoxia may not immediately be present, many of these patients have prolonged hospital stays, often requiring mechanical ventilation at some juncture. It is often the case that the timing of the cardiac and pulmonary pathologies coincides.

Differential hypoxia, also known as Harlequinn Syndrome or North–South Syndrome, is a process of cardiac recovery for patients on V-A ECMO. As the heart recovers, it will begin to eject more and more blood that has traversed the cardiopulmonary system. If the patient is still on lung protective ventilation settings or has a pulmonary pathology such as pneumonia, the ejected blood going through the native circulation may be hypoxic. This hypoxic "blue" blood mixes with the arterialized "red" blood that is still flowing retrograde from the V-A ECMO circuit. This shunt physiology creates a mixing cloud somewhere within the aorta, putting the patient at risk for hypoxemia, namely, within the coronary and innominate vessels.

The innominate vessel, which gives rise to the right common carotid and right subclavian vessels, is therefore the first major vessel affected by differential hypoxemia. Therefore, differential hypoxemia can be monitored by assessing pulse oximetry on the right upper extremity or via invasive arterial blood pressure monitoring with arterial blood gas sampling in the same limb.

There are several ways in which a treatment team can treat differential hypoxia. The first would be to treat any underlying pulmonary pathology or adjust ventilator settings if still utilizing ultra-lung rest settings. Decreasing the shunt physiology in the lungs would be the primary way of treating differential hypoxia. Another strategy would be to increase the RPMs of the ECMO circuit, thus increasing flow. This increase in retrograde flow would displace the mixing cloud back toward the aortic root. The major downside of this is that the newly recovering heart is now ejecting against an even higher afterload, possibly impeding recovery. Another consideration would be to reduce the patient's native cardiac output, forcing more blood through the ECMO circuit and again reducing shunt physiology. Reducing cardiac output could result in the way of increasing sedation, possibly paralysis or using a beta blocker. The final, most invasive strategy would be to convert to a new support platform. This would come in the form of introducing a new outflow cannula into the venous system, creating a V-AV ECMO circuit. Now, arterialized blood is returning to the right side of the heart, eliminating shunt physiology. As the heart continues to recover, the arterial limb can be spliced from the circuit, leaving the patient on a simple V-V ECMO platform.

Conclusion

ECMO is an increasingly used tool to help improve oxygenation during an acute severe illness where routine mechanical ventilation and circulatory support have failed. ECMO is truly an old process that has had improved technology. Although ECMO does not improve the underlying pathology, it is a means to improve arterial oxygenation to support life as a bridge to healing or transplantation. Future technology will continue to improve the safety and efficacy of ECMO. For now, it continues to help support ICU clinicians to deliver oxygen to sustain life. Other chapters in this book address a more geographic perspective on the availability of ECMO across North America and the world.

Declarations

Competing Interests The authors have no competing interests to declare that are relevant to the content of this manuscript.

Ethics Approval The authors declare that this manuscript does not include primary research with human participants.

The authors declare that this manuscript does not include primary studies involving animals.

Bibliography

1. Puri N, Baram M, Cavarocchi NC. Extracorporeal membrane oxygenation. Crit Care Clin. 2017;33(4):xi–xii. https://doi.org/10.1016/j.ccc.2017.07.002. PMID: 28887936. https://www.sciencedirect.com/science/article/pii/S0749070417300544?via%3Dihub.
2. Brogan TV, Lequier L, Lorusso R, MacLaren G, Peek GJ (Giles J.), editor. Extracorporeal life support: the ELSO red book. Extracorporeal Life Support Organization, issuing body. Ann Arbor: Extracorporeal Life Support Organization; 2017.
3. Merschel M. The chaotic beginnings of the tool that made heart surgery possible. American Heart Association; 2024. https://www.heart.org/en/news/2024/11/04/the-chaotic-beginnings-of-the-tool-that-made-heart-surgery-possible.
4. Hill JD, O'Brien TG, Murray JJ, Dontigny L, Bramson ML, Osborn JJ, Gerbode F. Prolonged extracorporeal oxygenation for acute post-traumatic respiratory failure (shock-lung syndrome). Use of the Bramson membrane lung. N Engl J Med. 1972;286(12):629–34. https://doi.org/10.1056/NEJM197203232861204. PMID: 5060491. https://www.nejm.org/doi/full/10.1056/NEJM197203232861204.
5. Bartlett RH. Esperanza: the first neonatal ECMO patient. ASAIO J. 2017;63(6):832–43. https://doi.org/10.1097/MAT.0000000000000697.
6. Zapol WM, Snider MT, Hill JD, Fallat RJ, Bartlett RH, Edmunds LH, Morris AH, Peirce EC 2nd, Thomas AN, Proctor HJ, Drinker PA, Pratt PC, Bagniewski A, Miller RG Jr. Extracorporeal membrane oxygenation in severe acute respiratory failure. A randomized prospective study. JAMA. 1979;242(20):2193–6. https://doi.org/10.1001/jama.242.20.2193. PMID: 490805. https://pubmed.ncbi.nlm.nih.gov/490805/.
7. Morris AH, Wallace CJ, Menlove RL, Clemmer TP, Orme JF Jr, Weaver LK, Dean NC, Thomas F, East TD, Pace NL, Suchyta MR, Beck E, Bombino M, Sittig DF, Böhm S, Hoffmann B, Becks H, Butler S, Pearl J, Rasmusson B. Randomized clinical trial of pressure-controlled inverse ratio ventilation and extracorporeal CO2 removal for adult respiratory distress syndrome. Am J Respir Crit Care Med. 1994;149(2 Pt 1):295–305. https://doi.org/10.1164/ajrccm.149.2.8306022. Erratum in: Am J Respir Crit Care Med 1994 Mar;149(3 Pt 1):838. PMID: 8306022. https://pubmed.ncbi.nlm.nih.gov/8306022/.
8. Peek GJ, et al. Efficacy and economic assessment of conventional ventilatory support versus extracorporeal membrane oxygenation for severe adult respiratory failure (CESAR): a multicentre randomised controlled trial. Lancet. 2009;374(9698):1351–63.
9. Combes A, Hajage D, Capellier G, Demoule A, Lavoué S, Guervilly C, Da Silva D, Zafrani L, Tirot P, Veber B, Maury E, Levy B, Cohen Y, Richard C, Kalfon P, Bouadma L, Mehdaoui H, Beduneau G, Lebreton G, Brochard L, Ferguson ND, Fan E, Slutsky AS, Brodie D, Mercat A, EOLIA Trial Group, REVA, ECMONet. Extracorporeal membrane oxygenation for severe acute respiratory distress syndrome. N Engl J Med. 2018;378(21):1965–75. https://doi.org/10.1056/NEJMoa1800385. PMID: 29791822.
10. Combes A, Fanelli V, Pham T, Ranieri VM; European Society of Intensive Care Medicine Trials Group and the "Strategy of Ultra-Protective lung ventilation with Extracorporeal CO2 Removal for New-Onset moderate to severe ARDS" (SUPERNOVA) investigators. Feasibility

and safety of extracorporeal CO_2 removal to enhance protective ventilation in acute respiratory distress syndrome: the SUPERNOVA study. Intensive Care Med. 2019;45(5):592–600. https://doi.org/10.1007/s00134-019-05567-4. Epub 2019 Feb 21. PMID: 30790030.
11. Barry PJ, Donaldson AL, Jones AM. Ivacaftor for cystic fibrosis. BMJ. 2018;361:k1783.
12. Schmidt M, Bailey M, Sheldrake J, Hodgson C, Aubron C, Rycus PT, Scheinkestel C, Cooper DJ, Brodie D, Pellegrino V, Combes A, Pilcher D. Predicting survival after extracorporeal membrane oxygenation for severe acute respiratory failure. The respiratory extracorporeal membrane oxygenation survival prediction (RESP) score. Am J Respir Crit Care Med. 2014;189(11):1374–82. https://doi.org/10.1164/rccm.201311-2023OC. PMID: 24693864.
13. Baram M, Awsare B, Merli G. Pulmonary embolism in intensive care unit. Crit Care Clin. 2020;36(3):427–35. https://doi.org/10.1016/j.ccc.2020.02.001. Epub 2020 May 11. PMID: 32473689.
14. Conrad S, Broman L, Taccone F, Lorusso R, Malfertheiner M, Pappalardo F, Di Nardo M, Belliato M, Grazioli L, Barbaro R, McMullan D, Pellegrino V, Brodie D, Bembea M, Fan E, Mendonca M, Diaz R, Bartlett R. The extracorporeal life support organization Maastricht treaty for nomenclature in extracorporeal life support. A position paper of the extracorporeal life support organization. Am J Respir Crit Care Med. 2018;198(4):447–51. https://doi.org/10.1164/rccm.201710-2130CP.
15. Bellezzo J. https://edecmo.org/chatter-causes-ivc-trauma/. 12 May 2014.
16. Toomasian J, Schreiner R, Meyer D, Schmidt M, Hagan S, Griffith G, Bartlett R, Cook K. A polymethylene fiber gas exchanger for long-term extracorporeal life support. ASAIO J. 2005;51(4):390–7. https://doi.org/10.1097/01.mat.0000169111.66328.a8.
17. MacLaren G, Brodie D, Lorusso R, Peek G, Thiagarajan R, Vercaemst L, editors. Extracorporeal life support: the ELSO Big Red Book. 6th ed. Ann Arbor: Extracorporeal Life Support Organization; 2022.
18. Lump A, Slinger P. Hypoxic pulmonary vasoconstriction physiology and anesthetic implications. Anesthesiology. 2015;122(4):932–46. https://doi.org/10.1097/ALN.0000000000000569.
19. Mahmood S, Pinsky M. Heart-lung interactions during mechanical ventilation: the basics. Ann Transl Med. 2018;6(18):349. https://doi.org/10.21037/atm.2018.04.29.
20. Grant C, Richards J, Frakes M, Cohen J, Wilcox S. ECMO and right ventricular failure: review of literature. J Intensive Care Med. 2021;36(3):352–60. https://doi.org/10.1177/0885066619900503.
21. Tonna J, Abrams D, Brodie D, Greenwood J, Mateo-Sidron J, Usman A, Fan E. Management of adult patients supported with venovenous membrane oxygenation (VV ECMO): guideline from the Extracorporeal Life Support Organization (ELSO). ASAIO J. 2021;67(6):601–10. https://doi.org/10.1097/MAT.0000000000001432.

ECMO in the Time of Pandemics

31

Michael Baram and Christine Stead

Introduction

The question is not whether there will be another pandemic. Instead, the question is when will there be another pandemic. The focus of this book is on oxygen, so naturally the focus of this chapter will be on respiratory pandemics such as the Spanish flu, H1N1, Polio, COVID, and near misses such as SARS and MERS. However, to better understand the nature of global health, other worldwide outbreaks such as cholera, Ebola, and HIV need to be included. Each of these viral illnesses posed a unique challenge to the world and created unique needs to which the world had to adapt. Before virology was a science in 1892, the world had to create basic tenets of public health to reduce and slow the spread of unidentified pathogens. As research and understanding evolved, organizations had to create methods for sharing knowledge and sharing technology [1].

Definitions in Epidemiology [2]

There are four important terms to consider when defining the status of an infection at a given time point: endemic, outbreak, epidemic, and pandemic [3]. An endemic infection would define a scenario where the expected number of cases is consistent with previous years' incidence of a disease. An outbreak is defined as a sudden rise in the incidence of a disease. It can be in a novel location or an increase in number.

M. Baram (✉)
Division of Pulmonary and Critical Care, Sidney Kimmel Medical College, Thomas Jefferson University, Philadelphia, PA, USA
e-mail: Michael.Baram@jefferson.edu

C. Stead
ELSO, Ann Arbor, MI, USA

G. C. Kane et al. (eds.), *Oxygen*, https://doi.org/10.1007/978-3-032-18934-9_31

But overall, it remains a low number. The next increase is epidemics that occur over a larger geographic area usually described by a country or neighboring countries. A pandemic would be defined by the continued spread of the disease to a global population. Current lifestyles with airplanes can spark infections that travel from country to country, continent to continent, in very short time frames. The effects of a pandemic can be viewed from both global and individual perspectives. This chapter will address this duality. Understanding the spread of respiratory pandemics and also understanding how ECMO can save lives from the individual perspective are the approaches this chapter will take.

Current dialogues now include noninfectious medical conditions as causes of epidemics and pandemics. It is well recognized that the effects of narcotics on the United States, Europe, and the rest of the world could be considered a pandemic, but this chapter will refer to classic infectious etiologies. The epidemic of gun violence in the United States continues to destroy lives. The root of this disease is not a microbiological infectious disease. Recognizing that these societal ailments are extremely important and equally lethal, these issues will not be covered.

History of Pandemics (with Emphasis on Respiratory Ailments)

Description of plagues can be read in the Old Testament as well as the New Testament. Most of the descriptions of these ailments were physical descriptions of boils and sores. As society became more agrarian and started residing in established cities, the descriptions changed more to outbreaks of cholera, Ebola, and flea-borne disease. With a mix of religion, early science, and folklore, societies began identifying patterns to avoid disease. As early as 1377, the City of Dubrovnik began quarantining visitors to be sure that they did not bring the plague to their city [4]. This was also used to isolate the infected who contracted the disease to avoid infecting others. Although plagues have existed as far back as written history, the Spanish flu pandemic of 1918 is one of the earliest pandemics that is well understood that truly caused respiratory ailment.

The Spanish flu is occasionally referred to as the forgotten flu due to its occurrence on the heels of World War I. There were more US casualties from the Spanish flu than the United States lost in World War I. With the tight military barracks and transport of troops to Europe, the virus spread. This relatively modern pandemic occurred in the twentieth century, and oxygen was already available, but not like today. Its delivery was improved during 1917 to help overcome toxic gases from trench warfare. The onset of the flu of 1918 was very rapid and often caused an alveolar hemorrhage that was lethal.

Polio, in contrast to flu and coronavirus pandemics that resulted in oxygenation issues, resulted in muscle weakness that created more of a ventilatory defect and failure of carbon dioxide clearance. This was addressed and highlighted by the lifesaving Iron Lung created by Dr. Drinker.

Severe Acute Respiratory Syndrome (SARS) was first recognized in 2003. It was a coronavirus as well that was mostly limited to Asia. With excellent public health, this virus, which carried a 10% mortality, was short lived [5]. The lethality and early containment caused the virus to burn out quickly. Although the SARS threat was short lived, it did spread to 37 countries. The rapid containment of this disease highlights the importance of groups such as the World Health Organization. Clear epidemiology work helped contain this pathogen. With its high mortality rate, this could have been more lethal than the recent COVID-19 outbreak.

COVID-19 with a Transition to ECMO

COVID-19 was a global pandemic, with rapidly spreading and mutating variants. The early wave with global impact began in Wuhan, China, affected the respiratory system, which advanced to Acute Respiratory Distress (ARDS). Different from other pandemics described above, this pandemic was approached with an international effort. Medication, education, and technology that were not previously available to healthcare providers were mobilized across the world. The story of COVID-19 is important to learn to help prepare for the next world pandemic. Early on, the latent period, which included an infectious period, often occurred. This asymptomatic phase contributed to this disease spreading like wildfire.

As this virus began spreading, medical professionals and public health officials began tracking its spread. The World Health Organization had been aware of a new outbreak with an unknown etiology in December 2019 in China. The Incident Management Support Team was activated on January 2, 2020 (all three levels: country, regional, and headquarters), and in mid-January the virus was named as the "2019 Novel Coronavirus" [6]. The virus was sequenced and posted online (GenBank) by Edward Holmes, University of Sydney, in cooperation with Yong-Zhen Zhang, Fudan University, Shanghai—a coordinated effort with the hospital, university, and CDC in Wuhan [7]. WHO would send members to meet with President Xi to better understand the situation and response, while screening for the virus began from those traveling from Wuhan to other countries in the region. On March 11, 2020, WHO declared COVID-19 a global pandemic [8].

Real-Time Communication

Colleagues from ELSO outside of Wuhan had been consulting colleagues in the region on the new cases and how best to apply ECMO for those who might benefit. Given the early results of patients on ECMO with COVID-19, there was a need for more collaboration and communication.

A WhatsApp group was established called "COVID-19 ECMO," which quickly reached a capacity of 400 at the time. Several other groups were created, but this was the go-to for real-time communication, where practitioners would offer advice and generally learn together in real-time as the virus made its way around the world.

Real-Time Data

The importance of real-time data could not be overstated, especially as clinicians were learning about the effects of COVID-19 and how best to treat it. Health equipment resources quickly became limited, including basics like PPE. As hospitals and countries made decisions about access to resource-intensive therapies, we believed this data was necessary to both improve outcomes and change access at multiple levels of decision-making (hospital, regional, provincial, and country).

The ELSO Registry was turned into a live registry where the summary statistics were publicly available. Our intent was to help practitioners in the field, but the public-facing Registry would be often inquired about by multiple news agencies throughout the pandemic, including *The Wall Street Journal* in Japan and *The New York Times*, along with local news agencies around the world. ELSO leadership was often asked to help explain what the data was showing to many kinds of institutions and people.

This global effort to collect and share data would come to change access to ECMO as it demonstrated improved efficacy for some COVID-19 patients, and centers got better at identifying when a patient might benefit from ECMO as a lifesaving option. Several countries changed their early position to allow access to ECMO care, thanks to the ELSO Registry and the public-facing outcomes for COVID-19.

ECMO Capacity

When the H1N1 virus began spreading in 2008, ELSO created an ECMO capacity map—a website where our ECMO centers could indicate whether they had the capacity to accept referrals for ECMO or not [9] (Fig. 31.1).

With so many factors affecting capacity restraints, ELSO made this system as simple as possible to encourage participation. The capacity map asked programs to identify their center's capacity status in the following categories: (green) available; (yellow) limited capacity; or (red) not available. Data were time-stamped when entered, which was also publicly available as a signal to reflect accuracy. More complexity may have allowed more data and studies, but the trade-off in participation was not worth more complexity (e.g., source of limitations). As a result, participation was reasonably good.

ECMO capacity was also made public and used by many—referring centers to ECMO centers, along with news agencies, public health entities, and patients and families. ELSO received many calls from those looking for ECMO capacity who were unable to find it in their region during waves of higher spread in communities around the world.

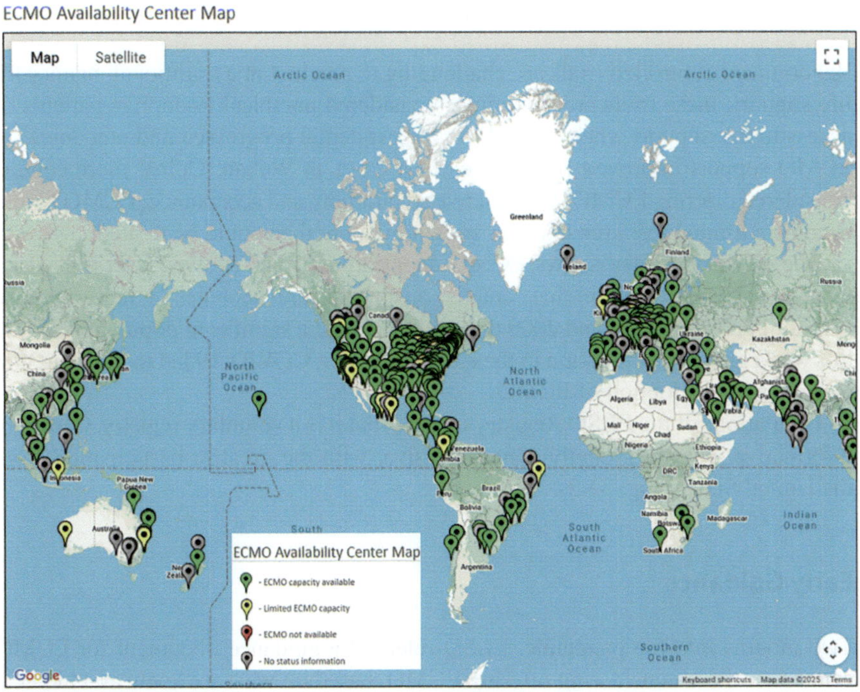

Fig. 31.1 ECMO capacity map as seen on July 26, 2025

Access to ECMO—FDA

Although many clinicians were aware of ECMO, few understood that ECMO was not approved for prolonged use. Its approved limit was only for a few days—this created a regulatory nightmare. On April 7, 2020, the FDA granted Emergency Use Authorization (EUA) for the use of ECMO to treat hospitalized COVID-19 patients [10]. Prior to the pandemic, there were very few devices (two oxygenators) that were approved by the FDA for use as ECMO. Device manufacturers did not readily pursue approval for this device, when devices were available as a mechanical circulatory support and approved as such. The FDA had to respond to this massive spike in ARDS incidence.

The FDA's EUA was important in improving access to ECMO in the United States. For countries that followed the FDA or used it as a pseudo-agency for themselves, this was sufficient to improve access during the pandemic in those areas. Some regions of the world had difficulties where ECMO did not have this kind of clearance. For example, in Europe, physicians assumed liability for devices used off-label. This became a risk in the region that was not resolved during the pandemic, except for by achieving CE-mark-approved status in the case of Europe.

ECMO as an Accepted Life Support

Randomized controlled trials are challenging to conduct in a traditional manner for life support; these trials are sometimes considered unethical to deprive patients of access to life support when needed. As the pandemic progressed and outcomes for ECMO support improved from the earliest cases in Wuhan, China, more centers considered offering ECMO. With increased publicity and acceptance, ECMO would become a limited resource that was sought by more than could be treated.

The ELSO Registry shows ECMO adoption as it has evolved over the years, from a fairly small amount that centered on children and neonates in the early days. Not until H1N1 in 2008 and 2009 did adults become a significant population. While this was a growing population in the ELSO Registry, COVID-19 led to much greater awareness and adoption of ECMO.

Limitations of the ELSO Registry include that it is a voluntary registry. Cases are informative, but not globally comprehensive, with the greatest participation from the United States (Fig. 31.2).

Early Guidance

Two months into the pandemic, ELSO released a guidance document for ECMO centers, or those considering offering ECMO, based on what we knew as a medical society at that time. In this document, we attempted to share guidance on whether COVID-19 patients should be considered for ECMO, under what circumstances,

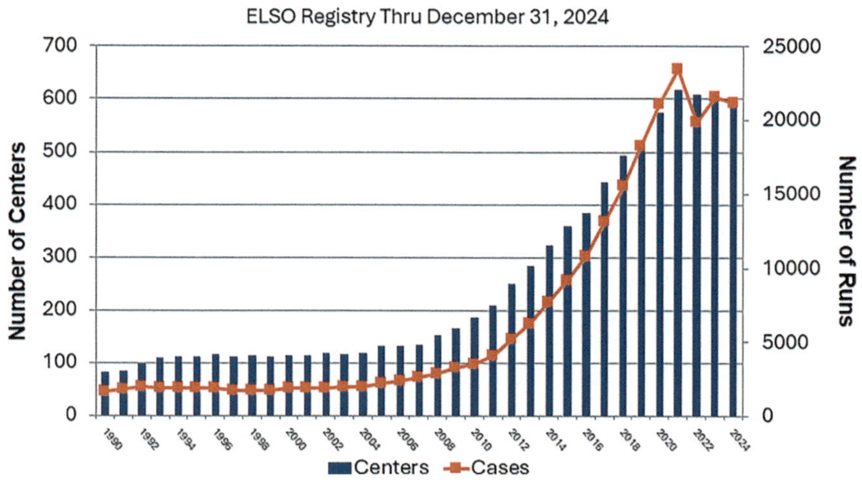

Fig. 31.2 ELSO Registry Data showing contributing centers and patient runs through December 31, 2024 [11]

and how to manage other patient ECMO candidates in the context of the pandemic [12].

In a year, ELSO would update this guidance document to be much more organized, including a tiered structure for candidacy considerations that mapped to resource constraints [13]. A year into this pandemic, centers had to increasingly make difficult decisions on access to resource-intensive care, such as ECMO. We felt it was important to provide an objective source that could be used at the local level, based on what we had learned at that time as a global medical society.

Early Findings

ELSO was able to release one of the largest data sets on ECMO experience with COVID-19 patients early in 2020. Data from 1035 patients from the ELSO Registry, contributed by 213 hospitals in 36 countries, with over 1500 contributing authors, showed that this early study had 37.4% in-hospital mortality at 90 days after ECMO initiation [14]. There were several important factors with this study:

- A large and diverse data set of ECMO COVID-19 patients showed efficacy of ECMO.
- While many studies were being published rapidly at the time, this data set was of relatively high quality.
- Results were similar to those of ARDS (Fig. 31.3).

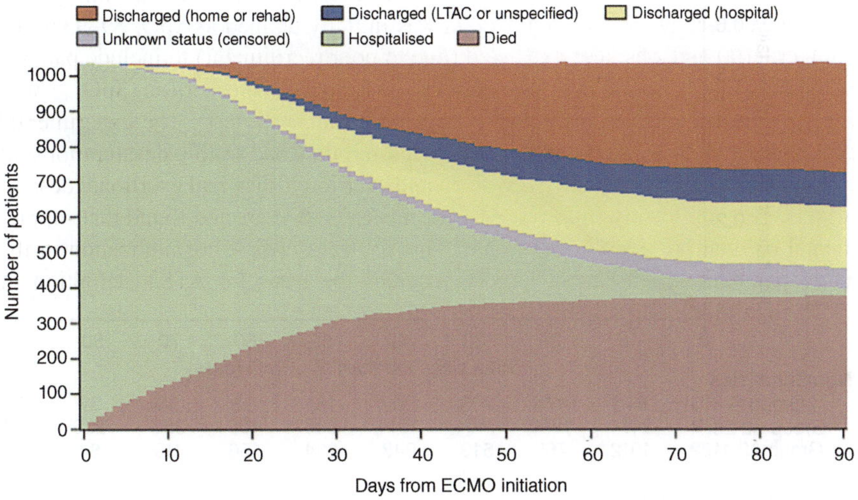

Fig. 31.3 Early results of COVID-19 patients on ECMO from the ELSO Registry [15]

Evolving Findings

Months later, the ELSO Registry was demonstrating worsening mortality rates in the COVID-19 data. This warranted a follow-up paper to our early paper quickly, with a different message: COVID-19 patients were not to be treated like typical ARDS patients, and patients did better in more experienced centers. Data included 4812 patients from 349 centers in 41 countries. In-hospital mortality after 90 days of the initiation of ECMO was 36.9% for early-adopting centers compared with 51.9% from May 1 to December 31, 2020, while late-adopting centers' in-hospital mortality was 58.9% [15] (Fig. 31.4).

Our charge began shifting to help improve education and training for late-adopting (or any) centers. The challenge, of course, was that we would need to provide something virtually and on a global scale.

Advancing Knowledge

Communication and collaboration were at a scale that made you believe in humanity—that people can rise to meet the crisis and support each other.

In July 2020, a team from Rush University published results on 40 patients showing the best outcomes of COVID-19 patients treated with ECMO that we were aware of at the time, with 15% mortality at the time of the study; several patients were still in hospital [17]. This study launched a series of webinars and speaking opportunities for this team, which started changing practice across many programs, specifically: prone positioning, early extubation, and ambulation on ECMO—not easy for every program to achieve with limited resources. Nonetheless, the

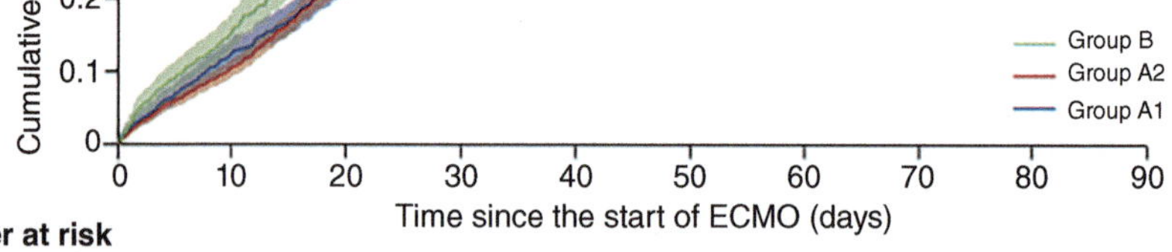

Number at risk

Group B 803	646	475	303	202	132	82	56	37	21
Group A2 2824	2471	1950	1404	1014	696	496	358	256	182
Group A2 1182	1012	765	513	348	234	156	110	84	60

Fig. 31.4 Early and late-adopting centers' outcomes during the pandemic for ECMO in COVID-19 [16]

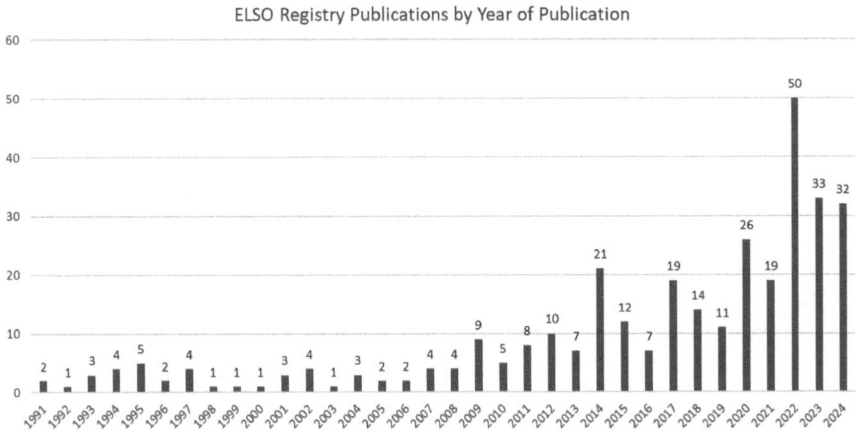

Fig. 31.5 Scientific publications based on data from the ELSO Registry

protocols used by this team challenged every program to consider adopting what they could.

Publications from the ELSO Registry doubled in the first year of the pandemic and peaked in its third year (2022 at 50 publications) [18]. This level of publications was important in advancing knowledge—coupled with free access to scientific publications related to COVID-19, which removed access barriers to those in more resource-constrained settings (Fig. 31.5).

Webinars were another means of advancing knowledge that was more real time than publications. ELSO hosted several of these and made the content available on our website thereafter (Fig. 31.6).

Advocacy

ELSO did what we could to make data available and worked with any institution or media outlet that was trying to improve access and outcomes for patients. We met with regulatory agencies, other medical societies, and others to advocate for better access to ECMO, where possible.

We also worked with many different journals and media organizations. Several articles were published in mainstream media, which helped with general awareness. One example from *The New York Times* journalist Sheri Fink went a long way toward this end, published in July 2021 and highlighting the challenges of access to ECMO at that time [19].

Further, we became adept in the power of social media for releasing information, newly published scientific evidence, and other content that we hoped would help programs better serve communities.

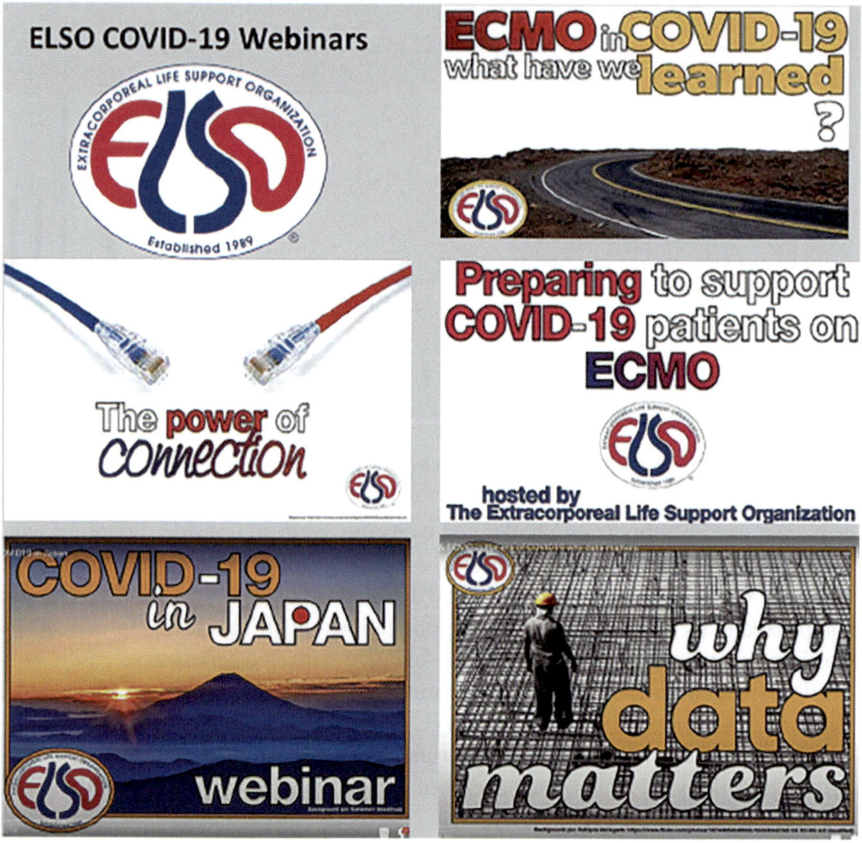

Fig. 31.6 Snapshot of ELSO Webinar series from 2020

In addition, advocating for the medical teams taking care of these patients became important. We would highlight how some teams were supporting their healthcare workers if it helped to share those ideas.

One example, which we incorporated into our 2021 Annual Report, was the work the Schwartz Center was doing to help support medical teams process trauma and high-stress situations—which was every day during the pandemic [20].

Scientific Conference During a Pandemic—Free, Globally Available, Virtual

ELSO made participation in our scientific conference free and virtually available everywhere. Collaboration and knowledge-sharing were paramount as we were all learning about this virus and its evolving effects on people around the world.

We were able to have speakers participate from everywhere and provide dedicated sessions on what we were learning about COVID-19.

Participation in this conference was ten (10) times that of the prior year, with 12,344 participants. The United States had its lowest percentage at an ELSO conference at that time: 55%. Broad global participation during this conference changed the trajectory of the annual ELSO conference from a regional focus to a global one and solidified the importance of making the program virtually available, which continues.

Collaboration

COVID-19 Critical Care Consortium started as ECMOCARD, led by John Fraser at Monash University in Brisbane, Australia. To deliver on a collaboration, ELSO worked with Oxford University from the United Kingdom and Monash University in Australia to create a Data Sharing Agreement among the participants that would allow data to be shared with this collaborative, which included the ISARIC data platform (Fig. 31.7).

Oxygen Delivery: India—The Last Mile

Through the COVID-19 Critical Care Consortium we met and had a wide variety of topics to share. One featured a discussion about the lack of oxygen in India. John Fraser invited a colleague from India to share the issue with this consortium. What was insightful about this discussion was that the issue was not oxygen production

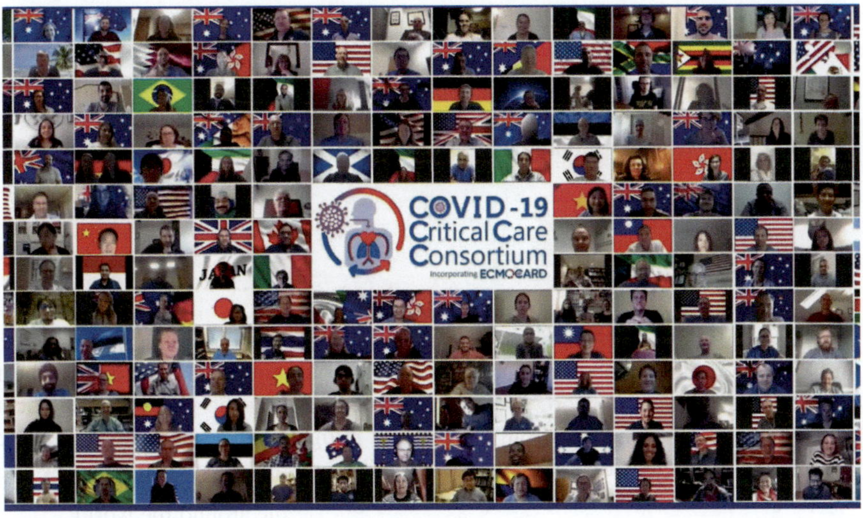

Fig. 31.7 COVID-19 Critical Care Consortium participation on a zoom call during the pandemic [21]

but oxygen delivery—what became known as "The Last Mile." Logistics to get oxygen to hospitals and clinics were difficult from production to a useful site.

There were oxygen production issues in other parts of the world, including Los Angeles, United States, at one point. Communities struggled with different resource constraints at different periods of time, including the production and delivery of oxygen, since the demand was so high.

Access to Care Across Regions

When access to care was exhausted in a region, ELSO was asked to help connect patients to access outside of a region or super-regional area, well beyond practitioners' typical network of referring centers.

Some regions took the initiative to coordinate care across multiple states, as was done well in the Pacific Northwest, where center leaders met weekly to review access to ECMO.

In addition, desperate patients and families would reach out directly to ELSO leadership during the pandemic when they were seeking access to ECMO but unsuccessful in their region. ELSO began fielding calls from patients or their families regularly for some time.

In the end, ELSO was unable to establish a tiered mechanism to help patients, families, and referral centers understand the scope of programs related to their ECMO services. This has led to the development of ELSO's Center Certification program, which will provide clarity of scope of services and operationalize a regional hub-and-spoke model with Level 1 centers committed to receiving referrals.

Access to ECMO Equipment

There were many times during the pandemic when more ECMO equipment was needed. ELSO eventually spent a year developing a supply exchange, which was intended to solve local supply chain issues when normal access was not working (Fig. 31.8).

Education and Training

We had a different problem on our hands during the pandemic: normal access to in-person training was no longer possible. Teams could train their own teams, but if they needed external support, this was not viable during the pandemic. Medical teams were often prohibited from traveling to mitigate spread and try to preserve their own workforce. However, demand for ECMO has never been higher. New and old programs needed a means to expand training.

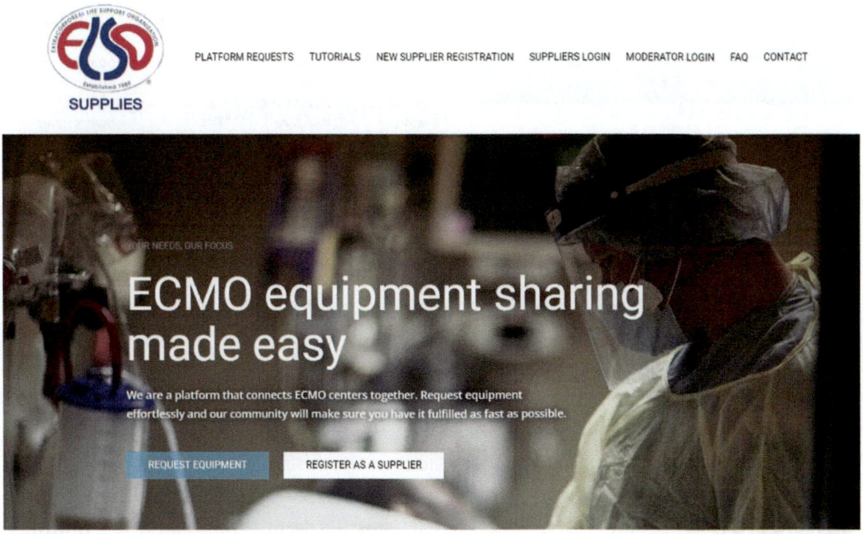

Fig. 31.8 ELSO supply exchange

Early on, ELSO put on training courses that were 2-day virtual programs. These helped with didactic training. We have long envisioned developing a didactic program. The pandemic pushed us into this being mission critical.

Approximately 100 experts from around the world were involved in a consensus-based methodology to create the first global standard in foundational ECMO education—something we call: ELSO Foundations. We started with the adult patient population because adults were more affected by the pandemic than children. We took a leap of faith and signed a resource-intensive contract with a program developer to create a virtual program that would be available globally. We were able to launch the ELSO Foundations Adult ECMO training course in December 2021, followed by the certification exam months later: E-AEC. Certification indicated foundational knowledge (didactic and simulation) along with clinical hours, which became valuable as practitioners began traveling to centers that needed ECMO support.

Participation in ELSO Foundations (Fig. 31.9)

Medical societies can be the platform for an escalated response to a pandemic which can impact outcomes, access to care, and policy at all levels of organizations on a global scale. This was ELSO's experience during the COVID-19 pandemic. So many groups came together to help overcome this pandemic.

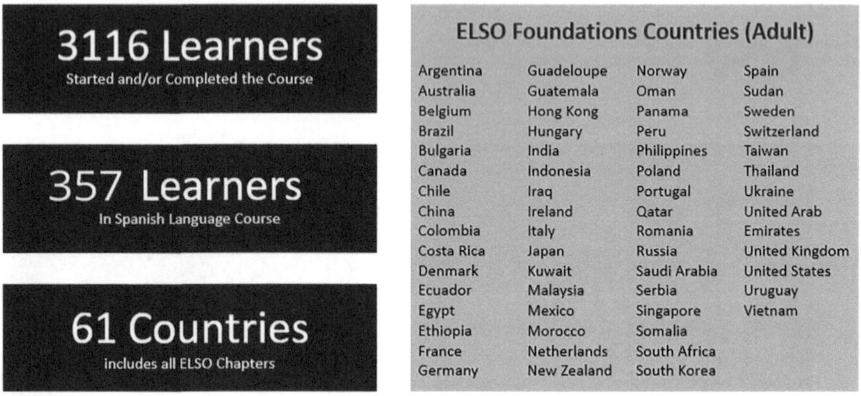

Fig. 31.9 Participation in ELSO Foundations Adult Training Course through July 2025

Conclusion

Through the recent COVID-19 pandemic much was learned, or perhaps more accurately relearned. It is inevitable that there will be other pandemics. We cannot control that pandemics will occur again. We can control our response. So, hopefully, by learning our history lessons and partnering with motivated, talented, and skilled healthcare providers, we can deliver the best outcomes with the least amount of suffering. Although pandemics caused significant suffering and death, there were heroes who emerged. Whether they were nurses who kept coming to work each day, or people who did the best to deliver food to those in need, some people stepped up to the plate. Together striking a balance of shared skills and knowledge, hopefully the next pandemic will be less challenging.

References

1. https://www.who.int/data/sets/global-excess-deaths-associated-with-covid-19-modelled-estimates.
2. Sampath S, Khedr A, Qamar S, Tekin A, Singh R, Green R, Kashyap R. Pandemics throughout the history. Cureus. 2021;13(9):e18136. https://doi.org/10.7759/cureus.18136. PMID: 34692344; PMCID: PMC8525686. https://pmc.ncbi.nlm.nih.gov/articles/PMC8525686/.
3. Grennan D. What is a pandemic? JAMA. 2019;321(9):910. https://doi.org/10.1001/jama.2019.0700. https://jamanetwork.com/journals/jama/fullarticle/2726986.
4. Mackowiak PA, Sehdev PS. The origin of quarantine. Clin Infect Dis. 2002;35(9, 1):1071–2. https://doi.org/10.1086/344062. https://academic.oup.com/cid/article/35/9/1071/330421?login=true.
5. Smith RD. Responding to global infectious disease outbreaks: lessons from SARS on the role of risk perception, communication and management. Soc Sci Med. 2006;63(12):3113–23. https://doi.org/10.1016/j.socscimed.2006.08.004. Epub 2006 Sep 15. PMID: 16978751; PMCID: PMC7130909.
6. https://www.who.int/emergencies/diseases/novel-coronavirus-2019/interactive-timeline.

7. Zhang YZ, Holmes EC. A genomic perspective on the origin and emergence of SARS-CoV-2. Cell. 2020;181(2):223–7. https://doi.org/10.1016/j.cell.2020.03.035. Epub 2020 Mar 26. PMID: 32220310; PMCID: PMC7194821.
8. https://www.who.int/emergencies/diseases/novel-coronavirus-2019/interactive-timeline#!.
9. https://elso.org/membership/ecmoavailabilitymap.aspx.
10. https://www.raps.org/news-and-articles/news-articles/2020/4/fda-offers-expanded-use-for-ecmo-cardiopulmonary-b; FDA page no longer available on July 26, 2025.
11. https://www.elso.org/registry/internationalsummaryandreports/internationalsummary.aspx.
12. Bartlett RH, Ogino MT, Brodie D, McMullan DM, Lorusso R, MacLaren G, Stead CM, Rycus P, Fraser JF, Belohlavek J, Salazar L, Mehta Y, Raman L, Paden ML. Initial ELSO guidance document: ECMO for COVID-19 patients with severe cardiopulmonary failure. ASAIO J. 2020;66(5):472–4. https://doi.org/10.1097/MAT.0000000000001173.
13. Badulak J, Antonini MV, Stead CM, Shekerdemian L, Raman L, Paden ML, Agerstrand C, Bartlett RH, Barrett N, Combes A, Lorusso R, Mueller T, Ogino MT, Peek G, Pellegrino V, Rabie AA, Salazar L, Schmidt M, Shekar K, MacLaren G, Brodie D. Extracorporeal membrane oxygenation for COVID-19: updated 2021 guidelines from the Extracorporeal Life Support Organization. ASAIO J. 2021;67(5):485–95. https://doi.org/10.1097/MAT.0000000000001422.
14. Barbaro RP, MacLaren G, Boonstra PS, Iwashyna TJ, Slutsky AS, Fan E, Bartlett RH, Tonna JE, Hyslop R, Fanning JJ, Rycus PT, Hyer SJ, Anders MM, Agerstrand CL, Hryniewicz K, Diaz R, Lorusso R, Combes A, Brodie D, for the Extracorporeal Life Support Organization. Extracorporeal membrane oxygenation support in COVID-19: an international cohort study of the Extracorporeal Life Support Organization registry. Lancet. 2020;396:1071–8.
15. Barbaro RP, MacLaren G, Boonstra PS, Combes A, Agerstrand C, Annich G, Diaz R, Fan E, Hryniewicz K, Lorusso R, Paden ML, Stead CM, Swol J, Iwashyna TJ, Slutsky AS, Brodie D, for the Extracorporeal Life Support Organization. Extracorporeal membrane oxygenation for COVID-19: evolving outcomes from the International Extracorporeal Life Support Organization Registry. Lancet. 2021;398:1230–8.
16. Barbaro R, MacLaren G, Boonstra P, et al. Extracorporeal membrane oxygenation for COVID-19: evolving outcomes from the International Extracorporeal Life Support Organization Registry. The Lancet. 2021;398:1230–8.
17. Mustafa AK, Alexander PJ, Joshi DJ, et al. Extracorporeal membrane oxygenation for patients with COVID-19 in severe respiratory failure. JAMA Surg. 2020;155(10):990–2. https://doi.org/10.1001/jamasurg.2020.3950.
18. https://www.elso.org/registry/elsoregistry-basedpublications.aspx.
19. https://www.nytimes.com/2021/07/12/us/covid-treatment-ecmo.html?smid=url-share.
20. https://www.theschwartzcenter.org/covid-19/.
21. https://www.ccrg.org.au/covid-critical.

Tracheostomy in the Intensive Care Unit

32

Jacob Woodroof, Shourjo Chakravorty,
Olugbenga Okusanya, Nathaniel R. Evans III,
and Frances Mae West

Introduction

Based on illustrations from ancient Egypt, tracheostomy creation has been described since around 3600 BC. However, the first scientific description of the procedure was not until the mid-sixteenth century, when Antonio Brasavola performed a tracheostomy to relieve an upper airway obstruction due to enlarged tonsils [1]. In the twentieth century, Chevalier Jackson refined the technical aspects of the tracheostomy procedure, making it much safer [2]. This prompted its use throughout the polio epidemic for airway management. The history and evolution of tracheostomy are discussed in a later chapter.

A tracheostomy may be created in cases of upper airway obstruction but is now more commonly used for facilitation of management and weaning of mechanical ventilation, and for more effective pulmonary toilet. In this chapter, we will discuss tracheostomy in the ICU, including indications and timing for placement and the technical aspects of the procedure. This chapter will take special consideration of how technique and procedural planning affect oxygenation and ventilation throughout the procedure. Routine tracheostomy care, weaning, and planned decannulation will be discussed in a later chapter.

J. Woodroof · O. Okusanya · N. R. Evans III
Division of Thoracic Surgery, The Department of Surgery at the Sidney Kimmel Medical College of Thomas Jefferson University, Philadelphia, PA, USA

S. Chakravorty · F. M. West (✉)
The Korman Respiratory Institute and the Division of Pulmonary, Allergy, and Critical Care, The Department of Medicine at the Sidney Kimmel Medical College of Thomas Jefferson University, Philadelphia, PA, USA
e-mail: frances.west@jefferson.edu

G. C. Kane et al. (eds.), *Oxygen*, https://doi.org/10.1007/978-3-032-18934-9_32

Indications, Benefits, and Timing of Tracheostomy Creation

Tracheostomy creation for airway management is indicated in several emergent and elective scenarios, as listed in Table 32.1 [3, 4]. While there are many indications, the only absolute contraindications are active cellulitis of the anterior neck, uncontrolled coagulopathy, and prior neck surgery, which completely obscure or obstruct the anterior neck anatomy. Typically, patients are stable on mechanical ventilation with an endotracheal tube in place prior to consideration for placement of a tracheostomy. Additionally, there are a few specific patient populations with special considerations for tracheostomy creation (e.g., obesity, repeat tracheostomy, emergent cricothyroidotomy), which are detailed later in this section. While essential for upper airway obstruction, tracheostomy is also an important alternative to leaving an endotracheal tube in place for extended periods of time, with risks of laryngeal injury, subglottic stenosis, and added difficulty for weaning from mechanical ventilation.

The benefits of tracheostomy creation are widely cited in the literature [5] with the following being of mention:

- Reduced oropharyngeal and laryngeal trauma
- Reduced work of breathing (due to decreased dead space and upper airway resistance)
- Improved pulmonary toilet
- Decreased sedation requirements
- Fewer days on mechanical ventilation
- Decreased ICU and hospital length of stay

Table 32.1 Indications for creation of a tracheostomy

Indications for tracheostomy creation	
Emergent	Elective
Acute upper airway obstruction with failure to secure an endotracheal tube	Prolonged intubation
Post-cricothyroidotomy (for formalization)	Facilitation of weaning from mechanical ventilation
Penetrating laryngeal trauma	Pulmonary secretion clearance
LeFort III fracture	Difficult airway/inability to intubate
	Prophylaxis in indicated head/neck surgery cases
	Refractory obstructive sleep apnea
	Impaired GCS/failure to manage oral secretions
	Advanced neuromuscular conditions (e.g., AML)

Adapted from Refs. [3, 4]

The timing of performing a tracheostomy has been a controversial topic with extensive study [6]. Historically, there has been a push to perform tracheostomy within 5–7 days of intubation to reduce complications like subglottic stenosis [7] and improve patient comfort [8]. Several RCTs have been designed to answer the question of the optimal timing of tracheostomy in various patient populations. The definition of early vs. late tracheostomy has differed in the literature, with most groups using 10 days or more as the cutoff for late tracheostomy, and some studies using a cutoff as few as 4 days for early tracheostomy.

Early randomized controlled trials showed discordant evidence on the benefit of early compared with late tracheostomy in ICU patients. Terrangni et al. showed that early tracheostomy was associated with a reduction in ventilator days, pneumonias, and more successful weaning [9]. The following year, Trouillet et al. did not show a decrease in ventilator-free days, ICU days, or pneumonias [10]. Neither study showed a mortality benefit associated with early tracheostomy.

The TracMan trial [11] remains the largest clinical trial investigating the benefits of early tracheostomy. Approximately 900 patients were randomized to receive early tracheostomy (<4 days) or late tracheostomy (>10 days). There was no difference in the primary outcome of 30-day mortality, along with other secondary outcomes, which included mortality while in the critical care unit, hospital discharge at 1 and 2 years, length of stay in the critical care unit, and antimicrobial-free days in the critical care unit (a surrogate for hospital-acquired infections). Furthermore, the authors determined that around 33% of patients who were selected for late tracheostomy did not end up undergoing tracheostomy at all. For these reasons, they concluded that it may be reasonable to wait until around day 10 before making a final decision on tracheostomy creation. This recommendation also accounts for the poor ability of physicians to accurately predict who will require mechanical ventilation for greater than 10 days, with approximately 20% of patients successfully weaning and being extubated [9–12].

More recently, there have been several systematic reviews to evaluate more longitudinal multi-facility data. Some of these studies have shown improved outcomes for patients undergoing tracheostomy within 7 days of intubation. Specifically, benefits include reduced hospital-acquired pneumonia (HAP), decreased mortality, fewer days on mechanical ventilation, and decreased ICU length of stay [5, 13]. It should be noted that while some studies used oxygen parameters for inclusion and exclusion criteria and as a safety parameter, these studies did not assess oxygenation requirements as an outcome.

With the collection of different studies in mind, there are guidelines for specific patient populations. The Eastern Association of Surgical Trauma (EAST) recommends early tracheostomy for patients with severe traumatic brain injury and those requiring prolonged ventilator support [14]. The time for tracheostomy in these patients is 3–7 days after intubation. Early tracheostomy should be especially considered for patients with severe traumatic brain injury, spinal cord injury, or those requiring neurosurgical intervention. For non-trauma patients, tracheostomy creation at around 5–7 days post-intubation is recommended by various other organizations [5, 14].

Creating a Tracheostomy: Relevant Anatomy and Common Techniques

Anatomy

Regardless of technique, one must be familiar with the anatomy of the anterior neck and the corresponding external anatomical landmarks; see Figs. 32.1 and 32.2. The trachea is composed of a series of cartilaginous rings, which begin at the larynx and end at the level of the mainstem bronchi. The cricoid cartilage represents the first and only complete circumferential cartilaginous ring within the airway. The remainder of the cartilaginous rings are incomplete in the posterior aspect, and the posterior wall is shared with the esophagus. Anterior to the trachea are the strap muscles as well as the thyroid gland, which is usually found over the second through fourth tracheal rings. Lateral to the trachea are the laryngeal nerves and lymph nodes. Further lateral is the carotid sheath and its associated structures—the carotid artery, internal jugular vein, and the vagus nerve. More distally, the trachea is bordered anteriorly by the thymus and the anterior mediastinum.

Palpable external landmarks include the thyroid notch, which demarcates the superior aspect of the larynx; the cricoid cartilage, which represents the junction of the larynx and the trachea; and the sternal notch, which identifies the thoracic inlet. Palpation of the sternal notch may also help identify a high-riding innominate artery prior to performing a tracheostomy [3, 16, 17].

Techniques

The two most common techniques for creating a tracheostomy are open surgical tracheostomy (OST) and percutaneous dilatational tracheostomy (PDT). Since the introduction of PDT in the 1980s, the paradigm has shifted toward performing more

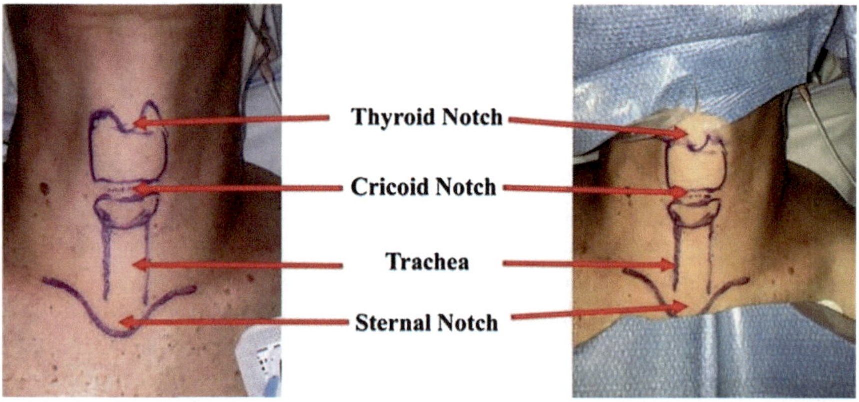

Fig. 32.1 Anatomical landmarks for tracheostomy creation

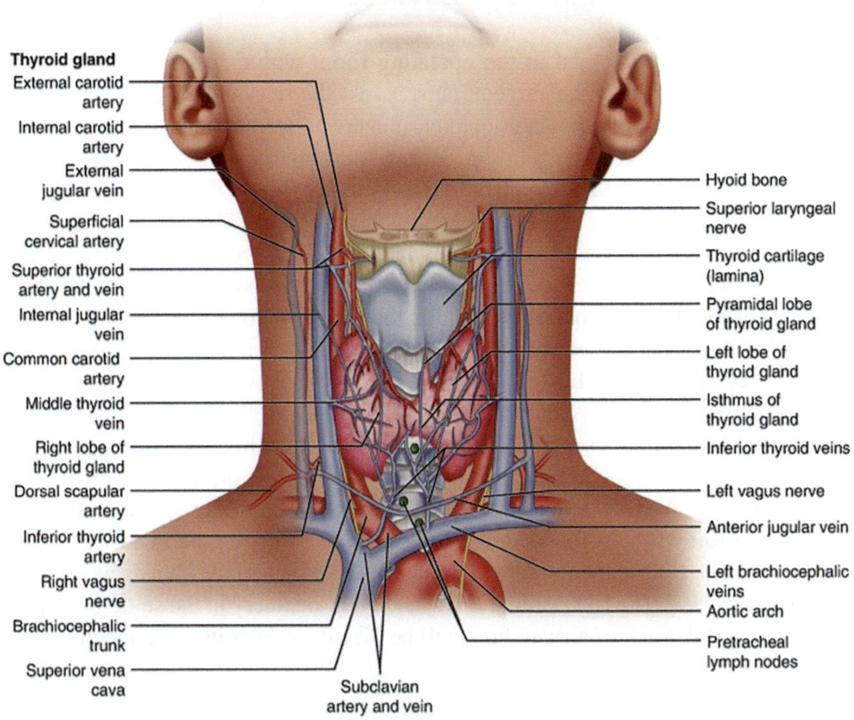

Fig. 32.2 Relevant anatomy of the anterior neck for tracheostomy creation. (Permission for use obtained via STM agreement [15])

procedures at the bedside in the ICU [18]. Bedside procedures can improve efficiency and reduce costs. This section will describe the different techniques for tracheostomy creation.

The type of technique should be decided on a case-by-case basis, though rates of PDT far exceed those of open tracheostomy in the modern era [5]. There have been numerous studies that confirm the validity and efficacy of PDT. Notably, PDT has been shown to result in decreased blood loss and infection rates. However, there are a few rare complications that may be seen with PDT, including aortic injury and esophageal perforation. As for indications for placement, please see the previously referenced Table 32.1. Additionally, there are some patients who may not meet the criteria for PDT and would be better served with OST. The relative contraindications include emergent access, difficult anatomy (aberrant vasculature, thyroid pathology), morbid obesity with a short neck, limited neck ROM or unstable cervical spine injury, and significant coagulopathy or thrombocytopenia [6].

Open Surgical Tracheostomy (OST) Procedure Details

OST is typically performed in the operating room with a full operating team. In preparation for the case, the surgeon must assess the relevant anatomic landmarks, including the thyroid cartilage, cricoid cartilage, and sternal notch. An overview of the key surgical steps is shown in Fig. 32.3. A marking for skin incision is generally made approximately 1–2 cm inferior to the cricoid cartilage. After the skin incision, the subcutaneous tissue is dissected, and the strap muscles are identified and retracted laterally to expose the thyroid gland and the cricoid cartilage. The isthmus of the thyroid may be retracted superiorly or divided, as indicated. The cricoid cartilage is then elevated with a hook to aid in the identification of the second and third tracheal rings. The surgeon then chooses a method for incision of the trachea between the second and third rings. While the space between the second and third tracheal rings may be incised horizontally, three other methods may be used. These include (1) removal of a segment of 1–2 rings of anterior tracheal cartilage, (2) vertical incision over 2 tracheal rings, and (3) creation of a Bjork flap (an inferior cartilage flap is created and sutured to the skin directly). Once the opening is created, the tracheostomy tube is inserted, connected to the ventilator, and end-tidal CO_2 is confirmed. The tube is then secured in place with sutures to the skin as well as transcervical ties [19]. The risks of high FIO_2 and electrocautery in the setting of tracheostomies, and the risk of airway fires will be discussed later in this chapter.

Introduction to Percutaneous Tracheostomy Creation

PDT was first described by Ciaglia et al. in 1985 [18]. The procedure combines bronchoscopy with a modified Seldinger technique and allows the patient to avoid being transported to the operating room. PDT is performed with a variety of techniques by a heterogeneous group of physicians, though commonly, it is performed with the single tapered dilator technique (SSDT). Some variations of PDT exist beyond SSDT, which are included in Table 32.2. The differences with respect to oxygenation and ventilation are discussed later in this section.

Looking to the future, there have been some promising new techniques with respect to tracheostomy creation. Notably, there is the use of an ETT-mounted camera as opposed to bronchoscopy to perform PDT. There are two non-inferiority trials [21, 22] which show that the use of an ETT-mounted camera may result in less hypercarbia and less hypoxia than traditional bronchoscope-guided PDT. Given that some patients have an inability to tolerate transient hypercarbia or hypoxia are contraindications to PDT, this is a promising technique to consider more patients for bedside tracheostomy placement.

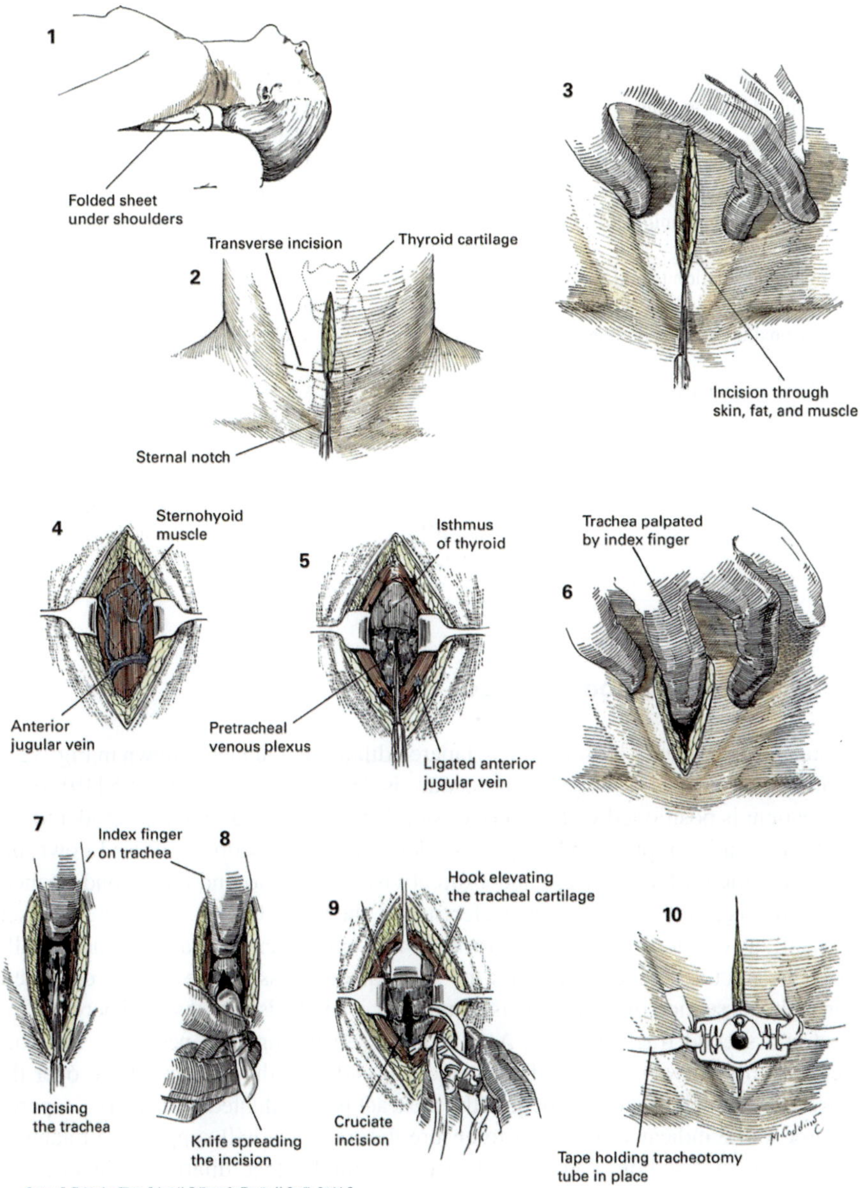

Fig. 32.3 Open surgical tracheostomy creation. (Permission for use obtained via STM agreement [19])

Table 32.2 Common methods for percutaneous tracheostomy creation

Methods of percutaneous tracheostomy creation		
Technique name	Discoverer, year	General technique
Multiple dilator technique (MDT)	Ciaglia et al., 1985	Antegrade, multi-step sequential dilation
Guide wire dilating forcep (GWDF)	Griggs, 1990	Antegrade dilation with special forceps
Translaryngeal technique (TLT)	Fanotni and Ripamonti, 1997	Retrograde, special cannula used as dilator and tracheostomy tube
Single-step dilation technique (SSDT)	Byhahn et al., 2000	Antegrade, single dilation with curved dilator and loading dilator
Rotational dilation technique (RDT)	Frova and Quintel, 2002	Antegrade, self-trapping screw
Balloon dilation technique (BDT)	Zgoda and Berger, 2005	Antegrade, similar to SSDT but includes balloon in the assembly
Ultrasound-guided percutaneous dilational tracheostomy (US-PDT)	Sustic et al., 1999	Similar to standard PDT but uses US guidance, avoids bronchoscopy
Endotracheal tube-mounted camera with pdt	Grensemann et al., 2017 Umutoglu et al., 2016	Antegrade, similar to standard PDT but with ETT mounted camera

Adapted from Refs. [6, 20]

Single-Stage Dilation Technique

A standard procedure kit for a single tapered dilator technique is shown in Fig. 32.4, while an overview of the typical procedure is demonstrated in Fig. 32.5 [19]. First, the patient is positioned with the neck extended, anatomic landmarks are identified, and the area is prepped and draped sterilely. A bronchoscope is passed down the ETT, and the ETT is retracted under direct visualization to find the second tracheal ring. At this point, based on the preference of the proceduralist, the skin is incised to facilitate dilation with a scalpel for around 2 cm, either vertically or horizontally over the intended access area, and the subcutaneous tissues are bluntly dissected. Once the dissection of the airway is completed, a needle is then inserted between the first and second tracheal rings. A wire is passed through the needle to maintain access to the airway. The needle is removed, and then the tract is dilated over the wire with a small dilator. Subsequently, the tract is then dilated with a large, tapered dilator to the indicated markings to ensure the tract size will support the tracheostomy tube. A less common alternative to the single-stage dilation technique is a multi-step dilatational technique. Instead of using a single, large, tapered dilator, a series of non-tapered dilators of increasing size is used in sequence to dilate the soft tissue and tracheal opening to the desired diameter. Once dilation is completed, the tracheostomy tube is inserted into the airway over the wire, and the wire is removed. The bronchoscope is then removed from the ETT and advanced down the tracheostomy to ensure adequate positioning. Once the position is confirmed, the balloon is inflated, and the ventilator is switched to the tracheostomy. In most cases, the

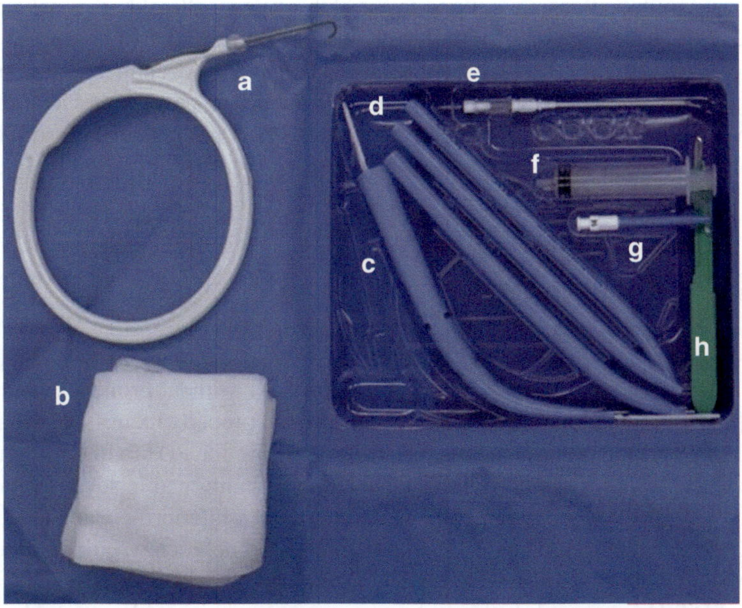

Fig. 32.4 Common items included for PDT; bedside procedure kit (**a**) wire, (**b**) gauze, (**c**) curved graduated dilator, (**d**) insertion dilators for tracheostomy tube, (**e**) access needle and sheath, (**f**) syringe, (**g**) initial access dilator, and (**h**) 15-blade. (Permission for use obtained via STM agreement [23])

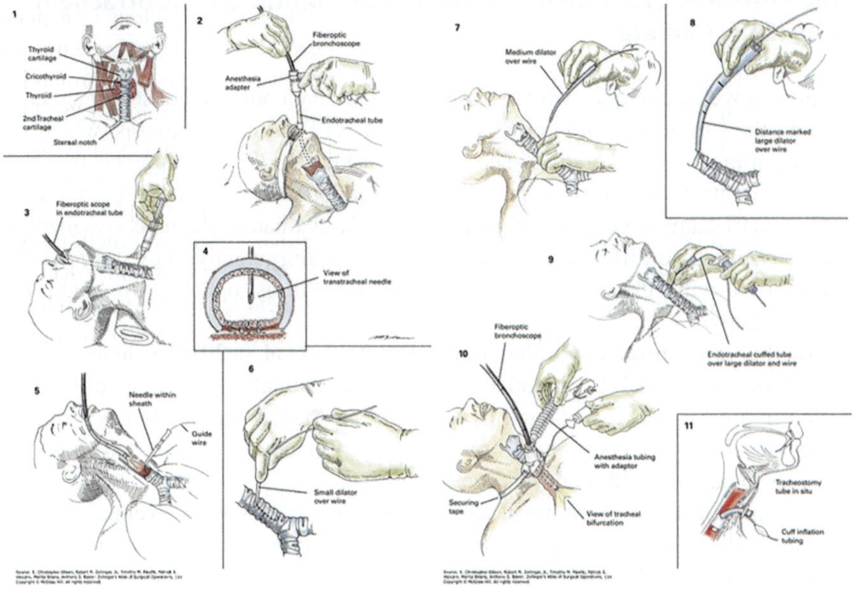

Fig. 32.5 Percutaneous dilatational tracheostomy creation, general steps. (Permission for use obtained via STM agreement [19])

tracheostomy tube flaps are sutured to the skin using small-caliber, nonabsorbable suture at the four corners. This aids with any oozing from the subcutaneous space and helps to secure the tracheostomy from accidental early decannulation. A protective foam dressing placed underneath a flexible flange can prevent pressure wounds. Following this, the patient is orally extubated [19, 20, 24], and the procedure is completed. After a period of 1–2 weeks, the sutures can be cut from the tracheostomy tube flaps.

Ultrasound-Guided PDT

USG-PDT was first described by Sustic et al. In 1999, two patients who had undergone anterior cervical spine surgery underwent PDT without bronchoscopic guidance [25]. In this technique, an ultrasound is used to properly identify key anatomic landmarks and the anterior trachea in order to allow for PDT without the use of bronchoscopy. The feasibility of this technique was confirmed in several follow-up studies [26, 27]. More recently, a randomized non-inferiority trial, named the TRACHUS trial, randomized 118 patients to bronchoscopy-guided PDT vs. US-guided PDT. They determined that US-guided PDT is non-inferior to bronchoscopic PDT. However, while this technique appears promising, there are other techniques that use mounted cameras on the endotracheal tube to provide visualization of the posterior tracheal wall [28].

Tracheostomy Creation in the Setting of a Mounted Endotracheal Tube (ETT) Camera

A more novel technique, which allows for percutaneous tracheostomy creation without the use of bronchoscopy, is the use of ETT-mounted cameras, which has been examined in a few studies. The VivaPDT trial [21, 29] was a prospective, randomized-control trial; 46 ICU patients were randomized to bronchoscopy-guided PDT vs ETT camera-guided PDT. They primarily evaluated adequate visualization and determined no difference between the groups. Importantly, they did note less hypercarbia with the ETT camera-guided method as opposed to traditional bronchoscopy.

Another randomized controlled trial by Umutoglu et al. in 2016 evaluated the use of ETView, a similar ETT-mounted camera, in 26 patients [22]. Their results suggested improved hypercarbia and hypoxia during PDT, with maintenance of adequate visualization of key structures, and recommended this as a procedure to consider in patients with poor pulmonary reserve.

In summary, these more novel techniques provide promising avenues for proceeding with PDT with less concern for hypoxia, hypercarbia, cuff rupture, or loss of airway, given the lack of use of bronchoscopy.

Oxygenation, Ventilation, and Airway Management During Tracheostomy Creation

During OST, the patient must remain on the mechanical ventilator, with maintenance of oxygenation and ventilation throughout the procedure. It is important to keep this in mind to avoid hypoxia, hypercarbia, and any associated intraoperative complications such as an airway fire, which has been reported [30]. The goal of the anesthesia team is to pre-oxygenate well during the pre-tracheostomy period and to administer as low FiO_2 as possible once the airway is incised. The surgical team must be careful to avoid the use of thermal energy devices, particularly when working near the airway. Unless on ECMO, there is no available method of maintaining oxygenation during OST, which completely eliminates the risk of airway fire. The most important factor is clear communication among the teams in the operating room in order to result in a safer, more coordinated effort.

During PDT, careful consideration must be taken to ensure adequate oxygenation and ventilation. The ventilator should typically be put in a control mode of ventilation. The patient is administered analgesia and amnestic sedatives. Neuromuscular blockade is often used, but is not required for every patient. The respiratory therapist will typically pre-oxygenate the patient to 100% and set an adequate positive end-expiratory pressure (PEEP). Importantly, during the procedure, when the balloon is deflated, there is a loss of positive end-expiratory pressure (PEEP), which can affect oxygenation. Once the procedure is started, the bronchoscope is kept within the oral endotracheal tube to ensure control of the airway. Clear communication and coordination are necessary between the bronchoscopist, proceduralist, and respiratory therapist to prevent accidental extubation. Careful monitoring of minute ventilation and end-tidal carbon dioxide is crucial in ensuring appropriate ventilation. End-tidal carbon dioxide is very useful in confirming placement of the tracheostomy tube once the tracheostomy cuff is inflated and connected back to the circuit. Direct visualization by bronchoscopy via the new tracheostomy can be done to confirm placement within the airway. These steps are critical prior to removal of the oral endotracheal tube [24].

Although the patient remains ventilated during the procedure with either a mechanical ventilator or with bag valve mask ventilation, hypercarbia has been described as a complication following percutaneous tracheostomy using bronchoscopic guidance [31].

In a study comparing 25 patients in a surgical ICU undergoing percutaneous tracheostomy with bronchoscopic guidance, ultrasound Doppler guidance, and standard open tracheostomies, the patients undergoing percutaneous tracheostomy experienced more severe hypercapnia and respiratory acidosis than the other two groups. A maximum delta $PaCO_2$ of 24 ± 3 mmHg and delta pH of -0.16 ± 0.02 were observed with continuous bronchoscopy compared to a maximum delta $PaCO_2$ of 8 ± 2 mmHg and delta pH of -0.07 ± 0.02 with ultrasound Doppler guidance, and a maximum delta $PaCO_2$ 3 ± 1 mmHg and delta pH of -0.04 ± 0.01 in the open tracheostomy group [32]. Patients in this study undergoing percutaneous tracheostomy with bronchoscopy were ventilated on volume-cycled ventilation with FiO_2

1.0 through an ETT tube; they noted that ventilator alarms and settings, including the minute ventilation, were not adjusted during the procedure.

The reason for hypercarbia is that the bronchoscope will partially obstruct the endotracheal tube during the procedure. If a ventilator is used to ventilate the patient, high airway pressure alarms need to be adjusted, as the presence of the bronchoscope in the airway will trigger the pressure alarms, and the machine will not deliver a breath. By virtue of increased airway resistance through the endotracheal tube with a limited lumen due to the presence of the bronchoscope, minute ventilation is often reduced during the procedure. Temporally increasing the high airway pressure alarms to the maximum limitation, often 70–100 cm H_2O, is necessary to maintain ventilation during the procedure [33]. It is important to understand that the pressure in the trachea and beyond is not elevated, since the resistance drops once beyond the endotracheal tube.

Patient Populations with Special Considerations

It is important to note a few patient populations of particular interest regarding PDT. Historically, there was particular concern about tracheostomy creation in morbidly obese patients and in patients who are undergoing repeat tracheostomy [34]. Both adequate positioning with neck extension and subcutaneous tissue dissection have been shown to facilitate safe tracheostomy creation with PDT. For these patients, one should also consider exchanging the current tracheostomy tube for a tracheostomy tube with a proximal extended-length during a future tracheostomy change. Use of an extended-length tracheostomy (XLT) tube is often required due to increased subcutaneous tissue. A meta-analysis of 1355 patients from 18 studies has shown that obese patients are more prone to complications, with 4% of patients experiencing serious complications, with intraoperative hypoxemia and accidental loss of airway being the most common [35].

Historically, there was concern that a previous tracheostomy was a contraindication for PDT; however, newer studies and commentary have shown that PDT may still be reasonable in this population and suggest that patients should not be excluded from consideration for PDT for this singular reason [34].

Patients requiring emergency surgical airways pose unique situational challenges, as oxygenation, ventilation, or both are often significantly impaired. Emergency cricothyroidotomy is a rare procedure that has long been considered a last-resort technique for establishing an airway in patients with a failed airway and without other available options [36]. Specific indications for cricothyroidotomy are listed below:

- Acute upper airway obstruction with failed endotracheal intubation (foreign body, angioedema, infection, anaphylaxis)
- Post-cricothyrotomy (if a cricothyrotomy has been placed, it should be immediately formalized into a tracheostomy once an airway has been secured)

- Penetrating laryngeal trauma
- LeFort III fracture

To perform a cricothyroidotomy, the standard technique has a number of reported variants, but the general concept is the same. Typically, the standard technique employs the use of a scalpel, dilator, hemostat, tracheal hook, and tracheostomy tube. The operator will palpate the thyroid and cricoid cartilages in order to make a vertical incision along the area of the cricoid membrane. A combination of blunt and sharp dissection aids in the identification of the cricoid membrane. This membrane is then incised horizontally before undergoing dilation (by dilator or by 90-degree rotation of a scalpel handle), followed by tracheostomy tube placement [36].

Two notable variations of the standard technique are the rapid, four-step technique (RFST) and the bougie-assisted cricothyroidotomy technique (BACT) [36–38]. RFST requires three items: a scalpel, a tracheal hook, and a tracheostomy tube (typically a #6 Shiley). The four steps are as follows:

1. *Palpation of landmarks.* Identify the cricoid cartilage.
2. *Incision.* A horizontal stab incision of the skin and cricoid membrane.
3. *Hook.* The tracheal hook is applied inferiorly to the skin/membrane.
4. *Tube placement.* A tracheostomy tube is inserted into the airway.

BACT is like the traditional technique, except that once the cricoid membrane is incised, a bougie is first passed distally to maintain access to the airway prior to advancement of a tracheostomy tube over the bougie. Waveform capnography is critical in this scenario to confirm tracheal ventilation and a successful airway.

Acute Complications Related to Tracheostomy Creation

There is some inherent risk in placing a tracheostomy tube. Major immediate complications include airway irritation and bleeding, pneumothorax, subcutaneous emphysema, injury to the recurrent laryngeal nerve, and local infection, though a more detailed list is included in Table 32.3. A small amount of bleeding is expected during a tracheostomy procedure, usually from the adjacent local vascular structures. A patient with severe bleeding should undergo bronchoscopy for suspected laryngotracheal stenosis or a tracheoesophageal fistula. Bleeding may also occur in the setting of airway trauma due to frequent or improper suctioning. It is important to note that the tracheostomy tube may obstruct the view of the bleeding source. If the tracheostomy is fresh, removal of the tube raises a significant risk.

Bleeding from a tracheostomy is a common occurrence, and a small amount may be physiological shortly after insertion or after tracheostomy changes. Further, irritation of the tracheal mucosa from the tracheostomy can also cause minor bleeding. Improper insertion of a tracheostomy tube can result in a false passage where the tip of the tracheostomy rests in a false passage outside of the trachea,

Table 32.3 Complications of tracheostomy creation

Complications of tracheostomy creation		
Immediate complications	Early complications	Late complications
Hemorrhage	Hemorrhage	Tracheal stenosis
Tracheal injury	Cannula displacement	Granulation tissue
Aspiration	Pneumothorax	Tracheomalacia
Airway loss	Pneumomediastinum	PNA
Hypercarbia	Skin ulceration	Aspiration
Hypoxemia	Dysphagia	Tracheoinnominate fistula
Air embolus	Stoma infection	Tracheoesophageal fistula
Respiratory failure	Subcutaneous emphysema	Dysphagia
Death		Tube dislodgement

which impedes ventilation and oxygenation. Another feared complication of tracheostomy is the creation of a fistula between the trachea and the brachiocephalic artery, which occurs in about 0.6% of cases [39]. Generally, this emergency occurs within 3–4 weeks after tracheostomy creation and is often heralded by a sentinel bleeding event, which may spontaneously resolve. Risk factors for developing a tracheal-brachiocephalic fistula include overinflated cuffs leading to mucosal injury, a high-riding brachiocephalic artery, low tracheostomies, and soft tissue friability due to chronic corticosteroid use and local radiation therapy. As up to 25% of the total cardiac output goes through the brachiocephalic artery, a tracheal-brachiocephalic fistula is fatal in most instances; however, cuff overinflation, digital compression of the brachiocephalic artery along the posterior sternal surface (Utley maneuver) and endotracheal intubation may purchase some time in order to plan surgical correction [40].

Summary

There is a wide array of patients in the ICU who will ultimately require tracheostomy creation. It is important to consider the timing and indications for all patients with prolonged mechanical ventilation. PDT has largely replaced open surgical tracheostomy in intensive care units due to its safety, efficacy, and cost-effectiveness. Ensuring proper oxygenation and ventilation during the procedure is necessary to prevent complications. Waveform capnography remains the gold standard for confirmation of airway placement.

Declarations
Competing Interests The author(s) have no competing interests to declare that are relevant to the content of this manuscript.

Ethics Approval The author(s) declare that this manuscript does not include primary research with human participants.

The author(s) declare that this manuscript does not include primary studies involving animals.

References

1. Goodall EW. On infectious diseases and epidemiology in the Hippocratic collection: (Section of the history of medicine). Proc R Soc Med. 1934;27:525.
2. Jackson C. Tracheotomy. Laryngoscope. 1909;19:285–90.
3. De Leyn P, Bedert L, Delcroix M, Depuydt P, Lauwers G, Sokolov Y, Van Verhaeghe A, Van Schil P. Tracheotomy: clinical review and guidelines. Eur J Cardio-Thorac Surg. 2007;32:412–21.
4. Rana S, Pendem S, Pogodzinski MS, Hubmayr RD, Gajic O. Tracheostomy in critically ill patients. Mayo Clin Proc. 2005;80:1632–8.
5. Adly A, Youssef TA, El-Begermy MM, Younis HM. Timing of tracheostomy in patients with prolonged endotracheal intubation: a systematic review. Eur Arch Oto-Rhino-Laryngol. 2018;275:679–90.
6. Cheung NH, Napolitano LM. Tracheostomy: epidemiology, indications, timing, technique, and outcomes. Respir Care. 2014;59:895–919.
7. Pasick LJ, Anis MM, Rosow DE. An updated review of subglottic stenosis: etiology, evaluation, and management. Curr Pulmonol Rep. 2022;11:29.
8. Davis K, Campbell RS, Johannigman JA, Valente JF, Branson RD. Changes in respiratory mechanics after tracheostomy. Arch Surg. 1999;134:59–62.
9. Terragni PP, Antonelli M, Fumagalli R, et al. Early vs late tracheotomy for prevention of pneumonia in mechanically ventilated adult ICU patients: a Randomized Controlled Trial. JAMA. 2010;303:1483–9.
10. Trouillet JL, Luyt CE, Guiguet M, et al. Early percutaneous tracheotomy versus prolonged intubation of mechanically ventilated patients after cardiac surgery: a Randomized Trial. Ann Intern Med. 2011;154:373–83.
11. Young D, Harrison DA, Cuthbertson BH, Rowan K. Effect of early vs late tracheostomy placement on survival in patients receiving mechanical ventilation: the TracMan Randomized Trial. JAMA. 2013;309:2121–9.
12. Szakmany T, Russell P, Wilkes AR, Hall JE. Effect of early tracheostomy on resource utilization and clinical outcomes in critically ill patients: meta-analysis of randomized controlled trials. Br J Anaesth. 2015;114:396–405.
13. Hosokawa K, Nishimura M, Egi M, Vincent JL. Timing of tracheotomy in ICU patients: a systematic review of randomized controlled trials. Crit Care. 2015;19:1–12.
14. Holevar M, Dunham JCM, Brautigan R, et al. Practice management guidelines for timing of tracheostomy: the EAST practice management guidelines work group. J Trauma Injury Infect Crit Care. 2009;67:870–4.
15. Guillory W, Miller C, Kodumudi G, Ettarh R. Anatomy of the head and neck. In: Narayan D, Kapadia SE, Kodumudi G, Vadivelu N, editors. Surgical and perioperative management of patients with anatomic anomalies. Cham: Springer; 2021. https://doi.org/10.1007/978-3-030-55660-0_1.
16. Tracheostomy – StatPearls – NCBI Bookshelf. https://www.ncbi.nlm.nih.gov/books/NBK559124/. Accessed 30 July 2025.
17. Hansen JT, Netter FH, Machado CAG. Netter's clinical anatomy. Elsevier; 2019.
18. Ciaglia P, Firsching R, Syniec C. Elective percutaneous dilatational tracheostomy: a new simple bedside procedure; preliminary report. Chest. 1985;87:715–9.
19. Christopher EE, Milton ZR, Pawlik TM, Vaccaro PS, Marita B, Baker AS. Zollinger's atlas of surgical operations. 11th ed. McGraw-Hill Education; 2022.
20. Cabrini L, Monti G, Landoni G, Biondi-Zoccai G, Boroli F, Mamo D, Plumari VP, Colombo S, Zangrillo A. Percutaneous tracheostomy, a systematic review. Acta Anaesthesiol Scand. 2012;56:270–81.
21. Grensemann J, Eichler L, Kähler S, Jarczak D, Simon M, Pinnschmidt HO, Kluge S. Bronchoscopy versus an endotracheal tube mounted camera for the peri-interventional

visualization of percutaneous dilatational tracheostomy – a prospective, randomized trial (VivaPDT). Crit Care. 2017;21:1–10.
22. Umutoglu T, Bakan M, Topuz U, Yilmaz S, Idin K, Alver S, Ozturk E, Salihoglu Z. Comparison of EtView™ tracheoscopic ventilation tube and video-assisted fiberoptic bronchoscopy during percutaneous dilatational tracheostomy. J Clin Monit Comput. 2017;31:507–12.
23. Schellenberg M, Inaba K. Percutaneous tracheostomy. In: Demetriades D, Inaba K, Lumb P, editors. Atlas of critical care procedures. Cham: Springer; 2018. https://doi.org/10.1007/978-3-319-78367-3_2.
24. Ingelfinger JR, Tracheostomy P, Hashimoto DA, Axtell AL, Auchincloss HG. Percutaneous tracheostomy. N Engl J Med. 2020;383:383.
25. Šustić A, Župan Ž, Eškinja N, Dirlić A, Bajek G. Ultrasonographically guided percutaneous dilatational tracheostomy after anterior cervical spine fixation. Acta Anaesthesiol Scand. 1999;43:1078–80.
26. Rajajee V, Fletcher JJ, Rochlen LR, Jacobs TL. Real-time ultrasound-guided percutaneous dilatational tracheostomy: a feasibility study. Crit Care. 2011; https://doi.org/10.1186/CC10047.
27. Rezende-Neto JB, Oliveira AJ, Neto MP, Botoni FA, Rizoli SB. A technical modification for percutaneous tracheostomy: prospective case series study on one hundred patients. World J Emerg Surg. 2011;6:35.
28. Gobatto ALN, Besen BAMP, Tierno PFGMM, et al. Ultrasound-guided percutaneous dilational tracheostomy versus bronchoscopy-guided percutaneous dilational tracheostomy in critically ill patients (TRACHUS): a randomized noninferiority controlled trial. Intensive Care Med. 2016;42:342–51.
29. Grensemann J, Eichler L, Hopf S, Jarczak D, Simon M, Kluge S. Feasibility of an endotracheal tube-mounted camera for percutaneous dilatational tracheostomy. Acta Anaesthesiol Scand. 2017;61:660–7.
30. Gorphe P, Sarfati B, Janot F, Bourgain JL, Motamed C, Blot F, Temam S. Airway fire during tracheostomy. Eur Ann Otorhinolaryngol Head Neck Dis. 2014;131:197–9.
31. Gemma M, Cozzi S, Cipriani A, Reilly PM, Anderson HL. Hypercarbia during tracheostomy (multiple letters) [5]. Intensive Care Med. 1998;24:279.
32. Reilly PM, Sing RF, Giberson FA, Anderson HL, Rotondo MF, Tinkoff GH, Schwab CW. Hypercarbia during tracheostomy: a comparison of percutaneous endoscopic, percutaneous Doppler, and standard surgical tracheostomy. Intensive Care Med. 1997;23:859–64.
33. Veelo DP, Dongelmans DA, Middelhoek P, Korevaar JC, Schultz MJ. Adaptive support ventilation with percutaneous dilatational tracheotomy: a clinical study. Anesth Analg. 2008;107:938–40.
34. Ernst A, Critchlow J. Percutaneous tracheostomy – special considerations. Clin Chest Med. 2003;24:409–12.
35. Roy CF, Silver JA, Turkdogan S, Siafa L, Correa JA, Kost K. Complication rate of percutaneous dilatational tracheostomy in critically ill adults with obesity: a systematic review and meta-analysis. JAMA Otolaryngol Head Neck Surg. 2023;149:334.
36. Langvad S, Hyldmo PK, Nakstad AR, Vist GE, Sandberg M. Emergency cricothyrotomy – a systematic review. Scand J Trauma Resusc Emerg Med. 2013;21:1–14.
37. Brofeldt BT, Panacek EA, Richards JR. An easy cricothyrotomy approach: the rapid four-step technique. Acad Emerg Med. 1996;3:1060–3.
38. Hill C, Reardon R, Joing S, Falvey D, Miner J. Cricothyrotomy technique using gum elastic bougie is faster than standard technique: a study of emergency medicine residents and medical students in an animal lab. Acad Emerg Med. 2010;17:666–9.
39. Ogawa K, Nitta N, Sonoda A, Takahashi M, Suzuki T, Kitamura S, Hanaoka J, Tezuka N, Murata K. Tracheo-brachiocephalic artery fistula after tracheostomy associated with thoracic deformity: a case report. J Med Case Rep. 2011;5:595.
40. Joshi KD, Singh A, Singh DK, Gupta V, Saxena S, Hota A, Girdhar S, Singhavi HR, Thapa S, Leelakanth K. Tracheo-innominate artery fistula: a systematic review of diagnostic and management strategies. Otolaryngol Head Neck Surg (United States). 2025; https://doi.org/10.1002/OHN.1333.

Ethics of Life-Sustaining Care and Withdrawing Mechanical Ventilation

33

David Oxman

Introduction

Perhaps the best way to begin the conversation about ethics in the intensive care unit (ICU) is with a case:

> A 70-year-old woman with advanced pancreatic cancer is admitted to the intensive care unit for septic shock and respiratory distress. Prior chemotherapy, over the last four months, has not led to a favorable response. She is placed on a ventilator for respiratory support and treated with antibiotics and vasopressors. Over the next two days, her condition stabilizes but does not improve significantly. She is unconscious, and her lungs are showing signs of acute respiratory distress syndrome. She requires maximum support from the ventilator, and her kidneys are beginning to fail. It is clear to her family and the treating physicians that while the ventilator can keep her alive temporarily, she will ultimately not survive, and she is suffering in the meantime. Moreover, her family relates to the intensive care physician that the patient made it clear to her family in the past that she never would have wanted prolonged life support therapies before her death.
>
> Later that day, the patient's family gathers at her bedside to say their goodbyes. She remains unconscious as the respiratory therapist removes her endotracheal tube. She continues to breathe on her own, but after a minute, she begins to struggle, and her breaths become rapid and shallow. Her nurse administers a small dose of intravenous morphine, and her breathing becomes slower and less labored. Over the course of the next hour, while her family holds her hand and sits vigil at her bedside, her respiratory rate declines further until it stops altogether, and she dies.

D. Oxman (✉)
The Korman Respiratory Institute and the Division of Pulmonary, Allergy and Critical Care, The Department of Medicine at the Sidney Kimmel Medical College of Thomas Jefferson University, Philadelphia, PA, USA
e-mail: david.oxman@jefferson.edu

G. C. Kane et al. (eds.), *Oxygen*, https://doi.org/10.1007/978-3-032-18934-9_33

Historical Perspective

Decisions to forgo or limit the use of life-sustaining treatments are common in a modern American intensive care unit. In fact, most deaths that occur in the ICU happen after a decision to stop or limit life support therapies, such as mechanical ventilation [1]. The ethical basis for removing life support is grounded in two foundational principles: the right of patients to decide for themselves which medical treatments they wish to undergo and which they do not (autonomy), and the physician's responsibility to put the patient's interests first and limit unnecessary suffering (beneficence). Moreover, over the last fifty years, the legal basis for these actions has been firmly established and affirmed [2].

Yet, despite the clear ethical and legal basis for removing life support at the end of life, questions may still arise. Is the removal of life support *causing* death, or merely allowing a terminal disease to run its natural course? Are there any limits that should be placed on a patient or their surrogate's right to refuse or withdraw life support therapies? And what does the law have to say about these cases?

The Emergence of the Legal and Ethical Grounds for the Withdrawal of Life Support Therapies

By the early 1970s, mechanical ventilation outside of the operating room and inside newly created intensive care units was becoming common, with seriously ill patients being placed on life support increasingly frequently. Similarly, the new technique of closed chest cardiac massage—or cardiopulmonary resuscitation (CPR)—was perfected and applied to more patients—including hospitalized patients who were at the end of life. While these techniques had the potential to save many lives, they also could inadvertently prolong the suffering and death of many more. And it was not clear to physicians and society in general how to decide when to deploy these life support measures and under what circumstances patients or their doctors could decide not to.

Relatively quickly, the right to refuse the initiation of life support therapies was established [3]. Patient-initiated directives like "Do Not Resuscitate" orders became common and were nearly universally respected. However, situations in which life support therapies were already initiated, but then no longer desired by patients or their families, caused much more controversy. It raised questions like: "Is a physician who removes a terminally ill patient from a ventilator to limit suffering intentionally causing their death?" and "was this process even legal?" Sadly, it took years and two tragic and well-publicized cases involving young women who suffered devastating neurological injuries in the prime of their lives to establish the norms and laws surrounding the withdrawal of life support therapies that we have today.

> Karen Ann Quinlan was just twenty-one years old in 1975 when she unintentionally overdosed on alcohol and prescription medications and suffered a severe anoxic brain injury. After months of life support in a New Jersey hospital's intensive care unit, it was clear to

Karen's parents that there was no hope for meaningful neurological recovery and that she would be left in a permanent minimally conscious state. Yet when Karen's parents asked her doctors to remove her from life support and let her die with "grace and dignity," the doctors and the hospital refused, claiming that it would be akin to murder.

In court, the Quinlans argued that continued life support, when there was no realistic hope for meaningful recovery, was not consistent with Karen's values. And since Karen was unable to speak for herself, as her parents—the ones who knew her better than anyone—they had a duty, and the right, to make the decision to stop it. Initially, the lower courts disagreed and ruled that Karen's parents could not force the doctors to remove Karen from life support, because it would, in effect, directly cause Karen's death. But the Quinlans persisted and took the case to the New Jersey Supreme Court, which ruled that the right to refuse medical treatment was part of a person's fundamental right to privacy. The court also ruled that there would be no liability for health care personnel involved in removing Karen from life support and that, in the future, resolving these kinds of cases was squarely in the domain of medical professionals and patients and that courts should not be involved [4, 5].

Another tragic case, the one of Nancy Cruzan, further established the norm in the United States that patients and their doctors could legally make decisions to terminate life support therapies when it could no longer reasonably be expected to be consistent with the wishes of a patient. Nancy Cruzan was a young woman left in a persistent vegetative state after an automobile accident. While she was not dependent on a ventilator, she relied on artificial nutrition through a feeding tube. After several years with no neurological recovery, her family asked the doctors to stop tube feedings and begin comfort-based care to allow her to have a dignified death. The hospital refused, and a Missouri court stated that without "clear and convincing evidence" [6] of Nancy's wishes, her surrogates could not make this decision for her. Eventually, the case went to the United States Supreme Court, which affirmed the right of individuals to refuse unwanted medical treatments but allowed states to put restrictions on the rights of surrogates to exercise these wishes on a patient's behalf. This ruling, in turn, brought national attention to the issue of advance care planning and advance medical directives.

Moral Justification for Withdraw of Life Support

The ethical justification for removing a patient at the end of life rests on two foundational principles of medical ethics. They are duty-bound to facilitate patient autonomy, and they have the duty to limit suffering and to put the patient's needs first. This is true even in situations when the removal of life support will undoubtedly hasten death.

A related moral justification rests on the "principle of double effect." This principle provides a way to guide individuals through actions that may be questioned as having both positive and negative effects [6]. The principle of double effect states that even if an action has foreseeable negative effects, it is permissible if the underlying motives of the action are good and the negative effect is proportional to the positive effect [7].

In the case of the removal of life support in a patient with a terminal illness, the underlying intention is to relieve suffering and further a patient's autonomy. And even though the act may foreseeably lead to death, the underlying intentions are positive and therefore permissible, particularly when one considers that in the case of a patient with a terminal illness, the underlying cause of death is the illness itself, not the act of removal of life support.

Medical Aid in Dying

A topic that is adjacent, but very separate from ethical questions surrounding the withdrawal of life support therapies, is the debate about medical aid in dying or so-called physician-assisted suicide. And it is crucial to distinguish the act of life support removal from these practices.

Medical aid in dying (MAID)—or as it is sometimes referred to, "physician-assisted suicide"—is a practice in which a physician helps a patient with a terminal illness end their life by giving them a prescription for a lethal dose of a drug, which the patient then may self-administer. As of 2025, MAID is currently legal in 12 states and the District of Columbia. But unlike Canada and several European countries, where practices around medical aid in dying are more expansive, in the United States, physicians are forbidden from participating in the administration of medication to intentionally end a patient's life [8].

In the United States, the question of whether patients facing the end of life or unremitting suffering should have the option to end their own life remains controversial. Many see the option as part of a patient's right to bodily autonomy. Others fear that the practice will lead to abuse and run directly counter to a physician's duty to preserve life. But whatever one's position on medical aid in dying, it is important to understand that this is a separate issue from the matter of consensually withdrawing life support.

Conflict Over the Use of Life Support

A different kind of ethical conflict surrounding the use of life support may occur when there is disagreement between clinicians and patients about the benefit of its use. This most commonly happens at the end of life or in the case of devastating neurological injuries, when clinicians may come to believe that life support therapies, such as prolonged mechanical ventilation, offer no meaningful benefit to a patient, and their surrogate decision makers nonetheless want to continue their use. Consider the following case:

> A 72-year-old man recently suffered a cardiac arrest and sustained devastating neurological injuries, leaving him in a persistent vegetative state. He is now admitted to the intensive care unit from a nursing home with acute kidney failure. In the six months since his arrest, he has shown no signs of neurological recovery and is not expected to. The medical team caring for him tells the family that while renal replacement therapy (dialysis) could temporar-

ily address his renal failure, it would not change his long-term prognosis and therefore offer no meaningful benefit. Despite the doctor's recommendations to forgo dialysis and focus on comfort-based care, the family insists that the ICU team initiate dialysis. What should the doctors do?

This case sets up an ethical conflict for the clinician who, on the one hand, wants to limit unnecessary suffering but, on the other hand, feels compelled to honor a patient's wish to choose which medical care they want to receive. Further complicating these conflicts is the fact that life support therapies are expensive and can only be provided in specialized facilities such as intensive care units, which adds to the ethical concern of the proper stewardship of limited resources.

While physicians are under no ethical obligation to provide a treatment of any kind that they believe is ineffective or harmful [8], withdrawing life support or refusing to provide CPR against the explicit request of a patient or their family is problematic. It can escalate conflict, undermine trust, and potentially expose clinicians to legal liability [2, 9]. For these reasons, experts in these conflicts recommend that clinicians engage in intensive communication and negotiations with patients or their families rather than just directly proceeding to unilateral decision-making. Fortunately, with time and patience, most of these conflicts can be resolved, and it is the minority where conflict becomes intractable [2, 8, 9].

Advice on Shared Decision-Making to Support Ethical Conversations

The practical aspects of withdrawing care are important to review. For patients who are likely to experience imminent death within a few days, many experts recommend discontinuing non essential medications and focusing on palliative therapies alone. Occasionally, long-standing therapies can be emotionally important to families or individual patients, and there is ample room for discussion and even negotiation with regard to these steps. With the widespread use of cardiac pacers, defibrillator devices, dialysis, and inotropes, the status of these devices must be addressed and adjusted after informing patients and their families of the practical aspects of their function and mitigating against shocks or pacer spikes during the dying process. Since the goal is to allow for patient autonomy and to completely remove artificial respiratory support, it is recommended that patients have the endotracheal tube and mechanical ventilation withdrawn promptly and replaced with simple supplemental oxygen. Based on family wishes, oxygen can be withheld since patients will have access to ambient air. While noninvasive ventilation might reduce the work of breathing, withholding this option will avoid prolonging the dying process or the period of suffering. It is important to recognize that oxygen and support are provided for comfort. These are titrated for patient comfort and not for routine physiological parameters. This use of oxygen to relieve the sense of dyspnea is a compassionate action. Other medications, such as opioids and anxiolytics, can be used to help further reduce any dyspnea or discomfort caused by the transition

Table 33.1 Practical aspects of palliative extubation [8, 12]

Patients and their families/legally designated representatives are at the center of discussions
Discussions and decisions should involve nursing and social work
The full care team in the ICU should be debriefed (including pastoral care)
Attention to pacer defibrillator should be provided and managed according to pt/family wishes
Essential medications should be maintained/nonessential medications discontinued
Program of comfort medications should be adjusted or initiated based on plan
Patient comfort should be confirmed
A second debriefing is recommended to assure timing of extubation is understood and accepted
Palliative extubation to simple oxygen or ambient air should occur with all necessary staff
Family should be provided prompt visitation (or be present during extubation if possible)
Comfort care measures should be adjusted to assure patient is comfortable
Maximize privacy for patient and family and assure pastoral care
Follow-up visits from nursing and physician staff are strongly suggested to support patient/ family and avoid a sense of abandonment

off life support. Enabling a compassionate death requires as much attention to detail as it takes to continue life support actions. The authors strongly suggest active engagement at the bedside to avoid abandonment during this critical phase of life [10].

The actual process of removing the mechanical ventilator should be carefully orchestrated with nursing, respiratory care, and the family so that this team works in concert with one another to assure that the steps are carried out with minimal suffering for the patient and maximum visitation for family and loved ones [11]. Nonmedical considerations should be included: timing, engagement with clergy, effects on younger children, music, the role of therapy/personal pets, or any other personal issues that are of importance to the dying person and the family.

Table 33.1 reviews suggested practical steps in the process.

The process, as outlined above, is challenging even for experienced ICU physicians and APCs. It is important that during the process, palliative extubation based on poor prognosis and patient/family preference is distinguished from active euthanasia. The two are entirely distinct. Transitioning from a curative care plan to a focus on comfort is well supported by legal and ethical experts. Focusing on comfort as patients are undergoing the dying process is an important role for the health care team [11–13].

Conclusion

The ethical justifications for removing patients from life support in certain situations align with a physician's duty to promote patient autonomy and safeguard their best interests. Nonetheless, clinicians must be attuned to the complex moral and emotional responses that it may provoke in families of patients and even other health care personnel [8–11, 13]. It is also essential that we pay careful attention to caregivers during these critical periods. The experience of caring for somebody at the end of life in the ICU can be emotionally draining and lead to depression or accelerated burnout [15, 16]. Clinicians must be sensitive and offer support while reminding them that although withdrawal of life support and systems of oxygen delivery at the end of life may hasten death, it is the underlying disease process and not the act of withdrawal that is the underlying cause. Additionally, supporting a patient's decision not to undergo or continue life support before death should be seen as consistent with patient autonomy and self-determination [11, 13, 14].

References

1. Orban JC, Walrave Y, Mongardon N, Allaouchiche B, Argaud L, Aubrun F, Lambiotte F. Causes and characteristics of death in intensive care units. Anesthesiology. 2017;126(5):882–9.
2. Luce JM, Alpers A. Legal aspects of withholding and withdrawing life support from critically ill patients in the United States and providing palliative care to them. Am J Respir Crit Care Med. 2000;162(6):2029–32.
3. Withdrawing Life Support. How is the decision made? JAMA. 1995;273(9):738–9. https://doi.org/10.1001/jama.1995.03520330068040.
4. Horan DJ. The Karen Ann Quinlan case. JAMA. 1976;235(17):1839–40.
5. Kennedy IM. The Karen Quinlan case: problems and proposals. J Med Ethics. 1976;2(1):3–7. PMID: 957371; PMCID: PMC2495105.
6. The Nancy Cruzan Case. N Engl J Med. 2010;324(8):561–2. https://doi.org/10.1056/NEJM199102213240812.
7. The Principle of Double Effect and Proportionate Reason. J Ethics. American Medical Association. Access 23 Oct 2025.
8. Lo B. Beyond legalization – dilemmas physicians confront regarding aid in dying. N Engl J Med. 2018;378(22):2060–2. https://doi.org/10.1056/NEJMp1802218.
9. Auriemma CL, Harhay MO, Haines KJ, Barg FK, Halpern SD, Lyon SM. What matters to patients and their families during and after critical illness: a qualitative study. Am J Crit Care. 2021;30(1):11–20. https://doi.org/10.4037/ajcc2021398. Erratum in: Am J Crit Care. 2021;30(2):144. doi:10.4037/ajcc2021507. PMID: 33385204; PMCID: PMC8101225.
10. Hernández-Fernández C, Meneses-Falcón C. Nobody should die alone. Loneliness and a dignified death during the COVID-19 pandemic. OMEGA J Death Dying. 2021;88(2):550–69. https://doi.org/10.1177/00302228211048316. (Original work published 2023).
11. American Thoracic Society Bioethics Task Force. Withholding and withdrawing life-sustaining therapy. Am Rev Respir Dis. 1991;144:726–31.
12. Withholding or Withdrawing Life-Sustaining Treatment | AMA-Code. Accessed 23 Oct 2025.
13. MacIntyre N. Discontinuing mechanical ventilatory support. Chest. 2007;132(3):1049–56.
14. Greco PJ, Schulman KA, Lavizzo-Mourey R, Hansen-Flaschen J. The Patient Self-Determination Act and the future of advance directives; 1991.
15. Linzer M, Visser MR, Oort FJ, Smets EM, McMurray JE, de Haes HC. Predicting and preventing physician burnout: results from the United States and the Netherlands. Am J Med. 2001;111:170–5. https://doi.org/10.1016/s0002-9343(01)00814-2.
16. Meier DE, Back AL, Morrison RS. The inner life of physicians and care of the seriously ill. JAMA. 2001;286:3007–14. https://doi.org/10.1001/jama.286.23.3007.

Part V

Lung Recovery

Tincture of Time: Recovery of the Lung After Injury

34

Susanna Betti and Michael Baram

Pathophysiology of Acute Lung Injury and ARDS

The concept of acute lung injury (ALI) has evolved over time. Initially, it was a descriptive term for a severe inflammatory lung syndrome, which accounts for 200,000 critical care admissions in the United States annually [1]. Since ALI was recognized to be a mild form of the more severe acute respiratory distress syndrome (ARDS), the use of its name has decreased, but the principal concepts remain the same. ARDS occurs as a secondary response to underlying conditions such as pneumonia, viral infections, pancreatitis, sepsis, or stress from trauma or aspiration. This triggers a cascade of pro-inflammatory cytokines and neutrophils, which damage endothelial cells, increase vascular permeability, and injure the alveolar epithelial barrier. This generates significant pulmonary edema and loss of surfactant, both of which contribute to pulmonary infiltrates, hypoxemia, and a rapid reduction in lung compliance. ARDS is defined as the presence of non-cardiogenic pulmonary edema, bilateral pulmonary infiltrates, and hypoxemia all within one week. ALI/ARDS is categorized by PaO_2/FiO_2 <300 mm Hg as mild, PaO_2/FiO_2 <200 mm Hg but greater than 100 mm Hg as moderate, and PaO_2/FiO_2 <100 mm Hg as severe [2]. This severity score mirrors mortality data.

The pathophysiology of ARDS can be grouped into three categories: the exudative phase in the first week, the proliferative phase in the second and third weeks, and the fibrotic phase from the fourth week onwards. These phases are

S. Betti
Internal Medicine, Thomas Jefferson University Hospital, Philadelphia, PA, USA
e-mail: Susanna.Betti@jefferson.edu

M. Baram (✉)
The Korman Respiratory Institute and the Division of Pulmonary, Allergy and Critical Care, The Department of Medicine at the Sidney Kimmel Medical College of Jefferson University, Philadelphia, PA, USA
e-mail: Michael.Baram@jefferson.edu

G. C. Kane et al. (eds.), *Oxygen*, https://doi.org/10.1007/978-3-032-18934-9_34

generalizations, but less predictable, is the rate of recovery. The exudative phase is characterized by destruction of the alveolar epithelium and fibrin deposition. A prominent histological finding in the first phase is the collection of extravascular fluid in the alveoli and the interstitial space. This physiology impedes oxygen's ability to be absorbed from the alveoli and into the blood. Failure to control inflammation at this time has been associated with worse outcomes for pulmonary recovery [3]. The proliferative stage is characterized by intra-alveolar and interstitial exudates and the early stages of fibrosis. Invasion of inflammatory cells can be seen on microscopy and further reduces oxygen diffusion. At this point, decreased lung compliance is a major contributor to mortality. Once a patient enters the fibrotic phase, the accumulation of fibroblasts and deposition of collagen rapidly progresses. This further decreases the ability of oxygen to diffuse into the blood, which is often seen as residual hypoxemia. This phase can have the most lasting effects on the recovery of pulmonary function and overall quality of life following the acute phase, but it also heralds the return of functional lung [4].

The Role of Ventilation and Supplemental Oxygen

Mechanical ventilation is a mainstay of ARDS lung support. Over the last thirty years, there has been a focus on lung-protective strategies using a low tidal volume strategy. A lower tidal volume reduces distension of the alveoli to minimize further damage to the lungs [5]. Decreased tidal volume will increase carbon dioxide levels in the blood, resulting in hypercapnia. The dangers of hypercapnia include respiratory acidosis and organ collapse, but this is balanced by the benefit of reduced cytokines caused by high-pressure ventilation. In ARDS, permissive hypercapnia with close monitoring is used to avoid over-distending the lungs [6]. High positive expiratory end pressure (PEEP) recruits collapsed alveoli, prevents further collapse, and has been associated with improved outcomes compared to low PEEP [7]. Both of these strategies have been shown to reduce mortality. Mechanical ventilation won't address the cause of ALI, but it provides supportive care for lung recovery, which generally follows if the patient can be supported successfully with limited complications.

Optimal ventilation strategies are still debated, as each has risks and benefits. Although controversial, recent trends in critical care suggest the use of humidified high flow oxygen instead of mechanical ventilation [8]. High flow can provide up to 60 liters of oxygen per minute via a large-bore nasal cannula and, in select patients, may provide enough support to avoid intubation. High flow may potentially avoid invasive **ventilation** by providing adequate oxygen support and improving lung recruitment.

In those who require mechanical ventilation, the duration of support is dependent on the clinical severity. In the mild stage, patients will spend an average of 6 days on a ventilator. With more moderate or severe ARDS, studies show that time on the ventilator is closer to two to three weeks [9]. Complications from prolonged ventilation are common, which include the development of nosocomial infections, critical care myopathy, ICU delirium, and more. Spontaneous breathing trials (SBT) are done daily in an effort to extubate as soon as clinically viable. In these SBTs, ventilator settings are typically switched to a minimal PEEP and a pressure support mode, in which the patient initiates their own breath while the ventilator provides support thereafter. Once a patient demonstrates the ability to breathe with minimal support, they can be liberated from the ventilator. At this point, non-invasive ventilation or additional oxygen can be introduced. Non-invasive ventilation, such as continuous positive airway pressure (CPAP) or bilevel positive airway pressure (BiPAP), keeps the airways patent to ease the transition off of mechanical ventilation. These modes may also decrease the risk of reintubation.

Supplemental oxygen is delivered through a nasal cannula and may help with dyspnea. By increasing the oxygen content in the blood, more oxygen is delivered to the muscles, which helps in delaying the onset of anaerobic metabolism and muscle fatigue. Anaerobic metabolism results in lactic acid formation, which requires an increased work of breathing to compensate. Supplemental oxygen also promotes lung recovery via oxygen delivery to the diaphragm to promote strengthening while decreasing an overactive respiratory drive [10].

There is more literature surrounding the evolution and progression of ARDS compared to its recovery process. From a clinical standpoint, there is a simple scoring system called the Murray score. It classified the degree of lung injury based on hypoxemia, PEEP levels, chest X-ray findings, and lung compliance [11]. The Murray score incorporates the physiological stress of ARDS by incorporating oxygenation, compliance, and radiographic perimeters. As the disease progresses, the Murray score worsens. During recovery, lung physiology improves. Ventilation deficits will typically resolve faster than oxygen deficits. The diffusion gradient of carbon dioxide from venous blood to the alveoli is slightly greater than 1, but that of oxygen from the alveoli to the blood is 2.5 [12]. While oxygen has a higher diffusion gradient, carbon dioxide is twenty times more soluble than oxygen, so it diffuses faster. In addition, damaged lungs hinder oxygen diffusion, further explaining why the resolution of ventilation deficits is quicker than oxygen recovery [13]. As lungs recover, compliance increases, eventually to the point of liberation from mechanical ventilation. As ARDS resolves, the Murray score returns to normal. Through monitoring ventilation requirements in real time, teams can continuously assess lung recovery in ARDS, transitioning patients from mechanical ventilation to passive oxygen delivery systems such as face masks and nasal cannulas.

Monitoring Oxygen Levels

Monitoring oxygen levels is necessary to assess recovery and prevent oxygen toxicity. As the lung recovers, if a patient is exposed to oxygen levels significantly higher than required, they may develop acute toxicity with central nervous system manifestations such as small muscle twitching, ear ringing, or nausea. If unchecked, acute toxicity can progress to chronic toxicity, which manifests as primarily pulmonary complaints. It is hard to quantify the effects of oxygen over supplementation, though clinicians should try to minimize oxygen use to avoid the inflammatory effects and the cost of unnecessary oxygen. Over oxygenated patients with underlying chronic obstructive lung disease can also lead to V/Q mismatching and worsening oxygenation saturations. Oxygen produces free radicals, which can damage the pulmonary lining, inactivate surfactant, and damage cellular membranes, leading to alveolar collapse [14]. When the alveoli are filled with pure oxygen, there is little nitrogen in the alveoli. The high oxygen alveolar gas creates a large diffusion gradient between the alveoli and capillaries. This drives more oxygen into the blood, leaving less gas in the alveoli. As a result, lungs can become atelectatic and have collapsed areas, which subsequently decreases the ventilation capacity of the lung. Hence, reducing oxygen overexposure leaves unabsorbed nitrogen in the alveoli to prevent atelectasis.

Frequent surveillance to avoid over- and under-oxygenating is key, and there are several options for adequate monitoring. While hospitalized, patients are placed on a pulse oximeter to help monitor their oxygen levels. This device is small enough to fit over a fingertip and emits a light that passes through the finger onto a sensor on the other side. The sensor detects the amount of light that is not absorbed by blood and is able to calculate the oxygen saturation of the blood. This is an inexpensive and non-invasive way to monitor oxygen levels continually, but it does have some drawbacks. It is less precise than other methods, with the reported oxygen levels may be off as much as 4% from the true value [15]. Newer generations of devices are being created to minimize the effects of different skin pigmentation. In addition, it is also prone to being moved or damaged, further causing inaccurate readings. Another method of oxygen monitoring is via an arterial blood gas. A needle is inserted into an artery, usually in the wrist, to remove a small amount of blood. This method is more invasive but highly accurate and can provide information on both oxygen and carbon dioxide levels in the blood. For many critically ill patients, these arterial blood samples are the gold standard and can be drawn off preexisting arterial catheters placed for hemodynamic monitoring.

During ARDS recovery, oxygenation and ventilation improve. The rate of improvement can vary between patients, but often ventilation will improve faster than oxygenation. Hence, patients who are liberated from the ventilator often have oxygen requirements. It is hard to predict when patients will be free of oxygen supplementation. The following sections review a few areas that speed up recovery from ARDS. It takes a tincture of time.

The Impact of Early Mobilization and Pulmonary Toilet in Recovery

Critically ill patients, especially those with ARDS, develop ICU-acquired muscle weakness due to deconditioning, use of sedatives, neuromuscular blocking agents, and corticosteroid-induced myopathy [16, 17]. Early mobilization of critically ill patients, ideally within 48 hours of diagnosis, improves recovery, increases independence at discharge, reduces time on mechanical ventilation, and decreases the length of the hospital and intensive care unit (ICU) stay. Once patients start exercising, they need to generate more spontaneous breaths in order to increase oxygen and decrease carbon dioxide levels in their blood. Spontaneous breathing provides a more uniform distribution of air compared to that in immobile patients. Mobilization improves oxygenation by aerating all areas of the lung, especially those that have been collapsed due to lying flat. This improved air distribution recruits more lung and decreases collapsed areas, which start producing surfactant again to improve other collapsed areas. With this cycle, spontaneous breathing triggers the recruitment of the healthy lung.

An important target for mobilization includes deep breathing exercises to force the diaphragm to generate negative pressure and avoid reliance on accessory respiratory muscles. Patients may perceive an increased work of breathing due to diaphragmatic muscle weakness despite their pulmonary function not being impaired [18]. Diaphragmatic weakness can occur from prolonged ventilation, so proper exercise combined with aggressive pulmonary toileting can increase successful extubations and recovery [16]. Pulmonary toilet is a term that encompasses deep breathing exercises, coughing, and chest physiotherapy. Studies have shown that early and aggressive pulmonary toilet reduces the risk of pneumonia and other pulmonary complications [19]. It improves oxygenation by clearing the airways of any secretions, reducing atelectatic lung, and decreasing ventilation-perfusion mismatch.

Once a patient has been tolerating some exercise, there are a few studies that can be done to assess cardiopulmonary recovery. The most common and achievable is the 6-minute walk test (6MWT). The patient's baseline heart rate and oxygen saturation are measured, along with their dyspnea level (assessed by a validated scale). The patient is then monitored while walking for a full six minutes, and their end heart rate, oxygen saturation, and dyspnea level are assessed. Most healthy individuals can achieve 400–700 m walking distance. The 6MWT is easy to complete, safe for most patients, and proven to assess the degree of functional impairment and disease severity in cardiopulmonary recovery and is especially useful to assess oxygen dependency during exercise. In fact, poor performance on the 6MWT has been directly correlated with lower quality of life, poor respiratory recovery, and decreased survival [20].

Long-Term Effects of ARDS

Recovery from ARDS is a lengthy process, with many patients still feeling the effects years later. Several studies have demonstrated long-term impairment in physical strength, exercise capacity, cognitive function, and quality of life. For most survivors, it takes a minimum of twelve months for pulmonary function to return to normal [21]). Any lingering fibrosis and microvascular changes in the lungs will often result in persistent hypoxemia and impaired oxygen transfer. Unfortunately, up to one-third of patients will have a permanent obstructive ventilatory defect despite lung volume and spirometry measurements recovering fully [5]. The diffusion capacity of the lung for carbon monoxide (DLCO) measures how well oxygen can transfer from inhaled air to the blood. Structural changes in the lungs caused by ARDS, such as increased fibrosis and thickened alveolar septa, interfere with this capacity, and decreased DLCO has been reported in over 80% of patients at least six months after ARDS [7].

Studies have also reported ARDS survivors having decreased quality of life scores. Interestingly, the poor quality of life is directly related to physical rather than emotional or psychological complaints, with rates similar to those of patients who suffer from long-term, chronic illness. Complaints include both pulmonary symptoms, like cough and dyspnea, and non-pulmonary symptoms, such as generalized weakness and nerve injury [18]. Levels of physical exercise are also reduced and comparable to those with chronic respiratory diseases, despite normalization of most pulmonary function. Part of this is from residual fibrosis impairing oxygen transfer, corticosteroid-induced and critical-illness myopathy, and fatigue. About 50% of all patients return to work one year after discharge, with those unable to work citing causes such as stress, physical restraints from the job, and persistent fatigue [20]. In summary, survivors of ARDS can expect the first few years to be marked by the return of pulmonary function, but with marked functional disability leading to decreased physical strength and oxygenation compared to their healthy counterparts [6].

The Role of Steroids in Recovery

The first week of ARDS has been shown to be a critical time for disease outcomes, with failure to control inflammation being a major predictor of poor outcome [3, 22]. Glucocorticoids, with their ability to downregulate systemic inflammation and minimize fibroproliferative progression, have been shown across multiple trials to reduce inflammation, dependence on mechanical ventilation, and ICU length of stay [22–26]. By dampening inflammation, they reduce alveolar–capillary membrane permeability, which limits the buildup of edema and improves oxygenation. The current recommendations favor low-dose methylprednisolone initiated within seventy-two hours of ARDS diagnosis. Methylprednisolone is typically administered with a 1 mg/kg loading dose, followed by a slow taper over several weeks [22].

Low-dose steroids have largely been preferred to higher doses, as they have been associated with earlier liberation from mechanical ventilation [27] and a decreased risk of secondary infections, psychosis, and residual muscle weakness [28]. Recent trials in ARDS patients suggest a decreased hospital length of stay, ICU requirements, and mechanical ventilation with methylprednisolone [25]. Methylprednisolone has been shown to have a higher concentration in the lungs compared to other corticosteroids due to its larger volume of distribution. Mineralocorticoids, like hydrocortisone, increase effective circulating volume, worsen pulmonary edema, and prolong the time on mechanical ventilation [26]. The decision of which corticosteroid and when to initiate should be based on the clinical judgment of the healthcare team and should factor in patient-specific considerations.

A Word on Multi-organ Failure

ARDS has been associated with a remarkably high mortality rate of 60% despite advances in lung-protective mechanical ventilation. Hypoxemia-related mortality in ARDS patients accounts for only about 15% of cases, with the rest attributed to multi-organ failure. While poor oxygenation is associated with negative outcomes, improvement has not been associated with improved outcomes. Conversely, reversing multi-organ failure has been linked to improved survival in ARDS patients [29]. It is important for the clinician to remember that in ARDS patients, the greatest threat is not respiratory failure, but rather multi-organ failure.

Pulmonary Hypertension as a Complication

One of the central processes involved in ARDS, as described earlier, is a damaged alveolar epithelial barrier leading to pulmonary edema. This edema and subsequent surfactant dysfunction contribute to ventilation-perfusion mismatch, which can be clinically observed as hypoxemia. This mismatch occurs when the ratio of oxygen entering the lungs and oxygen passing into your blood vessels is imbalanced. This can be due to either poor ventilation or poor perfusion. Low oxygen levels have a vasoconstrictive effect on pulmonary vessels, which attempt to mediate this ventilation-perfusion mismatch by shunting blood away from diseased airspaces [29]. Vasoconstriction occurring in response to pro-inflammatory cytokines released during stress or infection, in addition to vessel obliteration and microthrombi caused by endothelial cell damage, increases pulmonary vascular resistance (PVR) and is an underlying mechanism for the development of pulmonary hypertension (PH) in patients with ARDS.

PH is an increase in PVR leading to right ventricular dysfunction. A right heart catheterization demonstrating a mean pulmonary artery pressure of over 20 mmHg is required to make a diagnosis. Vascular remodeling in the subacute phases of ARDS will often continually elevate the PVR. Chronic phases characterized by fibrosis further obliterate the microvasculature, disrupt blood flow, and elevate PVR. Studies have demonstrated that PH is prevalent in 92% of ARDS patients, and the prevalence of right-sided heart failure is as high as 20% [30]. Administering vasodilators to target pulmonary hypertension in patients with ARDS may blunt the hypoxic pulmonary vasoconstrictive process and worsen oxygenation [30]. Supplemental oxygen is an effective tool to reduce PH, as it promotes pulmonary vasodilation to decrease PVR.

As discussed previously, the Murray score is a generalized severity score. It can also be used to assess improvement. As the oxygenation improves, the score improves. As markers of severity in the Murray score improve, the pulmonary hypertension improves as well. As described above, as oxygenation improves, PH improves. As PEEP is reduced, PH improves. Again, these are gross scoring levels, but they highlight how the lung heals, both acutely and over a year-long period [31].

The Role of Immunizations Following ARDS

While there is no standardized protocol for immunizing patients following ARDS, vaccinating eligible patients plays a large role in preventing secondary infections such as bacterial pneumonia and influenza. These secondary complications would cause further injury to the lungs and either blunt or worsen oxygenation in lungs that are recovering from ALI. Vaccines are a major preventative tool available for reducing the risk of these infections and have been shown to decrease admission duration, severe complications, and mortality [32].

Streptococcus pneumoniae results in over 500,000 cases of community-acquired pneumonia, 50,000 cases of bacteremia, 3000 cases of meningitis, and 40,000 deaths annually in the United States. Safe and effective immunization has been demonstrated in countless studies, and current Advisory Committee on Immunization Practices (ACIP) guidelines recommend vaccination in all patients aged 65 years and above, or those younger but with increased risk (including congestive heart failure, chronic respiratory illness, or diabetes). Similarly, the influenza virus is responsible for 114,000 hospitalizations and 20,000 deaths annually in the United States. Influenza infection is also a major risk for developing secondary bacterial pneumonia. The current ACIP guidelines recommend vaccination of those 50–64 years of age and patients at increased risk of complications (including those with chronic respiratory problems). It is crucial to prevent further complications and improve oxygenation in those recovering from ARDS, and reducing the risks of secondary infection, such as influenza and *Streptococcus pneumoniae*, is paramount in decreasing the risk of subsequent bacterial superinfection and recurrence of ARDS [33].

Nutrition

Patients with ARDS are at high risk for malnutrition because of an increased pro-inflammatory state and caloric expenditure, as well as mechanical ventilation dependence, which impedes typical oral access [33]. Higher rates of cytokine release can lead to an increased daily energy requirement of 20%, elaborating on the importance of adequate nutritional support. In fact, respiratory muscle strength starts to deteriorate after just a few days of failing to meet nutritional goals [33, 34].

Malnutrition has been associated with a higher likelihood of hypercapnia than that in well-nourished critically ill patients due to decreased respiratory muscle mass and contractility, altered respiratory drive, and decreased surfactant production [4]. Early nutritional support is paramount in overall recovery.

Determining appropriate nutrition goals should be patient-specific and involve expert consultation, as underfeeding fails to provide adequate support for pulmonary recovery and weakens immune strength, but overfeeding may contribute to hypercapnia and delayed ventilator weaning. Enteric feeds should ideally be given directly into the small bowel to minimize the risk of aspiration. Special care should be taken in patients with ARDS, as their respiratory function is already compromised. With complications of sepsis being a leading cause of mortality in ARDS patients, reducing the chances of aspiration pneumonia is paramount [34].

Conclusion

ARDS mortality is frequently discussed, and it is commonplace to discuss how ARDS can progress to multi-organ failure. It is important to recognize that most patients do survive ARDS. Tracking patient oxygenation and ventilation can give important clues on patient status. There are few concrete references that focus on recovery, and even fewer patient/family-directed literature. More research and attention need to be focused on healing and recovery. This chapter focuses on the acute phases of recovery; there is another chapter that covers post-ICU recovery and longer-term recovery.

References

1. Elicker BM, Jones KT, Naeger DM, Frank JA. Imaging of acute lung injury. Radiol Clin North Am. 2016;54(6):1119–32.
2. Yao S, Zeng L, Wang F, Chen K. Obesity paradox in lung diseases: what explains it? Obes Facts. 2023;16(5):411–26.
3. Meduri GU, Yates CR. Systemic inflammation-associated glucocorticoid resistance and outcome of ARDS. Ann N Y Acad Sci. 2004;1024:24–53.
4. Mizock BA. Nutritional support in acute lung injury and acute respiratory distress syndrome. Nutr Clin Pract. 2001;16(6):319–28.
5. Palakshappa JA, Krall JTW, Belfield LT, Files DC. Long-term outcomes in acute respiratory distress syndrome: epidemiology, mechanisms, and patient evaluation. Crit Care Clin. 2021;37(4):895–911.
6. Cooper AB, Ferguson ND, Hanly PJ, Meade MO, Kachura JR, Granton JT, et al. Long-term follow-up of survivors of acute lung injury: lack of effect of a ventilation strategy to prevent barotrauma. Crit Care Med. 1999;27(12):2616–21.
7. Neff TA, Stocker R, Frey HR, Stein S, Russi EW. Long-term assessment of lung function in survivors of severe ARDS. Chest. 2003;123(3):845–53.
8. Pérez-Nieto ORG-GM, Deloya-Tomas E, Ñamendys-Silva SA. Prone positioning combined with high-flow nasal cannula in severe noninfectious ARDS. Crit Care. 2020;24(1):114.
9. Force ADT, Ranieri VM, Rubenfeld GD, Thompson BT, Ferguson ND, Caldwell E, et al. Acute respiratory distress syndrome: the Berlin Definition. JAMA. 2012;307(23):2526–33.
10. Ekstrom M, Ahmadi Z, Bornefalk-Hermansson A, Abernethy A, Currow D. Oxygen for breathlessness in patients with chronic obstructive pulmonary disease who do not qualify for home oxygen therapy. Cochrane Database Syst Rev. 2016;11(11):CD006429.
11. Murray JF, Matthay MA, Luce JM, Flick MR. An expanded definition of the adult respiratory distress syndrome. Am Rev Respir Dis. 1988;138(3):720–3.
12. Molnar C, Gair J. Concepts of biology. 1st Canadian ed. BC Campus; 2015.
13. Speller J. Gas exchange: Teach Me physiology; 2025. Available from: https://teachmephysiology.com/respiratory-system/gas-exchange/gas-exchange/.
14. Cooper JS, Phuyal P, Shah N. Oxygen toxicity. Treasure Island: StatPearls; 2025.
15. Medicine Y. Pulse oximetry. Available from: https://www.yalemedicine.org/conditions/pulse-oximetry.
16. Jang MH, Shin MJ, Shin YB. Pulmonary and physical rehabilitation in critically ill patients. Acute Crit Care. 2019;34(1):1–13.

17. Latronico N, Eikermann M, Ely EW, Needham DM. Improving management of ARDS: uniting acute management and long-term recovery. Crit Care. 2024;28(1):58.
18. Orme J Jr, Romney JS, Hopkins RO, Pope D, Chan KJ, Thomsen G, et al. Pulmonary function and health-related quality of life in survivors of acute respiratory distress syndrome. Am J Respir Crit Care Med. 2003;167(5):690–4.
19. Cassidy MR, Rosenkranz P, McCabe K, Rosen JE, McAneny D. I COUGH: reducing postoperative pulmonary complications with a multidisciplinary patient care program. JAMA. 2013;148(8):750–45.
20. Matos Casano HA, Anjum F. Six-minute walk test. Treasure Island: StatPearls; 2025.
21. Herridge MS, Cheung AM, Tansey CM, Matte-Martyn A, Diaz-Granados N, Al-Saidi F, et al. One-year outcomes in survivors of the acute respiratory distress syndrome. N Engl J Med. 2003;348(8):683–93.
22. Meduri GU, Golden E, Freire AX, Taylor E, Zaman M, Carson SJ, et al. Methylprednisolone infusion in early severe ARDS: results of a randomized controlled trial. Chest. 2007;131(4):954–63.
23. Meduri GU, Annane D, Confalonieri M, Chrousos GP, Rochwerg B, Busby A, et al. Pharmacological principles guiding prolonged glucocorticoid treatment in ARDS. Intensive Care Med. 2020;46(12):2284–96.
24. Group WHOREAfC-TW, Sterne JAC, Murthy S, Diaz JV, Slutsky AS, Villar J, et al. Association between administration of systemic corticosteroids and mortality among critically ill patients with COVID-19: a meta-analysis. JAMA. 2020;324(13):1330–41.
25. Villar J, Ferrando C, Martinez D, Ambros A, Munoz T, Soler JA, et al. Dexamethasone treatment for the acute respiratory distress syndrome: a multicentre, randomised controlled trial. Lancet Respir Med. 2020;8(3):267–76.
26. Landolf KM, Lemieux SM, Rose C, Johnston JP, Adams CD, Altshuler J, et al. Corticosteroid use in ARDS and its application to evolving therapeutics for coronavirus disease 2019 (COVID-19): a systematic review. Pharmacotherapy. 2022;42(1):71–90.
27. Thompson BT, Ranieri VM. Steroids are part of rescue therapy in ARDS patients with refractory hypoxemia: no. Intensive Care Med. 2016;42(5):921–3.
28. Steinberg KP, Hudson LD, Goodman RB, Hough CL, Lanken PN, Hyzy R, et al. Efficacy and safety of corticosteroids for persistent acute respiratory distress syndrome. N Engl J Med. 2006;354(16):1671–84.
29. Del Sorbo L, Slutsky AS. Acute respiratory distress syndrome and multiple organ failure. Curr Opin Crit Care. 2011;17(1):1–6.
30. Price LC, McAuley DF, Marino PS, Finney SJ, Griffiths MJ, Wort SJ. Pathophysiology of pulmonary hypertension in acute lung injury. Am J Physiol Lung Cell Mol Physiol. 2012;302(9):L803–15.
31. Revercomb L, Hanmandlu A, Wareing N, Akkanti B, Karmouty-Quintana H. Mechanisms of pulmonary hypertension in Acute Respiratory Distress Syndrome (ARDS). Front Mol Biosci. 2020;7:624093.
32. Shorr AF. Preventing pneumonia: the role for pneumococcal and influenza vaccines. Clin Chest Med. 2005;26(1):123–34.
33. Braunschweig CA, Sheean PM, Peterson SJ, Gomez Perez S, Freels S, Lateef O, et al. Intensive nutrition in acute lung injury: a clinical trial (INTACT). JPEN J Parenter Enteral Nutr. 2015;39(1):13–20.
34. Turner KL, Moore FA, Martindale R. Nutrition support for the acute lung injury/adult respiratory distress syndrome patient: a review. Nutr Clin Pract. 2011;26(1):14–25.

Pulmonary Rehabilitation

35

Rafael Perez

Introduction

Pulmonary rehabilitation was developed and has been refined over the years with the ultimate goal of improving the functional status of individuals physically impaired by chronic lung diseases. The pulmonary impairment causes varying levels of disability that handicap the affected person in a way that he or she cannot achieve their desired level of social functioning. While the pulmonary impairment is essentially fixed, the disability and handicap are malleable and can be improved by a well-designed pulmonary rehabilitation program. Pulmonary rehabilitation is defined by the American Thoracic and European Respiratory Societies as "…a comprehensive intervention based on a thorough patient assessment followed by patient-tailored therapies that include, but are not limited to, exercise training, education, and behavior change, designed to improve the physical and psychological condition of people with chronic respiratory disease and to promote the long-term adherence to health-enhancing behaviors" [1]. Pulmonary rehabilitation programs employ various approaches that combine physical training, education, and behavioral changes to improve the overall quality of life for individuals living with chronic lung diseases. This chapter provides an overview of the rationale for and development of pulmonary rehabilitation programs to improve the lives of persons with chronic lung diseases.

Key "take-home" points about pulmonary rehabilitation are discussed herein. First, the majority of studies on pulmonary rehabilitation have been performed in individuals with chronic obstructive pulmonary disease (COPD). The knowledge gained from COPD studies has been applied to other chronic lung diseases, notably

R. Perez (✉)
The Korman Respiratory Institute and the Division of Pulmonary, Allergy and Critical Care, The Department of Medicine at the Sidney Kimmel Medical College of Thomas Jefferson University, Philadelphia, PA, USA
e-mail: rafael.perez@jefferson.edu

G. C. Kane et al. (eds.), *Oxygen*, https://doi.org/10.1007/978-3-032-18934-9_35

interstitial lung disease (ILD) and pulmonary hypertension, which have distinctly different pathophysiological mechanisms. Second, the improvements in physical and behavioral status are transient unless the individual maintains a level of activity and continues to implement behavioral changes to sustain the progress made during the rehabilitation sessions. Third, the availability and barriers to enrollment, adherence, and the cost of traditional outpatient pulmonary rehabilitation are such that only a small percentage of individuals who would benefit from it enter and complete a program.

A Brief History of Pulmonary Rehabilitation

The concept of rehabilitation techniques designed to enhance physical status and quality of life in patients with chronic obstructive pulmonary disease (COPD) emerged around the mid-twentieth century [2, 3]. None other than Dr. Alvan Barach, who pioneered the use of hospital and ambulatory oxygen therapy, promoted the benefits of interventions to improve the overall well-being of individuals with COPD [3]. Dr. Thomas Petty soon thereafter performed an uncontrolled yet comprehensive "proof-of-concept" two-year program enrolling 182 participants with COPD. The program demonstrated that a combination of disease education, breathing techniques, and physical training improved exercise tolerance and enhanced social participation in the majority of participants who completed the program [4]. Ries and colleagues later studied 119 men and women with COPD, randomized 1:1 to an intervention group receiving physical training and education vs. a control group receiving education alone over 8 weeks [5]. The intervention group showed significant improvements in maximal exercise tolerance, exercise endurance, and reduced dyspnea compared with the control group, which received education only. However, there were no significant differences in quality-of-life measures. The investigators followed the subjects for 72 months. They noted that the effects of exercise training diminished over the course of one year, and there were no significant differences in survival or hospitalizations between the groups. Nevertheless, this study formed the basis for subsequent studies that, over the years, refined the delivery of pulmonary rehabilitation to achieve improvements in quality of life, lower healthcare costs, and enhanced exercise abilities [6, 7].

Pulmonary Pathophysiology and Its Impact on Exercise Ability

Chronic lung diseases of the airways and parenchyma, including the lung interstitium and pulmonary vasculature, present with irreversible pathophysiology of varying severity [6, 8, 9]. Treatments for these diseases aim to prevent, at least, worsening and, at best, to recover some lung function. Examples are bronchodilator therapy in COPD, immune-modulating and anti-fibrotic drugs in ILD, and vasodilator medications in pulmonary hypertension. Despite treatment, both airway and parenchymal lung diseases lead to increased work of breathing through mechanisms that affect airflow, elastic properties, and ventilation-to-perfusion relationships (Fig. 35.1). Derangements and destruction of airways and the terminal gas exchange surface in COPD result in overdistension and increased dead space, leading to dynamic hyperinflation and air trapping during exertion. Fibrosis and "stiffening" of the lungs, accompanied by increased elastic recoil in ILD, result in small lung volumes, an increased respiratory rate, and a decreased surface area for gas exchange. The mechanical and gas exchange derangements across the spectrum of airway and parenchymal lung diseases lead to increased work of breathing and decreased oxygen delivery to working muscles. The early onset of lactic acidosis further increases the work of breathing, resulting in more exercise limitation and deconditioning.

Advanced chronic lung diseases are often accompanied by cardiac dysfunction caused by persistent increases in pulmonary vascular resistance [10]. Pulmonary vascular resistance increases with the destruction of pulmonary arteries and vasoconstriction in response to hypoxemia. Right heart overload ensues with ventricular distention and the manifestations of pulmonary hypertension. Impingement of the

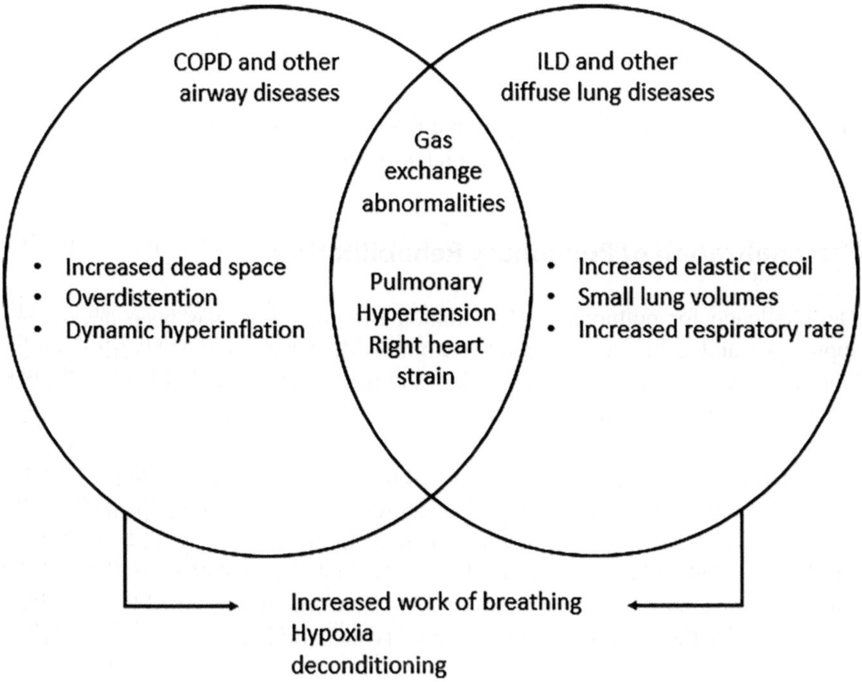

Fig. 35.1 COPD and other airway diseases are characterized by the destruction of supporting lung tissue along the branching airways, including respiratory bronchioles and acinar structures. The result is increased lung compliance, accompanied by increased dead space, overdistension, and dynamic inflation during exertion. In contrast, ILD and other diffuse lung diseases have a course characterized by increased deposition of interstitial matrix proteins, leading to fibrosis and obliteration of acinar structures. The result is decreased lung compliance, with small lung volumes and increased respiratory rate on exertion. Both airway and lung parenchymal diseases compromise pulmonary vessels, which contribute to gas exchange abnormalities and pulmonary hypertension

left ventricle from a deviated intraventricular septum and rhythm abnormalities also impede cardiac output to working muscles. Thus, in addition to the underlying pulmonary disease, cardiac impairment also contributes to exercise limitation and overall deconditioning.

Pulmonary Rehabilitation Program Design and Requirements

The accrediting agency for pulmonary rehabilitation in the United States is the American Association for Cardiovascular and Pulmonary Rehabilitation (AACVPR) [11]. The core of a pulmonary rehabilitation program requires a medical director who is responsible for ensuring that participants are medically stable and suitable for undergoing pulmonary rehabilitation. The director ensures the effectiveness of the program by recommending the appropriate training intensity for each individual participating in it. Other responsibilities include maintaining optimal training site space and equipment, supervising training personnel, and ensuring the implementation and maintenance of safety protocols, such as infection control. A program coordinator with rehabilitation training and knowledge of the regulatory and operational aspects of PR is on-site, working with participants and supervising other healthcare professionals. These other professionals may include respiratory therapists trained in pulmonary rehabilitation, occupational therapists, nutritionists, and social workers. The personnel number and mix depend on the program's size and local resources.

Personalization of Pulmonary Rehabilitation

The challenge for pulmonary rehabilitation over the years has been developing approaches and techniques tailored to each individual, based on the severity of their lung disease, informed by comorbidities, and their goals for social interaction [7]. The personalized prescription for pulmonary rehabilitation begins with a thorough assessment that focuses on a participant's cardiopulmonary status and any coexisting systemic and musculoskeletal abnormalities. The assessment includes exercise testing that determines the parameters of exercise for a given participant. Exercise testing establishes their maximal work capacity and identifies any musculoskeletal problems, including balance issues. Abnormal changes in vital signs and symptoms during exercise may indicate potential safety concerns that need to be addressed before exercise training, or they may disqualify the individual from participating in pulmonary rehabilitation.

Physical limitations in individuals evaluated for pulmonary rehabilitation are often accompanied by feelings of anxiety, depression, and fear of exercising [7]. Recognition of these feelings, at the very least, and collaboration with mental health experts as needed, improve an individual's chance of completing a pulmonary rehabilitation program successfully.

Approximately half of the individuals referred to a pulmonary rehabilitation program will not enroll or complete it [12]. Barriers to enrolling and adhering to a pulmonary rehabilitation program include socioeconomic factors such as living alone, the extent of comorbidities, smoking, and the "enthusiasm" of the referring provider [13, 14]. Hayton and colleagues performed a retrospective analysis of 711 subjects with COPD referred to pulmonary rehabilitation [14]. Around one-third did not enroll, with the main reasons being difficulty with transportation, a perception that the disease was either too severe or not severe enough to enroll, and failure to present for unknown reasons. Another third of the subjects were non-adherent (defined as attending less than 60% of exercise sessions), mainly because of COPD exacerbations, transportation problems, new limiting conditions, hospitalizations, or simply dropping out. The referring provider and the patient should thoroughly discuss the barriers to attending a pulmonary rehabilitation program and work together to alleviate them in the best way possible.

Exercise Training Initiation and Outcome Measures

Exercise training is the foundation of pulmonary rehabilitation, emphasizing techniques to improve endurance, strength, and flexibility for participants. The techniques employ a balance of frequency, intensity, time, and type (FITT) of exercise to obtain the best physical outcome [7, 15, 16]. Notably, participants in pulmonary rehabilitation tend to be middle-aged to elderly, and the effects of aging become more pronounced in this population. Decreased muscle mass and cardiopulmonary function must be taken into consideration when designing individualized FITT regimens. Exercise that is too intense or lasts too long increases the chance that the participant will drop out of the program. Notably, exercise training benefits both men and women with some nuanced differences beyond the scope of this chapter.

The initial evaluation includes some form of exercise testing that establishes the participant's starting level of exercise. Cardiopulmonary exercise testing (CPET) using a treadmill or cycle ergometry is ideal, as it yields the most accurate assessment of an individual's work capacity [17]. Another advantage of CPET is that it identifies issues such as cardiac dysrhythmias, abnormal blood pressure elevations, exercise-induced bronchoconstriction, and musculoskeletal limitations that may prevent participation in pulmonary rehabilitation. The limitation of CPET is that it is costly and requires specialized equipment and expertise to perform and interpret the test results.

The 6-minute walk test (6MWT) is a standardized assessment of ambulatory endurance [18]. The 6MWT is performed indoors on level ground, walking around cones or markers that are 30 m apart for precisely 6 min. Blood pressure and heart rate are taken at the beginning and end of exercise. The primary outcome is the distance walked at the individual's selected pace. Pulse oximetry is commonly performed at the beginning and end of exercise, along with an assessment of dyspnea using the Borg scale of perceived exertion [19]. The advantages of the 6MWT are that it can be easily performed in a clinic setting and requires minimal equipment. The 6MWT is performed even when CPET is available, as it is a more cost-effective method for measuring improvements in exercise ability. For example, an improvement in walk distance of 24–45 m (depending upon patient characteristics) after rehabilitation is considered a minimal clinically important difference for persons with idiopathic pulmonary fibrosis (IPF) [20].

Frequency, Intensity, Time, and Type (FITT) of Exercise Training

Pulmonary rehabilitation guidelines and procedures have been developed to optimize the frequency, intensity, and duration of improvement in individuals participating in pulmonary rehabilitation programs [7, 15, 16]. The type of training speaks to the specific outcome desired. For example, endurance involves whole-body exercise such as treadmill walking or cycling. Walking and cycling are individualized to allow participants to sustain exercise intensity between 60% and 70% of their maximal work capacity, as determined by exercise testing, for at least 20 min at a time [21]. Some individuals may develop intolerable dyspnea with constant exercise, as found in persons with COPD and substantial dynamic hyperinflation. They can exercise instead in short, intense intervals with rest in between to relieve the dyspnea. The benefits of endurance training can be measured after three sessions per week over 8 to 12 weeks, and are manifested as an overall improved activity level, accompanied by better aerobic capacity and reduced dyspnea.

Resistance training, done by exerting muscle groups against a load, improves strength. The load can take the form of exercise equipment, free weights, or the participant's body weight [21]. The intensity of strength training, light, moderate, or hard, is determined by the fraction of a load that can be performed only once. For example, a person who can lift 100 pounds only once trains with light-intensity lifting repetitions of 40 pounds or hard-intensity lifting repetitions of 80 pounds. Two to four sets of 8 to 12 repetitions, two to three days per week, improve strength. Strength training also improves endurance at repetitions of 15 or more per set.

Inspiratory muscle training (IMT) is specifically designed to enhance inspiratory muscle endurance and strength [7]. Devices that impose a resistive load on the sternocleidomastoid, intercostal, and diaphragmatic muscles improve oxidative capacity and decrease muscle fatigue. As a stand-alone modality, IMT can improve dyspnea, exercise capacity, and quality of life; however, these improvements are not observed when IMT is combined with other modes of exercise training [22]. Some pulmonary rehabilitation programs include IMT, but there is no specific recommendation in the latest American Thoracic Society clinical practice guidelines regarding the incorporation of IMT as part of the exercise regimen [6].

Education and Breathing Exercises

Comprehensive pulmonary rehabilitation programs typically include an education component that varies depending on the available expertise and program design. There are no specific recommendations on the types of education to offer, making it difficult to prove its efficacy [6]. Nevertheless, experts in pulmonary rehabilitation recommend incorporating education into the exercise program. The medical director may lead a discussion in lay terms about participants' disease pathophysiology and pharmacology. Social workers and occupational therapists may provide guidance on self-management and offer a broad range of lifestyle advice. The American Lung Association and COPD Foundation provide easily understandable information on lung disease and pulmonary rehabilitation on their websites [23, 24].

Breathing retraining is a crucial component of pulmonary rehabilitation. Breathing exercises were developed around the concept of dynamic hyperinflation with exercise in COPD [1]. Exhaling through tightened lips, creating a small orifice called "purse-lips breathing," causes airflow resistance at the mouth and creates a back pressure into the pulmonary airways. The effect is to slow breathing and decrease hyperinflation during exertion.

Unlike individuals with COPD, who have destruction of elastic lung tissue and airway collapse, causing airflow limitation, persons with ILD have increased deposition of elastic and fibrotic elements that splint open the airways relative to reduced lung volumes. They do not develop hyperinflation during exercise, so training in pursed-lips breathing is of questionable benefit in these diseases [25]. The airflow resistance caused by pursed-lip breathing, as taught for COPD, may add to the increased elastic resistance in those with ILD. However, a moderated pursed-lips breathing regimen to decrease the breathing rate during exercise may be beneficial in selected cases of ILD.

Pulmonary Rehabilitation in Interstitial Lung Disease

Pulmonary rehabilitation interventions for ILD, including IPF, came later than interventions for COPD. It was not clear until more recently that programs designed based on the experience with COPD could benefit individuals with ILD. A Cochrane analysis of 21 randomized controlled trials encompassing a range of ILD diagnoses and disease severities showed improvements in exercise capacity, dyspnea, and quality of life measures [26]. Notably, there were a few adverse events during rehabilitation, and four deaths were reported as unrelated to the exercise limitations. The quality of the evidence was low to moderate, and bias in the form of selection, blinding, and intent-to-treat was prominent.

Nevertheless, sensitivity analysis using the highest quality studies appeared to support the benefits of pulmonary rehabilitation in ILD. An assessment of 7 systematic reviews of randomized controlled trials on pulmonary rehabilitation in IPF also indicated improvements in exercise, quality of life, and even lung function [27]. However, there were profound levels of low methodological quality and high levels of bias among the studies.

A combined analysis of two randomized trials involving 188 subjects with ILD examined the effects of pulmonary rehabilitation on survival over 10 years [28]. The intervention group underwent 8 weeks of pulmonary rehabilitation. The intervention significantly improved survival at 5 years; however, the gap in survival closed thereafter, and no differences were observed at 10 years. The authors speculate that the sample sizes of the groups were too small to see a sustained effect on survival at 10 years. Other interventions in the control subjects, such as later participation in pulmonary rehabilitation, may have also contributed.

The American Thoracic Society clinical practice guidelines provide a strong recommendation for pulmonary rehabilitation in ILD, despite low to moderate evidence of benefit [6]. The Society holds that the benefits outweigh any undesirable effects of pulmonary rehabilitation and that the participants' self-management skills and disease knowledge are improved.

Pulmonary Rehabilitation in Pulmonary Hypertension

Pulmonary hypertension is defined by a broad range of diseases that produce a mean pulmonary arterial pressure of 20 mmHg or more [29]. Diseases that result in pulmonary hypertension are classified into five groups depending on the pathophysiology that increases pulmonary arterial pressure. For example, COPD and ILD, where the pulmonary vasculature is compromised by lung destruction or fibrosis, are found in group 3; left heart failure and valvular disease comprise group 2; chronic thromboembolic disease dominates group 4. The disease course, therapeutic management, and outcomes vary widely among the groups. This wide variability makes the development of pulmonary rehabilitation regimens for pulmonary hypertension a challenging task.

Panels from the American Thoracic Society and the European Respiratory Society reviewed a mix of randomized controlled trials, controlled trials, and cohort studies for a total of 1355 subjects with pulmonary hypertension [6, 30]. Subjects were included from all of the pulmonary hypertension groups, and they had mild to severe impairment of functional status. There was much heterogeneity among the studies. Nevertheless, there was consensus that the studies, taken together, demonstrated that pulmonary rehabilitation improves exercise capacity and health-related quality of life in individuals with pulmonary hypertension. As a result, the American Thoracic Society gives a conditional recommendation for individuals with pulmonary hypertension to participate in a pulmonary rehabilitation program. Studies on the development of pulmonary rehabilitation techniques tailored to each type of pulmonary hypertension may improve outcomes. Techniques added from experience in cardiac rehabilitation may also be considered, especially for individuals with group 2 pulmonary hypertension.

Pulmonary Rehabilitation and Supplemental Oxygen

Supplemental oxygen is recommended for pulmonary rehabilitation participants who have qualifying oxygen desaturation at rest, with exercise, or both [6]. There is no guidance or recommendation to use oxygen with exercise to improve exercise endurance, functional capacity, or quality of life. However, oxygen with exercise does produce immediate physiological benefits, whether or not the participant experiences oxygen desaturation. Individuals with COPD who exercise with oxygen experience a reduction in minute ventilation and dynamic hyperinflation, even if they do not exhibit oxygen desaturation [7, 31]. For subjects with COPD who experience oxygen desaturation during exercise, supplemental oxygen also reduces lactate accumulation. These benefits may be attributed to a lower ventilatory drive resulting from chemoreceptor inhibition and lower lactate levels, which contribute to improved exercise tolerance. One study found that supplemental oxygen at the beginning of a 12-week pulmonary rehabilitation program increased exercise tolerance in subjects with COPD who had no oxygen desaturation [31]. Exercise cycling on oxygen at 75% of each person's maximum workload increased exercise duration by 75 s compared with exercising on air alone. Exercise training for 12 weeks without oxygen increased exercise duration on a cycling ergometer by 28 s when performed on room air but by 153 s when the subjects were placed on oxygen. The investigators concluded that exercise training augmented the benefits of supplemental oxygen on exercise capacity.

While exercise training improves the immediate benefits of oxygen, the question remains whether training while on oxygen improves outcomes. The few studies on this question vary in their designs, and a meta-analysis of the pooled data is of low quality [32]. To date, no significant differences have been found in exercise capacity and quality of life measures between using oxygen during exercise and not using oxygen [7].

Smoking and Pulmonary Rehabilitation

Individuals who smoke tobacco during pulmonary rehabilitation still derive exercise benefits from participation similar to those of ex-smokers. However, they are less likely to attend a pulmonary rehabilitation program when referred and are less adherent than non- or ex-smokers [33]. A retrospective study of 711 subjects with COPD from 2 pulmonary rehabilitation programs in the United Kingdom found that 57% of current smokers initiated pulmonary rehabilitation compared with 75% of ex-smokers [14]. Of the 557 patients who started rehabilitation, 45% of the smokers were adherent (attended six or more sessions) compared with 80% of the ex-smokers. The question, then, is how to approach ongoing smokers who might otherwise benefit from a pulmonary rehabilitation program.

Around one-third of pulmonary rehabilitation programs in the United States prohibit current smokers from attending until they have demonstrated total smoking cessation, and less than 10% of programs allow smokers to participate [33]. Importantly, smokers who attend a program with smoking cessation management strategies have around a sixfold greater chance of stopping smoking than smokers who are not in pulmonary rehabilitation. Smokers covered by Medicare may enter a pulmonary rehabilitation program as long as there is a smoking cessation intervention included [33].

Vaping and the smoking of marijuana expose the lungs to injurious toxins that may have implications for pulmonary rehabilitation [34]. Moreover, vaping and smoking marijuana are often done concomitantly with tobacco smoking. While vaping as a nicotine replacement therapy may make it easier to stop smoking [34], concomitant smoking of tobacco and marijuana makes it more challenging to quit either product. There is no discussion, and there are no recommendations on vaping or using marijuana during pulmonary rehabilitation in the current guidelines [6, 35, 36].

Home-Based Innovations for Pulmonary Rehabilitation Delivery

Conventional supervised pulmonary rehabilitation was modeled as an in-person therapy in a group setting, and current guidelines for the delivery of pulmonary rehabilitation were developed based on this model. For reasons described earlier, the requirement to be physically present can present barriers to participation for many individuals who qualify for pulmonary rehabilitation. There has been a growing interest in home-based pulmonary rehabilitation, driven in large part by the COVID-19 pandemic and the availability of technologies that enable pulmonary rehabilitation to be delivered in the home [34]. These technologies include real-time telehealth training, mobile applications, and virtual reality approaches.

Reyschler and colleagues systematically reviewed 13 randomized clinical trials of pulmonary rehabilitation delivered via telerehabilitation compared with usual care or conventional supervised pulmonary rehabilitation [37]. Telerehabilitation was defined as any technology that offered visual contact with the subject in the home setting. There were 957 subjects, mostly with moderate to severe COPD, and two studies were done using individuals with IPF. Exercise capacity improved similarly in both telerehabilitation and conventional pulmonary rehabilitation compared with usual care. Some quality of life measures, including depression and anxiety, were improved with telerehabilitation compared with usual care. Dyspnea did not improve but was assessed with instruments of low sensitivity. The authors note that their findings were driven by the high numbers of individuals with COPD and may not apply to other chronic lung diseases like IPF.

Pulmonary rehabilitation has entered the mobile application space to provide access for individuals who are unable, or as an alternative, to participate in a conventional program. A systematic review and meta-analysis of 10 studies on the effectiveness of self-directed mobile applications in pulmonary rehabilitation compared with conventional pulmonary rehabilitation showed similar improvements in various outcomes [38]. The studies recruited a total of 1050 individuals with COPD in the sixth and seventh decades of life, representing a broad spectrum of disease severity. Outcomes in the domains of exercise capacity, quality of life measures, hospitalizations, and symptom scores improved with both approaches. The analysis did not address adherence to the mobile application programs as an important feature of success. In this regard, a study of 278 individuals with COPD found that only 40% of those using the mobile application were adherent to 3 or more sessions per week needed to demonstrate an increase in exercise capacity. The exercise capacity of non-adherent subjects did not improve [39]. Non-adherence is a key barrier to overcome for mobile applications to achieve optimal benefit.

Virtual reality (VR) is an interactive, computer-generated, immersive sensory experience in 3-dimensional space, with potential applications in pulmonary rehabilitation [40]. Investigations to date have explored the feasibility and possible effectiveness of VR, especially in older individuals who are most likely to be referred to pulmonary rehabilitation. The studies reveal that immersive VR experiences are engaging and motivational [41]. Moreover, VR is well-suited to incorporate biofeedback into the training experience, making users more aware, for example, of breathing patterns and how to better regulate them.

Of the remote technologies described here, only telerehabilitation, driven mainly by the isolation caused by the COVID-19 pandemic, has demonstrated that it is an alternative with outcomes similar to those of in-person pulmonary rehabilitation. The Telehealth Modernization Act of 2024 [42] was introduced based on the success of telerehabilitation during the pandemic, aiming to continue reimbursement for this remote service. Mobile applications and VR to provide pulmonary rehabilitation training appear to be promising approaches that need further investigation.

Concluding Remarks

Pulmonary rehabilitation improves exercise capacity, functional ability, and quality of life for those with chronic lung diseases and decreases hospitalizations and mortality for individuals with COPD [6]. A candidate will obtain the benefits of pulmonary rehabilitation if they are fully committed to the time and effort of participation. Barriers to participation should be thoroughly discussed between the participant and the referring provider, and accommodations should be made to ensure adherence to the rehabilitation program. Telerehabilitation may be an option for those who cannot participate in person, but reimbursement for this approach is still under review.

The benefits individuals derive from pulmonary rehabilitation tend to decrease over 6–12 months after participation in a program. Investigations on maintenance pulmonary rehabilitation therapy are limited and vary in study design. As a result, the American Thoracic Society guideline on Pulmonary Rehabilitation for Adults with Chronic Respiratory Disease provides a limited recommendation to offer maintenance pulmonary rehabilitation or usual care for individuals with COPD [6]. Nevertheless, the guidelines encourage graduates of a pulmonary rehabilitation program to continue regular exercise and lifestyle changes learned during the program.

References

1. Spruit MA, Singh SJ, Garvey C, ZuWallack R, Nici L, Rochester C, et al. An official American Thoracic Society/European Respiratory Society statement: key concepts and advances in pulmonary rehabilitation. Am J Respir Crit Care Med. 2013;188(8):e13–64.

2. Nici L, Goldstein RS. Pulmonary rehabilitation: the development of a scientific discipline. In: Donner CF, Ambrosino N, Goldstein RS, editors. Pulmonary rehabilitation. 2nd ed. Boca Raton: CRC Press; 2020. Preceded by Pulmonary rehabilitation/Claudio F. Donner, Nicolino Ambrosino, Roger Goldstein. 2005. CRC Press; 2020. p. 11–9.
3. Casaburi R. A brief history of pulmonary rehabilitation. Resp Care. 2008;53(9):1185–9.
4. Petty TL, Nett LM, Finigan MM, Brink GA, Corsello PR. A comprehensive care program for chronic airway obstruction. Methods and preliminary evaluation of symptomatic and functional improvement. Ann Intern Med. 1969;70(6):1109–20.
5. Ries AL, Kaplan RM, Limberg TM, Prewitt LM. Effects of pulmonary rehabilitation on physiologic and psychosocial outcomes in patients with chronic obstructive pulmonary disease. Ann Intern Med. 1995;122(11):823–32.
6. Rochester CL, Alison JA, Carlin B, Jenkins AR, Cox NS, Bauldoff G, et al. Pulmonary rehabilitation for adults with chronic respiratory disease: an official American thoracic society clinical practice guideline. Am J Respir Crit Care Med. 2023;208(4):e7–e26.
7. Troosters T, Janssens W, Demeyer H, Rabinovich RA. Pulmonary rehabilitation and physical interventions. Eur Respir Rev. 2023;32(168):1–14.
8. Hogg JC, Timens W. The pathology of chronic obstructive pulmonary disease. Annu Rev Pathol. 2009;4:435–59.
9. Thannickal VJ, Toews GB, White ES, Lynch JP, Martinez FJ. Mechanisms of pulmonary fibrosis. Annu Rev Med. 2004;55:395–417.
10. Borek I, Birnhuber A, Voelkel NF, Marsh LM, Kwapiszewska G. The vascular perspective on acute and chronic lung disease. J Clin Invest. 2023;133(16):1–16.
11. American Association for Cardiovascular and Pulmonary Rehabilitation (AACVPR) [Internet]. [cited 2025 July 8]. Available from: https://www.aacvpr.org/Program-Certification
12. Arnold E, Bruton A, Ellis-Hill C. Adherence to pulmonary rehabilitation: a qualitative study. Respir Med. 2006;100(10):1716–23.
13. Young J, Jordan RE, Adab P, Enocson A, Jolly K. Interventions to promote referral, uptake and adherence to pulmonary rehabilitation for people with chronic obstructive pulmonary disease (COPD). Cochrane Database Syst Rev. 2017;10:CD012813.
14. Hayton C, Clark A, Olive S, Browne P, Galey P, Knights E, et al. Barriers to pulmonary rehabilitation: characteristics that predict patient attendance and adherence. Respir Med. 2013;107(3):401–7.
15. Burnet K, Higgins S, Kelsch E, Moore JB, Stoner L. The effects of manipulation of Frequency, Intensity, Time, and Type (FITT) on exercise adherence: a meta-analysis. Transl Sports Med. 2020;3:222–34.
16. Chodzko-Zajko WJ, Proctor DN, Fiatarone Singh MA, Minson CT, Nigg CR, Salem GJ, et al. American College of Sports Medicine position stand. Exercise and physical activity for older adults. Med Sci Sports Exerc. 2009;41(7):1510–30.
17. Task Force ERS, Palange P, Ward SA, Carlsen KH, Casaburi R, Gallagher CG, et al. Recommendations on the use of exercise testing in clinical practice. Eur Respir J. 2007;29(1):185–209.
18. ATS Board of Directors. ATS statement: guidelines for the six-minute walk test. Am J Respir Crit Care Med. 2002;166:111–7.
19. Crisafulli E, Clini EM. Measures of dyspnea in pulmonary rehabilitation. Multidiscip Respir Med. 2010;5(3):202–10.
20. Du Bois RM, Weycker D, Albera C, Bradford WZ, Costabel U, Kartashov A, et al. Six-minute-walk test in idiopathic pulmonary fibrosis: test validation and minimal clinically important difference. Am J Respir Crit Care Med. 2011;183(9):1231–7.
21. Ewing Garber C, Blissmer B, Deschenes MR, Franklin BA, Lamonte MJ, Lee IM, et al. Quantity and quality of exercise for developing and maintaining cardiorespiratory, musculoskeletal, and neuromotor fitness in apparently healthy adults: guidance for prescribing exercise. Med Sci Sports Exercise. 2011 Jul;43(7):1334–59.

22. Ammous O, Feki W, Lotfi T, Khamis AM, Gosselink R, Rebai A, et al. Inspiratory muscle training, with or without concomitant pulmonary rehabilitation, for chronic obstructive pulmonary disease (COPD). Cochrane Database Syst Rev. 2023;1(1):CD013778.
23. American Lung Association education programs [Internet]. [cited 2025 July 8]. Available from: https://www.lung.org/help-support/education-programs
24. What is pulmonary rehabilitation? [Internet]. [cited 2025 July 8]. Available from: https://www.copdfoundation.org/Learn-More/Pulmonary-Rehabilitation/What-is-Pulmonary-Rehabilitation.aspx
25. Kenn K, Gloeckl R, Behr J. Pulmonary rehabilitation in patients with idiopathic pulmonary fibrosis – a review. Respiration. 2013;86(2):89–99.
26. Dowman L, Hill CJ, May A, Holland AE. Pulmonary rehabilitation for interstitial lung disease. Cochrane Database Syst Rev. 2021;2(2):CD006322.
27. Song S, Feng Z, Liu W, Li J. The role of pulmonary rehabilitation in idiopathic pulmonary fibrosis: an overview of systematic reviews. PLoS One. 2023;18(12):e0295367.
28. Dowman LM, Vainshelboim B, Holland AE. Impact of pulmonary rehabilitation on survival in people with interstitial lung disease. Chest. 2025;167(6):1696–704.
29. Mocumbi A, Humbert M, Saxena A, Jing Z-C, Sliwa K, Thienemann F, et al. Pulmonary hypertension. Nat Rev Dis Primers. 2024;10(1):1–20.
30. Grünig E, Eichstaedt C, Barberà J-A, Benjamin N, Blanco I, Bossone E, et al. ERS statement on exercise training and rehabilitation in patients with severe chronic pulmonary hypertension. Eur Respir J. 2019;53(2):1–28.
31. Voduc N, Tessier C, Sabri E, Fergusson D, Lavallee L, Aaron SD. Effects of oxygen on exercise duration in chronic obstructive pulmonary disease patients before and after pulmonary rehabilitation. Can Respir J. 2010;17(1):e14–9.
32. Nonoyama ML, Brooks D, Lacasse Y, Guyatt GH, Goldstein RS. Oxygen therapy during exercise training in chronic obstructive pulmonary disease. Cochrane Database Syst Rev. 2007;2007(2):CD005372.
33. Coleman SRM, Menson KE, Kaminsky DA, Gaalema DE. Smoking cessation interventions for patients with chronic obstructive pulmonary disease: a narrative review with implications for pulmonary rehabilitation. J Cardiopulm Rehabil Prev. 2023;43(4):259–69.
34. Connell JW, Humason SA, Panos RJ, Burkes R. Future considerations and areas for innovation for pulmonary rehabilitation in chronic obstructive lung disease patients. Semin Respir Crit Care Med. 2024;45(5):605–10.
35. Man W, Chaplin E, Daynes E, Drummond A, Evans RA, Greening NJ, et al. British Thoracic Society Clinical Statement on pulmonary rehabilitation. Thorax. 2023;78(Suppl 4):s2–s15.
36. Ries AL, Bauldoff GS, Carlin BW, Casaburi R, Emery CF, Mahler DA, et al. Pulmonary rehabilitation: joint ACCP/AACVPR evidence-based clinical practice guidelines. Chest. 2007;131(5 Suppl):4S–42S.
37. Reychler G, Piraux E, Beaumont M, Caty G, Liistro G. Telerehabilitation as a form of pulmonary rehabilitation in chronic lung disease: a systematic review. Healthcare (Basel). 2022;10(9):1–19.
38. Chung C, Lee JW, Lee SW, Jo M-W. Clinical efficacy of mobile app-based, self-directed pulmonary rehabilitation for patients with chronic obstructive pulmonary disease: systematic review and meta-analysis. JMIR Mhealth Uhealth. 2024;12:e41753.
39. Gloeckl R, Spielmanns M, Stankeviciene A, Plidschun A, Kroll D, Jarosch I, et al. Smartphone application-based pulmonary rehabilitation in COPD: a multicentre randomised controlled trial. Thorax. 2024;0:1–9.
40. Pittara M, Matsangidou M, Pattichis CS. Virtual reality for pulmonary rehabilitation: comprehensive review. JMIR Rehabil Assist Technol. 2023;10:e47114.
41. Colombo V, Aliverti A, Sacco M. Virtual reality for COPD rehabilitation: a technological perspective. Pulmonology. 2022;28(2):119–33.
42. H.R.7623: Telehealth Modernization Act of 2024and S.3967: Telehealth Modernization Act [Internet]. [cited 2025 July 8]. Available from: https://www.congress.gov/bill/118th-congress/house-bill/7623

Oxygen Use in Chronic Respiratory Failure

36

Simrin Kooner and John C. Madara

Introduction

The prescription of long-term oxygen therapy is commonplace in the United States. One study showed that of the more than five million Medicare beneficiaries with COPD, approximately 25% of them received supplemental oxygen therapy [1]. Chronic respiratory failure falls into two broad categories: chronic hypoxemic respiratory failure and chronic hypercapnic respiratory failure.

Chronic Respiratory Failure from Chronic Lung Disease

Oxygen supplementation has a long history in medical practice, first starting with the discovery of a chemical process for its production in the late 1700s, progressing to the first documented medical use of continuous oxygen supplementation in 1890. Not long after, in 1917, John Scott Haldane published "The Therapeutic Administration of Oxygen," defining fundamentals of oxygen physiology that are still relied on today [2]. Another step forward in time brings us to two studies in the 1970s that provided the basis for modern oxygen supplementation in patients with COPD. These studies were the continuous or nocturnal oxygen therapy in hypoxemic chronic obstructive lung disease (NOTT) [3] and long-term domiciliary therapy in chronic hypoxic cor pulmonale complicating chronic bronchitis and

S. Kooner
Penn State Health, Milton S. Hershey Medical Center, Hershey, PA, USA
e-mail: skooner@pennstatehealth.psu.edu

J. C. Madara (✉)
Medical Intensive Care Unit, Hershey Medical Center, Penn State Health, Milton S. Hershey Medical Center, Hershey, PA, USA
e-mail: jmadara@pennstatehealth.psu.edu

G. C. Kane et al. (eds.), *Oxygen*, https://doi.org/10.1007/978-3-032-18934-9_36

emphysema (MRC) [4]. Our modern definitions of chronic hypoxemic respiratory failure stem from the inclusion criteria of these two studies. The American Thoracic Society (ATS) has combined the definitions for severe hypoxemia from these two studies [PaO_2 </= 55 mm Hg or $PaO_2 \leq 59$ mm Hg, plus one of the following: edema, hematocrit $\geq 55\%$, or P pulmonale on ECG; vs. PaO_2 40–60 mm Hg] as they considered either definition valid as both the above studies demonstrated a mortality benefit. Interestingly, both studies defined the chronicity of respiratory failure differently. The NOTT study defined chronicity as a subject meeting severe hypoxemia criteria on at least two occasions more than 1 week apart over a course of 3 weeks. The MRC study required subjects to meet the severe hypoxemia criterion on two repeated measurements at least 3 weeks apart. Currently, ATS has removed the requirement for recurrent testing and instead defines chronic hypoxemia as resting hypoxemia in the absence of a reversible cause [5]. They considered the removal of the requirement for repeat measurements to allow for easier implementation of this definition. These recommendations are quite inclusive of a wide range of patients; there is a lack of consensus regarding definitions among international professional societies. Despite the impact of these studies on modern practice, they encompassed a total of only 290 subjects.

Two of the most common causes of chronic resting hypoxemia are COPD and Interstitial Lung Disease. In COPD patients with chronic severe resting hypoxemia, at least 15 h per day of supplemental oxygen is recommended. This recommendation is partially based on the design of the above two studies. It is not clear whether 24-h supplemental oxygen offers superior benefits for mortality, and in a more recent study, Long-Term Oxygen Therapy for 24 vs. 15 h per day in severe hypoxemia, 15 h of supplemental oxygen per day was shown to be noninferior to 24 h [6]. The evidence for oxygen supplementation in patients with severe resting hypoxemia in interstitial lung disease (ILD) is quite limited and is extrapolated from the current data for COPD. As such, when patients with ILD are found to have chronic resting hypoxemia, they should also be initiated on supplemental oxygen.

The NOTT and MRC studies characterized chronic and severe resting hypoxemia, though they did not address or characterize those patients with a moderate level of resting hypoxemia. There has been quite limited data in this area. One study cited by the ATS in the development of its guidelines, a randomized trial of long-term oxygen for COPD with moderate desaturation (LOTT), evaluated the effect of long-term oxygen supplementation on time to death and later composited with time to first hospitalization in COPD patients with moderate resting hypoxemia [7]. In that study, moderate resting hypoxemia was initially defined as SpO_2 89–93% (no PaO_2 criteria) and was later expanded (due to poor recruitment) to include patients with no hypoxemia at rest but who did have desaturations on exertion ($SpO_2 \geq 80\%$ for ≥ 5 min and $< 90\%$ for ≥ 10 s during the 6-min walk test). The experimental group received 24 h of oxygen supplementation if they had resting desaturations, or oxygen supplementation only with sleep and exertion if they had exertional desaturations. They ultimately followed 738 patients for 1–6 years and found that supplemental oxygen provided no change in time to death or first hospitalization in the study population. This study largely provides the basis for ATS's definition of moderate hypoxemia, defined as SpO_2 89–93%, and their recommendation against long-term oxygen therapy in patients with COPD and moderate resting hypoxemia [5].

Once it is determined that a patient would benefit from supplemental oxygen, it must subsequently be determined how the oxygen should be delivered. The two broad categories of oxygen supplementation are invasive and noninvasive. For the discussion of ambulatory oxygen supplementation, the focus will be on the latter. Noninvasive supplemental oxygen can further be subdivided into low- and high-flow supplementation, which is defined by the ability of the delivery device to provide the patient's complete inspiratory demand or minute ventilation. Low-flow devices are capable of providing much less than a patient's total inspiratory demand, and the remaining flow is entrained from ambient air. High-flow devices can provide sufficient flow to meet a patient's inspiratory demand, though if the patient's minute ventilation is able to overcome the provided oxygen flow, these systems can also provide a relatively low flow unless adjusted.

The most common low-flow oxygen delivery device is a nasal cannula, which is a flexible tube with two prongs inserted into a patient's nose, and it offers the advantage of comfort and maintenance of functional status in a spontaneously breathing patient. This device can deliver up to 6 Liters per minute (Lpm), though as patients' minute ventilation increases, the entrained ambient air will dilute this concentration. This is the most likely device to be encountered in a patient with chronic hypoxemic respiratory failure [8].

While Haldane's 1917 paper did not specifically address the mechanisms of carbon dioxide retention, he had previously, in 1914, described an increase in the capacity of deoxygenated blood to carry carbon dioxide, a property that would eventually be attributed to him as the Haldane Effect. At this point, his writings most closely attributed hypercapnia in respiratory failure solely to decreased alveolar ventilation, and it was not until much later that writers such as John B. West began to refine this concept. The increased carbon dioxide retention in those with underlying lung disease would ultimately be attributed to a mismatch in ventilation–perfusion, similar to oxygen [9]. This laid the basis for our modern understanding of hypercapnic respiratory failure, both acute and chronic. Chronic hypercapnic respiratory failure is defined by persistent elevation of $PaCO_2$ (>45 mmHg). Over 3–5 days, this elevation results in a compensatory increase in renal HCO_3- production as a buffer and, importantly, near normalization of arterial pH.

Common causes of chronic hypercapnic respiratory failure include obesity hypoventilation syndrome (OHS), severe COPD, and restrictive thoracic disease. Obstructive or central sleep apneas have traditionally not been thought to be the sole drivers of daytime hypercapnia. Instead, daytime hypercapnia in these apneas is seen as an indicator of the coexistence of one of the previously outlined conditions.

Once chronic hypercapnic respiratory failure is diagnosed, the mainstay of chronic management is positive pressure ventilation (PPV), which, in a spontaneously breathing patient without a tracheostomy, is delivered via a mask. PPV can be delivered to the patient in one of two overarching methods, continuous positive airway pressure (CPAP) and noninvasive positive pressure ventilation (NIPPV), which can then be subdivided into bilevel positive airway pressure (BIPAP) and the more recent average volume-assured pressure support (AVAPS). CPAP is conceptually the simplest form of PPV; the ventilator provides constant airway pressure regardless of the timing of the respiratory cycle. This can improve oxygenation and overcome physical obstruction in a chronic condition like obstructive sleep apnea. However, this delivery method does not increase minute ventilation and will not treat chronic hypercapnic respiratory failure. BIPAP differs from CPAP in that, in this mode, the constant expiratory positive airway pressure (EPAP) is augmented by increased inspiratory positive airway pressure (IPAP), the difference between these two representing a driving pressure [10]. This mode aims to improve minute ventilation and V/Q mismatch, addressing common underlying causes of chronic hypercapnic respiratory failure. AVAPS is a newer mode and is conceptually different from either of the preceding modes of NIPPV. In this mode, a target tidal volume is set, and IPAP will automatically vary from breath to breath to deliver this target volume. EPAP can either be set as a constant or can also be set to vary to meet this target tidal volume. This should result in increased minute ventilation and improve ventilation to perfusion (V/Q) mismatch, similar to BIPAP mode. There has been data to indicate that this mode is more efficient at decreasing $PaCO_2$ in the acute setting [11], though more research is needed to determine superiority as compared to BIPAP in stable hypercapnic respiratory failure.

The data for the prescription of NIPPV in patients with COPD remains controversial. One randomized control trial did show mortality benefit and longer time to readmission at 12 months when NIPPV was added to patients who were hospitalized with COPD exacerbation and demonstrated persistent hypercapnia ($PaCO_2 > 53$ mmHg) [12]. However, prior studies have shown discrepancies. There is no clear evidence to prescribe NIPPV to stable COPD patients without other underlying conditions. In regard to OHS, the American Thoracic Society recommends initiation of CPAP alone for patients with an overlap of OSA and OHS [13]; however, there was less certainty in those patients with OHS alone. In a follow-up review article, both CPAP and NIPPV were considered equally effective at improving gas exchange and symptoms. Therefore, they recommended initial management of OHS with CPAP, citing lower barriers of cost and initial titration [14].

When discussing long-term respiratory failure, it is important to recognize that patients may experience acute insults that lead to lung damage, leading to the need for long-term oxygen therapy and other long-term morbidities.

Respiratory Failure Post Acute Illness

Acute lung injuries of many etiologies converge in acute respiratory distress syndrome (ARDS), an acute, severe, and bilateral process that is life-threatening, often requiring an ICU-level of care. Though much of the concern in the acute phase revolves around oxygenation and improving survival, there is evidence that as soon as 24 h into this syndrome, a runaway fibroproliferative cascade starts to occur, which is a hallmark of the fibrotic phase of ARDS [15]. This fibrotic phase is traditionally considered a late finding presenting two weeks after the initial insult, though there is evidence suggesting it starts much earlier. Additionally, it does not happen to all survivors. The CT findings of this fibroproliferative phase are numerous. Traction bronchiectasis is common and is thought to develop earlier, whereas findings such as persistent ground-glass opacities, reticulations, and cysts/bullae are thought to develop later. The most severe findings of fibrosis are classically more prominent in the anterior part of the lung fields, possibly due to ventilator-induced lung injury and reactive oxygen species. This classic distribution is only seen in one-third of cases [16]. The presence of fibrotic ARDS is associated with a poor prognosis (increased mortality and ventilator dependence) as well as decreased quality of life.

In 2010, the Society of Critical Care Medicine (SCCM) coined the term post intensive care unit syndrome (PICS), thus labeling a phenomenon of long-standing impairments which had been recognized and studied in ICU survivors over the prior decades. They defined PICS as new onset or worsening of physical, cognitive, and/or mental health that develops after hospitalization in the ICU and persists after discharge. In the United States, over five million patients are admitted to an ICU per year. Advances in treatment and management of common ICU diagnoses, including acute respiratory failure, cardiogenic shock, and septic shock, have emerged and decreased mortality. This has led to an increase in ICU survivorship and in more patients with symptoms of PICS. It has been estimated that in the early 2000s, there were several hundred thousand patients who reached survivorship, and this number continues to grow [17]. With increasing survivorship comes an increasing need to care for these patients. The emergence of more PICS survival and recovery clinics across the United States and the world has helped address this deficit, but it certainly has not met the demand for services for these patients.

Several papers have looked at the long-term implications of these acute processes for pulmonary disease. One of the first was published in the *New England Journal of Medicine* (NEJM) in 2003. Herridge et al. aimed to follow survivors of acute respiratory distress syndrome (ARDS) and describe the long-term respiratory complications seen in these patients. One year after discharge, several abnormalities were noted to persist on patients' pulmonary function testing. Forced vital capacity (FVC) and forced expiratory volume in one second (FEV1) recovered only to 85% of predicted. A more significant decline was noted in the diffusion capacity of the lungs for carbon monoxide (DLCO), which at one year only recovered to 75% of predicted. They also noted that patients had persistent functional limitations with six-minute walk tests performed at 12 months, which only demonstrated recovery to 66% of predicted values [18]. Quality of life was significantly limited in these patients, as seen in evaluations with a short-form general health survey (SF-36). One year after survival, scores related to physical functioning, mental health, and general health were all reduced compared to age and sex-matched controls. This is further reflected in the fact that only 29% of these patients were able to return to work at one year. This group continued with a follow-up study in 2011, in which patients were followed for 5 years. At the end of the study, these patients still demonstrated significant reductions in 6MWT, scores on the SF-36, and the number who had returned to work full-time [19].

After the COVID-19 pandemic, there has been increased recognition of the long-term complications following acute illness. In 2021, the World Health Organization (WHO) described post–COVID-19 condition as individuals with a history of probable or confirmed SARS-CoV-2 infections, usually three months from the onset of COVID-19, with symptoms that lasted for at least 2 months and could not be explained by alternative diagnoses [20]. It is estimated that 6.2% of patients who had an acute COVID-19 infection developed symptomatic post–COVID-19 condition. 3.7% of patients had persistent respiratory symptoms, representing another large cohort of patients who have developed chronic respiratory issues after an acute insult [21].

Oxygen Supplementation in Sleep Apnea and ILD

Obstructive or central sleep apneas have been associated with nocturnal hypoxemia, and multiple sequelae of these conditions (increased cardiovascular risk, hypertension, daytime symptoms, etc.) have in the past been partially attributed to nocturnal hypoxemia. It is logical to assume that addressing this nocturnal hypoxemia with supplemental oxygen would benefit these patients; however, multiple studies have shown minimal benefit with supplemental nocturnal oxygen versus treatment with standard CPAP. In one randomized controlled study in 1980, it was found that, as compared to CPAP, nocturnal oxygen supplementation showed a greater improvement in nocturnal oxygenation, though it was not associated with a reduction in the apnea–hypopnea index, nor was it associated with improvement in daytime hypersomnolence [22]. Subsequently, a 2014 randomized controlled trial showed that supplemental nocturnal oxygen was not associated with decreased 24-h mean arterial pressure (MAP) as compared to CPAP [23]. Sleep apnea is not an independent indication for supplemental nocturnal oxygen unless there is persistent nocturnal hypoxia after initial treatment with CPAP. Obstructive and central sleep apneas have traditionally not been thought to be the sole drivers of daytime hypercapnia. Instead, daytime hypercapnia in these apneas is seen as an indicator of the coexistence of one of the previously outlined conditions.

Interstitial lung disease (ILD) is commonly associated with both resting and exertional hypoxemia. ILD can be derived from multiple etiologies, such as occupational/environmental exposures, and autoimmune illnesses, however, the causes are often difficult to identify and are frequently considered idiopathic. Regardless of cause, interstitial thickening and fibrosis drive hypoxia through decreased diffusion capacity and, in some cases, V/Q mismatch. Resting hypoxemia is more prevalent in patients whose ILD has progressed to a fibrotic phase. This phase is associated with an increased burden of symptoms such as dyspnea and earlier mortality. However, there is little high-quality data regarding resting oxygen supplementation in ILD, and thus, the effects of oxygen supplementation in this patient population are unknown. Similarly, there is no high-quality data to support supplemental oxygen for exertional hypoxemia in ILD. One randomized crossover study, Effect of ambulatory oxygen on quality of life for patients with fibrotic lung disease (AmbOx), showed that patients with ILD and isolated exertional hypoxia reported improvement in health-related quality of life with the addition of supplemental oxygen. Albeit this was in a relatively small sample size of 84 patients [24]. This study was part of the basis for the ATS recommendation for the prescription of supplemental oxygen for exertional hypoxemia in ILD. However, with the lack of even poor-quality evidence for resting hypoxemia, ATS guidelines generalized the evidence from resting hypoxemia in COPD and came to the same conclusion and recommended supplemental oxygen for resting hypoxemia in ILD. Hypercapnia can occur in ILD in advanced stages of the disease process, which is theorized in part to be due to decreasing tidal volumes and an increasing degree of physiologic dead space, particularly with exertion. There have been small retrospective studies suggesting an association between daytime hypercapnia and increased mortality in this patient population; however, this is an area that requires more study. Similarly, there is limited evidence as to the benefit of NIPPV, which does not alter the underlying pathology in ILD patients with chronic hypercapnia.

Oxygen Supplementation in Other Diseases

In patients with neuromuscular weakness, nocturnal hypoxia may develop as their disease process progresses, which is associated with nocturnal hypoventilation as well as daytime hypercapnia. Generally, resting daytime hypoxia is an indicator of very advanced disease and profound diaphragmatic/chest wall weakness, which is unlikely to be seen in isolation as an initial presentation. The predominant research in this area is in ALS patients due to their relative prominence. In their clinical practice guidelines, the American College of Chest Physicians found low certainty of evidence regarding the use of NIPPV in patients with NMD; however, it still recommended its use in patients who were symptomatic and had PFT findings of restriction, reduced inspiratory/expiratory forces, positive polysomnography, or daytime hypercapnia [25].

Another possible driver of hypoxemia is passive pulmonary congestion, primarily seen in the setting of heart failure with reduced ejection fraction (HFrEF). This can occur both in acute and chronic settings of heart failure; in either case, a major driver of hypoxemia is decreased diffusion capacity, though sufficient interalveolar fluid can result in the development of shunt physiology. The presence of fluid effectively increases the thickness of the alveolar wall, which is compounded by a relative loss of surface area for gas exchange. Removing or decreasing this interalveolar fluid will improve oxygenation. Peripheral hypoxia occurs in heart failure patients due to this diffusion limitation, as well as decreased cardiac output, limiting oxygen delivery to end organs, and is compounded by a decreased rate of lung perfusion. It is no longer recommended to prescribe supplemental oxygen for heart failure patients who have resting dyspnea without resting hypoxemia, as hyperoxia has been recognized to have detrimental hemodynamic effects in these patients.

However, in patients with resting hypoxemia, oxygen therapy is still often prescribed both in acute and chronic settings [26].

As seen in the NOTT trial, there has been a long-standing question regarding the benefits of nocturnal oxygen supplementation in COPD, and this question now applies to many pathologies. Recommendations regarding nocturnal hypoxia are very much dependent on the underlying pathology and are discussed in depth in the individual sections regarding these pathologies (COPD, ILD, OSA, etc.). Often, nocturnal hypoxia is driven by multiple underlying pathologies and must be assessed and evaluated in a stepwise fashion based on the individual patient presentation.

Other Considerations in Chronic Respiratory Failure

For many patients who suffer from chronic respiratory failure, treatment beyond supplemental oxygen therapy and ventilatory support must be targeted to the patient's specific disease state. Specific treatment strategies for each lung disease will not be discussed; general concepts and considerations for patients with chronic lung diseases will be explored.

Pulmonary Rehabilitation

In the 1960s, Thomas Petty, widely considered the father of pulmonary rehabilitation (PR), developed a multidisciplinary team focused on addressing the systemic effects that patients with COPD suffered. He subsequently published his findings, suggesting that a regimen of patient education, exercise, and breathing techniques (among others) led to significant improvement in patients' exercise tolerance and respiratory symptoms. Widespread recognition of the necessity for PR did not come until 1974, when the American College of Chest Physicians published its opinion reflecting the importance of developing tailored multidisciplinary approaches for patients to help them return to their "highest possible functional capacity." Many studies were published over the following two decades that evaluated outcomes of patients with COPD and the benefits of exercise and a structured PR program. The American Thoracic Society in 1999 released a statement paper that acknowledged that a comprehensive PR program showed improvement over standard medical management alone in increasing exercise tolerance and decreasing patient dyspnea. However, it was not until the early 2000s that PR became standard of care after several guidelines, including the Global Initiative for COPD (GOLD), recommended PR as part of their management plans [27]. The standard practice guidelines from the ATS, ACCP, ERS, and GOLD now recommend that a comprehensive multidisciplinary team approach should be offered to patients with COPD and other chronic lung diseases. While initially used by Petty in the 1960s for COPD patients, PR is now considered beneficial in multiple lung conditions, including diffuse parenchymal disease, bronchiectasis, cystic fibrosis, and pulmonary hypertension.

Several studies have demonstrated improvement in symptoms and overall quality of life for patients with these multiple conditions.

Vaccinations

Pulmonary infection is a common initiating factor in the pathway leading to chronic respiratory failure. A cornerstone in the reduction of these rates of infection is preventative vaccination. Most published guidelines are targeted toward specific disease states such as COPD or asthma. However, others, including CDC recommendations, are based on the presence of "heart or lung disease" rather than a specific individual diagnosis [28]. Many of the guidelines have variances in the specific disease states, age cutoffs, and individual vaccines addressed, which result in providers relying on local guidelines to determine which patients are eligible for specific vaccines and which vaccines should be considered in patients with chronic respiratory failure.

The 2024–25 CDC guidelines recommend pneumococcal vaccination in all adults aged 50 years or older (depending on previous vaccination status). In adults aged 19 to 49 years old, these guidelines recommend pneumococcal vaccination for patients with chronic medical conditions and specifically cite COPD and asthma as qualifying conditions. In general, a single dose of a 20-valent pneumococcal conjugated vaccine (PCV20) or a 21-valent PCV (PCV21) is appropriate in this patient population if the patient has never been vaccinated or is only partially vaccinated [29]. Regarding influenza vaccination, 2024–25 CDC guidelines continue to recommend 1 dose of any appropriate influenza vaccine for adults aged 19 years or older. Adults with chronic pulmonary disorders (including asthma) are considered at higher risk for medical complications attributable to severe influenza. Trivalent inactivated influenza vaccines (IIV3) and trivalent recombinant influenza vaccines (RIV3) are considered suitable for these patient populations [30]. Thorough clinical guidance is available through the CDC.

Lung Transplantation

In patients with end-stage lung disease, lung transplantation may be offered as a therapeutic option. The first lung transplant was performed by James Hardy at the University of Mississippi in 1963, in a patient with lung cancer and a pulmonary abscess. This patient survived 18 days post-procedure. The first double lung transplantation was almost 20 years later, in 1981, by Bruce Reitz at Stanford University in a patient with primary pulmonary hypertension [31]. The many advances in technical procedures, allocation scores, and indications have resulted in 2743 lung transplants performed in the United States in 2022. The most common diagnoses leading to lung transplant are restrictive lung diseases such as DPLD, followed by obstructive lung diseases such as COPD, and then pulmonary hypertension [32].

There continues to be a gradual increase in the number of lung transplants performed for patients with chronic respiratory failure, with over 3000 performed in the United States in 2023.

Conclusion

From Haldane's first description of oxygen delivery for patients with low oxygen levels to lung transplantation, there have been many advancements in our understanding and management of patients with chronic respiratory failure. While there are many unique management strategies for the individual diseases that cause chronic hypoxia and chronic retention of carbon dioxide, it is important to understand the underlying principles and pathophysiology of these disease states and their treatment strategies. Supplemental oxygen delivery and noninvasive ventilation are used to maintain levels of oxygen saturation and carbon dioxide at or near physiological levels, but it is frequently challenging to recognize these diseases, and definitions are not universal. Often, mild levels of these diseases may be asymptomatic and not be readily apparent on initial patient evaluations. Screening for comorbid conditions and disabilities is paramount to offering therapeutics targeting the reduction of symptoms and the mitigation of risks.

References

1. Duan KI, Obara E, Wong ES, Liao JM, Sabbatini AK, Donovan LM, et al. Supplemental oxygen use, outcomes, and spending in patients with COPD in the medicare competitive bidding program. JAMA Intern Med. 2024;184(12):1457–65.
2. Grainge C. Breath of life: the evolution of oxygen therapy. J R Soc Med. 2004;97(10):489–93.
3. NOCTURNAL OXYGEN THERAPY TRIAL GROUP*. Continuous or nocturnal oxygen therapy in hypoxemic chronic obstructive lung disease: a clinical trial. Ann Intern Med. 1980;93(3):391–8.
4. Leggett RJ, Cooke NJ, Clancy L, Leitch AG, Kirby BJ, Flenley DC. Long-term domiciliary oxygen therapy in cor pulmonale complicating chronic bronchitis and emphysema. Thorax. 1976;31(4):414–8.
5. Jacobs SS, Krishnan JA, Lederer DJ, Ghazipura M, Hossain T, Tan AYM, et al. Home oxygen therapy for adults with chronic lung disease. An Official American Thoracic Society Clinical Practice Guideline. Am J Respir Crit Care Med. 2020;202(10):e121–41.
6. Ekström M, Andersson A, Papadopoulos S, Kipper T, Pedersen B, Kricka O, et al. Long-term oxygen therapy for 24 or 15 hours per day in severe hypoxemia. N Engl J Med. 2024;391(11):977–88.
7. The Long-Term Oxygen Treatment Trial Research Group. A randomized trial of long-term oxygen for COPD with moderate desaturation. N Engl J Med. 2016;375(17):1617–27.
8. Rengasamy S, Nassef B, Bilotta F, Pugliese F, Nozari A, Ortega R. Administration of supplemental oxygen. N Engl J Med. 2021;385(3):e9.
9. West JB. Causes of carbon dioxide retention in lung disease. N Engl J Med. 1971;284(22):1232–6.
10. Kelly CR, Higgins AR, Chandra S. Noninvasive positive-pressure ventilation. N Engl J Med. 2015;372(23):e30.

11. Saunders H, Shrestha R, Khadka S, Beesetty M, Helgeson S, Jonna S. Comparing average volume-assured pressure support to bilevel positive airway pressure in the treatment of acute hypercapnic respiratory failure. Chest. 2023;164(4):A4996.
12. Murphy PB, Rehal S, Arbane G, Bourke S, Calverley PMA, Crook AM, et al. Effect of home noninvasive ventilation with oxygen therapy vs oxygen therapy alone on hospital readmission or death after an acute COPD exacerbation: a Randomized Clinical Trial. JAMA. 2017;317(21):2177–86.
13. Mokhlesi B, Masa JF, Brozek JL, Gurubhagavatula I, Murphy PB, Piper AJ, et al. Evaluation and management of obesity hypoventilation syndrome. An Official American Thoracic Society Clinical Practice Guideline. Am J Respir Crit Care Med. 2019;200(3):e6–24.
14. Soghier I, Brożek JL, Afshar M, Kakazu MT, Wilson KC, Masa JF, et al. Noninvasive ventilation versus CPAP as initial treatment of obesity hypoventilation syndrome. Ann Am Thorac Soc. 2019;16(10):1295–303.
15. Burnham EL, Janssen WJ, Riches DWH, Moss M, Downey GP. The fibroproliferative response in acute respiratory distress syndrome: mechanisms and clinical significance. Eur Respir J. 2014;43(1):276–85.
16. Zompatori M, Ciccarese F, Fasano L. Overview of current lung imaging in acute respiratory distress syndrome. Eur Respir Rev. 2014;23(134):519–30.
17. Iwashyna TJ, Cooke CR, Wunsch H, Kahn JM. Population burden of long-term survivorship after severe sepsis in older Americans. J Am Geriatr Soc. 2012;60(6):1070–7.
18. Herridge MS, Cheung AM, Tansey CM, Matte-Martyn A, Diaz-Granados N, Al-Saidi F, et al. One-year outcomes in survivors of the acute respiratory distress syndrome. N Engl J Med. 2003;348(8):683–93.
19. Herridge MS, Tansey CM, Matté A, Tomlinson G, Diaz-Granados N, Cooper A, et al. Functional disability 5 years after acute respiratory distress syndrome. N Engl J Med. 2011;364(14):1293–304.
20. Soriano JB, Murthy S, Marshall JC, Relan P, Diaz JV. A clinical case definition of post-COVID-19 condition by a Delphi consensus. Lancet Infect Dis. 2022;22(4):e102–7.
21. Global Burden of Disease Long COVID Collaborators. Estimated global proportions of individuals with persistent fatigue, cognitive, and respiratory symptom clusters following symptomatic COVID-19 in 2020 and 2021. JAMA. 2022;328(16):1604–15.
22. Phillips BA, Schmitt FA, Berry DTR, Lamb DG, Amin M, Cook YR. Treatment of obstructive sleep apnea. Chest. 1990;98(2):325–30.
23. Gottlieb DJ, Punjabi NM, Mehra R, Patel SR, Quan SF, Babineau DC, et al. CPAP versus oxygen in obstructive sleep apnea. N Engl J Med. 2014;370(24):2276–85.
24. Visca D, Mori L, Tsipouri V, Fleming S, Firouzi A, Bonini M, et al. Effect of ambulatory oxygen on quality of life for patients with fibrotic lung disease (AmbOx): a prospective, open-label, mixed-method, crossover randomised controlled trial. Lancet Respir Med. 2018;6(10):759–70.
25. Khan A, Frazer-Green L, Amin R, Wolfe L, Faulkner G, Casey K, et al. Respiratory management of patients with neuromuscular weakness: an American College of Chest Physicians Clinical Practice Guideline and Expert Panel Report. CHEST. 2023;164(2):394–413.
26. Sepehrvand N, Ezekowitz JA. Oxygen therapy in patients with acute heart failure. JACC Heart Fail. 2016;4(10):783–90.
27. Kaur A, Oo H, ZuWallack RL. History, current initiatives, and future directions of pulmonary rehabilitation for the patient with chronic obstructive pulmonary disease. Med Res Arch [Internet]. 2024;12(10) Available from: https://esmed.org/MRA/mra/article/view/5993
28. CDC. Vaccines & Immunizations. 2025 [cited 2025 Aug 1]. Adult Immunization Schedule by Medical Condition and Other Indication (Addendum updated July 2, 2025). Available from: https://www.cdc.gov/vaccines/hcp/imz-schedules/adult-medical-condition.html
29. Kobayashi M. Expanded recommendations for use of pneumococcal conjugate vaccines among adults aged ≥50 years: recommendations of the Advisory Committee on Immunization Practices – United States, 2024. MMWR Morb Mortal Wkly Rep [Internet]. 2025;74. Available from: https://www.cdc.gov/mmwr/volumes/74/wr/mm7401a1.htm

30. Grohskopf LA. Prevention and control of seasonal influenza with vaccines: recommendations of the advisory Committee on Immunization Practices – United States, 2024–25 Influenza Season. MMWR Recomm Rep [Internet]. 2024;73. Available from: https://www.cdc.gov/mmwr/volumes/73/rr/rr7305a1.htm
31. Panchabhai TS, Chaddha U, McCurry KR, Bremner RM, Mehta AC. Historical perspectives of lung transplantation: connecting the dots. J Thorac Dis [Internet]. 2018;10(7) Available from: https://jtd.amegroups.org/article/view/22674
32. Valapour M, Lehr CJ, Schladt DP, Smith JM, Swanner K, Weibel CJ, et al. Lung – Scientific Registry of Transplant Recipients [Internet]. 2025; Available from: https://srtr.transplant.hrsa.gov/ADR/Chapter?name=Lung&year=2022#fig:LUtx-counts-diag

A Breath of Fresh Air: How Lung Transplants Give Oxygen the Pink Slip

37

Neeraj Sinha

Introduction

The lungs, those delicate, spongy organs nestled in our chest, are our lifeline to the outside world. With every breath, they fill our blood with oxygen and clear it of carbon dioxide, making them essential to life. When diseases such as emphysema, cystic fibrosis, or pulmonary fibrosis turn these vital organs into scarred or unworkable tissue, a lung transplant may be the only hope to restore gas exchange—and thereby life itself. In this chapter, we take you on a journey through the fascinating evolution, intricate science, and life-changing potential of lung transplantation.

The Evolution of Lung Transplantation: From Pipe Dream to Reality

Early Attempts and Setbacks

Lung transplantation lies at the intersection of innovation and necessity. The earliest experimental attempts in the mid-twentieth century were on animal models. Anastomosis breakdown, infection, and rejection led to repeated failures. Advances in transplant sciences improved the foundation for lung transplant research. The first human lung transplant was performed in 1963 by James Hardy in Mississippi. The patient survived for only 18 days, succumbing to kidney failure, but the door had been opened [1]. The challenges were numerous: poorly understood immunology, rudimentary preservation techniques, and inadequate surgical tools. Recipients

N. Sinha (✉)
The Korman Respiratory Institute and the Division of Pulmonary, Allergy and Critical Care, The Department of Medicine at the Sidney Kimmel Medical College of Thomas Jefferson University, Philadelphia, PA, USA
e-mail: neeraj.sinha@jefferson.edu

G. C. Kane et al. (eds.), *Oxygen*, https://doi.org/10.1007/978-3-032-18934-9_37

often died due to infection or rejection within weeks [2]. One of the unique challenges of lung transplant is that the lungs are constantly exposed to environmental antigens with each breath. It is also unfortunate that the innate blood supply to the airways leads to slow healing and risk of anastomosis failure. Over time, improved surgical techniques and improved immunosuppression opened more opportunities for lung transplant success. There were areas for improvement, both from the donor side and in the protocols, to improve the recipient's care.

Breakthroughs and Milestones

The first lasting success came in the 1980s. Advances in immunosuppressive therapy, particularly the introduction of cyclosporine, transformed the field. In 1982, the first successful heart–lung transplant was performed at Stanford by Bruce Reitz [3]. Dr. Joel Cooper, while at Toronto, completed the first single-lung transplant, after which the patient survived for years. Credit for his success was attributed to increased attention to the vascular supply by attaching or wrapping the omentum at the anastomosis site. This added blood supply allowed improved blood flow and increased healing of this delicate surgical airway anastomosis [4, 5]. The first double transplant was accomplished 3 years later, also by Dr. Cooper's team. By the 1990s, single- and double-lung transplants became increasingly viable options for a growing list of end-stage lung diseases [5, 6]. The two major obstacles of airway healing and organ rejection were being overcome.

Modern Era and Ongoing Challenges

Today, lung transplantation is not only possible but also routine in specialized centers. About 4000 lung transplants are performed annually worldwide [7]. Roughly 3000 of these lung transplants occur in the United States, and the number is still rising [8] (Fig. 37.1). Still, the road ahead remains tough. Without constant monitoring, fine-tuned immunosuppression, and proactive management of complications, patient outcomes can quickly decline.

The Physiology of Lung Transplantation: Breathing New Life into Patients

Vascular Anastomoses: Connecting the Dots

Successful lung transplantation requires seamless vascular integration. Surgeons must carefully connect the pulmonary artery and veins from the donor lung to the recipient's heart. These vascular anastomoses restore perfusion, allowing blood to receive oxygen and expel carbon dioxide—a process that must be flawless to prevent thrombotic events or bleeding.

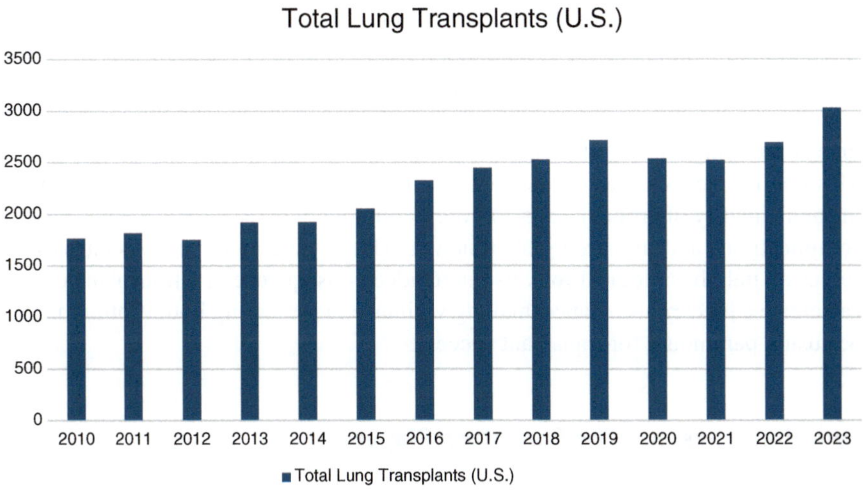

Fig. 37.1 Trends in total United States lung transplants 2010–2023

Bronchial Arteries: The Unrepaired Lifeline and Nature's Secret Detour

A fascinating quirk of lung transplantation is that the systemic bronchial arteries, which normally carry oxygen-rich blood to nourish the airways, are not reconnected during surgery [9]. While their absence raises valid concerns, particularly for airway ischemia and impaired healing, the body harbors a backup plan designed by nature itself. In all mammals, a network of minuscule pulmonary-to-systemic veno–venous anastomoses exists at the venular level [10, 11]. These act as detour routes: After transplantation, as the direct supply from the bronchial arteries is lost, the capillary beds feeding the airways—from the delicate terminal bronchioles right up to the mainstem bronchial anastomoses—become "back-supplied" by pulmonary venular blood shunted through these venovenous anastomotic connections. This hidden circulation, though less robust than the native arterial flow, sustains airway viability and remains essential for bronchial anastomotic healing.

Oxygen on a Tightrope: Ventilation, Perfusion, and the Double-Edged Sword of Hypoxic Vasoconstriction

Optimal gas exchange in the transplanted lung hinges on a delicate matchmaking of airflow (ventilation) and blood flow (perfusion) at the alveolar–capillary interface. Normally, regional variations in oxygenation are balanced by hypoxic pulmonary vasoconstriction—a reflex that shunts blood away from poorly ventilated alveoli to better-aerated regions, safeguarding overall oxygen delivery [12].

However, in the posttransplant lung, this finely tuned response comes at a price. Since systemic bronchial arteries are not reanastomosed, the airways and bronchial anastomotic sites rely on backflow of pulmonary venular blood. When hypoxic pulmonary vasoconstriction is triggered—whether by infection, fluid overload, or mucus plugging—blood flow is preferentially diverted away from these regions. This not only reduces gas exchange efficiency but may further jeopardize the healing and integrity of bronchial anastomoses, compounding risks for ischemia, airway complications, and impaired graft function. Thus, while hypoxic vasoconstriction serves a vital physiological role, its unintended consequence in a transplanted lung can create a precarious balance, making vigilance in preserving both ventilation and perfusion paramount for transplant success.

Lymphatic System: The Forgotten Player

Often overshadowed, the lymphatic circulation of the lung significantly influences posttransplant inflammation and rejection. However, donor lungs are typically transplanted without lymphatic reconnection, increasing susceptibility to edema and impaired immune resistance [13, 14].

Innervation: A Nervous Situation

Transplanted lungs are not reinnervated. Recipients lose the cough reflex temporarily, which impairs their ability to clear airway secretions [15]. This makes subtle signs of infection or early rejection harder to detect and manage. There continues to be research about the effect of aspiration, worsened by a lack of cough, on chronic lung rejection.

Immunology of Lung Transplantation: The Body's Defense Gone Awry

The immune system is primed to protect the body from foreign invaders. However, in transplant medicine, it becomes the villain. The body sees the donor lung as non-self and launches an attack—unless this aggressive response is systematically suppressed.

Three stages of rejection can occur:

1. Hyperacute Rejection: Minutes to hours postsurgery, usually due to preformed donor-specific antibodies.
2. Acute Cellular Rejection: Common in the first year, recipient T cells infiltrate the lung tissue.
3. Chronic Rejection: Manifests as bronchiolitis obliterans syndrome (BOS), a progressive narrowing of the airways.

Immune activation involves both innate and adaptive arms, with antigen-presenting cells, T lymphocytes, and a cytokine firestorm playing central roles [16]. Newer research is focusing on regulatory T cells (Tregs) and their potential to promote immune tolerance [17].

Pretransplant Care

Identifying the Right Candidates

Not every patient with advanced lung disease is eligible for transplantation—patients must fall within a critical "window of severity": sick enough to require a transplant but healthy enough to benefit from and withstand the procedure [18]. Over time, the specific lung transplant scoring systems have evolved (and are further discussed below). The essence of lung transplant eligibility depends on several key factors:

- Disease severity
- Failure to improve despite maximal medical therapy
- Absence of major extrapulmonary contraindications (like active malignancy or severe cardiac disease)
- High motivation and psychosocial stability

Common Diseases Leading to Lung Transplantation

The most frequent underlying diseases requiring lung transplantation include restrictive, obstructive, and vascular diseases. The following charts help better delineate the pulmonary pathology that drives transplants [7, 8, 19] (Figs. 37.2 and 37.3). Restrictive diseases include idiopathic pulmonary fibrosis (IPF) and other forms of pulmonary fibrosis (65%); obstructive lung diseases include chronic obstructive pulmonary disease (COPD)/emphysema (20%); pulmonary vascular disease (10%); CF and other diseases (3%); and retransplant (2%). These percentages can shift slightly from year to year, but pulmonary fibrosis and COPD remain the predominant indications. It is very exciting to see that advances in cystic fibrosis have reduced the need for young patients to undergo lung transplants. Data reviewed over time show a steep decline in transplants for cystic fibrosis, which peaked at 287 in 2016 and has now decreased to just 40 in 2025, attributed to improvements in cystic fibrosis therapeutics [8]. It is of interest to note that in recent years, more patients have been transplanted with diseases that are not specified, referred to as "other" or "other lung disease" in national databases, as these patients may have complex mixed diagnoses or be otherwise difficult to characterize [8].

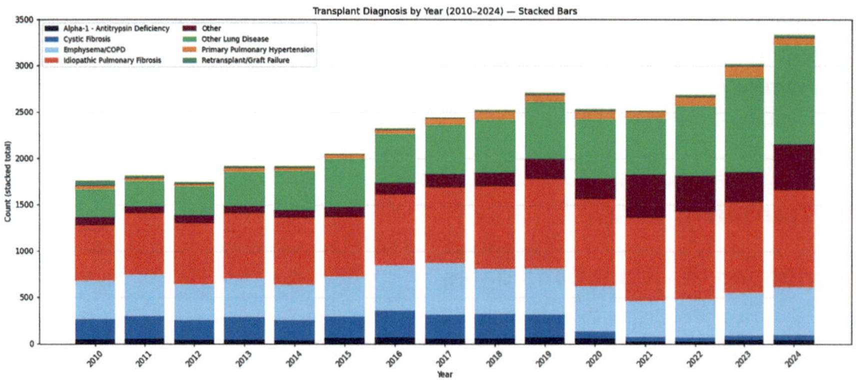

Fig. 37.2 Diagnosis of lung leading to transplant 2010–2024. (Sourced from OPTN data accessed November 2025 [8])

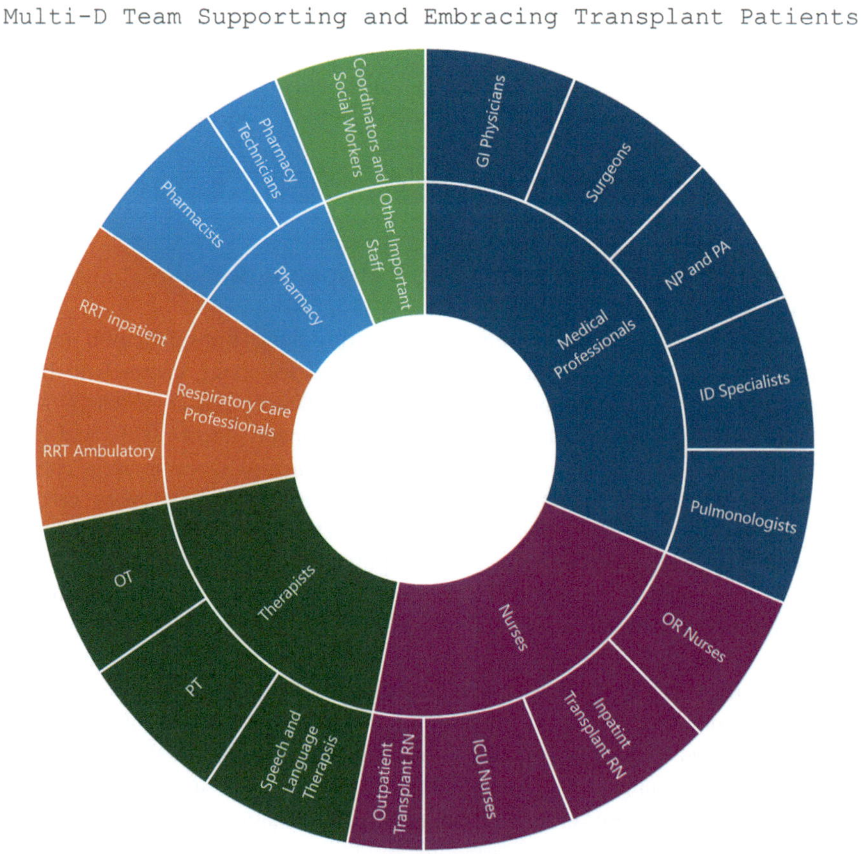

Fig. 37.3 Multidisciplinary (Multi D) nature of lung transplant program

Lung Allocation Score (LAS) and Composite Allocation Score (CAS)

Introduced in the United States in 2005, the Lung Allocation Score (LAS) revolutionized how organs are distributed to patients by quantifying who is most likely to benefit and face imminent death without a transplant [20]. LAS was calculated based on factors like:

- Pulmonary function (FEV1, oxygen needs)
- Age
- Diagnosis
- Other clinical parameters (right heart hemodynamics, 6-min walk distance, renal function, total bilirubin level)

Recently, the system has evolved further with the Composite Allocation Score (CAS), which incorporates all LAS metrics and adds additional considerations such as [20]:

- Medical urgency
- Posttransplant survival probability
- Anti-human leukocyte antigen sensitization (antibody profile)
- Broader equity criteria (extremes of height, ABO blood type)
- Pediatric priority
- Candidate's proximity to the donor hospital (geography)

The CAS is a more comprehensive framework that aims to optimize both patient outcomes and fairness in organ distribution. This system has evolved to prioritize net-survival benefit to provide transplants to those who need them most and are most likely to survive through transplantation. The new framework also prioritizes children (age 17 years or less) and corrects disadvantages arising due to blood type and extremes of height.

Waitlist Management

Candidates approved for lung transplantation are closely monitored on the waitlist for any changes in status. Even once approved, there is an active process to maximize transplant success [21, 22]. A structured multidisciplinary team can help with nutritional support to optimize weight and encourage physical rehabilitation and conditioning. Preventive actions such as vaccination and prompt attention to infections minimize clinical decompensation. Regular communication among transplant centers, the patient, and their family is critical to ensure a timely transplant and optimal outcomes during this uncertain and highly dynamic waiting period.

Perioperative Care

Donor Selection and Organ Preservation: Choosing the Perfect Match

Ideal donor lungs are from individuals less than 55 years old with no active infection, lung trauma, or prolonged mechanical ventilation. The donor-recipient match considers [23]:

- ABO blood type
- Size (to ensure proper chest fit)
- Crossmatching to screen for antibody incompatibility

Once accepted, lungs are flushed with cold preservation solutions and transported under hypothermic conditions, with ischemic times ideally under 6–8 h. There are ex vivo lung perfusion devices to provide nutrients and air movement into the lungs to preserve the health and function of the explanted lung prior to transplant into the recipient.

Surgical Techniques: Cutting-Edge Approaches

Depending on the disease, either single or bilateral lung transplantation is performed. Common incisions include a clamshell (transverse thoracosternotomy) or a posterolateral thoracotomy. The new lung is sequentially attached to the recipient lung's pulmonary artery, pulmonary veins (via an atrial cuff), and bronchus [24].

Intraoperatively, extracorporeal membrane oxygenation (ECMO) may support circulation [25].

Immediate Posttransplant Management: The Critical Hours

ICU care is intense and multidisciplinary [24]. Much of the care of a lung transplant revolves around some of the basic tenets of critical care, but there are some unique considerations. Some of the standard critical care practices include lung-protective ventilation to reduce the risks of barotrauma, volutrauma, and biotrauma [26]. Due to the sensitive anastomosis, hemodynamic monitoring is critical. In addition, minimizing blood product utilization and avoiding pulmonary edema improve outcomes. A unique characteristic of the postoperative period is monitoring for primary graft dysfunction (PGD), the major early complication. Primary graft dysfunction typically occurs by posttransplant day 3. It shares many characteristics with ARDS in that there is hypoxemia and diffuse infiltrates. Management is supportive with lung-protective strategies and potentially ECMO if severe. Careful attention to volume overload is critical.

Postoperative Care: The Road to Recovery

Early Postoperative Complications: Navigating the Stormy Seas

The concern for primary graft dysfunction (PGD) has already been mentioned. The greatest risk is during the first 72 h, resembling acute respiratory distress syndrome. Improved organ procurement and management have reduced the incidence and severity of this complication. Since lung transplant recipients are postoperative patients, they also carry the risk of hemorrhage, supraventricular arrhythmias, and airway complications such as dehiscence or stenosis [25, 27, 28]. Aggressive supportive care and bronchoscopy-guided assessment are often necessary.

Immunosuppression: Walking the Tightrope

Lung recipients typically receive a triple-drug maintenance regimen [29]:

1. Calcineurin inhibitors (e.g., tacrolimus): the backbone of therapy but associated with nephrotoxicity.
2. Antimetabolites (e.g., mycophenolate mofetil): to inhibit lymphocyte proliferation.
3. Steroids: administered in high doses initially, then gradually tapered over months.

For induction at the time of transplant, a hefty steroid dose, tapered over a few days, remains the mainstay, but the addition of basiliximab—a monoclonal antibody targeting the IL-2 receptor—serves as a valuable adjunct. By blunting early T-cell activation, basiliximab induction allows for a more gradual, gentler uptitration of tacrolimus, helping to safeguard against early postoperative nephrotoxicity as clinicians carefully navigate the stormy seas of the immediate posttransplant period [30].

Finding the balance between suppressing rejection and overexposing the patient to infections or malignancy is a dynamic process.

Therapeutic Drug Monitoring: Hitting the Sweet Spot

Regular drug level monitoring and dose adjustments are non-negotiable to ensure drugs like tacrolimus remain within a target range—too low invites rejection and too high causes toxicity. Emerging personalized pharmacogenomics (e.g., CYP3A polymorphisms for tacrolimus metabolism) promise improved tailoring of immunosuppression based on drug-metabolizing enzyme profiles [31].

Rehabilitation and Long-Term Follow-Up: The Marathon, Not the Sprint

Physical Rehabilitation

Patients often enter transplantation in a deconditioned state. Posttransplant rehab focuses on the same pretransplant issues: ambulation, strength training, and good pulmonary hygiene [32].

Gains in exercise capacity correlate with long-term survival.

Routine Monitoring

After surgery, patients remain under vigilant care. Transplant medicine requires a constant watch for infections, rejection, and complex drug–drug interactions. The following list is part of common outpatient follow-up protocols [33, 34].

- Pulmonary function testing (PFTs)
- Daily home spirometry and exercise oximetry logs
- Molecular monitoring: monthly blood tests for cell-free DNA and donor-specific antibodies
- Immunosuppressive drug level monitoring
- For-cause (as opposed to surveillance) transbronchial biopsies (for molecular, physiological, and/or clinical decline)
- Chest imaging
- Surveillance of organ function (renal, hepatic, glucose)
- Screening for recurrence such as sarcoidosis, chronic thromboembolic pulmonary hypertension (CTEPH), bronchiectasis, etc.
- Assessing for posttransplant lymphoproliferative disorder (PTLD) and appropriate Epstein–Barr virus (EBV) monitoring

Chronic and Acute Rejection: The Ongoing Battle

Acute Rejection: The Early Threat

Detected via transbronchial biopsy, this occurs in up to 80% of patients within the first year. If untreated, it can progress to chronic rejection. Symptoms may be subtle—cough, fatigue, and decline in spirometry—and often respond well to steroid pulse therapy [35].

Chronic Lung Allograft Dysfunction (CLAD): The Long-Term Enemy

CLAD is the leading cause of long-term graft failure. The most recognized form is bronchiolitis obliterans syndrome (BOS), characterized by fixed airflow obstruction. This irreversible fibrosis destroys terminal bronchioles and is minimally responsive to therapy, though azithromycin and extracorporeal photopheresis show promise [36].

Infection Risk: The Price of Immunosuppression

Common Pathogens: The Usual Suspects

Infection is the second leading cause of death in lung recipients (after CLAD). The risk varies over time [37]:

- First month: Bacterial and fungal infections (nosocomial)
- 1–6 months: Opportunistic infections like CMV (cytomegalovirus)
- Beyond 6 months: Community-acquired infections or reactivation of latent infections (e.g., TB)

Prophylactic medications include the following:

- Trimethoprim-sulfamethoxazole: For Pneumocystis
- Valganciclovir: CMV suppression
- Antifungal Agents (e.g., isavuconazole): For invasive mycosis (*Aspergillus*, *Mucor*)

Vaccinations, patient education, and frequent monitoring are crucial.

The Multidisciplinary Nature of Lung Transplantation

From initial referral to long-term follow-up, lung transplantation is the archetype of multidisciplinary care. Every aspect of inpatient and outpatient care is carefully orchestrated among a team of physicians and surgeons. It is crucial to recognize that lung transplant involves more than just physicians—it is a multidisciplinary process. Figure 37.3: Regular team meetings align treatment plans, address psychosocial needs, troubleshoot complex complications, and communicate with referring physicians and families. Many transplant recipients single out the ongoing guidance, empathy, and vigilance of this vast team as essential to their survival and quality of life—a true testament to collaborative medicine in action [38]. In addition to the health care team, the importance of the patient support team cannot be underestimated.

Conclusion: Breathing Easy into the Future

Breathing is something most take for granted. For lung transplant recipients, every breath is a triumph—a literal gift of life. Lung transplantation has evolved from an audacious experiment to a cornerstone of treatment for end-stage pulmonary disease. Despite significant hurdles—rejection, infection, and lifelong medication—many patients enjoy added years of life and improved functional status with a renewed sense of well-being [39]. As research blazes forward with improved immunosuppressants, xenotransplantation, ex vivo lung perfusion, and immune tolerance strategies, the prospect of truly long-lasting graft function is becoming increasingly attainable.

References

1. Hardy JD, Webb WR, Dalton ML Jr, Walker GR Jr. Lung Homotransplantation in man. JAMA. 1963;186:1065–74.
2. Wildevuur CR, Benfield JR. A review of 23 human lung transplantations by 20 surgeons. Ann Thorac Surg. 1970;9(6):489–515.
3. Reitz BA, Wallwork JL, Hunt SA, Pennock JL, Billingham ME, Oyer PE, Stinson EB, Shumway NE. Heart-lung transplantation: successful therapy for patients with pulmonary vascular disease. N Engl J Med. 1982;306(10):557–64.
4. Meyers BF, Lynch J, Trulock EP, Guthrie TJ, Cooper JD, Patterson GA. Lung transplantation: a decade of experience. Ann Surg. 1999;230(3):362.
5. Kaiser LR, Pasque MK, Trulock EP, Low DE, Dresler CM, Cooper JD. Bilateral sequential lung transplantation: the procedure of choice for double-lung replacement. Ann Thorac Surg. 1991;52(3):438–45.
6. Mal H, Andreassian B, Pamela F, Duchatelle JP, Rondeau E, Dubois F, Baldeyrou P, Kitzis M, Sleiman C, Pariente R. Unilateral lung transplantation in end-stage pulmonary emphysema. Am Rev Respir Dis. 1989;140(3):797–802.
7. Singh TP, Hsich E, Cherikh WS, Perch M, Hayes D Jr, Lewis A, Dellgren G, Cogswell R, International Society for Heart and Lung Transplantation. The International Thoracic Organ Transplant Registry of the International Society for Heart and Lung Transplantation: 2025 annual report of heart and lung transplantation. J Heart Lung Transplant. 2025;25:S1053-2498(25)01920-5.
8. The SRTR Lung chapter reports national US lung transplant waitlist, transplant activity, and outcome statistics using registry data. Accessed 25 Nov 2025.
9. Stewart KC, Patterson GA. Current trends in lung transplantation. Am J Transplant. 2001;1(3):204–10.
10. Baile EM. The anatomy and physiology of the bronchial circulation. J Aerosol Med. 1996;9(1):1–6.
11. Aviado DM, Daly MD, Lee CY, Schmidt CF. The contribution of the bronchial circulation to the venous admixture in pulmonary venous blood. J Physiol. 1961;155(3):602–22.
12. Robin ED, Theodore J, Burke CM, Oesterle SN, Fowler MB, Jamieson SW, Baldwin JC, Morris AJ, Hunt SA, Vankessel A, et al. Hypoxic pulmonary vasoconstriction persists in the human transplanted lung. Clin Sci (Lond). 1987;72(3):283–7.
13. Cui Y, Liu K, Lamattina AM, Visner G, El-Chemaly S. Lymphatic vessels: the next frontier in lung transplant. Ann Am Thorac Soc. 2017;14(Supplement_3):S226–32.
14. Dashkevich A, Heilmann C, Kayser G, Germann M, Beyersdorf F, Passlick B, Geissler HJ. Lymph angiogenesis after lung transplantation and relation to acute organ rejection in humans. Ann Thorac Surg. 2010;90(2):406–11.

15. Duarte AG, Terminella L, Smith JT, Myers AC, Campbell G, Lick S. Restoration of cough reflex in lung transplant recipients. Chest. 2008;134(2):310–6.
16. Kreisel D, Goldstein DR. Innate immunity and organ transplantation: focus on lung transplantation. Transpl Int. 2013;26(1):2–10.
17. Liao M, Wang C, Zhang M, Qiao K. Insight on immune cells in rejection and infection post-lung transplant. Immun Inflamm Dis. 2023;11(7):e868.
18. Leard LE, Holm AM, Valapour M, Glanville AR, Attawar S, Aversa M, Campos SV, Christon LM, Cypel M, Dellgren G, Hartwig MG, Kapnadak SG, Kolaitis NA, Kotloff RM, Patterson CM, Shlobin OA, Smith PJ, Solé A, Solomon M, Weill D, Wijsenbeek MS, Willemse BWM, Arcasoy SM, Ramos KJ. Consensus document for the selection of lung transplant candidates: an update from the International Society for Heart and Lung Transplantation. J Heart Lung Transplant. 2021;40(11):1349–79.
19. https://optn.transplant.hrsa.gov/media/p0ynumsn/continuous_distribution_of_lungs-public_comment.pdf.
20. Tsuang WM, Lease ED, Budev MM. The past, present, and near future of lung allocation in the United States. Clin Chest Med. 2023;44(1):59–68. 19. Chamogeorgakis T, Mason DP, Murthy SC, Thuita L, Raymond DP, Pettersson GB, Blackstone EH. Impact of nutritional state on lung transplant outcomes. J Heart Lung Transplant 2013;32(7):693–700.
21. Singer JP, Peterson ER, Snyder ME, Katz PP, Golden JA, D'Ovidio F, Bacchetta M, Sonett JR, Kukreja J, Shah L, Robbins H, Van Horn K, Shah RJ, Diamond JM, Wickersham N, Sun L, Hays S, Arcasoy SM, Palmer SM, Ware LB, Christie JD, Lederer DJ. Body composition and mortality after adult lung transplantation in the United States. Am J Respir Crit Care Med. 2014;190(9):1012–21.
22. Arjuna A, Mazzeo AT, Tonetti T, Walia R, Mascia L. Management of the potential lung donor. Thorac Surg Clin. 2022;32(2):143–51.
23. Subramanian M, Meyers BF. Lung transplant procedure of choice: bilateral transplantation versus single transplantation complications, quality of life, and survival. Clin Chest Med. 2023;44(1):47–57.
24. Expert Consensus Panel, Hartwig M, van Berkel V, Bharat A, Cypel M, Date H, Erasmus M, Hoetzenecker K, Klepetko W, Kon Z, Kukreja J, Machuca T, McCurry K, Mercier O, Opitz I, Puri V, Van Raemdonck D. The American Association for Thoracic Surgery (AATS) 2022 expert consensus document: the use of mechanical circulatory support in lung transplantation. J Thorac Cardiovasc Surg. 2023;165(1):301–26.
25. Natalini JG, Clausen ES. Critical care management of the lung transplant recipient. Clin Chest Med. 2023;44(1):105–19.
26. Kao CC, Parulekar AD. Postoperative management of lung transplant recipients. J Thorac Dis. 2019;11(Suppl 14):S1782–8. https://doi.org/10.21037/jtd.2019.05.60. PMID: 31632755; PMCID: PMC6783721.
27. Natalini JG, Diamond JM. Primary graft dysfunction. Semin Respir Crit Care Med. 2021;42(3):368–79.
28. Crespo MM, McCarthy DP, Hopkins PM, Clark SC, Budev M, Bermudez CA, Benden C, Eghtesady P, Lease ED, Leard L, D'Cunha J, Wigfield CH, Cypel M, Diamond JM, Yun JJ, Yarmus L, Machuzak M, Klepetko W, Verleden G, Hoetzenecker K, Dellgren G, Mulligan M. ISHLT consensus statement on adult and pediatric airway complications after lung transplantation: definitions, grading system, and therapeutics. J Heart Lung Transplant. 2018;37(5):548–63.
29. Patterson CM, Jolly EC, Burrows F, Ronan NJ, Lyster H. Conventional and novel approaches to immunosuppression in lung transplantation. Clin Chest Med. 2023;44(1):121–36.
30. Shagabayeva L, Osho AA, Moonsamy P, Mohan N, Li SS, Wolfe S, Langer NB, Funamoto M, Villavicencio MA. Induction therapy in lung transplantation: a contemporary analysis of trends and outcomes. Clin Transpl. 2022;36(11):e14782.
31. Thervet E, Loriot MA, Barbier S, Buchler M, Ficheux M, Choukroun G, Toupance O, Touchard G, Alberti C, Le Pogamp P, Moulin B, Le Meur Y, Heng AE, Subra JF, Beaune P, Legendre

C. Optimization of initial tacrolimus dose using pharmacogenetic testing. Clin Pharmacol Ther. 2010;87(6):721–6.
32. Montgomery E, Macdonald PS, Newton PJ, Chang S, Wilhelm K, Jha SR, Malouf M. Reversibility of frailty after lung transplantation. J Transp Secur. 2020;2020:3239495.
33. Odisho AY, Liu AW, Maiorano AR, Bigazzi MOA, Medina E, Leard LE, Shah R, Venado A, Perez A, Golden J, Kleinhenz ME, Kolaitis NA, Maheshwari J, Trinh BN, Kukreja J, Greenland J, Calabrese D, Neinstein AB, Singer JP, Hays SR. Design and implementation of a digital health home spirometry intervention for remote monitoring of lung transplant function. J Heart Lung Transplant. 2023;42(6):828–37.
34. Halverson LP, Hachem RR. Antibody-mediated rejection: diagnosis and treatment. Clin Chest Med. 2023;44(1):95–103.
35. Todd JL, Neely ML, Kopetskie H, Sever ML, Kirchner J, Frankel CW, Snyder LD, Pavlisko EN, Martinu T, Tsuang W, Shino MY, Williams N, Robien MA, Singer LG, Budev M, Shah PD, Reynolds JM, Palmer SM, Belperio JA, Weigt SS. Risk factors for acute rejection in the first year after lung transplant. A multicenter study. Am J Respir Crit Care Med. 2020;202(4):576–85.
36. Beeckmans H, Bos S, Vos R, Glanville AR. Acute rejection and chronic lung allograft dysfunction: obstructive and restrictive allograft dysfunction. Clin Chest Med. 2023;44(1):137–57.
37. Magda G. Opportunistic infections post-lung transplantation: viral, fungal, and mycobacterial. Clin Chest Med. 2023;44(1):159–77.
38. O'Grady JG, Asderakis A, Bradley R, Burnapp L, McPake DM, Perrin M, Russell S, Watson AR, Watson CJ, Wray J, Wilson LC. Multidisciplinary insights into optimizing adherence after solid organ transplantation. Transplantation. 2010;89(5):627–32.
39. Lamas DJ, Lakin JR, Trindade AJ, Courtwright A, Goldberg H. Looking beyond mortality in transplantation outcomes. N Engl J Med. 2018;379(20):1889–91.

Part VI

Special Physiological Circumstances

38 Under the Sea: Principles of SCUBA and Understanding Decompression Sickness, Barotrauma and Nitrogen Narcosis

Gregory C. Kane

Something, most certainly, happens to a diver's emotions underwater.

—Barry Lopez.

The etymology of the self-contained underwater breathing apparatus (SCUBA) dates to the early 1950s, when an American naval serviceman, Christian J. Lambersen, who had been involved in developing oxygen rebreathers for the first "frogmen" during World War II, went on to patent a free-swimming oxygen rebreather in 1952 [1]. A modification of the original device is named "SCUBA," the acronym for self-contained underwater breathing apparatus, and quickly became a generic English word for diving equipment that allowed for free swimming. While the acronym is SCUBA, conventional utilization in the English language, in both written and spoken usage, is with the word "scuba" (all lower case). We will follow this usage throughout this chapter. It is interesting to note that early rebreather devices led to oxygen toxicity, which ultimately led to revisions of devices and the use of simple air (a standard mixture of 79% nitrogen and 21% oxygen as is present in atmospheric air) in modern scuba tanks [2]. Today, scuba, which colloquially refers to both the activity of utilizing such equipment and the equipment itself, is practiced by both professionals and recreational divers to explore at least the superficial depths of oceans, seas, and inland bays and rivers across the globe.

It is important for the medical practitioner to understand the physiology of diving for the purpose of advising patients on safe practices and for diagnosing and treating

G. C. Kane (✉)
The Korman Respiratory Institute and the Division of Pulmonary, Allergy and Critical Care, The Department of Medicine at the Sidney Kimmel Medical College of Thomas Jefferson University, Philadelphia, PA, USA
e-mail: gregory.kane@jefferson.edu

G. C. Kane et al. (eds.), *Oxygen*, https://doi.org/10.1007/978-3-032-18934-9_38

people who experience respiratory ailments while engaging in this activity. In this chapter, we will discuss the physiology of diving and utilize the gas laws (reviewed in earlier chapters) to understand the peculiar challenges that emerge from breathing compressed air at depths of up to three atmospheres or more. The illnesses of diving using scuba gear are unique to scuba itself. Free divers, skin divers, and diving mammals generally do not experience decompression illness because they do not breathe compressed air at an increased pressure during their dives. We will offer a detailed explanation of this physiology later in this chapter.

Some Early Clues to Illness Related to Breathing Compressed Air

It is surprising that more than 75 years before the introduction of scuba, the first cases of decompression sickness were being described across the United States as civil engineering marvels took shape across broad rivers. To cross a river with a major bridge, it is essential for workers to work in submerged caissons in order to excavate the riverbeds down to bedrock, so that piers can be created out of stone or concrete to support the towers which will, in turn, support the suspension cables (Fig. 38.1). Caissons, essentially steel and wood compartments, are shaped like upside-down boats, and they can be sunk to the bottom of the river. If positive pressure is applied, it will keep the water out so that workers can descend through a series of holds and locking chambers in order to clear and shovel away sand, stone,

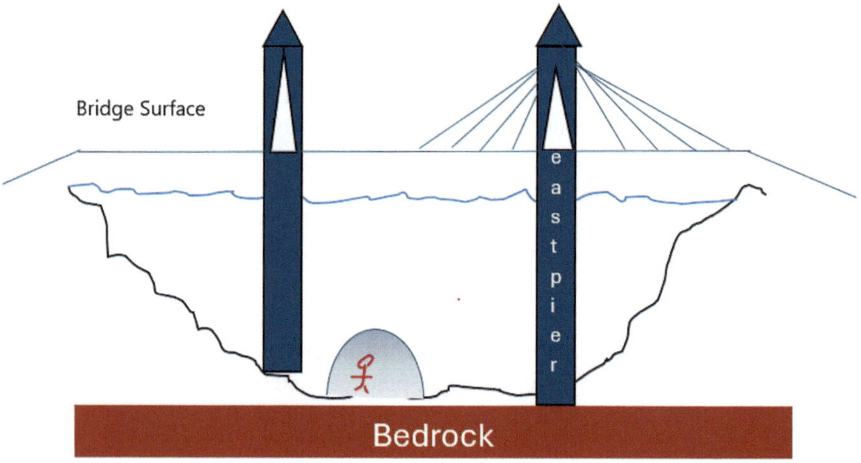

Fig. 38.1 A schematic showing key elements of a suspension bridge, such as the Brooklyn Bridge. Note that the west pier is on a sandy bottom and not all the way to bedrock, while the east pier is on bedrock. The caisson is shown as well, but without the connecting pressurized hoses that allow workers to enter and exit. At the bottom of the river, inside the caisson, ready to begin shoveling the last few feet of sandy material, is a single worker delineated as a red stick figure. The suspension cables are shown only for the east pier, which is completed and resting on bedrock

and muck. At the extreme depths, workers may be exposed to markedly increased (several atmospheres) pressure, which increases the dissolved nitrogen in the blood of these unsuspecting workers. In the nineteenth century, most of these workers were immigrants.

In his "Epic story of the building of the Brooklyn Bridge," David McCullough describes the first deaths among workers on the site as a direct result of entering the caissons and exiting them at the end of the workday. In April 1862, 50-year-old Patrick McKay of Ireland died unexpectedly after a shift in the caisson being used to excavate the footing for the western pier in the East River. He had been working on the job for nearly 4 months with no ill effects. However, on the afternoon of his demise, he stayed down in the caisson an extra 30 min [3]. It was during this added 30 min that additional dissolved nitrogen entered his blood. There, the nitrogen under pressure was awaiting future release as McKay came to the surface—his body now a demonstration project much like the opening of a can of Diet Coke. As workers exposed to high pressure (3 atmospheres or 2280 mmHg) for longer periods of time returned to the surface, they were now exposed to only one atmosphere of pressure (1 atm of 760 mmHg). When this process happens rapidly, bubbling of nitrogen out of the solution and into the blood can occur—just like opening a soda in a can or bottle form—releasing dissolved gas with the sudden reduction of applied pressure. These open bubbles could then create ischemia by blocking small blood vessels and denying distal tissues oxygen, also referred to as tissue ischemia. When this occurs in the extremities, severe pain ensues. In the brain, this would cause a major stroke or seizures. Typical patients would be twisted and bent over from the gnarly pain in the abdomen, joints, and extremities; thus, the name "the bends" was coined for this illness in this era. Mr. McKay rapidly became unconscious, experienced seizures, and passed away. Only later would physicians recognize that Dr. Andrew Smith, an ENT physician and the attending doctor for the building of the Brooklyn Bridge, would come so close to solving the mystery. He was able to observe that the suffering of the caseworkers was precisely the same in intensity and type, and he did go on to contend "that the amount of pressure" and "the length of time down below" were important factors, as was the "problem of rapid decompression" [4]. If only Dr. Smith could have convinced the workers to spend more time in the lock; but at the end of the day, in the dark, damp caisson, workers were highly motivated to escape the confines of the caisson as quickly as possible. They were not at all willing to follow the doctor's instructions and spend more time in an intermediate chamber enroute to the surface. Indeed, Dr. Smith was very close, as the mysterious ailment threatening the lives of so many caisson workers was a disease that had a risk generated directly by the amount of time and the degree of pressure in the caisson. Further, the acute phase of decompression illness in caisson workers was directly related to how quickly the pressure was released on ascent to the surface. The reader will see that scuba divers, breathing from a pressurized tank, mitigate against the risk of decompression illness by limiting the time of dives or the depths of dives and ascending slowly [5].

Here is a more detailed discussion: When in a caisson at 3 atmospheres of pressure (which would be 3 × 760 mmHg or 2280 mmHg), all workers will be exposed to the increased pressure of both oxygen and nitrogen. It is essential to understand that a pressure equal to the water pressure at any specific depth is needed to keep water out of the caisson, thus permitting work to progress and keeping the caisson from filling up with river water. Breathing under these conditions, the partial pressure of both of these gases will build up in the serum and tissues of the body in exposed persons. The gas entering the caisson is simple air, and so in a caisson at 3 atmospheres of pressure, the partial pressure of nitrogen would be 1801 mmHg, and the partial pressure of oxygen would be 479 mmHg in the worker's serum and over time in the tissues. It is important to note that this fulfills Dalton's law since the sum equals 2280 mmHg [5]. In addition, this process is consistent with Henry's law, which states that the concentration of a gas in the liquid (capillary blood traveling through the pulmonary circuit in the lungs) will gradually rise to match the partial pressure in the alveoli (Fig. 38.2) [6]. We remember here that the alveolar gas equation described in this chapter will help us predict how alveolar nitrogen and oxygen pressures are slightly reduced because of humidifying the inspired air and the exchange for carbon dioxide at the alveolar level when consuming a normal diet. Furthermore, the content of a gas in solution is directly proportional to the partial pressure of the applied gas. Thus, over time men working in the caisson will see their partial pressure of nitrogen rise from 553 mmHg before descent to 1753 mmHg after descent over time. At the bottom of the caisson, while remaining under pressure, this gas will remain dissolved in solution. In persons who rapidly ascend, and particularly those who do not "blow off" a large volume of exhaled gas in the process or do not take a pause for a more gradual process of equilibration, the high pressure of dissolved nitrogen in the blood, suddenly exposed to normal ambient pressure, leads to a rapid escape of gas from the solution. The phenomenon can also be understood when considering a "twist off plastic bottle of Diet Coke." When the cap is rapidly unscrewed, the carbon dioxide dissolved in the beverage container rapidly bubbles out of the soda liquid, creating the fizz or effervescence. The phenomenon can be mitigated substantially by very gently unscrewing the cap and briefly tightening it back to restore pressure. This is analogous to a gradual emergence from a caisson (such as by waiting in the hold chamber for an hour or so) or adding a "safety stop" while ascending upon completing a scuba dive. Bubbling out of solution does not happen substantially with oxygen because the majority of oxygen in the blood is bound to hemoglobin as opposed to free oxygen in solution, and the tissues are continuously utilizing oxygen at the cellular level for metabolism. The diatomic molecule nitrogen, on the other hand, is relatively inert, and the nitrogen content in the serum can much more easily "bubble out" of solution as pressure is released when ascending too quickly, especially from dives of greater depth and of greater duration.

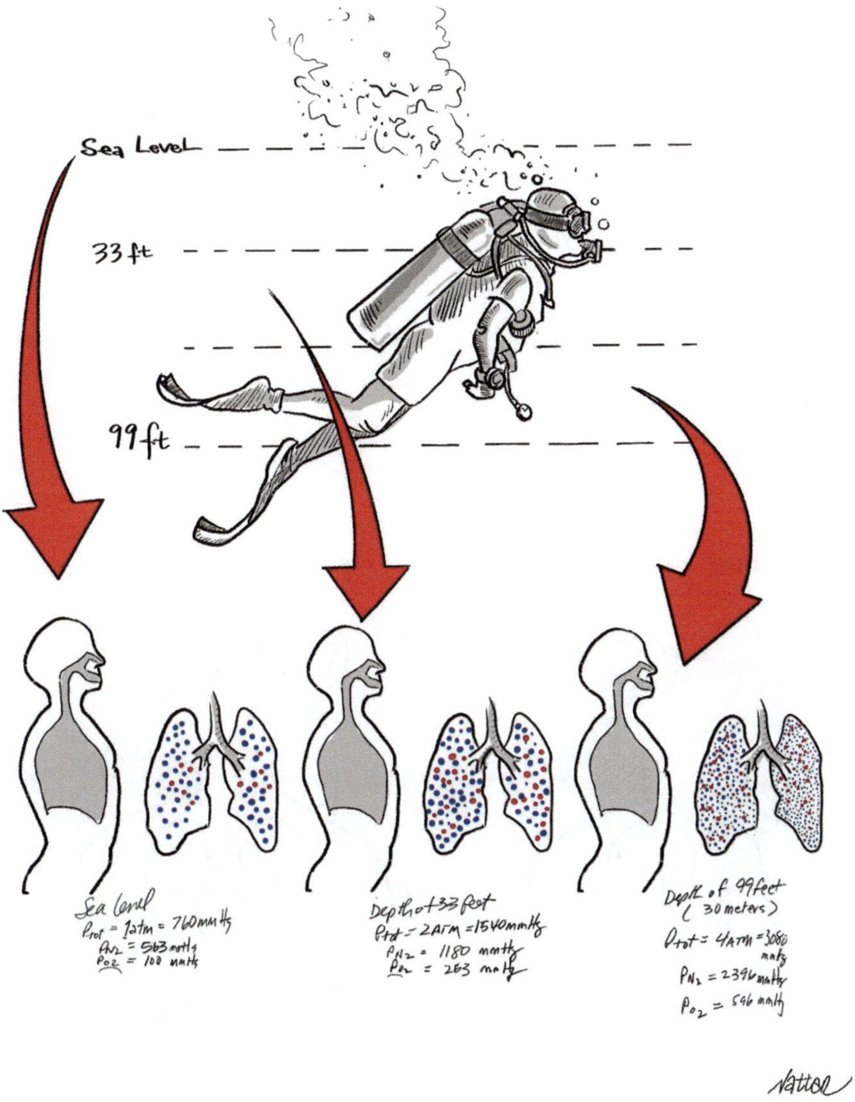

Fig. 38.2 A graphic representation of pressure in the lung at sea level, 33 feet of depth, and 99 feet of depth. Note that each representation is for a scuba diver using pressurized air. The lungs maintain their volume through breathing pressurized air, and to do this, the number of molecules increases proportionally. The increased number of molecules will play a role in creating the risk for barotrauma (see Fig. 38.3), and the greater pressure of nitrogen will create the risk for decompression illness and nitrogen narcosis. (The figure is courtesy of Michael Natter, MD, who provided this figure for use in this chapter)

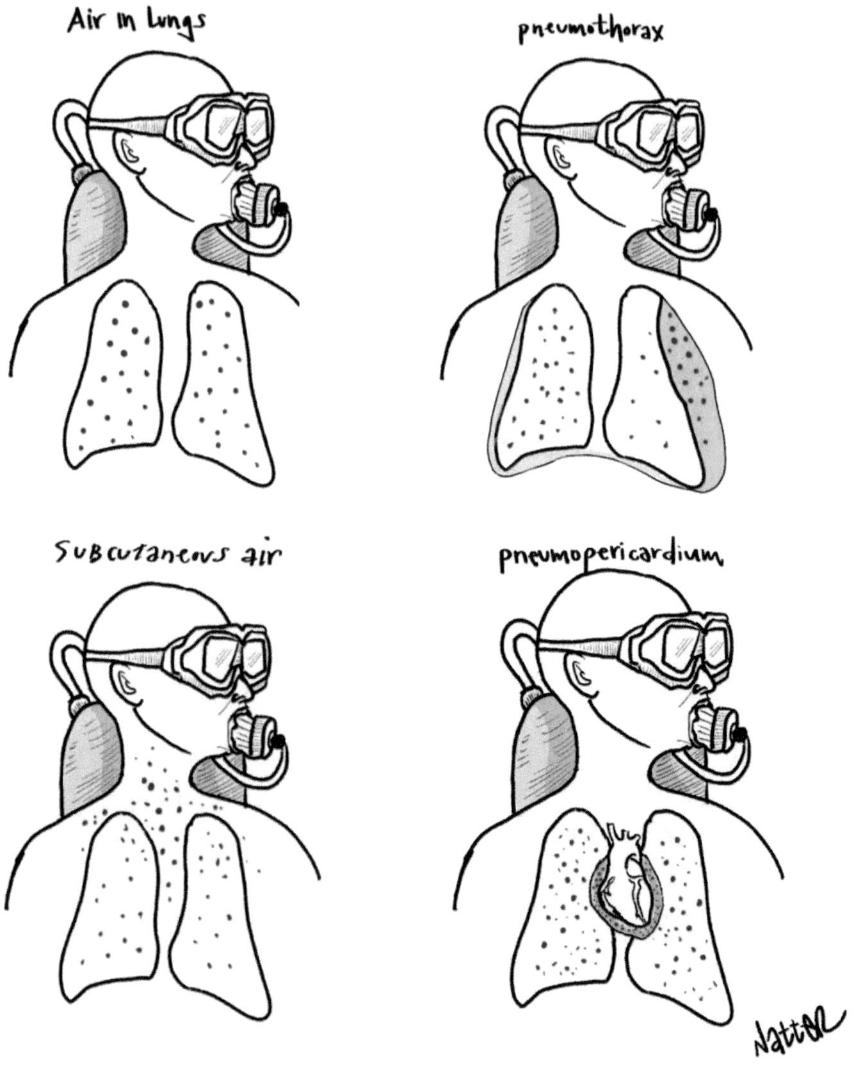

Fig. 38.3 The figure demonstrates the normal amount of air in the lung while using scuba, with each subsequent panel showing a specific form of pressure injury to lung tissue that occurs when the diver fails to exhale to reduce the pressure in the lungs along his or her ascent. When this happens, the large volume of air molecules at lower depths expands, and during expansion, it can tear through the pleural surface, alveoli, or bronchial walls. The type of injury created depends on exactly where the disruption of lung tissue occurs. (The figure is courtesy of Michael Natter, MD, who provided this figure for use in this chapter)

Conundrums of Undersea Medicine

There are a number of apparent conundrums when we move from caisson workers to the discussion of scuba and decompression illness in that context. The first conundrum, which requires some attention and thought, is what happens to diving mammals, including humans, who take their last full breath at the surface prior to diving to depths of 30 or 100 feet or even further, but without scuba equipment. Simply stated, the bends, or decompression illness, generally do not occur in this circumstance [5]. A physiological and physical chemistry approach to this analysis requires the understanding that if the partial pressure of nitrogen in a breath at sea level just before diving is 600 mmHg, then the pressure will certainly increase as the diving mammal descends to three atmospheres, but the total content of nitrogen in the blood will remain at the content it was at the surface when nitrogen was fully dissolved in body fluids and tissues. How could the total content of nitrogen change since the animal/human is not taking any breaths while submerged? Thus, ascent to the surface, where the pressure of inhaled nitrogen will be 600 mmHg, will mean that there will be no gradient that will drive nitrogen to bubble out into the circulation. There is, however, concern that nitrogen levels in diving mammals can become supersaturated in certain tissues, leading to the possibility that there can be some bubble formation on rapid ascent in selected tissues or body compartments [7]. This remains an important and mystifying aspect of mammalian physiology that continues to be under study across the globe [7], but in general, the bends are not a problem for diving mammals and humans capable of diving to significant depths during a free dive.

Physiology of Scuba

Scuba is different from free diving in one very important way that is linked to the three major illnesses that can arise from scuba diving. Remember that the scuba tank is not filled with oxygen but simply with air at a higher pressure and that it flows through a regulator before inhalation into the lungs [8]. The regulator works in a 2-step process where the highly pressurized air is reduced to a safer level in the first step and then finally to a level that matches the surrounding pressure in the second step [8]. This ingenious design allows the diver to descend with a substantial amount of air (in the tank) for a prolonged dive and assures that the pressure of each breath matches the surrounding water pressure, regardless of the depth at the time the breath is taken [8]. That is to say that if the diver has descended to 33 feet, which is 2 atmospheres, the air inhaled will be at two atmospheres of pressure, or 1540 mmHg [1].

There are three illnesses that can result from scuba diving; each will be important to discuss for clinicians who are focusing on the diver's health and safety. The first, decompression illness, we have already discussed in part. The second is barotrauma, which can result from holding one's breath on ascent (this includes alveolar gas embolism). The third can arise on prolonged dives when high levels of nitrogen accumulate in the blood and alter the sensorium. This is termed nitrogen narcosis. We will discuss each of these in succession.

Decompression Illness

It has been said that decompression sickness (DCS) is a manifestation of the "ever-present desire of humankind to explore new limits" [9]. This is certainly true. DCS, in brief, is a group of often severe symptoms, often life threatening that can develop after a "change in ambient pressure" [9]. This definition works since decompression illness can affect eighteenth-century caisson workers, nineteenth-century divers, and Caribbean undersea wreck explorers, and twenty-first-century astronauts who go on space walks after emerging from a pressurized space station [9]. The initial symptoms of mild (or Type I) disease include pain in the joints and extremities, so severe as to make affected individuals double over in pain. The large joints are susceptible to being the earliest involved body parts. More severe symptoms (or Type II), which can be deadly, arise in the central nervous system and can result in strokes, seizures, and loss of consciousness [9, 10]. The emergence of symptoms is related to the length of the dive or the duration of time that a subject's body is at increased pressure above ambient pressure, the difference in baseline and maximal pressure, and the rate of ascent. Surprisingly, symptoms often do not occur immediately but can start in the first few hours and usually have their onset within the first 48 h. Divers must be aware that not only the length, depth, and duration of a dive contribute to risk, but so does air travel within 48 h of the last dive. This should be avoided [10].

Treatment for decompression illness is twofold; recompression is the most important, but the administration of oxygen can help [11–15]. Recompression allows for a return to solution for gases that have bubbled out in the circulation, or at least a diminution of bubble size, reducing infarction size. Of course, once recompression is achieved, there will not be any further bubbling out of solution for any of the dissolved gases in the serum. Recompression is best accomplished with a recompression chamber, but in rare circumstances, recompression can be achieved in emergent circumstances through reimmersion, which is referred to as "in-water recompression" [16]. The process of recompression, otherwise involves a sealed chamber that can help apply a pressure, otherwise, of up to 2–6 atmospheres. When reintroduced to a pressurized atmosphere, not only is future bubbling out of solution stabilized, but air bubbles will also be reduced in size based on the application of Boyle's law [17]. This will decrease the area of ischemia and help facilitate reabsorption of gas in the bubbles. Once applied and patients improve, the pressure can be reduced gradually to allow for equilibration of N2 concentration without triggering recurrent bubbling out into the circulation. In addition, 100% oxygen is applied, which increases the gradient for exhaled clearance of nitrogen gas in the alveoli during exhalation. Administering oxygen also helps restore oxygen to ischemic tissues. Of course, these chambers tend to be located in hospitals or healthcare clinics near active dive centers [18]. More portable devices, called monochamber devices, can facilitate care at more remote locations [19].

Barotrauma

The second type of injury related to misadventure while scuba diving is barotrauma [20, 21]. This is just as important to understand because it, too, can prove fatal if not avoided. The pathogenesis is straightforward in scuba, and it is related to failure to breathe (or, more specifically, to exhale) during ascent (Fig. 38.3). Applying Boyle's law, the reader can imagine that the volume of air in the chest will increase with ascent into lower-pressure water as a diver approaches the surface [17]. This expansion of highly pressurized air will easily lead to disruption of lung tissues, allowing air to escape into the pleural space (pneumothorax), the mediastinum (pneumomediastinum), subcutaneous tissues (leading to subcutaneous emphysema), or alveolar gas embolism. The sudden development of a pneumothorax while diving can be fatal, and even after ascent to the surface, it is essential that rapid treatment include assessment for chest tube placement and the administration of oxygen [22, 23]. Clinically, pneumothorax occurs when there is a tear in the pleural surface, allowing air to leak into the space between the lung and the chest wall. This has several effects, including limiting the expansion of the lung, building up pressure, which further limits breathing (this can cause death from hypoxia), and potentially building up pressure in the thorax that prevents blood from entering the chest through the superior or inferior vena cava (this can cause death from cardiovascular collapse). Pneumomediastinum may be compelling to view on a radiograph but is typically well tolerated. Its importance for recognition is that it can be a precursor to pneumothorax. Alveolar gas embolism can be fatal as well and occurs when lung tissue is disrupted in ascent, allowing air under pressure to be forced into the bloodstream via disrupted pulmonary veins, which can create issues downstream, as the bubbles can cause strokes, heart attacks, or a "bends-like condition" where bubbles create tissue ischemia after passage through the left atrium, left ventricle, and into the systemic circulation [22, 23].

Of course, treatment modalities are vitally important, but the major approach to complications of scuba is one of prevention. Dive tables are an essential tool for safe diving. They guide the approach to ascent based upon the depth and duration of dive time. They also limit repetitive dives wherein cumulative time under pressure increases the level of dissolved N2 gas. They also help by describing limits at which no decompression stop is required (referred to as non-decompression limits (NDL)). When a diver is careful not to surpass the NDL, they can ascend freely. This is most typically achieved during shorter dives at shallow depths. For longer dives at more substantial depths of 10 feet or greater, scuba divers will need to carefully follow the dive tables in order to plan for rest stops during ascent. Beyond managing time at a particular depth or ascent, the dive table will also address repetitive dives, since divers who may dive multiple times throughout a day will also accumulate a higher pressure of nitrogen in their systems. How remarkable it is that one of the contributors to the history of understanding decompression illness, John Haldane, also made a remarkable contribution to the creation of dive tables [24]. These have been updated by the Navy, and dive computers are available for divers to customize their unique diving itineraries [26]. Many divers rely upon fixed, printed dive tables so as not to rely on whether a computer is working or able to be powered up [25].

A second key part of a safe ascent is continued breathing such that intrathoracic pressure does not build up and the diver is not at risk for barotrauma. This can be accomplished by maintaining the glottis in an open position and continually breathing to be sure that there is adequate exhalation. These preventive measures, by decreasing the risk of pneumothorax or barotrauma, will also limit the risk of alveolar gas embolism (AGL). Finally, there is evidence that pre-dive exercise may help reduce the risk of decompression illness and enhance the likelihood of a successful dive [26].

In the end, two (2) final rules prevail for recreational divers whose activity is limited to depths of 100 feet. First, always stop for a rest on ascent at 15–20 feet from the surface and stay at that depth for 3–5 min using a buddy check [27, 28]. There are several benefits of this approach. The stop allows a gradual reduction in nitrogen pressure to mitigate decompression illness. It also allows for additional time to breathe and avoid the possibility of barotrauma injury. The continuous breathing ensures that the glottis remains open (Fig. 38.4a, b). Third, the buddy check involves the entire dive crew in keeping each other safe by watching for bubbles and assuring that everybody pauses for the safety stop. Finally, during a safety stop, the divers can plan for their final ascent by noting the location of their dive boat, releasing a surface buoy to identify their location and avoid injury, and reminding the divers to go very slow during the final ascent and rise only 5 feet every 2–3 min.

In summary, the unique illnesses associated with scuba are related to the inhalation of pressurized gas below the surface that increases both the volume and pressure of the lungs. As a result, a large volume of dissolved nitrogen moves into the

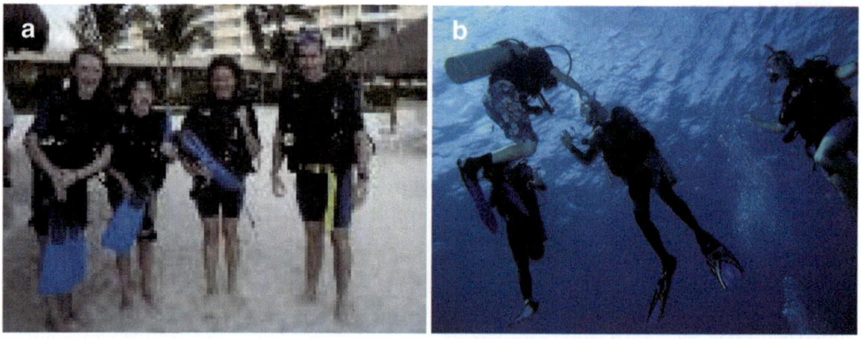

Fig. 38.4 (**a**) The author (far right) with (from left to right) Mary Bridget Kane, Brian Kane, and Jean Kane preparing for scuba instruction in Cozumel, 2006. (Photo courtesy of the author) (**b**) The author with his family (Brian, top left, and Mary Bridget, lower left in the background) making a safety stop, which affords greater time for nitrogen (N2) to move out of the body tissues gradually before reaching the surface. The safety stop also provides for a pause with continued breathing, which can be observed by noting bubbles from the regulators. This is a good sign that there is continued breathing with an open glottis, which prevents barotrauma. (Photo courtesy of the author)

serum and tissues of the body. Ascending too quickly can allow that nitrogen to move out of solution and bubble out into the circulation, leading to the bends, named for the pain that results from tissue infarction in the joints, extremities, and abdomen. This condition can be fatal. Not only does breathing compressed air increase the risk of decompression illness, but the increased number of molecules contained in the chest cavity can also create havoc if one ascends while holding their breath. Doing so can easily lead to pneumothorax, pneumomediastinum, alveolar gas embolus, or subcutaneous air [23, 27, 28].

Declarations

Competing Interests The author(s) has no competing interests to declare that are relevant to the content of this manuscript.

Ethics Approval The author(s) declares that this manuscript does not include primary research with human participants.

The author(s) declares that this manuscript does not include primary studies involving animals.

References

1. Vann RD. Lambertsen and O2: beginnings of operational physiology. Undersea Hyperb Med. 2004;31(1):21–31. PMID 15233157. Archived from the original on June 13, 2008.
2. Snyder MA. Exploring underwater with scuba. Arch Environ Health. 1966;13(6):690–4. https://doi.org/10.1080/00039896.1966.10664650.
3. The Great Bridge. Simon & Schuster; 2012. ISBN 9781451683233. Retrieved 29 Aug 2018.
4. The Great Bridge. Simon & Schuster; 2012. ISBN 9781451683233. Retrieved 29 Aug 2018 (page 308).
5. Chandan G, Cascella M. Gas laws and clinical application. [Updated 2023 Aug 28]. In: Stat Pearls [Internet]. Treasure Island: Stat Pearls Publishing; 2025. Available from: https://www.ncbi.nlm.nih.gov/books/NBK546592/.
6. Henry W. Experiments on the quantity of gases absorbed by water, at different temperatures, and under different pressures. Phil Trans R Soc Lond. 1803;93:29–43. https://doi.org/10.1098/rstl.1803.0004.
7. Hooker SK, Fahlman A, Moore SJ. Deadly diving? Physiological and behavioural management of decompression stress in diving mammals. Proc R Soc B. 2012;279:1041–50. https://doi.org/10.1098/rspb.2011.2088.
8. https://www.force-e.com/blogs/blog/scuba-regulators-explained/#:~:text=The%20regulator's%20first%20stage%20which%20attaches%20to,regulator%20hose%20to%20the%20regulator's%20second%20stage.&text=When%20the%20regulator%20is%20pressurized%20by%20opening,chamber%20until%20the%20intermediate%20pressure%20is%20reached. Accessed 19 May 2025.
9. Mahon RT, Regis DP. Decompression and decompression sickness. Compr Physiol. 2014;4:1157–75. https://doi.org/10.1002/j.2040-4603.2014.tb00566.x.
10. https://www.nasa.gov/reference/risk-of-decompression-sickness/#:~:text=When%20astronauts%20move%20from%20a,what's%20known%20as%20decompression%20sickness.
11. Francis TJ, Mitchell SJ. 10.6: manifestations of decompression disorders. In: Brubakk AO, Neuman TS, editors. Bennett and Elliott's physiology and medicine of diving. 5th Revised ed. Saunders; 2003. p. 578–99. ISBN 978-0-7020-2571-6. OCLC 51607923.

12. Feldman J, Cooper JS. Flying after diving. [Updated 2023 Nov 23]. In: StatPearls [Internet]. Treasure Island: StatPearls Publishing; 2025. Available from: https://www.ncbi.nlm.nih.gov/books/NBK499855/.
13. Toklu AS, Cimsit M, Yildiz S, Uzun G, Korpinar S, Sezer H, Aktas S. Decompression sickness cases treated with recompression therapy between 1963 and 1998 in Turkey: review of 179 cases. Undersea Hyperb Med. 2014;41(3):217.
14. Chin W, Joo E, Popa DA, Covington DB. Efficacy of the US navy treatment tables in treating DCS in 103 recreational scuba divers. Undersea Hyperb Med. 2017;44(5):399.
15. Yarbrough OD, Behnke AR. The treatment of compressed air illness using oxygen. J Ind Hyg Toxicol. 1939;21:213–8. ISSN 0095-9030.
16. Doolette DJ, Mitchell SJ. In-water recompression. Diving Hyperb Med. 2018;48(2):84–95. https://doi.org/10.28920/dhm48.2.84-95. PMID: 29888380; PMCID: PMC6156824.
17. West JB. The original presentation of Boyle's law. J Appl Physiol. 1999;87(4):1543–5.
18. Rendina C. A historical review of the US Navy's busiest recompression chamber in the Pacific theater with a current perspective on caring for civilian divers within its area of responsibility. Undersea Hyperb Med. 2018;45(2):183–9.
19. Clarke R. Monoplace chamber treatment of decompression illness: review and commentary. Diving Hyperb Med. 2020;50(3):264–72. https://doi.org/10.28920/dhm50.3.264-272. PMID: 32957129; PMCID: PMC7755460.
20. Russi EW. Diving and the risk of barotrauma. Thorax. 1998;53(suppl 2):S20–4.
21. Marcy TW. Barotrauma: detection, recognition, and treatment. Chest. 1993;104:578–84.
22. Moon RE. Treatment of diving emergencies. Crit Care Clin. 1999;15(2):429–56.
23. Mitchell SJ, Bennett MH, Moon RE. Decompression sickness and arterial gas embolism. N Engl J Med. 2022;386:1254–64. https://doi.org/10.1056/NEJMra2116554.
24. West JB. JS Haldane and some of his contributions to physiology. In: Integration in respiratory control: from genes to systems. New York: Springer New York; 2008. p. 9–15.
25. US Navy. US navy diving manual, 6th revision. Washington: US Naval Sea Systems Command; 2006.
26. Madden D, Barak O, Thom SR, Yang M, Bhopale VM, Ljubkovic M, Dujic Z. The impact of pre-dive exercise on repetitive SCUBA diving. Clin Physiol Funct Imaging. 2016;36(3):197–205.
27. Lucrezi S, Egi SM, Pieri M, Burman F, Ozyigit T, Cialoni D, et al. Safety priorities and under-estimations in recreational scuba diving operations: a European study supporting the implementation of new risk management programs. Front Psychol. 2018;9:383.
28. Melamed Y, Shupak A, Bitterman H. Medical problems associated with underwater diving. N Engl J Med. 1992;326:30–5. https://doi.org/10.1056/NEJM199201023260105.

Ascent into Thin Air: How Oxygen Is Reduced to the Elevation Due to Low Barometric Pressure

39

Gregory C. Kane

The wind is a musical instrument with a certain range of tones, beyond which in both directions we have an infinite silence.

—John Tyndall (1820–1893, Irish physicist and Mountaineer)

Climb high, sleep low.

—Mountaineer aphorism, not attributed

Introduction

A 13-year-old boy from Vineland, New Jersey, develops a cough and shortness of breath while skiing the Back Bowls at Vail (elevation of 11,200 feet). His pulse ox is 73%, and his heart rate is 160 bpm at the aid station. He states that he is "too tired to walk." By way of background, this young teenager grew up in South Jersey (elevation of 100 feet). He learned to ski at Blue Mountain just north of Allentown, Pennsylvania, by age 7, and his family had frequented Elk Mountain in northern Pennsylvania as well as Okemo in southern Vermont, where he had improved his skill even on the most challenging slopes. On this trip to Vail, his first out west with his family, they had landed in Denver, staying for just one night, and traveled by car directly to Vail early the next morning to get in a full day of skiing. The boy had not slept well in Denver and complained of some mild stomach upset en route. Based on this history and presentation, this teen, who had never been to this altitude, appears to be suffering from high-altitude pulmonary edema (HAPE). In this chapter, we will review the physiological challenges that contribute to the development of this disorder and others.

G. C. Kane (✉)
The Korman Respiratory Institute and the Division of Pulmonary, Allergy and Critical Care, The Department of Medicine at the Sidney Kimmel Medical College of Thomas Jefferson University, Philadelphia, PA, USA
e-mail: gregory.kane@jefferson.edu

G. C. Kane et al. (eds.), *Oxygen*, https://doi.org/10.1007/978-3-032-18934-9_39

Humans have longed to ascend to the highest peaks. Among these are many of the famous: from Mount McKinley in Alaska (20,308 feet), to Mount Whitney in the lower 48 US states (14,505 feet), to Kilimanjaro in Africa (19,341 feet) and Everest on the China–Nepal border, rising to 29,031 feet. The important physiological challenge of ascent on any of these peaks is hypoxia generated because of the fall in barometric pressure with each foot of elevation. The greatest air or barometric pressure (760 mmHg) is measured at sea level, and the lowest pressure on the Earth's surface is at the peak of Everest (253 mmHg) [1, 2]. Since the amount of oxygen molecules represents 21% of air at both sea level and altitude, the partial pressure of oxygen (PO2) at the summit of Everest falls to just 53 mmHg. Visualized as an "ocean of air" [3], one can imagine that the highest pressures are at the bottom of the ocean and the lowest pressures are toward the surface in the exosphere, where oxygen molecules may be so rare they can float into space without collision. Simply stated, the higher you go, the fewer air molecules there are in any unit of measure of the air, such as one square foot. That means there are fewer nitrogen and oxygen molecules as well with every step of elevation (Fig. 39.1).

In Chap. 5, we introduced the reader to the important gas laws that govern alterations in the partial pressure of oxygen [4]. In understanding how hypoxia can develop at altitude, it is essential to understand how the partial pressure of oxygen in the atmosphere translates into the relative PAO2 in the alveolus (or air sacs of the lung) where gas exchange occurs. This relationship can be explained by the alveolar gas equation. At sea level, the air that we breathe is at a pressure of 760 mmHg of mercury (mmHg) and represents the bottom of the "ocean of air." The higher one goes into the atmosphere, whether it be climbing on a mountain summit or ascending in a balloon or non-pressurized aircraft, the more limited is the column of air above, and thus, the corresponding ambient pressure is reduced.

The reasons for the reduction in atmospheric pressure are relatively simple: pressure is reduced as the air column above becomes thinner. Stated otherwise, there are

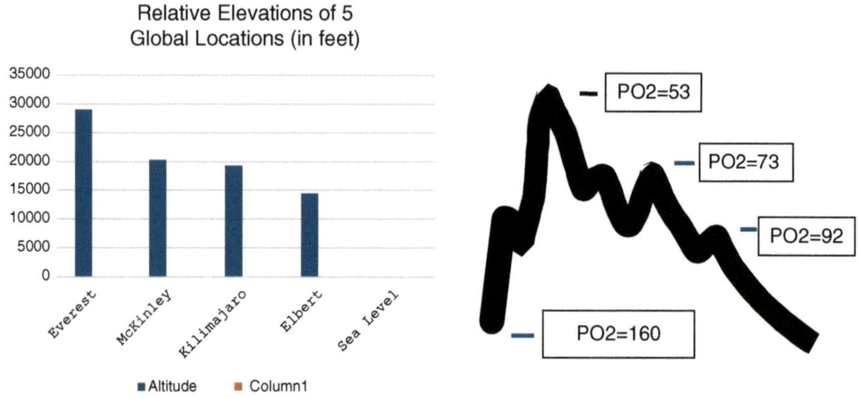

Fig. 39.1 This figure shows the relative altitude in feet for several mountain elevations across the globe, including Mount Everest on the border of Nepal and China, Mount McKinley in Alaska, Mount Kilimanjaro in Tanzania and Mount Elbert near Leadville Co. The corresponding relative atmospheric PO2 is displayed in the simulated elevations for each of these four peaks in the frame to the right

simply fewer molecules at the higher elevation, and these molecules are at lower pressure because they are not compressed by the same column of air above. The reason that hypoxia is so poorly tolerated is related to the long oxygen gradient between the alveolus and mitochondria, where oxygen is ultimately used to generate adenosine triphosphate or ATP (Fig. 39.2).

PO2 is easily calculated from atmospheric pressure because, uniformly throughout the atmosphere and regardless of elevation, oxygen composes 21% of all molecules in the atmosphere. At higher altitudes, the lower PO2 in the atmosphere contributes to hypoxemia, or low levels of oxygen in the bloodstream for humans at that level, which can be difficult for climbers to manage even in the absence of high-altitude pulmonary edema or high-altitude cerebral edema. Table 39.1 shows the relative variations in atmospheric pressure and PO2 at 4 selected altitudes. Altitudes below 14,000 feet were not selected because they are more easily tolerated. Altitudes below 5000–7000 feet generally do not require acclimatization.

Having reviewed and understood the partial pressure of oxygen that humans can breathe at various elevations, it is next important to understand how that reduced partial pressure translates into an even lower partial pressure in the alveolar sacs. There are three simple factors that contribute to this reduction (see Table 39.2). First, at a body temperature of approximately 98.6 °F, breathed air becomes humidified by the nasal passages, and the humidity pressure of water vapor is approximately 47 mmHg. Humidification prevents drying of the lower airways of the lungs and maintains the mucociliary blanket lining the airways. This humidification is added to the air that we breathe, but according to Dalton's law, the total of all these gases in the trachea, where air has been warmed, must continue to be equal to the barometric pressure. For example, at sea level, if the air we breathe is 760 millimeters in mercury in total and composed of 160 mmHg of oxygen and 500 mmHg of nitrogen; when we add humidification 47 mm of mercury, then the pressure of the nitrogen and oxygen components is reduced to a total of 713 mmHg: 563 mm of mercury of nitrogen and 150 mmHg of oxygen. The net effect is that in the trachea, where air has been warmed by our body's humidity, the partial pressure of oxygen falls to 150 mmHg.

As we move further through the major conducting airways and down toward the alveolar sacs, there is a second problem created by the gas laws, which is the presence of carbon dioxide, which is being excreted from the blood as a byproduct of metabolism. This carbon dioxide takes up additional space in the alveolus; it must be accounted for as a new gas entering this compartment. Again, Dalton's law requires that the summation of the partial pressure of nitrogen, oxygen, water vapor, and carbon dioxide must all still equal the total partial pressure (760 mmHg at sea level). These are generally accounted for arithmetically with one subtle exception, as the amount of carbon dioxide generated through metabolism is not always directly equal to the amount of oxygen consumed; rather, this ratio alters with our food intake and whether we utilize principally protein, carbohydrate, or fat for nourishment.

Oxygen (O_2) is not consumed 1-for-1 with an equal generation of carbon dioxide (CO_2) in a steady state, since the ratio of CO_2 produced varies slightly with the

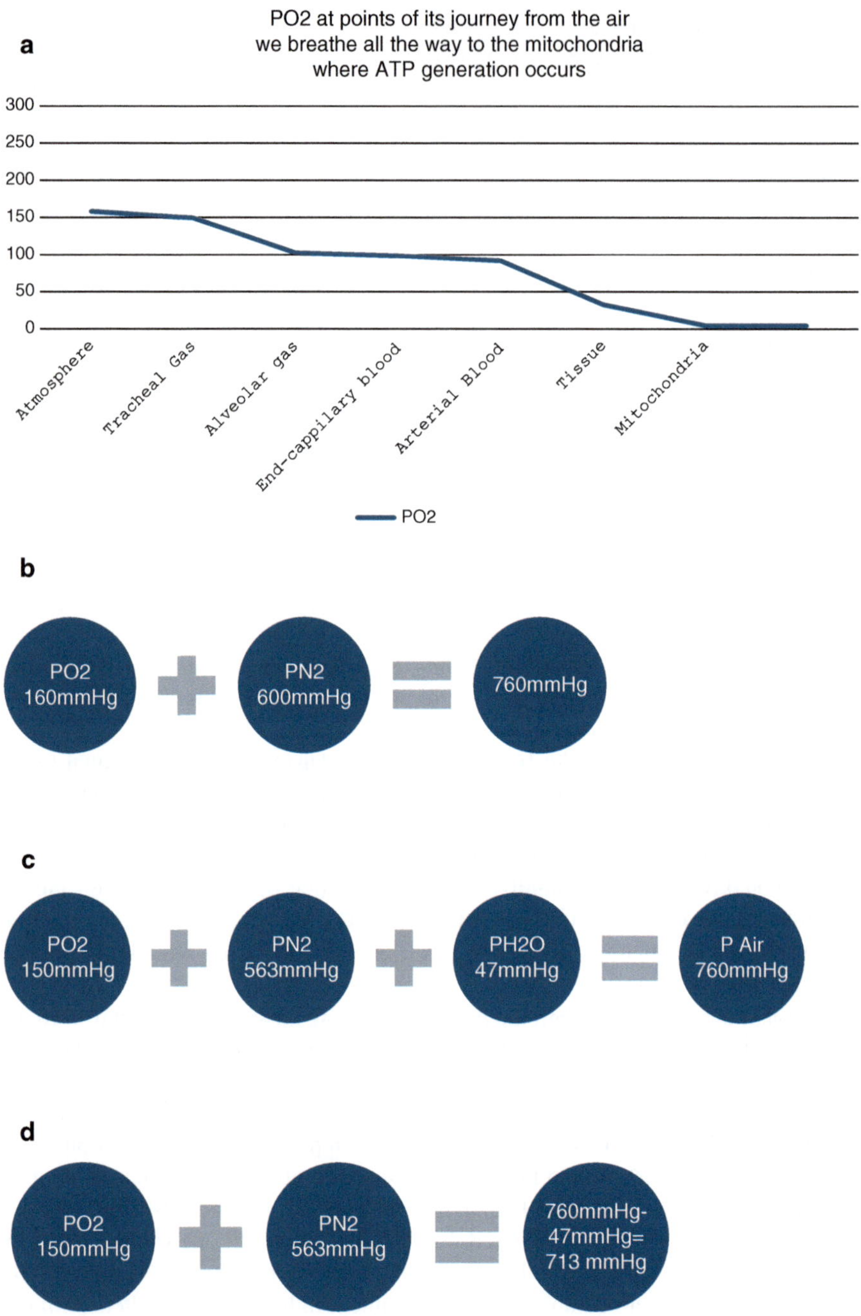

Fig. 39.2 (**a**) This figure displays the gradient for oxygen from the highest (atmospheric air) through the lung and ultimately to the tissues and mitochondria (where PO2 can be below 5 mmHg) (**b**) A representation of how Dalton's law applies to atmospheric air. There is very little carbon

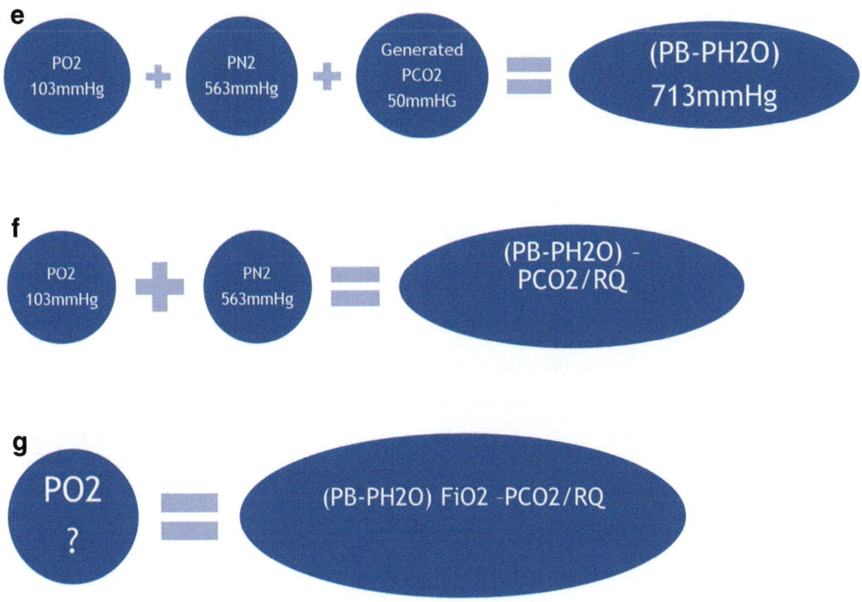

Fig. 39.2 (continued) dioxide in the atmosphere, and so the total partial pressure is principally made up of oxygen and nitrogen (**c**) Dalton's law at the level of the trachea. The function of the nasal passages and sinus cavities is to help humidify the air that we breathe to avoid excess drying of the tracheal mucosa, which can lead to mucus plugging and/or infections. The addition of water vapor, which is 47 mm of mercury at normal body temperature, must be accounted for in Dalton's law, and so both the PO2 and PN2 are proportionally reduced (**d**) This simplified equation shows how PO2 is reduced because of the impact of water vapor. We still have further to go to explore the PO2 at the level of the alveolus (**e**) Dalton's law applied to gases at the level of the alveolus. Note that when humans consume a balanced diet, they generate 120% of CO_2 molecules for every O_2 molecule consumed to generate ATP in the mitochondria. Because oxygen and carbon dioxide are exchanged into the red blood cell and in cellular metabolism, it is PO2 that is reduced at the alveolar level, while nitrogen remains relatively constant (this figure is for a normally breathing subject) (**f**) After rearranging the terms, we now have the alveolar gas equation, and the PO2 can be calculated based on (1) various barometric pressure measurements, (2) the degree of hyper- or hypoventilation and the attendant PaCO2, and (3) the dietary intake and resultant respiratory quotient (RQ) (**g**) At any altitude, a variation of the barometric pressure or an alteration of oxygen supply, this formula will allow the reader to calculate the PO2 in the alveolus. The result will fall with any altitude above sea level and will increase when supplemental oxygen is being utilized (as it would be for a patient or climber, for example). Two liters, for example, would increase FiO2 to approximately 28%, while the application of a high-flow nasal cannula might increase FiO2 all the way to 100%. CO_2 should also be measured by blood gas determination as well, and the PO2 can rise in hyperventilating subjects while falling in those who retain CO_2, as the higher CO_2 displaces oxygen at the level of the alveolus to fulfill Dalton's law

Table 39.1 Atmospheric pressure and the associated partial pressure of oxygen at various altitudes

Location	Elevation (m/ft)	Atmospheric pressure (mmHg)	PO_2 (mm Hg) (21% of total pressure)
Sea level	0 m/0 ft	760	159
Mt. Elbert	4401 m/14440 ft	450	94.5
Mt. Kilimanjaro	5895 m/19,341 ft	376	79
Mt. McKinley (Denali)	6190 m/20,310 ft	364	76.4
Mt. Everest	8848 m/29,029 feet	265	55.7

Table 39.2 Factors that lead to the reduction of PO2 from air to alveolus

Factor	Approximate reduction	Comment
Added humidity in airways/ trachea	47 mmHg	Water vapor is added to inspired air
Exchange of CO_2 f0r O_2 at the alveolus	50 mmHg = 40 mmHg/ respiratory quotient (RQ)	May vary with diet and the resultant RQ
Variation of PCO2 based on hyperventilation of hypoventilation	Can range from 10 mmHg to 80 mmHg (or more)	Still need to divide by the RQ

relative dietary intake and whether it is composed chiefly of protein, carbohydrate, or fat. In a standard balanced diet, the production of CO_2 molecules at the cellular level is approximately 120% more than the O_2 molecules that undergo combustion through aerobic metabolism via the Krebs cycle. Thus, in accounting for this in a calculation of how much the O_2 in the alveolus will be reduced, the calculation must reflect the 20% increase in CO_2 molecules that enter the alveolus in a steady state, compared with oxygen moving into the capillary blood. This is accomplished by dividing the CO_2 by the RQ—a factor that can be established for different types of diets but one that is typically 0.8 [5].

The alveolar gas equation is one important approach to understanding how atmospheric PO2 correlates with alveolar PO2 in the alveolar sacs of the lungs (typically referred to as PAO2 using a capital "A" to distinguish the alveolar partial pressure from the partial pressure in the arterial blood, which is referred to as PaO2 with a small "a"). From the perspective of Dalton and his gas law, which states that the partial pressures of each gas in a system must be equal to the total partial pressure, this adjustment is quite easy to understand. Since there is no valve or barrier between the upper trachea and the lower alveolus, the sum of these partial pressures must also be equal to 760 mm of mercury for a human at sea level. Thus, when humidity is added through the nasal passages, it would be most appropriate for the available partial pressure constituted by nitrogen and oxygen be reduced by 47 mm of mercury, which is exactly the partial pressure of humidity, or water vapor, at body temperature. The second part of this alveolar gas law is more complex, and this is because carbon dioxide and oxygen are not exchanged equally in the alveolus but vary depending on the diet, which contributes to the specific fuel that is metabolized at the cellular level. Depending on the fuel, there may be more or less CO_2 created for each mole of oxygen consumed. As such, the CO_2 entering the alveolus is adjusted to reflect its relative production and exchange for O_2 in a steady state by dividing the PaCO2 by the respiratory quotient (RQ) [4]. The alveolar gas equation takes into account the added gases to the system, which must somehow correspond to a reduction in both the partial pressure of nitrogen and oxygen in the trachea, as well as the reduction in O_2, more so at the level of the alveolus, since oxygen is in a direct change relationship with CO_2. Two final assumptions in generating this formula are that the alveolar and arterial CO_2 are essentially the same because of the more rapid diffusion of carbon dioxide related to its lower molecular weight, and that the use of this equation in clinical practice may require altering the FiO2 from its typical 21%, both at sea level and at altitude.

$$\text{PAO2} = (\text{PB} - 47\,\text{mmHg}) \times \text{FiO2}\,\text{minus}\;\; \text{PCO2}/\text{RQ}$$

An immediate and whimsical application of this formula occurs when using the barometric pressure at the summit of Mount Everest. To the uninitiated who might assume that the alveolar CO_2 will be normal at 40 mmHg, the alveolar gas equation would yield (assuming a standard diet and RQ of 0.8):

$$\text{PAO2} = (253\,\text{mmHg} - 47\;\;\text{mmHg}) \times 0.21\,\text{minus}\;\; \text{PCO2}/0.8$$

The barometric pressure at Everest is 253 mm of mercury, and the fraction of gas at that elevation, which is oxygen, is 21%.

$$\text{PAO2} = (206\,\text{mmHg}) \times 0.21\,\text{minus}\,40\,\text{mmHg}/0.08$$

This would yield the following:

$$\text{PAO2} = 43.26\,\text{mmHg} - 50\,\text{mmHg} = ??$$

In applying the alveolar gas equation to calculating the alveolar O_2 at the summit of Everest, the uninitiated would come to a preliminary conclusion that the alveolar O_2 would be a negative number. Recognizing that this is not possible, the reader will immediately realize that substantial hyperventilation will be expected of mountaineers approaching the summit of Mount Everest. If one might substitute hyperventilation of a factor of 4 (meaning that the increase in respiratory rate and tidal volume would be fourfold the normal level), then one would anticipate a PCO2 of approximately 10 mmHg.

$$\text{PAO2} = (206\,\text{mmHg}) \times 0.21\,\text{minus}\,10\,\text{mmHg}/0.08$$

$$\text{PAO2} = 43.26\,\text{mmHg} - 12\,\text{mmHg} = 31.26\,\text{mmHg}$$

In applying the alveolar gas equation to calculating the alveolar PO2 (PAO2) at the summit of Everest, with an expected degree of hyperventilation, we can see that alveolar O_2 actually might be 31 mmHg. The question is, can this or was this ever validated?

Proof of the validity of the calculations above has come in two forms. First, Reinhold Messner and Peter Habeler reached the summit of Everest without oxygen in the spring of 1978, demonstrating in quite an interesting way that this would be the highest altitude that humans could both theoretically and practically ascend to on the planet [5]. How remarkable that this happens to be the highest point of the Earth's elevation on any continent. More recently, a group of intrepid mountaineer scientists took actual measurements, but only at the last base camp before the final ascent on Everest [6]. In all, 4 subjects had measures of their blood gases with an average PO2 of 13 mmHg and a corresponding average PaO2 of 24.6 mmHg [7]. The validity of these measurements lies in their comparison to the expected alveolar O_2 in the alveolar gas equation of approximately 27 mmHg. These calculations also highlight the remarkable efficiency of the lungs in these fit mountaineers, with such a low difference between alveolar and arterial O_2. Corresponding partial pressures at various altitudes can be substituted in the alveolar gas equation to identify the hypoxic challenges at these altitudes. Indeed, on a personal note, this author experienced hypoxia on Mount Kilimanjaro. On the final day of ascent, still short of the summit, my O_2 saturation by pulse oximetry was 62%. This was no doubt due to pulmonary hypertension or early high-altitude pulmonary edema, in addition to the impact of reduced barometric pressure on the available atmospheric PO2. An attentive crew of guides offered supplemental oxygen for 20 min, such that I could regain energy and control of my breathing and ability to continue trekking, enabling me to summit. My son did not require supplemental oxygen and arrived at the summit well ahead of me (Figs. 39.3 and 39.4).

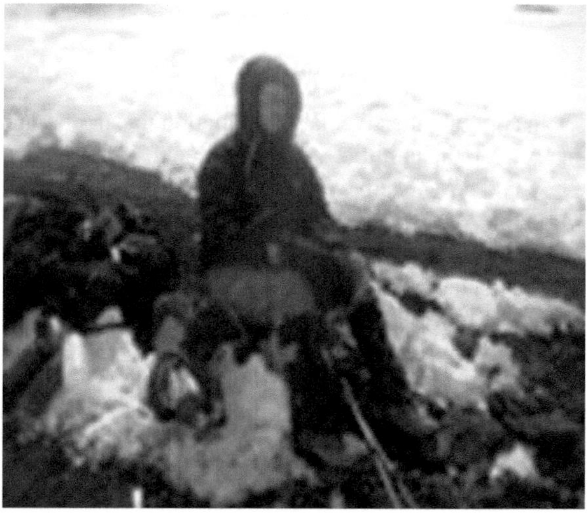

Fig. 39.3 The author takes a break in the snow-covered terrain of the final ascent at Kilimanjaro in the spring of 2012. While my O_2 saturation was approximately 62% prior to going on oxygen, it quickly rebounded to 88% after a few minutes. After about 15–20 min of rest utilizing the oxygen, I was able to make the summit without any ongoing supplemental oxygen support

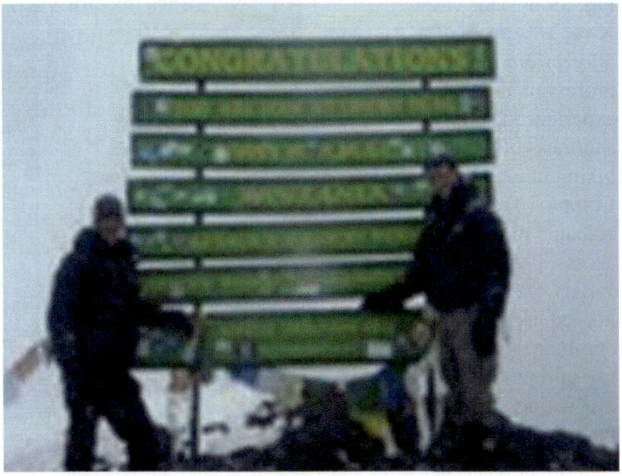

Fig. 39.4 The author with his son, Brian, at the summit of Kilimanjaro. The smile is perhaps at reaching the summit successfully, but also at the recognition that I could soon descend almost immediately after this picture was taken. Photo provided by the author

High-Altitude Pulmonary Edema

Some climbers are not so fortunate, and it appears that the most prominent risk factors for the development of high-altitude pulmonary edema (HAPE) are often related to having been born at or near sea level with limited travel in one's youth or early adulthood.

The mechanism of high-altitude pulmonary edema (HAPE) is complex but most likely related to pulmonary vasoconstriction from hypoxia in the lung with subsequent capillary leak into the alveolar sacs [8]. Afflicted individuals experience shortness of breath, cough, fatigue, and may appear to have bluish skin around the lips and fingers consistent with cyanosis. Of course, pulse oximetry or arterial blood gas measurements will confirm hypoxia with a widened alveolar–arterial O_2 gradient. Oxygen saturations can be as low as 40% and are often between 40% and 70% [8]. Symptoms can start anywhere from 2 to 5 days after the ascent and may be mitigated by acclimatization achieved by spending 1–2 days at a lower altitude prior to the final ascent [8]. If there are available clinical resources for radiology, the clinician will identify radiographic findings that include bilateral chest infiltrates without cardiomegaly (see Fig. 39.5). The diagnosis is often straightforward because few people will attempt to ascend to high altitudes when they are sick and might have pneumonia, though some might experience an exacerbation of asthma at altitude. People with preexisting heart or lung disease should be advised to avoid ascending to altitudes greater than 5000 feet to avoid such challenges. Persons with advanced heart and lung disease may experience worsening of symptoms, even ascending to 5000 feet (the elevation of Denver, Colorado). A clinical diagnosis of HAPE can be established for patients with recent ascents to high altitude, who have at least 2 signs and 2 symptoms from the criteria shown in Table 39.3 [8].

Children are also at risk for HAPE, but few studies have characterized clinical factors in these children. One cross-sectional study did establish that children may

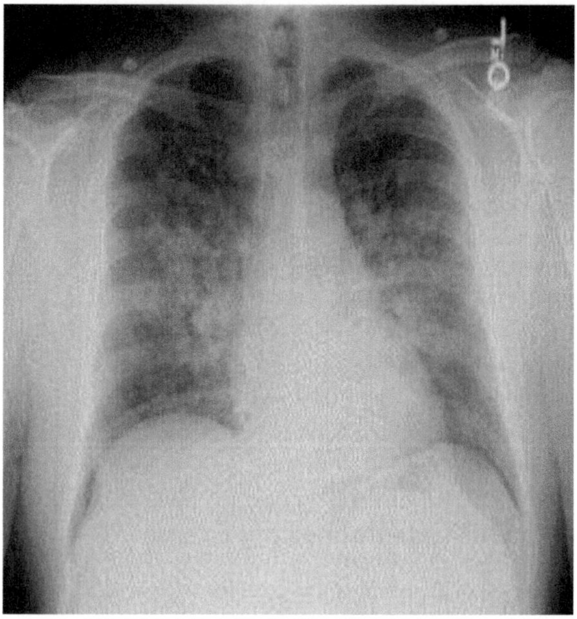

Fig. 39.5 This chest X-ray was taken of a 40-year-old medical professional who experienced sudden shortness of breath while hiking in Ecuador on the Cotopaxi Trek. This volcanic mountain is accessible to climbers of a variety of skills and does not require technical climbing skills such as the use of ropes. After evacuating down the mountain, this chest X-ray was taken at a local medical clinic. Treatment was with supplemental oxygen and rest. (Figure 39.5, courtesy of Dr. Gregory Kane)

Table 39.3 Lake Louise consensus criteria for clinical diagnosis of HAPE [8, 9]

Lake Louise consensus criteria	Signs	Symptoms
	Crackles or wheezing in at least one lung field	Weakness or decreased exercise performance
	Cyanosis	Dyspnea at rest
	Tachypnea	Cough
	Low oxygen saturation	Chest tightness or chest congestion
	Tachycardia	

commonly have upper lobe pulmonary edema on chest X-ray, and more than 40% may go on to have future episodes [11].

The primary treatment for HAPE is descent [10]. Supplemental oxygen, if available, is highly recommended until symptoms improve and the edema fluid reabsorbs, which can take several days. As one can imagine, there are relatively limited treatment trials, but one randomized trial published in the journal *High-Altitude Medicine and Biology* showed comparable outcomes in groups randomized to oxygen alone, oxygen plus dexamethasone, and oxygen plus nicardipine. Patients entered into this trial were identified over 1 1/2 years, and the authors started with 246 patients who were screened and met the Lake Louise criteria for high-altitude pulmonary edema [9]. This study was approved by a local IRB, and the authors stated that all protocols were consistent with the Helsinki Declaration on medical research involving human subjects. The important finding was that the authors found no difference in hospital stay or speed of recovery among the three groups.

Table 39.4 Preventive drug therapies for HAPE

Drug	Dose	Duration
Nifedipine	30 mg twice daily	6 days or duration of time at high altitude
Tadalafil	10 mg twice daily	6 days or duration of time at high altitude
Sildenafil	40 mg three times a day	6 days
Salmeterol	125 mcg twice daily	Duration of time at high altitude

Other treatments for HAPE have been examined independently [12]. A group of investigators at a military hospital in India examined the effect of nifedipine in 110 subjects with HAPE. The clinical measures that were collected included vital signs, symptoms, pulmonary auscultation findings, chest X-rays, EKG, and pulse oximetry. All the patients were treated with a reduction in altitude, plus supplemental oxygen and bed rest. In the nifedipine group, there was no more accelerated improvement compared to placebo in the normalization rate for oxygen saturations, the timing for resolution of pulmonary physical exam findings, the chest X-ray infiltrates, or the length of hospital stay. The average hospital stay overall was about 4 days and ranged from 2 to 6 days. Based on these two trials, it appears that once the edema occurs, descent and treatment with supplemental oxygen represent the best current treatment and that subjects should be prepared for a recovery that may take several days or up to a week [12].

Of course, the best approach to HAPE is prevention, and this can often be aided by acclimatization through gradual ascent with rest days and by a stop at a lower altitude prior to the final ascent. Taking this a step further, the aphorism, "climb high, sleep low," has been used by mountaineers for many years to mitigate against the risk of challenges at altitude. HAPE rarely occurs at elevations below 8000 feet [8]. One interesting observation is that the occurrence of HAPE does not appear to be related to physical fitness or exercise intensity during ascent [13]. A careful review of prior ascents to over 8, 000–10,000 feet is of particular benefit for people with prior episodes of HAPE, identifying those who should take particular precautions in future ascents [8, 13].

There are, fortunately, several pharmacological approaches for prevention, which are outlined in Table 39.4 [14–16]. These are most important for people who have previously experienced high-altitude pulmonary edema and have a personal commitment to continuing mountaineering activities.

Acute Mountain Sickness and the Spectrum of HACE

Acute Mountain Sickness [8, 17–19] is a neurological illness that can occur in up to 20% of individuals ascending to altitudes greater than 8000 feet and up to 40% of individuals ascending to altitudes greater than 10,000 feet [20]. One should think of acute mountain sickness (AMS) and high-altitude cerebral edema (HACE) as a spectrum of illness essentially affecting the central nervous system. While AMS is manifested by headache that occurs within 6–12 h of a rapid ascent, high-altitude cerebral edema (HACE) is associated with brain edema of a vasogenic cause and is associated with more profound symptoms of confusion, loss of consciousness, and altered mental status. Individuals are typically unable to sit up [8, 21].

AMS, which may be well recognized by readers who have ascended to altitudes of greater than 8000 feet, is characterized by headache but is often associated with nausea, dizziness, malaise, and sleep disturbance, either alone or in combination. The risk is greatest for those who ascend to these altitudes (>8000 feet) within 24 h. An example would be for individuals who fly to Denver from Boston and then drive directly to a mountain resort higher than 8000 feet. Typically, symptoms may be relieved by administration of aspirin or nonsteroidal anti-inflammatory agents and rest. In severe cases, affected individuals may need to descend to altitudes below 8000 feet or utilize supplemental oxygen.

The development of HACE may be easily confused with stroke or subarachnoid hemorrhage, other causes of sudden change in neurological status. It would be less likely to confuse HACE with other intracranial cranial pathology that are typically gradual in onset, because HACE is associated with rapid ascent and symptoms are relatively acute in nature. While for most patients the characterization of HACE as part of the spectrum of AMS certainly holds, in some rare situations, HACE may have a sudden onset without warning [21]. CNS imaging of affected individuals will show vasogenic edema and may also reveal microhemorrhages principally in the corpus callosum [22, 23].

The mechanisms of this illness are poorly understood, but it is clearly related to hypoxia, which leads to vasogenic edema that alters the blood–brain barrier [22]. Treatment is straightforward with descent and application of oxygen therapy but different from HAPE, the administration of dexamethasone plays an important role. Understandably, controlled clinical trials are not available for HACE, and the administration of this therapy (typically in doses of dexamethasone 4 mg every 6 h after a loading dose of 8 mg IV or IM) is based upon decades of clinical experience and the recognition that dexamethasone is effective in treating cerebral edema of multiple etiologies [23–25]. Oral therapy is an option when IV is not available, and it should not be delayed in remote areas [23]. Another factor supporting the use of dexamethasone in HACE is that there is clear evidence that it also helps in AMS, including circumstances of AMS induced in carefully controlled environments in a hyperbaric chamber with human volunteers at a simulated altitude of 14,200 feet [26].

Primary and secondary prevention steps are appropriate for HAPE and AMS; patients with HACE should avoid threatening altitudes due to the risk of neurological injury. Elite athletes are not protected because they too may experience symptoms at high altitude if they are not acclimatized [27, 28].

In summary, altitude and hypoxia can trigger common and troubling symptoms of AMS, but also potentially life-threatening HAPE or HACE. This chapter focuses on the presentation and treatment of these illnesses and on understanding how hypoxia plays the cardinal role in their pathogenesis.

Declarations

Competing Interests The author(s) have no competing interests to declare that are relevant to the content of this manuscript.

Ethics Approval The author(s) declare that this manuscript does not include primary research with human participants.

The author(s) declare that this manuscript does not include primary studies involving animals.

References

1. West JB. High-altitude medicine. Am J Respir Crit Care Med. 2012;186(12):1229–37.
2. Fenn WO, Rahn H, Otis AB. A theoretical study of the composition of the alveolar air at altitude. American Journal of Physiology-Legacy Content. 1946;146(5):637–53.
3. Walker G. An ocean of air: why the wind blows and other mysteries of the atmosphere. Harcourt; 2007.
4. James WS. The discovery of the gas laws. Sci Prog (Twentieth Cent). 1929;24(93):57–71. JSTOR, http://www.jstor.org/stable/43428731. Accessed 8 Apr 2025.
5. Westerterp KR. Food quotient, respiratory quotient, and energy balance. Am J Clin Nutr. 1993;57(5):759S–65S.
6. West JB. Human limits for hypoxia: the physiological challenge of climbing Mount Everest. Ann N Y Acad Sci. 2006. https://doi.org/10.1111/j.1749-6632.2000.tb06173.x.
7. Michael PW, Michael PW, Grocott MPW, Martin DS, Levett DZH, McMorrow R, Windsor J, Montgomery HE, For the Caudwell Xtreme Everest Research Group. Arterial blood gases and oxygen content in climbers on Mount Everest. New Engl J Med. 2009;360(2):140–9.
8. Bärtsch P, Swenson ER. Acute high-altitude illnesses. N Engl J Med. 2013;368(24):2294–302.
9. Yanamandra U, Nair V, Singh S, Gupta A, et al. Managing high-altitude pulmonary edema with oxygen alone: results of a randomized controlled trial. High Alt Med Biol. 2016;17:294–9. https://doi.org/10.1089/ham.2015.0120.
10. Hackett PH. High-altitude medicine. In: Auerbach PS, editor. Wilderness medicine. 6th ed. Philadelphia: Mosby; 2012. p. 2–43.
11. Kelly TD, Meier M, Weinman JP, Ivy D, Brinton JT, Liptzin DR. High-altitude pulmonary edema in Colorado children: a cross-sectional survey and retrospective review. High Alt Med Biol. 2022;23:119–24.
12. Deshwal R, Iqbal M, Basnet S. Nifedipine for the treatment of high altitude pulmonary edema. Wilderness Environ Med. 2012;23(1):7–10. https://doi.org/10.1016/j.wem.2011.10.003.
13. Bircher HP, Eichenberger U, Maggiorini M, Oelz O, Bärtsch P. Relationship of mountain sickness to physical fitness and exercise intensity during ascent. J Wilderness Med. 1994;5(3):302–11.
14. Maggiorini M, Brunner-La Rocca H-P, Peth S, et al. Both tadalafil and dexamethasone may reduce the incidence of high-altitude pulmonary edema: a randomized trial. Ann Intern Med. 2006;145:497–506.
15. Sartori C, Allemann Y, Duplain H, et al. Salmeterol for the prevention of high-altitude pulmonary edema. N Engl J Med. 2002;346:1631–6.
16. Richalet JP, Gratadour P, Robach P, Pham I, Déchaux M, Joncquiert-Latarjet A, et al. Sildenafil inhibits altitude-induced hypoxemia and pulmonary hypertension. Am J Respir Crit Care Med. 2005;171(3):275–81.
17. Roach RC, Bärtsch P, Hackett PH, Oelz O, Lake Louise AMS Scoring Consensus Committee. The Lake Louise acute mountain sickness scoring system. In: Sutton JR, Houston CS, Coates G, editors. Hypoxia and molecular medicine. Burlington: Charles S. Houston; 1993. p. 272–4.

18. Poudel KM, Poudel TR, Shah N, Bhandari S, Sharma R, Timilsina A, et al. Ascent rate and the Lake Louise scoring system: an analysis of one year of emergency ward entries for high-altitude sickness at the Mustang district hospital, Nepal. PLoS One. 2022;17(10):e0276901. https://doi.org/10.1371/journal.pone.0276901.
19. Singh I, Khanna PK, Srivastava MC, Lal M, Roy SB, Subramanyam CSV. Acute mountain sickness. N Engl J Med. 1969;280:175–84.
20. Simancas-Racines D, Arevalo-Rodriguez I, Osorio D, Franco JV, Xu Y, Hidalgo R. Interventions for treating acute high-altitude illness. Cochrane Database Syst Rev. 2018;6(12):CD009567. Schoene, Robert; Milledge.
21. Zelmanovich R, Pierre K, Felisma P, Cole D, Goldman M, Lucke-Wold B. High altitude cerebral edema: improving treatment options. Biologics. 2022;2(1):81–91. https://doi.org/10.3390/biologics2010007.
22. Hackett PH, Yarnell PR, Hill R, Reynard K, Heit J, McCormick J. High-altitude cerebral edema evaluated with magnetic resonance imaging. JAMA. 1998;280:1920–5.
23. Kallenberg K, Dehnert C, Dörfler A, et al. Microhemorrhages in nonfatal high-altitude cerebral edema. J Cereb Blood Flow Metab. 2008;28:1635–42.
24. Luks AM, Auerbach PS, Freer L, Grissom CK, Keyes LE, McIntosh SE, Rodway GW, Schoene RB, Zafren K, Hackett PH. Wilderness medical society clinical practice guidelines for the prevention and treatment of acute altitude illness: 2019 update. Wilderness Environ Med. 2019;30:S3–S18.
25. Jha SK. Cerebral edema and its management. Med J Armed Forces India. 2003;59:326–31.
26. Levine BD, Yoshimura K, Kobayashi T, Fukushima M, Shibamoto T, Ueda G. Dexamethasone in the treatment of acute mountain sickness. N Engl J Med. 1989;321:1707–13.
27. Campbell AD, McIntosh SE, Nyberg A, Powell AP, Schoene RB, Hackett P. Risk stratification for athletes and adventurers in high-altitude environments: recommendations for preparticipation evaluation. Wilderness Environ Med. 2015;26(4_suppl):30–9.
28. Derby R, deWeber K. The athlete and high altitude. Curr Sports Med Rep. 2010;9(2):79–85.

"The Oxygenator": A Key Component of the Heart–Lung Machine and More 40

Without Oxygen, We Die!

Louis Samuels

Personal Prologue

In the process of writing this section, I was evaluated and subsequently informed that I had surgical-type coronary artery disease and will require coronary artery bypass grafting. As a cardiac surgeon for three decades, I have taken for granted the operation and the equipment needed to perform it. Regarding the latter, I can now appreciate (more than ever) the work and commitment of those who laid the foundation for what we now consider "routine." The pump and oxygenator, the two featured components of the heart–lung machine, are marvels in bioengineering, and I thank all those tenacious pioneers who persevered through trials (and often failures) to take us to where we are today. As a faculty member at Thomas Jefferson University, it is particularly fortuitous that the machine about to be used to help perform my procedure was invented by another Jefferson faculty member over seventy years ago (Fig. 40.1). I am forever grateful.

The Heart–Lung Machine: Links to the Oxygenator

Willem Kolff

In 2002, a much younger version of me (1961–present) and a much older version of Willem Kolff (1911–2009) sat together on a couch at Hahnemann University in Philadelphia, PA. Dr. Kolff, often referred to as "The Father of Artificial Organs," came to discuss my research and clinical experience with the latest artificial heart at

L. Samuels (✉)
Jefferson-Einstein Medical Center Philadelphia, Sidney Kimmel School of Medicine, Thomas Jefferson University, Philadelphia, PA, USA
e-mail: Louis.Samuels@jefferson.edu

G. C. Kane et al. (eds.), *Oxygen*, https://doi.org/10.1007/978-3-032-18934-9_40

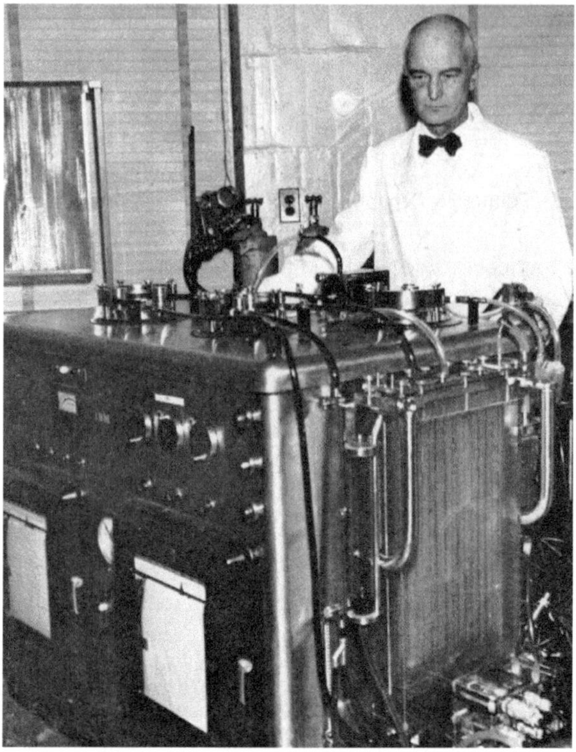

Fig. 40.1 John H. Gibbon, Jr. with the heart–lung machine he invented. (Courtesy Thomas Jefferson University Siegman Archive with permission)

that time, the AbioCor™ totally implantable electric unit (Abiomed, Inc., Danvers, MA) [1]. It was an honor to sit beside this surgical pioneer—a man who invented the artificial kidney (i.e., hemodialysis), an artificial heart, and an artificial lung (i.e., an oxygenator) [2]. He was a contemporary of another surgical giant, Denton Cooley (1920–2016), who placed the world's first total artificial heart in 1969 [3]. In addition, Dr. Kolff was the mentor to Robert Jarvik (1946–2025), a brilliant physician and engineer who developed the artificial heart of the 1980s, the Jarvik-7 (Symbion, Inc., Brentwood, TN) [4]. In my office, Dr. Kolff had with him a leather briefcase—its exterior worn and frayed over decades of use—within which were notes on his research regarding an artificial lung. He showed me the yellowed pages—drawings and concepts of his ideas to artificially replace the lungs *long term*—an extension of his earlier work and something that has yet to be achieved. He was hoping I would take over where he left off. I resisted the temptation to say yes and to photocopy these handwritten pearls—decisions that I regret to this day.

Dr. Kolff's contributions to the field of artificial technologies are noteworthy and have laid the foundation for future research and refinement of artificial organs. His development of the membrane for hemodialysis was the foundation upon which a similar membrane for oxygenation and carbon dioxide removal was based. Yet the story of the cardiopulmonary bypass machine in general and the oxygenator in particular began before Kolff and involved another remarkable yet unexpected individual—the aviator Charles Lindbergh (1902–1974).

Charles Lindbergh and Alexis Carrel

The origin of Charles Lindbergh's pursuit of a machine that could artificially oxygenate and circulate blood was personal. In the 1920s, his sister-in-law was diagnosed with rheumatic heart disease, and the prognosis was extremely poor. Partnering with the most famous surgeon of his day (and a Nobel Prize winner), Alexis Carrel (1873–1944), they designed an apparatus that could keep cells (and theoretically tissue) alive outside the body [5] (Fig. 40.2). Initial versions of the device were made in the 1930s and tested in the lab. Although more contemporary iterations of the technology were demonstrated in the 1960s, the device they invented was never used for the purposes intended. The pursuit of such a concept, however, led another individual to develop something that would change history forever—Dr. John H. Gibbon, Jr. (1903–1973) (Fig. 40.3).

John H. Gibbon, Jr.

Dr. Gibbon's "incentive" to develop the heart–lung machine began in the early 1930s when he was at the Massachusetts General Hospital in Boston under the guidance of Dr. Edward Churchill (1895–1972), another notable surgeon who performed the first pericardiectomy (1928) for the treatment of constrictive pericarditis, as well as researched extensively the consequences of acute and chronic pulmonary emboli (PE). In 1931, a patient on Dr. Churchill's service had suffered from an acute PE, and it was Dr. Gibbon's job to watch over her until her condition either improved or worsened, the latter scenario triggering an operation. As the woman's condition

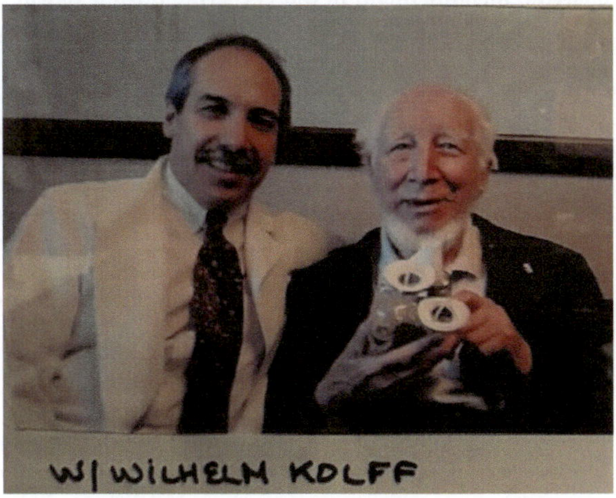

Fig. 40.2 Drs. Samuels and Kolff at Hahnemann Hospital (Philadelphia, PA) with AbioCor™ total artificial heart. (Abiomed, Inc., Danvers, MA). (Personal photo courtesy of Dr. Louis Samuels)

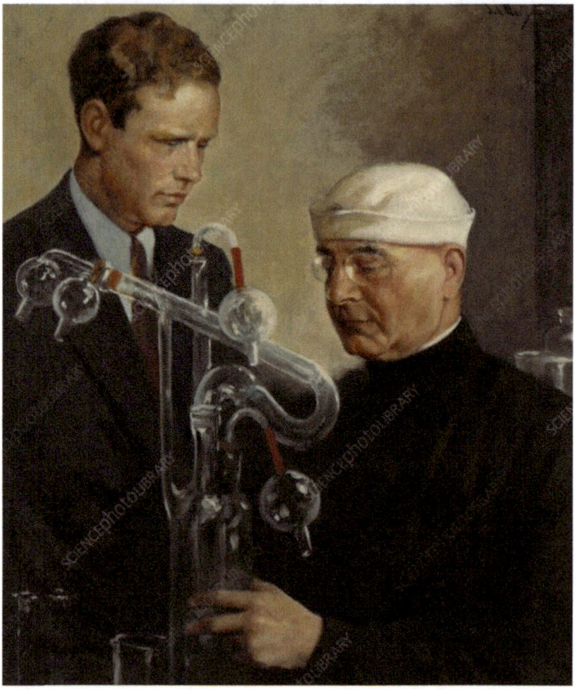

Fig. 40.3 Charles Lindberg, with Alexis Carrel, with a prototype "pump-oxygenator." (https://npg.si.edu/es/object/npg_NPG.87.TC2). (Courtesy National Portrait Gallery, Smithsonian Institution, USA)

deteriorated, an attempt at a pulmonary embolectomy failed, and the young woman expired. This event left an impression on Dr. Gibbon, who imagined the possibility of *successfully* operating with the aid of an extracorporeal circulatory device. Although his desire to research such an ambitious project began in Boston—where he met his wife, Mary Hopkinson (1905–1986), a technician in Dr. Churchill's research lab and key partner in the development of the heart–lung machine—he moved to Philadelphia, where he continued his experiments, interrupted for several years by his enlistment in the US Army during World War II. His early research on artificial oxygenation makes for fascinating reading and deserves some repeating (see below) [6]. Published in 1937, he wrote:

> *The apparatus designed to oxygenate the blood has already been described* [8]. *The essential feature of the apparatus is a vertical revolving cylinder* (Fig. 40.4). *The stream of blood is directed at a tangent to the inner surface of the cylinder at its upper extremity. The revolution of the cylinder results in the distribution of a thin film of blood over its inner surface. The film moves downward by gravity, and the blood is collected in a stationary cup (B) at the bottom. The greater part of the space within the revolving cylinder is occupied by a hollow, closed, stationary cylinder (C), through the center of which passes a metal tube (D). A mixture of 95 per cent oxygen and 5 per cent carbon dioxide is conveyed through this tube to the bottom of the oxygenator. From here the gas passes up between the stationery and the revolving cylinders over the film of blood and escapes at the top. The apparatus was designed to meet the requirements of this particular problem. The ratio between the amount of oxygen introduced per minute into the blood and the volume of blood contained in the oxygenator is higher than in other oxygenators which have been described* [8]. *It accom-*

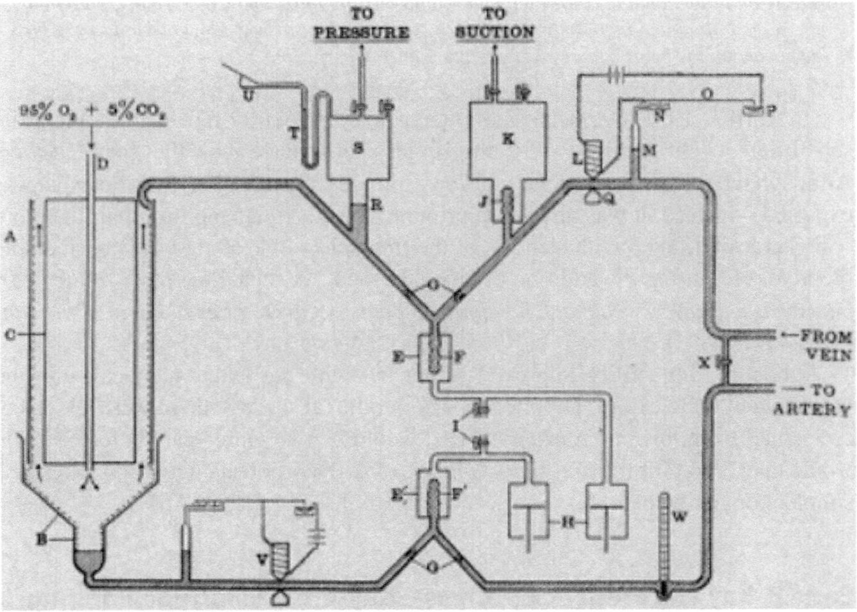

Fig. 40.4 A schematic of Gibbon's early prototype oxygenator as described in the referenced text. A diagram of the apparatus used to withdraw venous blood, introduce oxygen, and return the blood to the arterial system. (Courtesy Thomas Jefferson University Siegman Archives with permission)

> *modates a flow of blood of 500 cc. or more per minute, and large variations in the rate of flow do not produce foaming* [8]. *Gibbon, J. H., Jr.: An Oxygenator for Blood with a Large Surface Volume Ratio, to be published.)*

This apparatus was utilized in animal experiments throughout the 1930s and 1940s, modified by Gibbon and others along the way. It would take another decade before the clinical application of a heart–lung machine would be put to the test, and the first attempt (not by Dr. Gibbon) failed.

Clarence Dennis

In 1951, Clarence Dennis (1909–2005) of the University of Minnesota, using a modified Gibbon oxygenator and a Dale-Shuster pump, conducted several dog experiments in an attempt to utilize cardiopulmonary bypass to perform open-heart surgery. Dr. Dennis recognized the inadequacy of oxygenation with the rotating vertical cylinder pattern of Gibbon's device and developed a novel approach to artificial oxygenation using a series of screen discs. Quoting from his 1951 manuscript [7]:

> *Blood is pumped by modified Dale-Schuster pumps from the vena cava, through a flow meter, and to a system of jets which films it on several 38 cm. screen discs as they rotate*

slowly on a horizonal axis for exchange with a mixture of 02 and CO2. On dripping from the screen discs, the blood is pumped back to the femoral artery. Flow of blood from the vena cava to the heart is arrested by ligature during perfusions.

On April 1, 1951, Dr. Dennis admitted a six-year-old for repair of an interatrial septal defect. On April 5, 1951, the surgery took place with the "new" device. Although the unit performed well for forty minutes, the pathology was not what was expected—instead, it was an ostium primum defect. An attempt to repair the more complex lesion failed with stenosis of the tricuspid valve, along with considerable blood loss requiring the addition of citrated blood. As such, *"the force of the heart beats was extremely weak, and no vigorous beats occurred after removal of the cannulas."* [7]

Although contractility improved somewhat with the addition of calcium, the patient went on to expire. Despite the lack of clinical success, there were lessons to be learned from this initial experience. It would be two more years before Gibbon would take credit for the first *successful* use of extracorporeal circulation to repair a simpler congenital pathology—a secundum atrial septal defect (ASD).

Earle B. Kay and Frederick S. Cross—Kay-Cross Film-Type Rotating Disc Oxygenator

The concept of the rotating disc oxygenator was introduced by Viking Bjork (1918–2009) in 1948 and later modified by Earle Kay (1911–2000) and Frederick Cross (1920–2007), among others [8]. In 1956, these surgeons used their oxygenator at St. Vincent's Charity Hospital in Cleveland, Ohio, with application well into the 1970s. The unit, however, was cumbersome—heavy, difficult to sterilize, and required a large amount of blood to prime. Eventually, it fell out of use in favor of the bubble oxygenator.

Richard DeWall—Helical Reservoir Bubble Oxygenator

Richard DeWall (1926–2016), a Minnesotan, served a military internship during the Korean War, during which time he encountered a seaman with severe rheumatic valvular heart disease. There was no cure for the disease at the time. He pondered the problem and believed that a mechanical solution could be invented. Following his discharge from the Navy, he continued his training and career at the University of Minnesota, where he was fortunate to be mentored by two prominent surgeons. Beginning with the chief of heart surgery, Dr. Richard Varco (1912–2004), Dr. DeWall developed a prototype flutter valve made from plaster of Paris. Not knowing how to proceed further with the valve, he was assigned by Dr. Varco to work with another pioneering heart surgeon, C. Walton Lillehei (1918–1999). Dr. Lillehei, who was working on cross-circulation, suggested that Dr. DeWall pursue the development of a heart–lung machine and was advised, ironically, to avoid bubble oxygenator systems. (I had the pleasure of meeting Dr. Lillehei, along with Dr. Cooley, as a cardiac surgery trainee—it was the highlight of that year) (see Fig. 40.7).

Dr. DeWall worked for several years on a system that would avoid the pitfalls of previously designed oxygenators and eventually developed the helical reservoir pump-oxygenator, a bubble oxygenator. This device was first used clinically on May 13, 1955. The patient was a 3-year-old boy with a ventricular septal defect. The system worked well and became a useful tool in subsequent procedures. A wonderful reflection of this historical time was written by Dr. DeWall nearly 50 years afterwards [9]. DeWall's bubble oxygenator became popular for its simplicity and cost-effectiveness, particularly in comparison to the other oxygenators that were big, bulky, expensive, and difficult to operate. For decades, bubble oxygenators were in vogue and remained that way until the membrane oxygenator supplanted them.

Clinical Oxygenator "Success": *"In the Room Where It Happened" with Dr. Gibbon and Colleagues*

As previously described, the oxygenators of the 1930s and 1940s, with all their shortcomings, paved the way for the first successful use of extracorporeal circulation to repair an intracardiac defect (in an open-heart fashion) in 1953. Partnering with IBM, Gibbon designed three models of what was referred to as the "Gibbon-IBM" pump. Model I was used in the laboratory animal experiments. The original oxygenator was a large rotating cylinder that exposed oxygen to the blood. Although this concept worked on laboratory animals, such as cats and dogs, the required surface area for a human would be impossibly large.

Model II was the version used on May 6, 1953, when Dr. Gibbon repaired the secundum ASD in a teenage girl (Cecilia Bavolek) at Thomas Jefferson Hospital in Philadelphia, Pennsylvania. It was reported a year later in the 1954 *Minnesota Medicine* [10]. Model II (see Fig. 40.5a) was a heavy stainless-steel machine that weighed >2000 pounds and was very complex. Blood was propelled by 3 DeBakey roller pumps. The oxygenator was an enclosed battery of stainless-steel screens (Fig. 40.5b), each 40 cm tall and 25 cm wide. Blood flowed down each side of six screens while being exposed to oxygen. This provided a surface of $\approx 8\ m^2$ of exposed blood, far less than the $\approx 70\ m^2$ of alveolar surface of a normal lung, but enough to provide 100% oxygen saturation at flows up to 5 L/min.

The total bypass time was 45 minutes, and the circulation was supported completely for twenty-six of those minutes. It was a landmark moment that heralded the modern beginnings of open-heart surgery. An excellent manuscript describing Dr. Gibbon's work was published in 1982 by Dr. J. Donald ("Don") Hill, the surgeon who is credited with the first use of ECMO in 1971 [11, 12]. (On a personal note, it was Dr. Hill who invited me to participate on a panel of mechanical circulatory support experts as a young attending at the 44th Annual American Society for Artificial Internal Organs (ASAIO) Conference held in New York City from April 23–25, 1998.)

This "new" Model II unit (and subsequently Model III) allowed for adequate oxygenation in adult humans. The idea of using small strips of "screens" of material suspended in a cylinder and used as the surface for gas exchange (see Fig. 40.6a–c) was a feature introduced by Bernard J ("BJ") Miller, a surgical colleague in Dr. Gibbon's laboratory and in the operating room [13]. Dr. Miller, in conjunction with

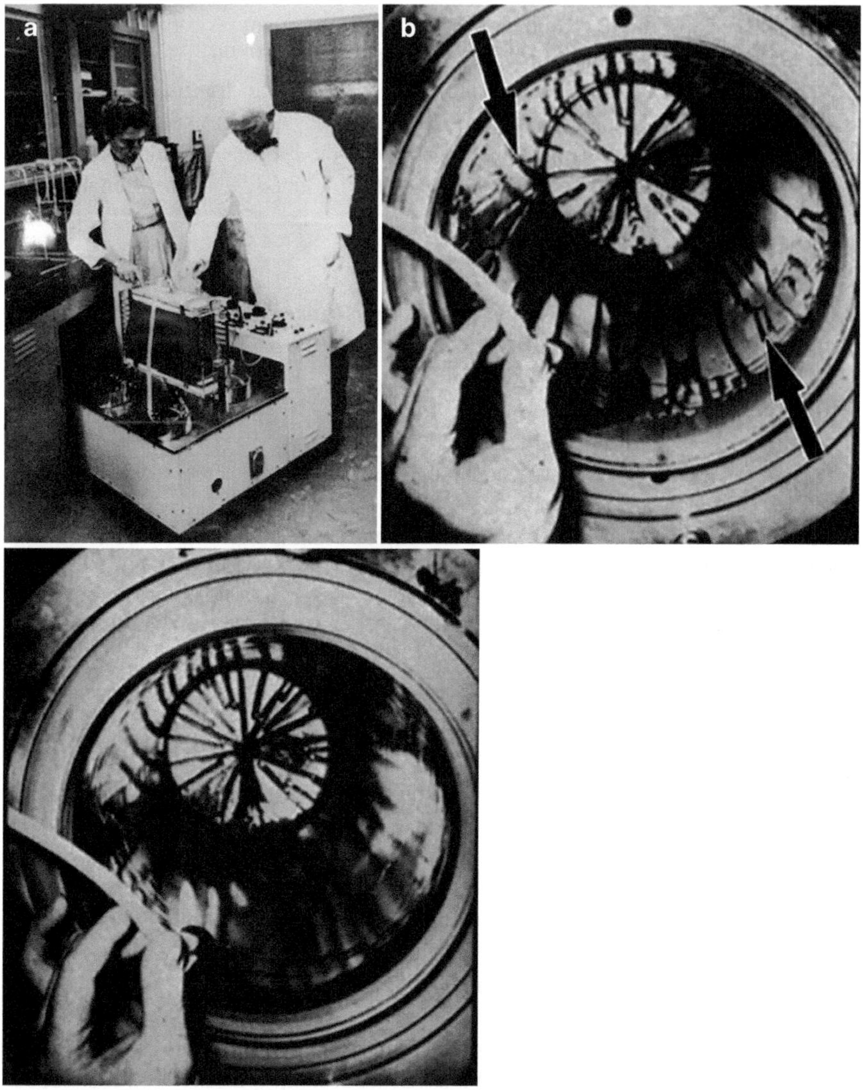

Fig. 40.5 (**a**) Dr. John Gibbon Jr's heart–lung machine (Mary Gibbon and Dr. John H Gibbon, Jefferson Medical College, 1927) with the 1964 heart–lung machine model. (Courtesy Thomas Jefferson University Siegman Archives with permission). (**b**) Dr. Gibbon's Cylinder Oxygenator. (Courtesy Thomas Jefferson University Siegman Archives with permission)

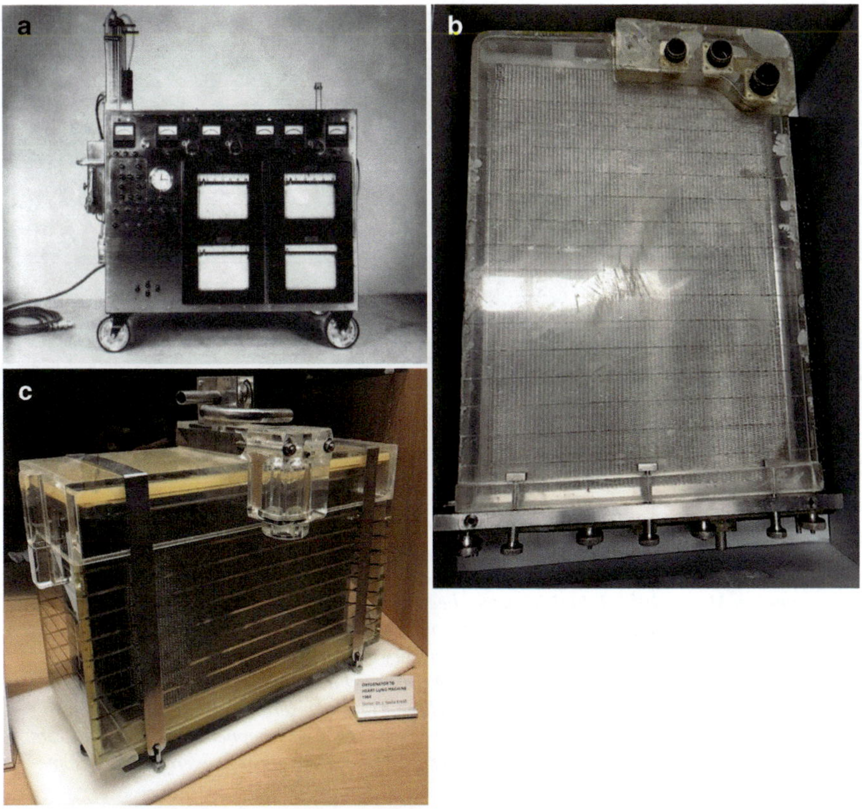

Fig. 40.6 (**a**) Model II Gibbon-IBM heart–lung machine used on May 6, 1953. (Courtesy Thomas Jefferson University Siegman Archives with permission). (**b**) A closer look at the oxygenator used for the 1953 Model II Gibbon-IBM heart–lung machine. (Courtesy Thomas Jefferson University Siegman Archives with permission). (**c**) A closer look at the oxygenator used for the 1964 Model III Gibbon-IBM heart–lung machine. This oxygenator provided more surface area than the one used in 1953. (Courtesy Thomas Jefferson University Siegman Archives with permission)

Dr. Stokes and Dr. Flick tested wire sizes, mesh sizes, and materials in the gas exchange of cow's blood. Finally, Mr. Gustav A. Malmrose—an IBM engineer—produced the idea of using a battery configuration for multiple screens in a large box, which led to the final design used in Model II. This design alleviated the low oxygenation levels of earlier models [14] (Fig. 40.7).

Ironically, the oxygenator failed during Gibbon's one (and only) successful case, with the need for creative solutions to avoid disaster. An account of that historic day was mentioned in an interview with the son (Dr. Stanton Miller) of Dr. Gibbon's colleague (Dr. Bernard J. Miller— "BJ") [15].

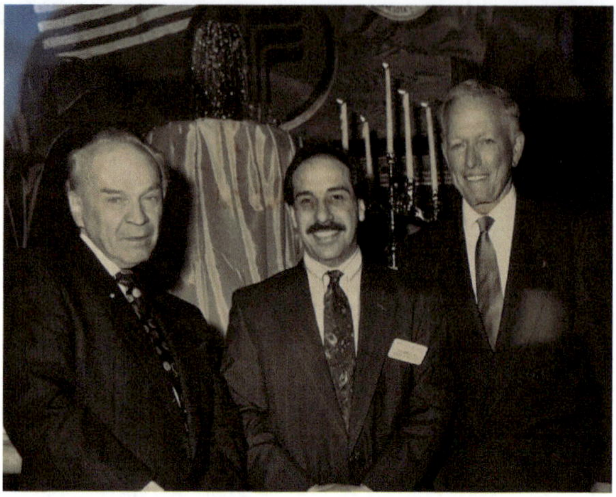

Fig. 40.7 Personal photo: Dr. C. Walton Lillehei and Dr. Cooley with author (L.S.) during photo op during tour of Medtronic, Inc. (Minneapolis, MN) facility (1995). (Personal photo courtesy of Dr. Louis Samuels)

Q: What was your father's involvement on the actual day of the first successful case and in the cases to follow?

A: My father participated and had a critical contribution to the famous case, the very first one, on May 6, 1953. I think it's never been a well-known fact that the machine actually clotted, and my dad, because of his thorough knowledge of the machine, hand-cranked the pumps the rest of the day during the surgery to ultimately get the patient successfully off of the bypass. That had been because the blood bank had not prepared the heparin concentration properly to prime the machine. He broke scrub to hand crank it the rest of the way. When it was evolving that that was what was happening, Gibbon's exact words per Dr. Victor Greco, a surgical resident present in the case, were, "BJ, do something." [15]

Additional descriptive details, absent from the original case report, were added at later dates [16, 17].

Meanwhile, as intended, oxygen-depleted blood flowed from Bavolek (the patient) and through a tube that served as her out-of-body artery. Propelled by the mechanical heart of four DeBakey roller pumps, the dark blood climbed to a clear, acrylic tower that housed the aluminum mesh screens. The blood then trickled down over the screens, gathering oxygen and turning bright red.

Everything went as planned, until it didn't.

At some moment during the 45 minutes in which the machine functioned as Bavolek's heart and lungs, her blood clotted. The clots first stuck in the mesh of the screens and then traveled down to the bottom of the artificial lung. There, the clots stoppered up the exit tubes. The incoming blood frothed. Bubbles rose.

Greco, who was operating the machine with Gibbon's head technician, Joan Carruthers, jumped up onto a stool and threw his arms on the lid of the lung's housing.

"I was afraid the pressure would blow the top of the artificial lung off," Greco recalls. "You'd have blood all over the operating room."

"BJ, get over there and do something!" Greco recalls Gibbon saying to Bernard J. Miller, MD, another assisting surgeon.

Dr. Miller, who had made crucial contributions in the machine's electrical design, dropped out of the surgery, cut the pumps, and operated the machine's pressure manually.

Gibbon had intended to close the defect with a patch, but time was up. Instead, he sewed the hole closed with a silk thread.

The team removed Bavolek from the machine, and Gibbon watched her heart. It was in spasm, fluttering rather than beating. Gibbon shocked it back into rhythm [16].

Another account verified the terrifying moment when the oxygenator failed and the aftermath of a heroic resolution.

The chest was opened through a transverse incision dividing the sternum. After being placed on cardiopulmonary bypass, a large atrial defect was closed with a continuous suture. The patient was on partial bypass for 45 minutes and total bypass for 26 minutes. There was 1 major problem with the heart-lung machine during the operation. Heparinized fresh blood had been used to prime the pump oxygenator. Each 500 mL of blood had received only 10 mg of heparin. Just as Gibbon was ready to close the defect, the oxygen saturation of the blood began to rapidly fall, and clots began to form on the oxygenator screens because of inadequate heparinization. Gibbon had planned to close the defect with a pericardial patch, but because of the drop in oxygenation, it was decided to close the defect as quickly as possible with a continuous suture and to end bypass as rapidly as possible. The patient had no adverse effect from this problem and was awake within an hour after the conclusion of the operation. Gibbon's operative note states that each 500 mL of blood should have received 25 mg of heparin. That evening he made 2 telephone calls, 1 to Alfred Blalock and the second to Clarence Crafoord, telling them the good news [17].

Reflecting on his work in the *American Journal of Surgery* in 1978, Dr. Gibbon commented:

I thought then, and it turned out later to be true, that the most difficult part of the extracorporeal circuit would be the construction of the artificial lung. [18]

Oxygenator Development Beyond Gibbon—General Categories

The early oxygenators were prone to clot formation and foaming, conditions that caused failure of the device and/or serious sequelae in the patient, including cerebral air embolization—"pump-heads." In an effort to remedy the problems associated with the existing oxygenators, scientists and clinicians developed alternative technologies that proved to be safer, simpler, and more dependable.

In a review article published in 2004, Iwahashi and others provided a past, present, and future description of oxygenators, broadly categorizing them into three types: Film-type oxygenators, Bubble-type oxygenators, and Membrane-type oxygenators [19].

Film-Type Oxygenators

Film-type oxygenators were designed to produce a thin blood film upon which gas exchange would take place. Because there is no mechanical introduction of gas into the blood, the blood trauma caused by this type of oxygenator is minimal. However, a large surface area and a high priming volume are necessary for this device. These were the devices that were initially developed in the earliest versions of oxygenators.

Bubble-Type Oxygenators

In the case of the bubble-type oxygenator, gas is introduced directly into the blood in the form of bubbles. The image of the porous stone in the fish tank with tiny bubbles emanating from it comes to mind. The oxygenation that takes place in this setting is highly effective due to the large surface area of the bubbles. In addition, as demonstrated in the fish tank analogy, these oxygenators are among the most effective and simplest to design, manufacture, and manage. However, because of the mechanical stress induced by air bubbles in the blood and because of the direct contact of the air bubbles with the blood, the trauma to the red blood cells is the highest among all the oxygenator types (Fig. 40.8).

Membrane-Type Oxygenators

The membrane oxygenator became the primary (and preferred) technology following the bubble oxygenator. Returning to Dr. Kolff, the success of dialysis rested upon the principles of diffusion across a membrane. It was simply a matter of applying this principle with the proper materials to allow for oxygen delivery and carbon dioxide removal. In the case of an oxygenator, blood is exposed to oxygen through a gas-permeable membrane. Because gas does not have any direct contact with the blood, trauma is minimal. As such, these oxygenators are the least traumatic to the blood of all the oxygenator types. However, the membrane introduces resistance to the permeating gases, which necessitates a large surface area. Consequently, a large priming volume is needed if the gas transfer rate of the membrane is to be optimized. Several types of membrane oxygenators were developed over the decades: plate-type membrane oxygenators, disposable coiled-membrane oxygenators, and hollow-fiber membrane oxygenators. Several companies from around the world created membrane oxygenators, focusing on the efficiency of gas exchange and durability. As extracorporeal circulation expanded to therapies beyond the duration of a surgical procedure (i.e., ECMO), the oxygenators needed to support days to weeks of cardiopulmonary support were of interest.

Artificial Heart Task Force (Including the Oxygenator)—*Counterpart to the NASA Moon Initiative*

Although we might be tempted to think of the heart and lungs as a pump and an oxygenator and something easily replicated in a laboratory, the reality is that mammalian evolution took millions of years to create these organs, and it is fanciful to imagine that we can imitate them in a matter of decades. Furthermore, the heart/

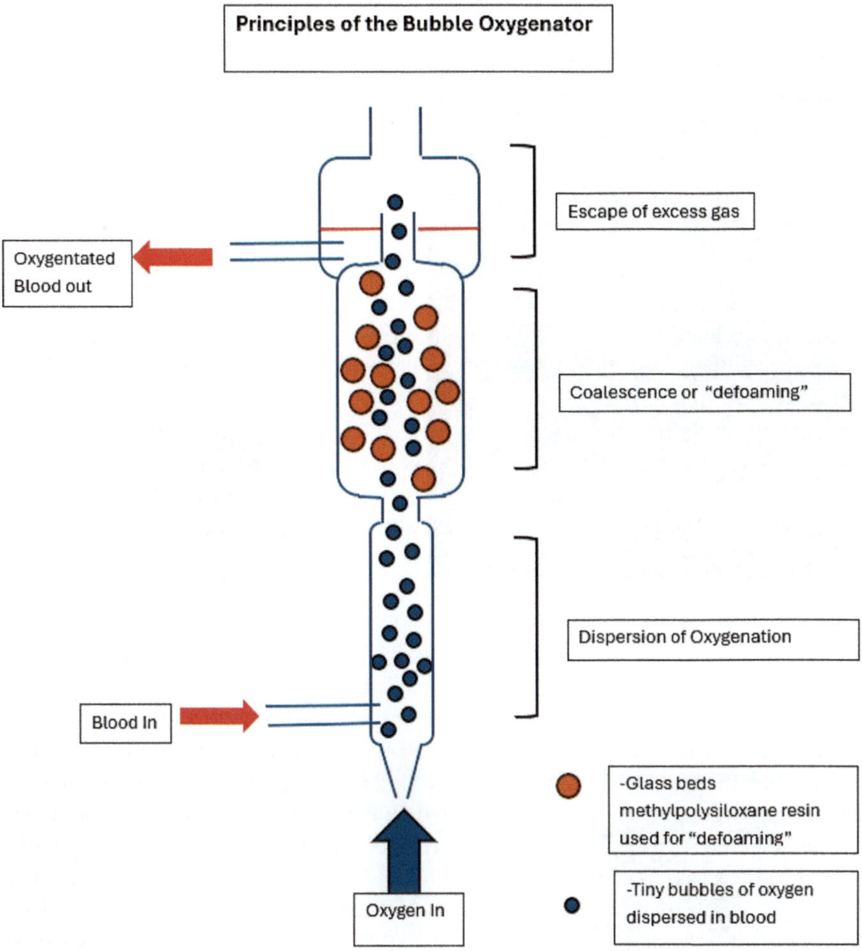

Fig. 40.8 A schematic of a bubble oxygenator for use in cardiac bypass surgery, prior to the advent of the membrane oxygenator

pump and lung/oxygenator do not work in a vacuum—instead, they work in a constantly changing dynamic state, influenced by a multitude of factors. In the same year (1969) that NASA successfully sent astronauts to the moon and back, an equally ambitious task force was assembled to develop artificial heart (and lung) technologies. Proceedings from the Artificial Heart Program Conference held in Washington, D.C. from June 9–13, 1969, by the US Department of Health, Education, and Welfare (a division of the National Institutes of Health), were published in a 1129-page book [20]. This book sits in my library, and reading its contents is daunting yet inspiring. Some examples of the book contents along with the titles, authors, and industries involved with oxygenator research are shown in Fig. 40.9a–c.

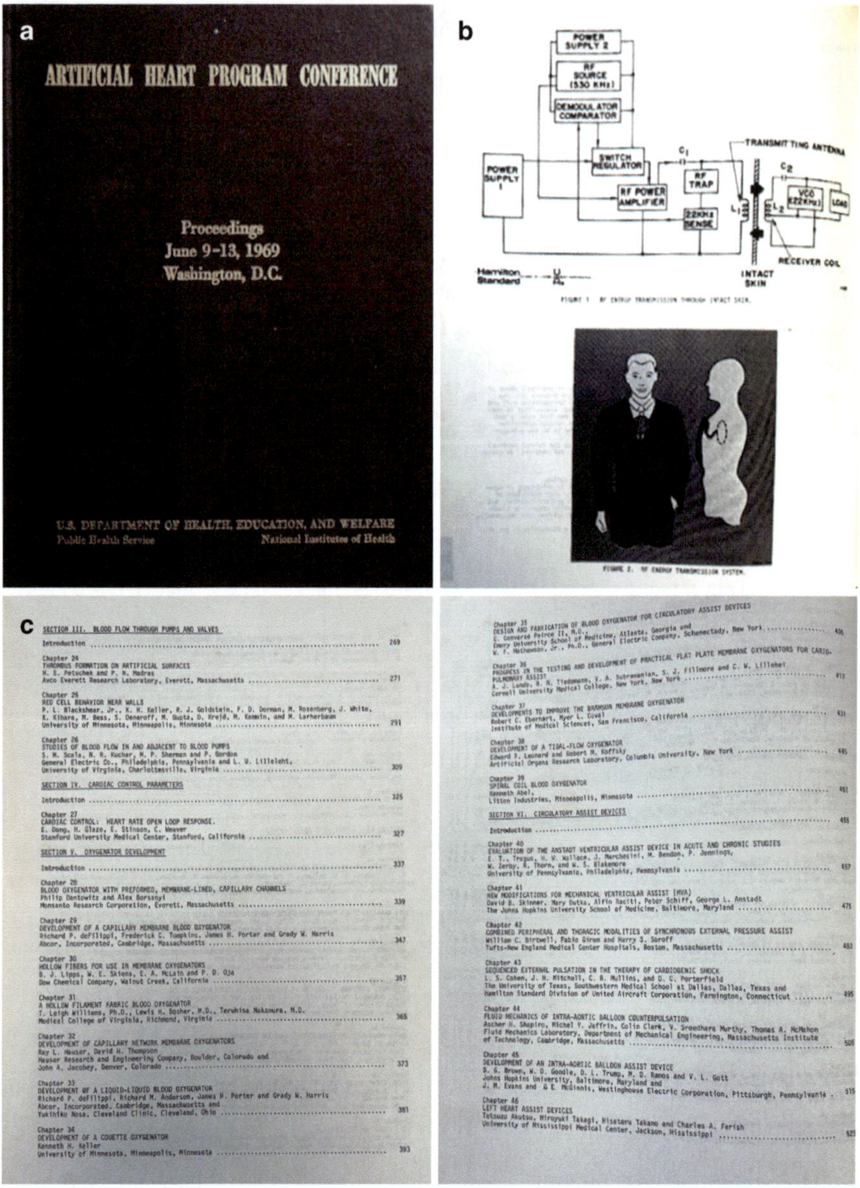

Fig. 40.9 (**a, b**) The Artificial Heart Program Conference—selected page showing transcutaneous energy transfer technology. (Official National Institute of Health (NIH) Publication). (**c**) Section V. Oxygenator Development—showing titles, authors, and companies involved. (Official NIH Publication)

The minds at work on this task force represented clinicians and bioengineers alike, working in collaboration with one another to develop a technology that could replicate the human heart and lungs. Reading through its contents, the forerunner of the modern-day oxygenator was conceived of, and further testing and clinical application were forthcoming—it was just a matter of time.

Modern-Day Oxygenator Technology

As the transition from screen to bubble and bubble to membrane oxygenation took place, additional design modifications were added to the safety, efficiency, and durability of the units we use today. In 1969, Robert L. Hewitt, a notable surgeon from Tulane University, was quoted as stating:

> *A suitable membrane oxygenator will make cardiopulmonary bypass more applicable to patients with failing hearts* [21].

Nearly 25 years later, William Haworth, presenting at a symposium for the 50th anniversary of Gibbon's historic event, commented on the following bioengineering advancement regarding the oxygenator and membrane oxygenator advances:

> *But probably the most far-reaching change was the introduction of microporous hollow fibers and the manufacture of oxygenators from these membranes. Hollow fibers had been used previously with blood flow inside the fiber and gas flow outside. This new design reversed this flow arrangement with the blood flowing over the outside of the fibers and the gas flowing down the fiber lumen. This is a significantly more efficient arrangement for gas transfer, so that smaller membrane area will provide adequate gas transfer capability...* [22].

Leonard, in the journal *Perfusion*, echoed Haworth's comments on the microporous hollow-fiber membrane oxygenator and added how numerous companies (in 2003) were competing to capture the market for this novel technology: Baxter (Deerfield, IL), Membrana (Wuppertal, Germany), COBE (Lakewood, CO), Shiley (Irvine, CA), Medtronic (Minneapolis, MN), among others [23].

In the past 20 years, membrane oxygenation has steadily grown, a product of open-heart surgery applications as well as the need for longer-term pulmonary support in patients requiring ECMO. The clinical expansion of oxygenator use became apparent during the two pandemics of the twenty-first century, the H1N1 flu (2009) and COVID-19 (2020–2023). A business report from Grand View Research in 2023 estimated the global membrane oxygenator market size valued at 125 million USD and expected it to grow at a rate of 2.2% from 2024 to 2030 [24].

How the Modern-Day Oxygenator Works

The modern-day oxygenator is part of a larger circuit and functions in concert with the pump and a heater-cooler unit, among several other connections and items. The actual unit in the operating room appears complicated but is simply an assembly of the component parts (Fig. 40.10).

Referring to the illustration below [25], gas flows inside the fibers, with blood flowing around them, with oxygen passing from gas to blood and carbon dioxide passing from blood to gas. Gas exchange occurs through the micropores via a protein film, which develops as blood comes into contact with the oxygenator at the initial phase of cardiopulmonary bypass. A gas blender allows control of pO_2 by altering FiO_2 (typically 0.4–0.8) and control of pCO_2 by altering gas flow (typically 2–4 L/min) through the oxygenator (Fig. 40.11).

It is clear from this reference (and others) that the bioengineering industry and clinicians desperate for a solution to respiratory failure have partnered over the decades to better understand and design a unit that allows for the short-term (hours-days) and intermediate-term (weeks–months) support of the lungs.

Future Endeavors

In 2020, a manuscript entitled "Toward a Long-Term Artificial Lung," by Arens and colleagues, described the challenges associated with the development of a long-term oxygenator [27]. In the article, they identified seven areas that require further investigation:

1. Research on new anticoagulation regimes and biomarker development
2. Analysis and design of biocompatible membrane and system surfaces
3. Analysis of inflammatory mechanisms and therapy for inflammatory processes induced by the artificial lung
4. Investigation of technical solution corridors for miniaturization, structural integration, and connection of the essential components of a lung support system
5. *In silico* and *in vitro* analysis of blood flow and gas exchange
6. *In vitro* verification and *in vivo* validation methods development for lung assist systems
7. Influence of long-term lung support on pathophysiology

Regarding item 3—inflammatory mechanisms—it has been known for decades that there is a considerable inflammatory response to blood passage through artificial surfaces, which, in the cardiopulmonary bypass circuit, includes the tubing of the circuit itself as well as the oxygenator. In 1993, for example, two notable publications highlighted this reaction [28, 29].

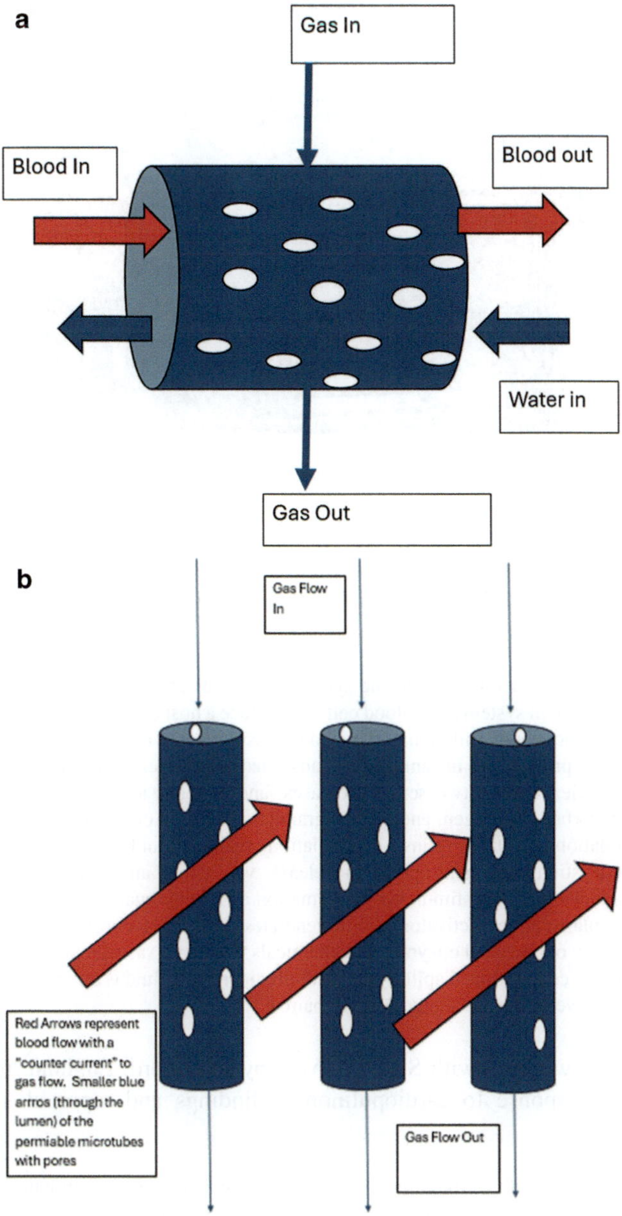

Fig. 40.10 (**a**) Modern-day oxygenator "anatomy" and "physiology" feature "hollow" permeable microtubules or fibers, with pores to facilitate gas transfer. In this depiction, blood flows through the microtubules of fibers with air moving over the fibers. This is further described by Vandewiele and Bouchez in Chap. 13 of a recently published book on cardiopulmonary bypass [26]. (**b**) Modern-day oxygenator "anatomy" and "physiology" feature "hollow" permeable microtubules or fibers with pores to facilitate gas transfer. In this depiction, blood flows over the microtubules or fibers with air moving through the hollow core. This is also further described by Vandewiele and Bouchez in Chap. 13 of a recently published book on cardiopulmonary bypass [26]

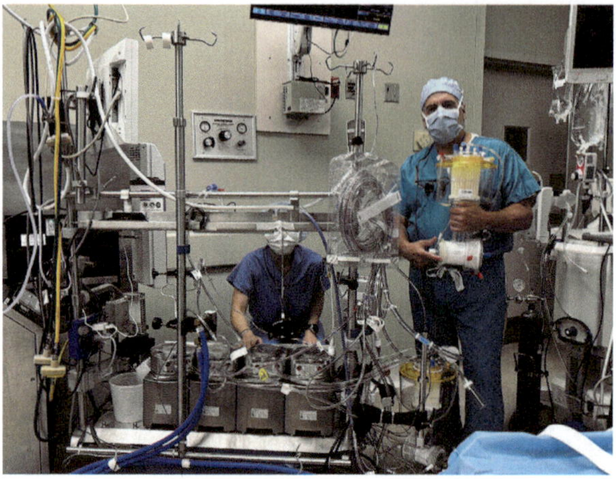

Fig. 40.11 A current heart–lung machine pictured with the author at the right of the image (holding oxygenator)

Research conducted by L. Henry Edmunds Jr. from the University of Pennsylvania, presented at the eighth International CardioStim Conference in 1992, highlighted the following in their abstract [28]:

> The interaction between blood and the synthetic surfaces of the heart-lung machine activates plasma protein systems and blood cells to produce a host of vasoactive substances that mediate the "whole body inflammatory response" associated with cardiopulmonary bypass (CPB). Plasma proteins are instantaneously adsorbed onto nonendothelial surfaces; plasma factor XII is cleaved into two serine proteases; and platelets are activated to aggregate, adhere to adsorbed fibrinogen, and release granule contents. Activation of factor XII initiates coagulation by the intrinsic coagulation pathway and activates complement. Complement stimulates neutrophils to release vasoactive and cytotoxic substances. Endothelial cells, perhaps stimulated by formation of minute quantities of thrombin, produce tissue plasminogen activator, which generates plasmin, a fibrolytic enzyme. Blood becomes a stew of powerful enzymes and chemicals that alters vascular smooth muscle and endothelial cell contraction. Capillary permeability increases, fluid is retained, and function of essentially every organ is temporarily impaired.

John Butler, working with Stephen Westaby in Oxford, England, reviewed the inflammatory response to cardiopulmonary findings and reported similar findings [29]:

> Cardiac operations with cardiopulmonary bypass cause a systemic inflammatory response, which can lead to organ injury and postoperative morbidity. Causative factors include surgical trauma, contact of blood with the extracorporeal circuit, and lung reperfusion injury on discontinuing bypass. Advances in immunological techniques have allowed measurement of both plasma and intracellular components of this multifaceted perioperative response. This includes activation of the complement, coagulation, fibrinolytic, and kallikrein cascades, activation of neutrophils with degranulation and protease enzyme release, oxygen radical production, and the synthesis of various cytokines from mononuclear cells (including tumor necrosis factor, interleukin-1, and interleukin-6).

Specific to the oxygenator, in addition to the inflammatory responses described above, there are mechanical aspects that derange the hematologic system that can have primary and secondary effects on organ systems. For example, deposition of blood elements (red cells, platelets, proteins) can not only result in oxygenator failure but also in secondary effects on remote end-organs (e.g., kidneys, lungs, liver, brain). While the photo below illustrates a profound deposition of blood elements on an oxygenator during ECMO, exposure of blood to the oxygenator during "routine" cardiopulmonary bypass is not completely benign. Variations in patient response follow a bell curve, with some patients reacting with few side effects and others with more malignant ones.

Summary

In summary, the development of the oxygenator is more than a century old in conception and design. Several of the early investigators took a personal and/or professional interest in its creation and persevered through the proverbial "trials and errors" of research until a breakthrough was accomplished on May 6, 1953. Since then, oxygenator technology has evolved to a level that is not only commercially available but also safe and reliable (for the most part). The challenge now, as it was when Dr. Kolff sat on my sofa in 2002, is a long-term (years) oxygenator—a true artificial lung. Until then, scientists and clinicians will continue to collaborate and innovate in an effort to replicate what took nature millions of years to do.

References

1. Samuels L. The AbioCor totally implantable replacement heart. Am Heart Hosp J. 2003;1(1):91–6.
2. Cooley DA. In Memoria: Willem Johan Kolff 1911-2009. Tex Heart Inst J. 2009;36(2):83–4.
3. Cooley DA, Liotta D, Hallman GL, Bloodwell RD, Leachman RD, Milam JD. Orthotopic cardiac prosthesis for two-staged cardiac replacement. Am J Cardiol. 1969;24(5):723–30.
4. DeVries WC, Anderson JL, Joyce LD, Anderson FL, Hammond EH, Jarvik RK, Kolff WJ. Clinical use of the total artificial heart. N Engl J Med. 1984;310(5):273–8.
5. Carrel A, Lindbergh CA. The culture of whole organs. Science. 1935;81(2112):621–3.
6. Gibbon JH Jr. Artificial maintenance of circulation during experimental occlusion of the pulmonary artery. Arch Surg. 1937;34(6):1105–31.
7. Dennis C, Spreng DS, Nelson GE, Karlson KE, Nelson RM, Thomas JV, Eder WP, Varco RL. Development of a pump-oxygenator to replace the heart and lungs; an apparatus applicable to human patients and application to one case. Ann Surg. 1951;134(4):709–21.
8. Bjork VO. Brain perfusions in dogs with artificially oxygenated blood. Acta Chir Scand. 1948;137(96):1–5.
9. DeWall RA. Origin of the helical reservoir bubble oxygenator heart-lung machine. Perfusion. 2003;18:163–9.
10. Gibbon JH Jr. Application of a mechanical heart and lung apparatus to cardiac surgery. Minn Med. 1954;37:171.
11. Hill JD. John H. Gibbon, JR. Part I. The development of the first successful heart-lung machine. Ann Thorac Surg. 1982;34(3):337–41.

12. Hill JD, Obrien TG, Murray JJ, Dontigny L, Bramson ML, Osborn JJ, Gerbode F. Prolonged extracorporeal oxygen for acute post-traumatic respiratory failure (shock-lung syndrome): use of the Bramson membrane lung. N Engl J Med. 1982;286(12):629–34.
13. Miller BJ. Recollections of my research in developing the heart-lung machine at Jefferson Medical College. Jefferson Biographies. 2005;12:1–24.
14. Bauer TM, Tchantchaleishvili V, Miller SB. Bernard J. Miller: MD, ScD. (Hon), FACS: life-long surgeon-scientist and critical contributor to the Gibbon heart-lung machine. ASAIO J. 2021;67:353–61.
15. Chen JR, Tchantchaleishvili V. Pioneer Interview with Stanton b Miller: Bernard J Miller's Role in the Development of the Gibbon Heart-Lung Machine Pioneer Editorials Artificial Organs Sep 25, 2024. https://icaot.org/pioneer-interview-with-stanton-b-miller-bernard-j-millers-role-in-the-development-of-the-gibbon-heart-lungmachine/
16. Parry T. Jefferson Alumni Magazine: Heart and Lung/Time Machine. Fall 2020, 11/09/20. https://magazine.jefferson.edu/issues/fall-2020/heart-and-lung.html#:~:text=In%20May%201953%2C%20John%20H,since%20saved%20millions%20of%20lives
17. Stoney WS. Evolution of cardiopulmonary bypass. Circulation. 2009;119(21):2844–53.
18. Gibbon JH Jr. The development of the heart-lung apparatus. Am J Surg. 1978;135:608–19.
19. Iwahashi H, Yuri K, Nose Y. Development of the oxygenator: past, present, and future. J Artif Organs. 2004;7(3):111–20.
20. Artificial Heart Program Conference. National Heart Institute. Artificial Heart Program. Frank W. Hastings, M.D. Chief. Lowell T. Harmison, Ph.D., Assistant Chief. Proceedings. Washington, DC, June 9–13, 1969. Edited by Ruth Johnsson Hegyeli, M.D.
21. Hewitt RL. Historic highlights of extracorporeal circulation. J Extracorp Circ Tech. 1969;1(3):5–10.
22. Hawthorth WS. The development of the modern oxygenator. Ann Thorac Surg. 2003;76:S2216–9.
23. Leonard RJ. The transition from the bubble oxygenator to the microporous membrane oxygenator. Perfusion. 2003;18:179–83.
24. https://www.grandviewresearch.com/industry-analysis/membrane-oxygenators-market
25. Bishop H, Middleton B. Cardiothoracic surgery I: cardiopulmonary bypass. Surgery. 2017;6(2):63–7.
26. Chapter 13 in Cardiopulmonary Bypass. January 2023. Korneel Vandewiele and Stefaan Bouchez. p. 189–222.
27. Arens J, Grottke O, Haverich A, et al. Toward a long-term artificial lung. ASAIO J. 2020;66:847–54.
28. Edmunds LH Jr. Blood-surface interactions during cardiopulmonary bypass. J Card Surg. 1993;8(3):401–10.
29. Butler J, Rocker GM, Westaby S. Inflammatory response to cardiopulmonary bypass. Ann Thorac Surg. 1993;55(2):552–9.

Part VII

Conclusions

Future of Lung Support

41

Michael Baram

Introduction

This chapter serves to discuss directions that researchers are exploring to improve oxygen delivery, including lofty ideas. Previous chapters discussed medical devices that we now take for granted, which surprisingly took decades to evolve. Even the endotracheal tube evolved over decades. Some devices took even longer, plus the work of many collaborating and even competing entities to make their products work. This will be no surprise to those familiar with science; there were significant failures along the path to success.

This chapter will review the science of creating lung replacements. Some of the technologies to be discussed will be refinements of current devices, such as smaller, miniaturized portable ECMO circuits to do the work of the lung, creating processes of lung repair by bioengineering, versus replacing lungs by artificial means. Lung transplant continues to be a growing field and is discussed elsewhere. Unfortunately, there continues to be a growing demand for lung transplants; hence, the need for innovative technology to support breathing when a transplant may not be feasible (Fig. 41.1).

More importantly, Fig. 41.2 highlights the need for creative solutions since lung transplant is not currently able to keep up with demand. The transplant rate is reflected in the death of patients while on the transplant list per 100 patient-years of waiting (Fig. 41.2). Every year, more people are dying waiting for transplants, indicating the ever-growing need for innovative technologies.

M. Baram (✉)
The Korman Respiratory Institute and the Division of Pulmonary, Allergy and Critical Care, The Department of Medicine at the Sidney Kimmel Medical College of Thomas Jefferson University, Philadelphia, PA, USA
e-mail: Michael.baram@jefferson.edu

G. C. Kane et al. (eds.), *Oxygen*, https://doi.org/10.1007/978-3-032-18934-9_41

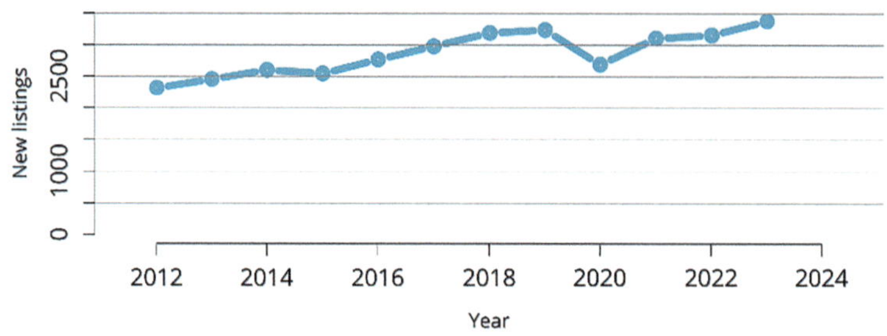

OPTN/SRTR 2023 Annual Data Report

Graph from Us Dept. Of Health source: https://srtr.transplant.hrsa.gov/annualdatareports

Fig. 41.1 New adult candidates on the lung transplant list

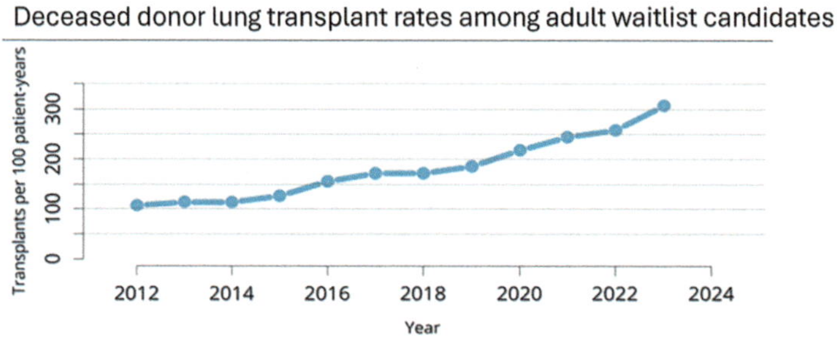

OPTN/SRTR 2023 Annual Data Report

Graph from Us Dept. Of Health source: https://srtr.transplant.hrsa.gov/annualdatareports

Fig. 41.2 Deceased donor lung transplant rates

The above figure highlights the need to advance technology. If transplant lungs are a scarce commodity and the survival of lungs as a transplanted organ is less than ideal, there is a need for artificial options. Perhaps "artificial" is not the correct term since some of the future options include organs from animals, hybrid biotechnology like organoids, or even modified human organs. Additionally, included in this chapter are wearable monitor devices to help alert patients to potential illnesses that may cause acute-on-chronic lung injury. The hope is that these devices will empower patients to get medical attention prior to further injury.

Prevention

Before diving into the topic of the future of lung support, respect should be given to the adage "prevention is better than cure." Preventing lung injury is a mechanism for reducing the need for lung repair. Watching the evolution of cystic fibrosis (CF) care has been exhilarating in this regard. Children born with this inheritable disease were on the path to requiring a lung transplant in their early adult years. Now, with medications such as cystic fibrosis transmembrane conductance regulator (CFTR) modulators, the mechanism of lung deterioration has been largely averted, and lung transplants are no longer necessary for the majority of patients. So, although it does not correct a genetic mutation, it has created a mechanism to overcome the pathological obstacle, thus allowing normal lung function. This class of medications has revolutionized the field. For some patients, they are not effective, and in other patients, their pre-CFTR modulator lung disease was too far advanced to avoid transplantation [1]. Because young adults will require fewer lung transplants, it has allowed patients with other forms of chronic lung disease to be allocated higher on the transplant list. What is even more exciting is that when the destructive process of CF is halted, even a compromised lung can heal, and improvements in gas exchange and function can be measured. Quality of life improves dramatically with CFTR modulator therapy.

Preventing lung destruction is one very tenable process to reduce the need for lung replacement. There are now preventative options to treat other genetic diseases. For example, there is a patented process to replace errors in the genetic sequencing of sickle cell disease [2]. Gene modification prevents the sequelae of hemoglobin sickling, which perpetuates acute chest syndrome and other forms of lung scarring. Clustered Regulatory Interspaced Short Palindromic Repeats (CRISPR) technology is being used to create gene sequence replacements [2]. It is expensive and time-intensive, but it is promising. The process has not yet been perfected but attempts to cure patients of sickle cell disease are underway. In that same theme, there are models designed to test gene therapy for cystic fibrosis to cure patients of their pulmonary disease prior to developing tissue damage [3]. A recent clinical trial to cure patients of their alpha-one antitrypsin deficiency was halted for futility, highlighting the challenges and difficulties in this field. It is hard to track success by days or weeks, but the United States health care system has been able to innovate and create worldwide changes. Only through vast networks and unifying infrastructure that includes the Department of Health and Human Services can these important advances be made. None of this progress will be low-cost or immediately revolutionary.

To expand the idea of "prevention is better than a cure," even Dr. Jenner recognized the benefits of vaccination back in the 1700s. The English physician recognized the benefits of mild viral exposures in preventing life-threatening disease. Using cowpox pustules, he showed that protection was offered against smallpox. To some, there remains doubt about the benefits of vaccines, but the facts are facts. A Lancet article in 2024 outlined the World Health Organization (WHO) efforts to improve worldwide vaccinations. Their modeling predicted that their 50-year efforts had saved 154 million lives [4]. If each averted death were converted to life-years saved, then 10.2 billion years of life were saved. True science confirms the benefits of vaccinations. Although many of these life-years saved are from averting childhood diseases such as measles, there are benefits to vaccinating older populations. Vaccinating patients with lung disease results in a 30% risk reduction in death from respiratory causes during flu season [5]. In addition to saving lives for patients suffering from lung disease, it is cost-effective to vaccinate patients since it reduces overall health care costs. It is imperative that health care departments continue to support, fund, and administer appropriate vaccinations to protect our vulnerable populations. Vaccination strategies continue to improve the range of ailments averted.

Although intuitive, it must be said that the greatest protector of lung function is smoking cessation. Smoking is known to reduce lung function, resulting in low oxygen levels and poor compliance in patients with chronic obstructive pulmonary disease (COPD). One of the greatest risk factors for idiopathic pulmonary fibrosis (IPF) is pack-years of smoking. Although vaping was considered a safer alternative, this has not been confirmed. Although there are some advantages to vaping over cigarettes, there remain significant risks that are being researched [6]. Creating more smoke-free environments will contribute to better lung function and reduce the need for future interventions. A reduction in smoking prevents many health risks, including risks of coronary artery disease, strokes, cancer, and COPD. To extrapolate further, lower smoking rates have resulted in 10% fewer forest fires, which have contributed to improved air quality [7]. There have been a range of national and community efforts to reduce smoking in public areas. Hopefully, worldwide, there will be a reduction in smoking-related lung injury and improved air quality.

Advances in Portable Lung Assistance

If lung injury is not prevented and/or is not preventable, and subsequently patients develop lung injury that requires oxygen support, new opportunities for support are on the horizon. To patients who need oxygen supplements, the world looks like a series of stepping stones. How do I keep the flow of oxygen going? How long does the tank last? Will there be oxygen at my final destination? This topic is covered extensively elsewhere (Chap. 18), but it is necessary to highlight this thought process. For hospital-based health care providers, oxygen is often unlimited. The oxygen wall supply flows like Niagara Falls. High flow oxygen delivery devices running at 60 liters per minute at 100% FIO_2 require 90,000 liters of room temperature oxygen per day. If an E-cylinder can provide 660 liters of oxygen, it would take over 125 E-cylinders of oxygen per day to provide high flow at this rate. Whereas standard portable ventilators can function on a standard E-cylinder for a time, the issue of limited oxygen supply applies to any form of future lung support. The device must either have a pure supply of oxygen, which is bulky, or have an oxygen concentrator, which is often heavy. Thinking back to how the lung must provide oxygen and create airflow to remove CO_2 produced by glycolysis and oxygen, the devices must be efficient. In the next few sections, such devices will be discussed, and all these devices are subject to the same liters per minute/canisters per hour limitations.

The technology and principles underlying ECMO have been reviewed in Chaps. 30 and 31. The most exciting part of ECMO is where it is going. The father of ECMO, Dr. Bartlett from the University of Michigan, received the Lifetime Achievement Award from the Society of Critical Care Medicine in 2019. What was most striking about his presentation was the refusal to accept the status quo (see https://www.youtube.com/watch?v=4ceeOdQRnaI). It was inspirational to see the evolution of ECMO presented as: ECMO development, ECMO version 1, ECMO version 2, and then to review his lab goals of creating more transportability. Despite a lifelong career of development, Dr. Bartlett recognized that there was still room to improve, inspiring us all.

With the first ECMO machines being the size of a room and now reduced to the size of a pushcart, the hope is to make ECMO portable and carriable. No different from cardiac assist devices, right ventricular assist device (RVAD), left ventricular assist device (LVAD), or artificial hearts, the hope is that ECMO devices will be backpack-sized and wearable. This level of portability should offer patients the freedom to live their lives. Not only does the circuitry have to be reduced, but the efficiency of gas exchange must also be considered. Portable ECMO machines still require an oxygen supply [8]. Oxygen and air blenders are used to sweep off CO_2 from the hemoglobin. Instead of wasting pure O_2, compressed air is used to sweep off CO_2, thus requiring less oxygen flow in the circuit and thereby reducing the need to transport as much oxygen. Most of the current devices are large. Prototypes are getting smaller and provide patients with more mobility options. Increasingly, these devices may be used as long-term supports and a bridge to transplant. If these devices can provide pathways for patients to ambulate and maintain their independence, they will contribute to improved quality of life and overall outcomes.

Portable ECMO still requires both internal and external components. The connection to the vascular supply requires cannulas, which will be both internal and external, and the pump and oxygenator will be external. This strategy offers easy component exchange, but it is still fraught with problems such as infection and size. There is an important fraction to consider when considering ECMO. In most scenarios, there remains some lung function. ECMO support is needed to oxygenate only a small portion of the cardiac output. This fraction of ECMO support will depend on each patient. Since chronic lung injury typically requires less support than acute respiratory distress syndrome (ARDS), there are options for smaller oxygen-providing devices. It follows, then, that the lower the oxygenation needs, the lower the power consumption of the pump (i.e., a smaller battery), and the smaller overall components. Pumpless systems are being developed that are better for ventilation than oxygenation, but they are improving. These smaller models are potentially partially implantable. These systems are considered paracorporeal since part of the devices are implanted, while other parts are still external. But importantly, these devices are being created to help the body oxygenate. The external nature of ECMO makes it an ideal option for a bridge to transplant or a bridge for lung recovery. The next section covers more durable products that may offer longer-term recovery and support options.

Intracorporal Options

Total Implantable Device

The creation of implantable lungs that can provide oxygen to the blood remains an elusive goal. Early models were created for mammals back in the 1970s, but they did not endure [9]. Whether these devices are bioengineered or fully artificial, there remain a few ideal traits. First, the flow through the device remains linked to cardiac function, so a pump or power supply is not required. Second, blood flow should be rapid enough to minimize clotting. Third, the device would require low resistance to allow for a low-pressure system. Fourth, an ideal device might be connected to the trachea to reduce the need for internal oxygen sources. Fifth, the device will need to offer a minimal risk of infection. There are a few proposed configurations, either in series or in parallel with native lungs. The hope is that over the next few years, paracorporeal systems that are prototypes now will soon come to human use. Thought leaders are hopeful that in a decade, a fully implantable artificial lung will be available [10].

In a similar fashion to cardiac disease, the device will be considered a bridge to transplant and destination therapy. Either way, it will need to have the characteristics mentioned above. The range of options from ECMO, to paracorporeal, to fully implantable will present with increasing levels of invasiveness.

Xenotransplantation

There has been a significant advancement in organ transplants from other species. Heart transplants from a genetically modified pig have already been completed [11]. The first two transplant recipients (2022 and 2023) lived for 2 months, and the other 6 weeks, respectively. Advances in genetic modification of animals have reduced the rejection rates of lungs transplanted from other species. For ethical reasons and infectious reasons, the focus of the donor has shifted from primates to pigs [12]. Removal of antigens from pig tissue has reduced the risk of antibody-associated rejection, which was the cause of acute transplant rejection. Using the same CRISPR technology used to modify human DNA, antigens have been removed from pig cells to create fewer antigens and thus allow xenotransplant to progress. Animal husbandry to create sterile environments is essential to reduce the risk of pig-to-human disease transmission, which remains a concern.

Part of the unique challenges of lung transplant are some of the physiological properties that make it so well-suited for oxygen absorption in a healthy state [13]. Lungs need to be able to tolerate large blood flows at very low pressure. This is specifically seen at the alveolar level, where active oxygen uptake occurs. In addition, unlike the kidney and heart, the lung is exposed to significant numbers of inhaled particles with each breath. These range from organic particulate matter to larger bacterial and viral particles and even aspirated food-sized particles. The lung needs to process this exposure as well. These challenges affect immunologic properties, coagulation properties, and flow properties of the blood. A heart transplant only needs to be connected to blood vessels, while lungs need to be connected to blood vessels and to airways that are constantly exposed to internal and external elements (or pollutants). These elements can be inhaled particles in the air, such as smoke or smog, gastric contents from micro or macro aspiration, or oropharyngeal contents, which may contain pathologic bacteria. Either way, these inhalations increase inflammation and present increased antigens and increase lung inflammation.

Lung Regeneration Therapies

The above section discussed the mechanical replacement of the lungs. These devices mirror hemodialysis machines that require mechanical pumps to create flows to allow blood to undergo diffusion. In dialysis, the diffusion is of solute waste; in lung devices, the diffusion is of oxygen onto hemoglobin. With the creation of efficient hardware, there has been success in creating devices, but they have limited durability and have few self-repair mechanisms. A novel approach is to bioengineer cells and tissues that repair or replace damaged organs.

Cellular Therapies

Stem cell therapy continues to carry the mystique of a fountain of youth cure. Although the field of heme malignancy has been revolutionized by this therapy, there remains a lot of controversy about other organ repairs. Textbooks could be created on just this field. But in brief, mesenchymal cells are already partially differentiated cells that innately provide a reservoir of repair cells for the host organ [14]. The pathways of cell migration and differentiation are increasingly studied, leading to a greater understanding of underlying repair mechanisms at the cellular and matrix level. How best to harvest and prime these cells to produce specific repairs is less understood. There remains a divide in the scientific community as to whether the harvesting and transplanting of these cells cause exocrine responses versus cellular transplant. Some experts believe that mesenchymal cells function as anti-inflammatory cells. There is a thought that the process of harvesting and infusing mesenchymal cells produces a reservoir of cytokines that reduce systemic inflammation [15]. There are others who believe that these cells mature and reimplant into organs and improve function. This latter concept is harder to prove. There continues to be low engraftment and low survival of these engrafted cells [14]. In an interesting paradox, engraftment into the lung should be the simplest to perform. One of the advantages of this therapy for lung disease is that nearly all venous blood passes through the lung, and the mesenchymal cells can collect there. Again, this is a field of investigation that offers promising scientific advancement.

Another pathway to use stem cells for lung regeneration is to collect pluripotent mesenchymal cells and encourage them to differentiate into the cells damaged by an ailment [16]. These cells can then function as repair cells to replace the injured cells. Targeting specific cellular lines reduces the need for total lung replacement.

The goal is to induce specific cellular lines to initiate repair or replacement of pathologic tissue. In vivo, Type II epithelial cells in the lung serve as a reproducing reservoir of repair cells. They can replicate and convert to Type I cells. In lungs severely damaged by acute respiratory distress syndrome (ARDS), there is a loss of Type I and II alveolar cells. The loss of these reserve cells means that there is a lack of Type I cells left to participate in oxygen exchange. Researchers are beginning to understand the mechanism by which cells migrate to damaged lungs [17]. The goal consists of harvesting these cells, inducing replication, then reinjecting patients with their own pluripotent cells to stimulate lung healing. One advantage of repopulating the lungs with cells is that all venous blood must first pass through the lungs. This allows the lungs to function as a filter/collection destination for all injections. Even if pluripotent cells are not used, it is possible to induce cell types and then inject the deficient cells. Targeting the specific cellular deficiency in a disease may be a focused method of repairing in situ cellular damage. For example, in pulmonary arterial hypertension (PAH), endothelial cells would be the replacement cell line of choice [16]. However, in pulmonary fibrosis, alveolar Type II cells would be the cells of interest [16]. Some of these cells are already being used in clinical trials to help reverse lung scarring.

Matrix Therapies

The lungs are extremely delicate organs. They are exposed to toxins with each breath and bathed in blood, which may carry oxidants, toxins, or carcinogens. Lung research has progressed from the dissection of tissues to the creation of organoids. These organoids are complex systems derived from stem cells [18]. This microsystem functions as a small unit that can be used to simulate in vivo cell reactions. These systems are more physiological when compared to in vitro models when used in experiments. This technology is leading researchers to create larger arrays of 3D printed structures. These structures can then be the skeleton, which can be coated with stem cells. The merger of 3D printing and stem cells may provide the structure for lung replacement in the future. As a less synthetically engineered lung, bioartificial lungs have growing potential that offers more lung replacement opportunities [19]. A human lung is removed from organ donors, and the cellular components are decellularized to create an extracellular matrix. This organic structure can then be repopulated with the recipient's stem cells to repropagate the cellular components [19]. This technology is not yet available, but advances by both industry and university programs are working to make these potential organ replacements a reality. This research is not without controversy; efforts have been undertaken to be sure that the ethical ramifications of this type of research are considered [20].

Continued Challenges

Relevant to all of these potential modalities, challenges regarding lung replacement therapies revolve around clotting, inflammation, and infection. These three intertwined pathways, which are essential for human life, are often an obstacle to artificial lungs. As previously mentioned, the large amount of blood flow through artificial tubes causes cytokine activation and clotting [21]. Any foreign body can potentially introduce infection, compounded by the immunosuppressive agents used. The fine balance of clotting vs. bleeding and immunosuppressive needs vs. the risk of infection are some of the challenges that all these ideas must overcome.

Monitors to Detect Airflow

This section fits better under prevention, but it was saved until the end for a holistic reason that connects many of the above themes. Monitoring devices provide the patient with control of their disease. They serve as a warning that can integrate both medical and nonmedical data. Self-advocacy provides another level of mind–body healing. All clinicians are familiar with vital sign monitoring and transmission to central services for monitoring. Now there are new generations of sensors that are specific to disease entities. Tools such as air quality monitors, often maintained by the Environmental Protection Agency (EPA), can help alert asthmatics to days when they may be more symptomatic, encouraging compliance with medication or initiating their steroidal inhalers early. Technology companies have created sensors to monitor lung sounds to help identify COPD exacerbations and help patients begin therapy for acute exacerbation of COPD (AECOPD). Imagine sending a patient home from the hospital with a digital sensor that can quantify and trend wheezing to be sure the patient is improving.

Home monitoring can include a gamut of devices. In a similar fashion, OSA devices have downloadable/transmittable data, and the same is true with a variety of lung-associated health care devices. Using patient-related data is the key to patient-specific care. For example, if there is measured data showing an increase in smog/pollution, a patient-focused algorithm can take effect. For example, if the smog is on the West Coast, patients with asthma could be warned to increase their inhaled steroids. Lung function could then be assessed with home spirometers. If lung function worsens and the medication automonitors indicate an increase in beta-agonist use, the patient can be warned to come in for a visit, or medications such as inhaled steroids need to be further escalated. But just as importantly, as environmental markers improve and the patient shows stability in their lung function, the medications can be reduced. Now imagine what if the recommendations are tailored not to smog but to specific triggers. If pollen counts are high, one prescriptive plan for seasonal allergy sufferers may increase anti-inflammatories. The trigger for another patient might be cold air induced, requiring a different plan. These plans can be tailored to each patient's unique needs. All of this technology is available now. The science behind asthma action plans has been proven and is available on public sites [22]. If this information can empower patients to tailor their health care needs, it provides an opportunity for patients to minimize medication usage when they are well and to ramp up medication usage based on their specific needs. Empowering patients to control/manage their own care can reduce emergency department visits and hospitalizations.

Imagine taking this one step further. Clinical experience has taught us that patients with chronic lung disease often have stepwise deteriorations of their lung function. Exacerbations often trigger declines, or more often, a failure to fully return to the previous status. There are models that show that lung inflammation from viral infections, bacterial infections, ARDS, or other stressors causes the death of alveolar cells, which results in the exposure of basement membranes that are then exposed to further inflammation, resulting in further lung destruction [23]. If home detection could trigger earlier care to reduce the severity of inflammation, such as in COPD or infections, perhaps long-term lung destruction could be slowed. These direct relationships have yet to be shown, but this is a growing field. With pattern recognition, patterns of change can be identified by computer software. Improvements in datasets, sensing technology, and computer algorithms could surely improve patient-focused treatment.

Conclusion

This chapter is not as fantastical as the futuristic ideas presented by Jules Verne because it draws on publications and ideas shared at pulmonary conferences and iterative gains in technology over the last half-century. Progress will not occur in silos, and the importance of shared ideas is pivotal. It is becoming clearer that sharing ideas must be more widespread than just among and within health care institutions. The platforms of change include technology, informatics, industry, patient advocacy, and any venue that can spark or trigger a revolution. Hopefully, collaborations between universities, health care entities, industry, and governments will create environments that inspire and nurture innovation and growth of lung support and replacement technologies.

Selected References

1. Huang W, Smith AT, Korotun M, Iacono A, Wang J. Lung transplantation in a new era in the field of cystic fibrosis. Life. 2023;13(7):1600. https://doi.org/10.3390/life13071600.
2. Ma L, Yang S, Peng Q, Zhang J, Zhang J. CRISPR/Cas9-based gene-editing technology for sickle cell disease. Gene. 2023;874:147480. https://doi.org/10.1016/j.gene.2023.147480. Epub 2023 May 12. PMID: 37182559.
3. Sun Y, et al. In vivo editing of lung stem cells for durable gene correction in mice. Science. 2024;384:1196–202. https://doi.org/10.1126/science.adk9428.

4. Shattock AJ, et al. Contribution of vaccination to improved survival and health: modelling 50 years of the Expanded Programme on Immunization. Lancet. 403(10441):2307–16.
5. Nichol KL, Baken L, Nelson A. Relation between influenza vaccination and outpatient visits, hospitalization, and mortality in elderly persons with chronic lung disease. Ann Intern Med. 1999;130(5):397–403. https://doi.org/10.7326/0003-4819-130-5-199903020-00003. PMID: 10068413.
6. National Academies of Sciences, Engineering, and Medicine. Public health consequences of e-cigarettes. Washington, DC: The National Academies Press; 2018. https://doi.org/10.17226/24952. https://nap.nationalacademies.org/catalog/24952/public-health-consequences-of-e-cigarettes
7. Butry DT, Prestemon JP, Thomas DS. Investigation of the decline in reported smoking-caused wildfires in the USA from 2000 to 2011. Int J Wildland Fire. 2014;23(6):790–8. 9 p
8. Griffith BP, Wu ZJ, Zhang J. Pasta for all: Abiomed Breethe extracorporeal membrane oxygenation system. JTCVS Open. 2021;8:108–13. https://doi.org/10.1016/j.xjon.2021.10.004. PMID: 36004106; PMCID: PMC9390355.
9. Shah-Mirany J, Head LR, Ghetzler R, Formolo AJ, Palmer AS, Bodell BR. An implantable artificial lung. Ann Thorac Surg. 1972;13(4):381–7., ISSN 0003-4975,. https://doi.org/10.1016/S0003-4975(10)64870-9.
10. Naito N, Cook K, Toyoda Y, et al. Artificial lungs for lung failure: JACC technology corner. JACC. 2018;72(14):1640–52. https://doi.org/10.1016/j.jacc.2018.07.049.
11. Chaban R, et al. Pig heart and lung xenotransplantation: present status. J Heart Lung Transplant. 41(8):1014–22.
12. Chaban R, Cooper DKC, Pierson RN 3rd. Pig heart and lung xenotransplantation: present status. J Heart Lung Transplant. 2022;41(8):1014–22. https://doi.org/10.1016/j.healun.2022.04.010. Epub 2022 May 13. PMID: 35659792; PMCID: PMC10124776.
13. Chaban R, Ileka IS, Pierson RN III. Lung xenotransplantation: status 2023. Eur J Transplant. 2023;1(3):217–25. https://doi.org/10.57603/EJT-311.
14. Nasri A, Foisset F, Ahmed E, Lahmar Z, Vachier I, Jorgensen C, Assou S, Bourdin A, De Vos J. Roles of mesenchymal cells in the lung: from lung development to chronic obstructive pulmonary disease. Cells. 2021;10(12):3467. https://doi.org/10.3390/cells10123467. PMID: 34943975; PMCID: PMC8700565.
15. Shi Y, Wang Y, Li Q, et al. Immunoregulatory mechanisms of mesenchymal stem and stromal cells in inflammatory diseases. Nat Rev Nephrol. 2018;14:493–507. https://doi.org/10.1038/s41581-018-0023-5.
16. Goecke T, Ius F, Ruhparwar A, Martin U. Unlocking the future: pluripotent stem cell-based lung repair. Cells. 2024;13(7):635. https://doi.org/10.3390/cells13070635. PMID: 38607074; PMCID: PMC11012168.
17. Chioccioli M, et al. Stem cell migration drives lung repair in living mice. Dev Cell. 59(7):830–840.e4.
18. Kühl L, Graichen P, von Daacke N, Mende A, Wygrecka M, Potaczek DP, Miethe S, Garn H. Human lung organoids-a novel experimental and precision medicine approach. Cells. 2023;12(16):2067. https://doi.org/10.3390/cells12162067. PMID: 37626876; PMCID: PMC10453737.
19. Ohata K, Ott HC. Human-scale lung regeneration based on decellularized matrix scaffolds as a biologic platform. Surg Today. 2020;50(7):633–43. https://doi.org/10.1007/s00595-020-02000-y. Epub 2020 May 4. PMID: 32363425; PMCID: PMC7305261.
20. de Jongh D, Massey EK, Cronin AJ, Schermer MHN, Bunnik EM, VANGUARD Consortium. Early-phase clinical trials of bio-artificial organ technology: a systematic review of ethical issues. Transpl Int. 2022;35:10751. https://doi.org/10.3389/ti.2022.10751. PMID: 36388425; PMCID: PMC9659568.
21. Kirupaharan P, Blazoski C, Hilton R, Feduska E, Leong R, Baram M. Systemic inflammatory response syndrome after extracorporeal membrane oxygenation Decannulation in COVID-19 patients. Cureus. 2023;15(3):e36436. https://doi.org/10.7759/cureus.36436. PMID: 37090372; PMCID: PMC10115560.

22. https://www.cdc.gov/asthma/living-with/index.html#:~:text=Create%20your%20own%20Asthma%20Action,fillable%20PDF%20for%20your%20use
23. Molyneaux PL, Maher TM. The role of infection in the pathogenesis of idiopathic pulmonary fibrosis. Eur Respir Rev. 2013;22(129):376–81. https://doi.org/10.1183/09059180.00000713. PMID: 23997064; PMCID: PMC9487348.

42 The Search for Oxygen in the Universe

Gregory C. Kane

"We are awfully lucky to be here—and by 'we', I mean every living thing. To attain any kind of life in this universe of ours appears to be quite an achievement. As humans we are doubly lucky, of course: We enjoy not only the privilege of existence but also the singular ability to appreciate it and even, in a multitude of ways, to make it better. It is a talent we have only barely begun to grasp.

We have arrived at this position of eminence in a stunningly short time. Behaviorally modern human beings—that is, people who can speak and make art and organize complex activities—have existed for only about 0.0001 percent of Earth's history. But surviving for even that little while has required a nearly endless string of good fortune.

We really are at the beginning of it all. The trick, of course, is to make sure we never find the end. And that, almost certainly, will require a good deal more than lucky breaks."

Bill Bryson (author and University President)

"Mars is there waiting to be reached."

Buzz Aldrin (Gemini 12 and Apollo 11Astronaut)

"Look again at that dot. That's here. That's home. That's us. On it everyone you love, everyone you know, everyone you ever heard of, every human being whoever was, lived out their lives. The aggregate of our joy and suffering, thousands of confident religions, ideologies, and economic doctrines, every hunter and forager, every hero and coward, every creator and destroyer of civilization, every king and peasant, every young couple in love, every mother and father, hopeful child, inventor and explorer, every teacher of morals, every corrupt politician, every

G. C. Kane (✉)
The Korman Respiratory Institute and the Division of Pulmonary, Allergy and Critical Care, The Department of Medicine at the Sidney Kimmel Medical College of Thomas Jefferson University, Philadelphia, PA, USA
e-mail: gregory.kane@jefferson.edu

G. C. Kane et al. (eds.), *Oxygen*, https://doi.org/10.1007/978-3-032-18934-9_42

'superstar,' every 'supreme leader,' every saint and sinner in the history of our species lived there-on a mote of dust suspended in a sunbeam."

Carl Sagan, Astronomer and author of The Pale Blue Dot

"It's a special time for us here on Earth. It's the first time in human history that we actually have the technological capability to find other Earths, to identify them as Earths, and to look for signs of life on the first handful or the first dozen or hundreds of exoplanets, and that's a special time in history. So, I'm trying to do what I can to make sure that happens now."

Dr. Sara Seager, Astronomer and Planetary Scientist at MIT

If there is a father of modern exploration of the universe, it would be Nicolaus Copernicus. Shockingly, Copernicus was born in February 1493 and received his education from the great universities of his age, including the University of Krakow, the University of Bologna, the University of Ferrara, and the University of Padua. Considered a Renaissance polyglot and polymath, Copernicus published his book "on the revolutions of the celestial spheres" just before his death at age 70, triggering the Copernican Revolution and making him a pioneer of the scientific revolution [4]. Just 500 years later, Voyager 1 and Voyager 2 were launched by NASA in 1977, originally designed to conduct close-up studies of Jupiter, Saturn, and Saturn's rings, as well as the larger moons of the two planets. While the spacecrafts were designed to last 5 years, the mission has continued (through to this writing in the Winter of 2026), and both are now considered interstellar probes, which are expected to leave our solar system. Three other probes are following, including Pioneer 10, Pioneer 11, and New Horizons. As of this writing, only Voyager 1 and Voyager 2 have reached interstellar space [5].

Through timing that can only be described as the best of luck, Voyager 1 and Voyager 2 have exploited a four planet layout of Jupiter, Saturn, Uranus, and Neptune which occurs once every 175 years, allowing Voyager 1 and Voyager 2 to perform a flyby of each planet and pick up a gravity assist, whereby each of the first three planets bent the spacecraft flight path and increased its velocity en route to the next catapult. Remarkably, Voyager 1 reached Jupiter on March 5, 1979, and Saturn on November 12, 1980. Voyager's path brought it as close as it would get to Neptune on August 25, 1989. Voyager 1 and Voyager 2 are now leaving the solar system and moving about 300 million miles each year [6].

Why space exploration? The Intergovernmental Panel on Climate Change (IPCC) provides regular reports and scientific assessments of climate change for policymakers and identifies potential future risks and strategies [6]. An essential argument has emerged, acknowledging that humans now enjoy the highest living standards in their history and the greatest life expectancy ever, but that the world around us is in crisis, creating for the first time in our history the very question as to whether or not humanity can continue to be successful on this planet [7, 8]. This certainly has contributed to the cause of space exploration, with the goal of finding other planets suitable for human life.

In this chapter, we will explore progress toward identifying life elsewhere, both in this solar system and beyond, and describe the key resources that will be required, such as oxygen, atmospheric gases, and water, that will be essential to support complex life forms. We have described how the great oxygenation event enabled the rise of complex multicellular organisms and, eventually, the existence of humans on this planet (see Chap. 1: The Emergence of Oxygen on Earth). It is likely, then, that Earth will need to serve as a template based on its remarkable combination of an atmosphere with abundant oxygen, a surface with abundant water, and a variety of fortunate circumstances that have allowed for the evolution of complex life to proceed over billions of years. We have described why oxygen is so important to the development of complex life forms, but this does not exclude the possibility that some other basis for life and energy might be identified. For humans, however, to travel to and inhabit an alternate planet, that planet will have to contain oxygen or a mechanism for generating oxygen from available sources.

Remember that our oxygen machines used to support people with chronic pulmonary disease simply scrub the oxygen from the atmosphere rather than manufacture it de novo. So, it goes without saying that to breathe and live elsewhere in the universe, we will need to have oxygen present or manufacture oxygen in that location.

Astronomers will have to prioritize identifying those planets with an oxygen-rich atmosphere, and this will be a daunting task. Among the first 5000 confirmed exoplanets, none promise the presence of oxygen for life as we know it. Oxygen, then, is our beacon and our hope.

There are four (4) terrestrial planets in our solar system, that is, planets with solid ground, as opposed to being composed of a gaseous core. Humans will most likely need a terrestrial planet for space colonization.

Mars requires a very detailed discussion, given the current interest in landing humans on Mars and the discussion of creating a colony there for human survival. Thus, in the discussion of our solar system's planets, we will start closest to our Sun. First is Mercury, too hot for life as we know it, primarily because of its proximity to the Sun. Moreover, its atmosphere is considered tenuous, of low pressure, and very thin by comparison to the Earth [9]. It is unlikely that we will be looking to Mercury for habitability.

Similarly, Venus is unsuitable for life due to an extreme temperature (464 degrees Celsius) and a lack of water [10, 11]. It does, however, have an atmosphere of carbon dioxide that theoretically could support plant life. Experts point out that an extrasolar planet (outside of our solar system) with Venus-like conditions could be a candidate for sustaining life if such a planet were at a suitable distance from its star and had water [11].

Beyond Earth and Mars, the gas giants (planets that are primarily made of gases) have a composition that is mostly hydrogen, helium, and other gases. The most important of these is Jupiter. Through NASA-sponsored space exploration, the Juno spacecraft arrived at Jupiter on July 4, 2016, after a 5-year journey covering more than 1700 million miles. The craft entered into a 53-day polar orbit and continues to send information back to Earth (Fig. 42.1). One recent major discovery is that one

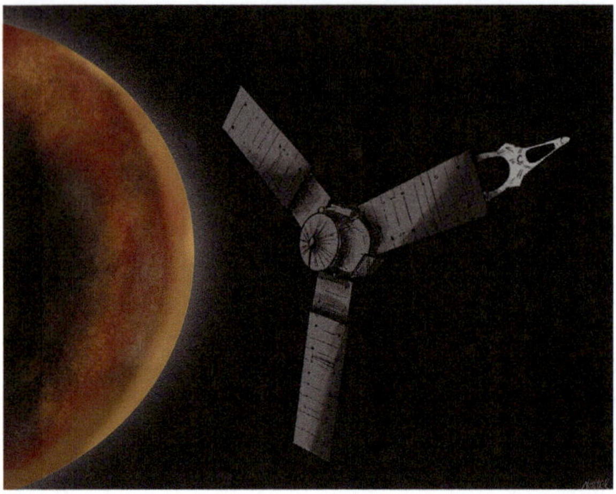

Fig. 42.1 Space exploration continues to identify important findings. The Juno spacecraft arrived at Jupiter on July 4, 2016, after a 5-year journey covering more than 1700 million miles. Still on a 53-day polar orbit, Juno continues to send information back to Earth, including the detection of an icy crust on Europa (one of Jupiter's moons that emits oxygen into its atmosphere). Pictured here is a rendering of the craft, Juno, with Jupiter in the background. (Courtesy of Michael Natter, MD)

of the moons of Jupiter, Europa, has an icy crust that releases a substantial amount of oxygen that theoretically could sustain a large population of humans [12, 13]. The Hubble Telescope has also detected oxygen on Saturn [14, 15].

Of all of our neighboring planets and moons, Mars has created much speculation about the prospect that it could support life. Mars does not currently have evidence of life [16]. Mars does have an atmosphere, and it appears to be composed principally of carbon dioxide, but also of nitrogen, argon, and traces of other gases. The atmosphere is much less dense than that of Earth, though it includes a lot of dust from the surface of the planet. Indeed, this dust has contributed to the hazy, rusty, red appearance of Mars from Earth. While this description of Mars' prospects is not encouraging, it is of interest to note that Mars may have had a thicker atmosphere in the past and that this thicker atmosphere may have allowed for the presence of liquid water on the surface. There remains much speculation about life on Mars. At this time, it is mostly about setting up a colony on Mars, which we will discuss [17–19].

If we were to colonize Mars, we would need to find a way to transport oxygen there or produce oxygen on the surface of that planet. If there were water, this could be accomplished in part by finding a way to cultivate plants suitable to grow on Mars' surface in the absence of water. Water, too, would have to be transported to the surface of the planet, in addition to an energy source, for work or activity to commence. I am reminded that, given the prospects of robotics, we may identify a way that robots can do much of this work.

The movie "The Martian," starring Matt Damon and based on the book by Andy Weir, surprisingly got a lot right [20, 21]. To grow plants on Mars, it would require enclosed greenhouses made of transparent polymers, which could control pressure, temperature, and humidity. Water could be harvested from melting ice underneath the surface of the Martian crust. Hydroponic and aeroponic methods could be employed, as they are already being employed on the International Space Station. If soil from Mars were to be used, there would have to be a way to clean away toxic chemicals, which are known to exist there, so that plants could survive and be consumed as food. Scientists would have to consider and trial a variety of plant species in order to identify successful candidates. This would augment the supply of oxygen for these settlements [22, 23]. Analyses still point out that certain aspects of a "mission to Mars" are left unsolved, such as shielding the astronaut-voyagers from solar radiation. Radiation exposure will need to be addressed on the surface of Mars, but it could be accomplished by covering dwellings with dirt.

Much of the technology to support such a colony is already in place and demonstrated by the success of the International Space Station [24–26]. We will discuss the three capabilities that are essential. These are outlined in Table 42.1:

The International Space Station (ISS) obtains its oxygen through a combination of methods: electrolysis of water, resupply from Earth, and in-flight generation using solid fuel generators, according to HowStuffWorks [17]. The International Space Station (ISS) can grow plants through a number of systems and must overcome a variety of challenges, such as limited gravity in an extraterrestrial environment and the need for LED lights [18, 19]. A final helpful system in space or a colonized Mars would be water reclamation, which would be essential, but this too can be achieved [20].

Based upon this discussion, this author believes that travel to Mars will indeed be possible in the near future. Indeed, since 2010, NASA has articulated and written about such a mission, with work on the International Space Station (ISS) serving as an important intermediate step. It is exciting to realize that already a fleet of robotic spacecraft and Rovers have either landed on or around Mars, increasing our understanding of the challenges in sending humans to the surface of Mars. This amazing feat, with some luck and a lot of planning, may well happen in the next 2 decades [26].

Based upon the detection of oxygen on Europa, one of Jupiter's moons, and on Saturn as well, it was reasonable to expect that we would identify a planet with an oxygen-rich atmosphere outside our solar system through Voyager or other exploration vehicles [13]. This, in fact, does exist, as scientists have most recently discovered the first exoplanet with oxygen—HD 209458b, also referred to as Osiris [27]. With the pace of progress and a flotilla of at least 80 probes and/or spacecraft, we have made startling discoveries of planetary oxygen in our very own solar system and in the atmosphere of an exoplanet located more than 150 light-years away, with

Table 42.1 What will be needed for cultivating life on Mars?

Necessary elements for life on Mars	Current NASA capability?
Water: This would need to be extracted or transported to the surface	Yes
Sunlight: Though Mars gets less sunlight than the Earth it is probably enough for photosynthesis	Yes
CO2: There is plenty on the surface of Mars though it may need to be pressurized in greenhouses in order to aid in photosynthesis and absorption	Yes

oxygen and carbon in the atmosphere [2]. With the foundation of these discoveries and recognition of the sheer size of the universe, several scientists have predicted that it is just a matter of time until we discover a planet that has just the right amount of luck—luck to support complex life forms. Whether we find life there remains the question [3]. Based on oxygen's remarkable reactivity, we should expect that oxygen will play a key role in this possibility.

Where does this leave us? Since Voyager 1 (Fig. 42.2) is in many ways responsible for the discoveries that led us to detect oxygen beyond our Earth, it is fitting and proper to close this chapter with a focus on an iconic image taken by Voyager 1 of Earth from 3.7 billion miles away. The image captures Earth as a tiny blue fleck in a band of light (Fig. 42.3).

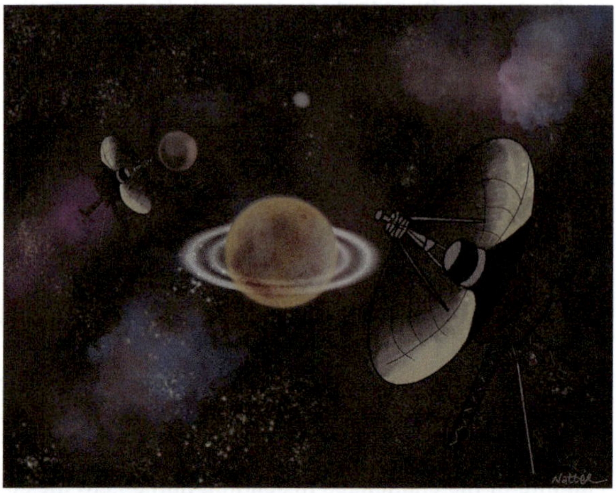

Fig. 42.2 Launched in 1977, and perhaps two of space exploration's most remarkable achievements, Voyager 1 and Voyager 2 continue to send data and pictures back to the Earth for half a century at the time of this publication. (Rendering courtesy of Michael Natter, MD)

Fig. 42.3 This iconic image of Earth from outer space was taken by NASA's Voyager 1 spacecraft. Suspended in the vertical beam of light is a tiny pale blue dot—our Earth. Image credit is to NASA consistent with NASA media usage guidelines

Carl Sagan published a book by this name in 1994. In Sagan's book [28], he captures the significance of our pale blue dot:

> Look again at that dot. That's here. That's home. That's us. On it everyone you love, everyone you know, everyone you ever heard of, every human being who ever was, lived out their lives. The aggregate of our joy and suffering, thousands of confident religions, ideologies, and economic doctrines, every hunter and forager, every hero and coward, every creator and destroyer of civilization, every king and peasant, every young couple in love, every mother and father, hopeful child, inventor and explorer, every teacher of morals, every corrupt politician, every "superstar," every "supreme leader," every saint and sinner in the history of our species lived there-on a mote of dust suspended in a sunbeam.
>
> The Earth is a very small stage in a vast cosmic arena. Think of the endless cruelties visited by the inhabitants of one corner of this pixel on the scarcely distinguishable inhabitants of some other corner, how frequent their misunderstandings, how eager they are to kill one another, how fervent their hatreds. Think of the rivers of blood spilled by all those generals and emperors so that, in glory and triumph, they could become the momentary masters of a fraction of a dot.
>
> Our posturings, our imagined self-importance, the delusion that we have some privileged position in the Universe, are challenged by this point of pale light. Our planet is a lonely speck in the great enveloping cosmic dark. In our obscurity, in all this vastness, there is no hint that help will come from elsewhere to save us from ourselves.
>
> The Earth is the only world known so far to harbor life. There is nowhere else, at least in the near future, to which our species could migrate. Visit, yes. Settle, not yet. Like it or not, for the moment the Earth is where we make our stand.
>
> It has been said that astronomy is a humbling and character-building experience. There is perhaps no better demonstration of the folly of human conceits than this distant image of our tiny world. To me, it underscores our responsibility to deal more kindly with one another, and to preserve and cherish the pale blue dot, the only home we've ever known.

Conclusion

Is there oxygen out there that could support human life? Yes. Could we create oxygen from water by electrolysis? Yes. Will we ultimately identify a planet with oxygen in the atmosphere capable of supporting complex life out in the cosmos somewhere? I believe we will.

But for now, the Earth is all we have. We'd better start thinking about how we can preserve this pale blue dot. Sure, a colony on Mars is not too far off, but how many people can we get there? For now, the Earth is where we will have to make our stand. And while we do that, we might as well treat each other with a little kindness and, in the process, avoid the self-destruction of our arrogance.

References

1. Lenton TM. The role of land plants, phosphorus weathering and fire in the rise and regulation of atmospheric oxygen. Glob Chang Biol. 2001;7(6):613–29.
2. https://science.nasa.gov/missions/hubble/oxygen-and-carbon-found-in-atmosphere-of-an-extrasolar-planet/#:~:text=The%20planet%20HD%20209458b%20is,atmosphere%20containing%20oxygen%20and%20carbon.
3. Seager S. The smallest lights in the universe: a memoir. New York NY: Crown; 2020.
4. Hartner W. Copernicus, the man, the work, and its history. Proc Am Philos Soc. 1973;117(6):413–22. http://www.jstor.org/stable/986460
5. Science.nasa.gov/mission/voyager/factsheet/#:~:text=Had%20the%20Voyager%20mission%20ended,planets%20in%20our%20solar%20system.
6. White PJ, Ardoin NM, Eames C, Monroe MC. Agency in the Anthropocene: supporting document to the PISA 2025 science framework. OECD Educ Work Pap. 2023;297:0_1–4.
7. Pinker S. Enlightenment now: the case for reason, science, humanism, and progress. New York NY: Viking; 2018.
8. IPCC. Climate change 2021: the physical science basis. In: Contribution of working group I to the sixth assessment report of the intergovernmental panel on climate change. Cambridge, UK/New York, NY: Cambridge University Press; 2021. https://doi.org/10.1017/9781009157896.
9. Balogh A, Giampieri G. Mercury: the planet and its orbit. Rep Prog Phys. 2002;65(4):529.
10. Cockell CS. Life on Venus. Planet Space Sci. 1999;47(12):1487–501.
11. Izenberg NR, Gentry DM, Smith DJ, Gilmore MS, Grinspoon DH, Bullock MA, et al. The Venus life equation. Astrobiology. 2021;21(10):1305–15.
12. Hall DT, Strobel DF, Feldman PD, McGrath MA, Weaver HA. Detection of an oxygen atmosphere on Jupiter's moon Europa. Nature. 1995;373(6516):677–9.
13. Szalay JR, Allegrini F, Ebert RW, et al. Oxygen production from dissociation of Europa's water-ice surface. Nat Astron. 2024;8:567–76. https://doi.org/10.1038/s41550-024-02206-x.
14. Noll KS, Roush TL, Cruikshank DP, Johnson RE, Pendleton YJ. Detection of ozone on Saturn's satellites Rhea and Dione. Nature. 1997;388(6637):45–7.
15. Maltagliati L. The Saturn–Enceladus watery link. Nat Astron. 2019;3:879. https://doi.org/10.1038/s41550-019-0912-y.
16. McKay CP. The search for life on Mars. Orig Life Evol Biosph. 1997;27(1):263–89.
17. Petrescu RV, Aversa R, Apicella A, Kozaitis S, Abu-Lebdeh T, Petrescu FI. There is life on Mars? Am J Eng Appl Sci. 2018;11(1):78–91.
18. Ely DR. Exploring Mars: the red planet revealed. David R Ely; 2024.
19. Neukart F. Towards sustainable horizons: a comprehensive blueprint for Mars colonization. Heliyon. 2024;10(4):e26180.
20. https://pubs.aip.org/physicstoday/online/12054/The-Martian-A-science-movie-review
21. Weir A. The Martian: a novel. Random House; 2014.
22. https://science.howstuffworks.com/oxygen-made-aboard-spacecraft.htm
23. https://www.nasa.gov/spacecraft-oxygen-recovery-scor/
24. Reed DW, Vanden Bosch CA. Engineering perspectives of growing plants in space. J Indian Inst Sci. 2023;103(3):797–805.
25. Bagdigian RM, Dake J, Gentry G, Gault M. International space station environmental control and life support system mass and crewtime utilization in comparison to a long duration human space exploration mission. In: 45th international conference on environmental systems. Texas Digital Library; 2015. p. 16.
26. https://science.nasa.gov/resource/nasas-human-path-to-mars/#:~:text=NASA%20is%20developing%20the%20capabilities,Policy%2C%20also%20issued%20in%202010.
27. Vidal-Madar A, Desert J-M, Lecavelier des Estang GH, Ballester GE, et al. Detection of oxygen and carbon in the hydrodynamically escaping atmosphere of the extrasolar planet HD209458b. Astrophys J. 2004;604:L69.
28. Sagan C, Druyan A. Pale blue dot: a vision of the human future in space. New York: Random House; 1994.

Conclusion

43

Michael Baram, Gregory C. Kane, and Urvashi Vaid

"Plant trees. They give us two of the most crucial elements for our survival: oxygen and books."

A. Whitney Brown, writer and comedian

The balance of our atmosphere is precarious at best. Made up primarily of four gases—nitrogen (78%), oxygen (21%), argon (0.93%), and carbon dioxide (0.43%)—the atmosphere is abundant in oxygen for life, and the balance of carbon dioxide and oxygen is relatively supported by the balance of plant and animal life on our planet [1, 2].

While oxygen has only been identified since the work of several brilliant observers of the atmosphere in the late 1700s, we have learned much about the use of oxygen in health and disease [3, 4]. Rapidly on the heels of Lavoisier, entering the age of biochemistry, we came to understand the high-octane metabolic potential for oxygen to create ATP—the specific fuel of complex mammalian life forms [3–5]. We learned in Chap. 3 that the three components of cellular metabolism for energy production include: glycolysis, the citric acid (or Krebs) cycle, and the Electron Transport Chain. Indeed, when cells have adequate access to oxygen (aerobic metabolism), thirty-two to thirty-six ATP are generally expected to be produced in the metabolism of glucose. This ATP is then the currency of cellular activities: molecule and ion transport across membranes, muscle contraction for locomotion and circulation, nerve impulse

M. Baram · G. C. Kane (✉) · U. Vaid
The Korman Respiratory Institute and the Division of Pulmonary, Allergy and Critical Care, The Department of Medicine at the Sidney Kimmel Medical College of Thomas Jefferson University, Philadelphia, PA, USA
e-mail: Michael.Baram@jefferson.edu; gregory.kane@jefferson.edu; urvashi.vaid@jefferson.edu

G. C. Kane et al. (eds.), *Oxygen*, https://doi.org/10.1007/978-3-032-18934-9_43

propagation and signaling, substrate phosphorylation, chemical synthesis, and assembling of proteins and nucleic acids. During these processes, oxygen combustion leads to the formation of heat and water, and carbon dioxide. The first two byproducts are beneficial to the subject. The latter is beneficial to plant life if produced in balance so as not to create an exaggerated greenhouse gas effect.

The reader can easily imagine how heart, lung, and blood diseases can limit the ability to deliver oxygen to the tissues and the brain; it is then that supplemental oxygen, in all its forms, can be deployed to support the patient. Table 43.1 shows some examples of medical conditions, and several are discussed in individual chapters throughout this book.

Kenneth Ludmerer captured the evolving age of the modern hospital with Intensive Care Units (ICUs) to support care, developing in the 1970s, as well as the

Table 43.1 An outline of potential clinical uses of supplemental oxygen for adult patients with or without pressurized delivery. The reader is encouraged to seek further information in specific chapters discussing several of these important topics in greater detail

Types of oxygen support depending on the clinical circumstances	Examples of clinical scenarios
Hospice:	
None or nasal cannula	Supportive care in hospice
Ambulatory:	
None	Healthy adult outside the hospital
Nasal cannula	Chronic obstructive pulmonary disease (COPD) or interstitial lung disease (ILD) with hypoxia
Nasal cannula	Chronic heart failure with hypoxia
Nasal cannula and/or continuous positive airway pressure (CPAP) or bi-level positive airway pressure (BiPap)	Obstructive or central sleep apnea
Hospital care:	
Nasal cannula, face mask, venturi mask, partial rebreather or non-rebreather	Acute illness with hypoxia such as pneumonia, pulmonary edema, inflammatory lung diseases
High flow nasal cannula	Acute pneumonia (viral or bacterial) including COVID-19 pneumonia
BiPAP	COPD with acute exacerbation, acute congestive heart failure (CHF), hypercarbic respiratory failure, post-extubation
Intubation with mechanical ventilation	Sepsis with adult respiratory distress syndrome (ARDS), severe pneumonia, cardiogenic shock
Intubation with mechanical ventilation with prone positioning	Sepsis with ARDS, severe pneumonia, COVID-19 pneumonia
ECMO	Sepsis with ARDS, severe pneumonia, cardiogenic shock when intubation with mechanical ventilation cannot reverse hypoxia or correct hypercapnia
Cardiopulmonary bypass pump with oxygenator	Use during cardiac surgery or heart and lung transplant

use of resident physicians to support staffing these units [6]. It is in these ICUs that many of these advanced techniques are applied as lifesaving therapies for critically ill patients. Less severely ill patients may be treated with simple supplemental oxygen (such as supplied through nasal cannulas using commercial oxygen supplied to the hospital) on general hospital wards, with or without telemetry monitoring dictated by the underlying illness. Our hope is that the reader will visit individual chapters for the nuance, detail, and methodology of using these remarkable techniques based on their interest and the focus of their daily work in Medicine. The reader is also reminded that the true understanding of these techniques cannot be grasped without a fundamental grasp of the Gas Laws and their application in specific circumstances. These chapters should be of great interest to our student readers; though we expect residents and fellows will also refer to these sections to refresh their understanding. The beauty of the amazing array of supportive oxygen delivery techniques and modalities described in this treatise is that when used for the right disease at the right time, they can allow the natural healing powers of the human body to regain natural function supported by the bridge of oxygen delivery techniques so carefully outlined herein. In chronic conditions such as COPD and Obstructive Sleep Apnea (see Part III contributions), research highlights that these diseases may be adversely impacting humans directly through the burden of hypoxia, and addressing this burden through reversing hypoxia might restore health and longevity. Finally, it is sobering to be reminded (see Chap. 7) that too much oxygen in routine healthcare can have negative consequences, reminding us that the symphony of our human physiology is quite carefully balanced and explicitly orchestrated.

Chapters on scuba diving and diving disorders, as well as altitude, remind the reader that healthy adults can find themselves in environmental conditions where breathing can be challenged or oxygen availability may be reduced. The chapters may be of interest to the recreational scuba diver or mountaineer but should also be of value to physicians caring for patients with illnesses resulting from participation in these activities.

Finally, it is worthwhile to comment on how oxygen may be manufactured for use in space, such as on the International Space Station (ISS), and man's ongoing search for oxygen and complex life outside our solar system. We hope you will enjoy this discussion. This chapter is not at all futuristic, as Voyagers 1 and 2 have both entered interstellar space and are expected to send data back to Earth through 2036, when they may be replaced by even more sophisticated space probes [7, 8].

In closing, complex life as we know it is dependent on the interconnected, balanced ecology of plant and animal life on this planet that maintains atmospheric oxygen at approximately 21% and creates the appropriate amount of carbon dioxide for plant-based photosynthesis. Already, we are seeing how human activities such as burning excessive fossil fuels and wildfires are altering the carbon dioxide side of this equation and contributing to global warming [9, 10]. At this juncture, the oxygen supply does not appear to be at risk. Hopefully, we can muster a belief in science among our democratic people so that we can use reason to address these challenges in time to avert a crisis [11]. Some might say the landscape for international collaboration is at an all-time low, but we must remind the reader that a precedent for such work has already been established. In September 1987, the Montreal Protocol was adopted and signed universally across the globe, endorsed by President Ronald Reagan, to regulate more than 100 man-made chemicals responsible for depleting the ozone layer, which protects us from the harmful rays of the sun and an accelerated risk of skin cancers, including melanoma. This unprecedented multilateral agreement is considered one of the most successful environmental agreements of all time and should inspire us to take action collectively to combat global warming for our children's children and generations to come [11, 12]. With that type of inspiration, a spirit of collaboration for a sustainable planet, using reason and data to chart the path, and mustering the courage to address climate and other challenges, we may have a fighting chance at continuing the run we are having on this breathtaking planet as a human species [13–15]. Let us hope we can.

References

1. Lenton TM. The role of land plants, phosphorus weathering and fire in the rise and regulation of atmospheric oxygen. Glob Chang Biol. 2001;7(6):613–29.
2. https://www.noaa.gov/jetstream/atmosphere. Accessed 3 July 2025.
3. Sternbach GL, Varon J. The discovery and rediscovery of oxygen. J Emerg Med. 2005;28(2):221–4., ISSN 0736-4679. https://doi.org/10.1016/j.jemermed.2004.10.012.
4. Severinghaus JW. Priestley, the furious free thinker of the enlightenment, and Scheele, the taciturn apothecary of Uppsala. Acta Anaesthesiol Scand. 2002;46:2–9.
5. Beretta M. The enlightenment of matter. The definition of chemistry from Agricola to Lavoisier. Canton: Science History Publications; 1993.
6. Lazerson M, Kenneth M, Ludmerer A. Time to heal: American medical education from the turn of the century to the era of managed care. New York: Oxford University Press; 1999. p. 514. Cloth $29.95. Hist Educ Q 2001;41(1):116–118. https://doi.org/10.1017/S0018268000016885.
7. https://science.nasa.gov/missions/hubble/oxygen-and-carbon-found-in-atmosphere-of-an-extrasolar-planet/#:~:text=The%20planet%20HD%20209458b%20is,atmosphere%20containing%20oxygen%20and%20carbon.
8. Seager S. The smallest lights in the universe: a memoir. New York: Crown; 2020.
9. White PJ, Ardoin NM, Eames C, Monroe MC. Agency in the anthropocene: supporting document to the PISA 2025 science framework. OECD Educ Work Pap. 2023;297:0_1–4.
10. IPCC. Climate change 2021: the physical science basis. In: Contribution of working group I to the sixth assessment report of the intergovernmental panel on climate change. Cambridge, UK/New York, NY: Cambridge University Press; 2021. https://doi.org/10.1017/9781009157896.
11. Gonzalez M, Taddonio KN, Sherman NJ. The Montreal protocol: how today's successes offer a pathway to the future. J Environ Stud Sci. 2015;5(2):122–9.
12. Birmpili T. Montreal protocol at 30: the governance structure, the evolution, and the Kigali amendment. Compt Rendus Geosci. 2018;350(7):425–31.
13. Whitesides G. Learning from success: lessons in science and diplomacy from the Montreal protocol. Learning. 2020;8:10.
14. Ruhl JB. Do Montreal! A review article. Polit Sci Q. 2025;140(1):105–19.
15. Pinker S. Enlightenment now: the case for reason, science, humanism, and progress. New York NY: Viking; 2018.

Index

G. C. Kane et al. (eds.), *Oxygen*, https://doi.org/10.1007/978-3-032-18934-9

GPSR Compliance

The European Union's (EU) General Product Safety Regulation (GPSR) is a set of rules that requires consumer products to be safe and our obligations to ensure this.

If you have any concerns about our products, you can contact us on ProductSafety@springernature.com

In case Publisher is established outside the EU, the EU authorized representative is:

Springer Nature Customer Service Center GmbH
Europaplatz 3
69115 Heidelberg, Germany

Batch number: 10726133

Printed by Printforce, the Netherlands